THE CIBA COLLECTION
OF MEDICAL ILLUSTRATIONS

Volume 7

Respiratory System

A compilation of paintings depicting anatomy and
embryology, physiology, pathology, pathophysiology,
and clinical features and treatment of diseases

Prepared by

Frank H. Netter, M.D.

Edited by

Matthew B. Divertie, M.D.

Alister Brass, M.D.
Directing Editor

Commissioned and published by

C I B A

Other published volumes of
THE CIBA COLLECTION OF MEDICAL ILLUSTRATIONS
Prepared by
Frank H. Netter, M.D.

Nervous System

Reproductive System

Upper Digestive Tract

Lower Digestive Tract

Liver, Biliary Tract and Pancreas

Endocrine System and
  Selected Metabolic Diseases

Heart

Kidneys, Ureters, and Urinary Bladder

See page 328 for additional information

First Printing, 1979
Second Edition, 1980

ISBN 0-914168-09-6
Library of Congress Catalogue No. 53-2151

Printed in U.S.A.

Color Engraving: The Case-Hoyt Corporation, Rochester, N.Y.
Text Typography: The Type Group Inc., New York, N.Y.
Printing: The Case-Hoyt Corporation, Rochester, N.Y.
Binding: Wm. F. Zahrndt & Son, Inc., Rochester, N.Y.

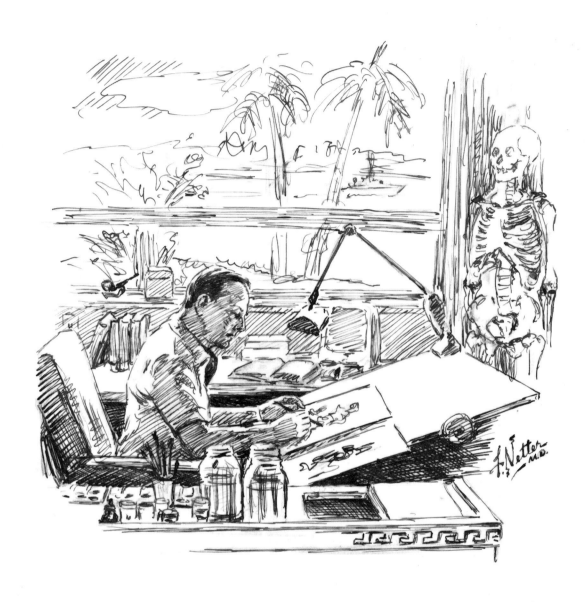

Self-portrait of the artist at work in his studio

The medical paintings of Dr. Frank Netter have received such wide acclaim from physicians the world over for so long that the image of the man himself has begun to take on mythical proportions. And, indeed, it is easy to understand how such a transformation could take place. Yet, Dr. Netter is a real human being who breathes, eats and carries on a daily routine just like the rest of us and who, for that matter, stands a little in awe of the image which is so often ascribed to him.

In order to help affirm his reality as a man, we asked Dr. Netter to make the accompanying self-portrait of himself at work in his studio. The sketch portrays a number of elements which may be familiar to those who have seen photographs of Dr. Netter's studio in previous volumes of THE CIBA COLLECTION OF MEDICAL ILLUSTRATIONS or in other publications—the man himself, the drawing board, the paints, the brushes, the skeleton and other accoutrements. The difference is in the background. No longer is it the skyline of New York, which could be seen from his former studio window. Now it is the open sunny landscape of southern Florida, with waving palm trees and a boat traversing the waters of the intracoastal waterway.

Nevertheless, the Netters' move south from their long established New York home does not signify an intention to wind down a highly productive work schedule. Florida has meant a change in location and climate, but the intensity of Frank Netter's commitment to what has become his life's work continues undiminished. He is usually in his studio by 7:00 AM, where he concentrates on the project before him until about two o'clock. The afternoons are mostly devoted to golf, to swimming in the sea or pool, to fishing, to time with his family or friends, or to other diversions. At times he takes a "postman's holiday" to paint a landscape or a portrait just for the fun of it.

But not all of Dr. Netter's work is done at the drawing board. Much of it consists of intensive study and wide reading, observation of physicians at work in the clinic, hospital or laboratory, and long hours of discussion with a collaborator. Even during his hours of relaxation the concept of the illustrations is germinating in his mind. After these preliminaries he makes pencil sketches, composing the details and layout of the various elements of the illustrations, positioning x-rays and photomicrographs, and determining the exact dimensions and placing of the legends in order to achieve the maximum teaching effect. Only after the sketches are checked, double checked, and revised for accuracy and detail does he proceed with the finished painting. Most of his paintings are in water color, but at times he has used other media including casein paint, chalks, acrylics or oils. He maintains, however, that the medium is not very important. Good pictures can be made in any medium. He prefers water color only because through long use he feels more at home with it and because he can express himself more directly and work more rapidly with it.

Dr. Netter's great facility and skill at representative painting, gift though it may be, did not come to fruition without dedicated study and training—not only in drawing and painting but in graphic design, composition and layout as well. From the time he was a little boy he wanted to be an artist. He studied intensively at the National Academy of Design, the Art Students League of New York and other outstanding schools as well as with private teachers. He won many honors and, indeed, became a successful commercial artist in the heyday of that profession. But then, partly because of his own interest and partly because of urging by his family to do "something more serious" he decided to give up art and initiate a new career in medicine. Once in medical school, however, he found that because of his graphic training he could learn his subjects best by making drawings. So his early medical illustrations were made for his own education. But it was not long before his drawings caught the eyes of his professors, who then kept him busy in what little spare time he had making illustrations for their books and articles. Netter graduated from New York University School of Medicine and completed his internship and surgical residency at Bellevue Hospital in the depths of the great depression. It soon became evident that his art commissions from publishers and pharmaceutical manufacturers were a better source of income than his depression-stifled medical practice, and he made the decision to be a full-time medical artist.

Dr. Netter's association with the CIBA Pharmaceutical Company began in 1938 with his creation of a folder cut out in the shape of a heart. Paintings of the anterior and posterior (basal) surface of the heart were printed on the front and back and sections of the internal anatomy were depicted on the inside. An advertising message was overprinted both inside and out. The immediate response of physicians to this piece was to request that it be produced without the advertising message. This was done to great success, and thus was born a series of anatomy and pathology illustration projects, the demand for which was so great that it eventually led, in 1948, to the publication of the first book of THE CIBA COLLECTION OF MEDICAL ILLUSTRATIONS. The year 1978, then, is not only the year of introduction of Volume 7, Respiratory System, but is also the thirtieth anniversary of the first book of THE CIBA COLLECTION OF MEDICAL ILLUSTRATIONS. Coincidentally, it is also the thirtieth anniversary of the first issue of the CIBA CLINICAL SYMPOSIA series.

Dr. Netter is still preparing well over 100 paintings a year for THE CIBA COLLECTION OF MEDICAL ILLUSTRATIONS and CLINICAL SYMPOSIA. Even now he is well into the task of illustrating a new atlas on the musculoskeletal system. Much has been said and written in the past about the Netter "genius." Perhaps the most impressive aspect of all is not his "genius," but the use this remarkable artist-physician-teacher makes of his gifts. His collective works are monumental, and they continue to grow.

PHILIP B. FLAGLER
DIRECTOR
MEDICAL EDUCATION

Introduction

Whenever a new atlas of mine appears, I feel as a woman must feel when she has just had a baby. The tediousness and travail of the long pregnancy and the pain of delivery are over, and it remains to be seen how my offspring will fare in the world.

In this case, there were a number of problems during the gestation. One of these was that interest in the respiratory system and its diseases has not only greatly increased in recent years but that its focus has been radically altered. The reasons for these changes are manifold. They include the great differences which have come about in the incidence of various lung diseases; the advent and better utilization of antibiotics; advances in radiologic technique and interpretation; the development of additional diagnostic techniques such as radioactive isotope scanning; expansion in the study of pulmonary physiology and application of pulmonary function tests; progress in understanding of pulmonary pathology; increased facility in thoracic surgery and the development of methods for predetermining operability, such as mediastinoscopy; the design or improvement of technical and diagnostic mechanisms such as oxygen and aerosol apparatus, mechanical ventilators, more efficient spirometers and surgical staplers; and alterations in the personal habits, environment and average age of the population.

All these factors, as well as others, are, however, interactive. For example, the great decrease in incidence of pulmonary tuberculosis is related to the advent of antibiotics; but it is also a consequence of improvement in living standards and habits, as well as of improved early diagnosis. These factors may also be responsible for the lesser incidence and morbidity of pneumococcal pneumonia. Whereas in former years these two diseases were major concerns of the chest physician, they are nowadays of much less significance. But this, on the other hand, has allowed more time and effort to be diverted to other lung disorders. The greatly increased incidence of lung cancer appears to have resulted in considerable measure from changes in personal habits (such as smoking), environmental pollution and occupational activity, and possibly also change in population age. But earlier discovery of tumors through greater public awareness and improved diagnosis, plus greater surgical facility, have led to increased interest in operability, and this in turn has stimulated study of pathologic classification in relation to malignancy. The increase in chronic bronchitis and emphysema, while largely real and attributable to the same etiologic factors as cancer, may to some extent be only apparent—due to better diagnostic methods and utilization of pulmonary function studies. But recognition of some of the etiologic factors and better understanding of the underlying pathologic processes, coupled with availability and utilization of such measures as aerosol medication, improved equipment for oxygen administration and mechanical ventilation, and postural drainage have greatly modified for the better the management of these distressing disorders. The current relatively high incidence of occupational diseases may likewise to some extent be only apparent, because of greater awareness and better diagnosis. Pulmonary embolus and infarction have also received increased attention in recent years as the common sources of emboli have been identified, and as the manifestations of pulmonary vascular obstruction have been more clearly defined.

In light of the foregoing examples of the changing emphasis in the field of pulmonary medicine, to which many more could be added, I have tried in this atlas to give to each topic its proper emphasis in relation to the subject as a whole, in accord with current concepts. In doing this, much consideration had to be given to space availability. A good public speaker must deliver the essentials of his message within the time allotted to him for if he rambles on and on, his audience is lost and his message ineffective. So, too, the artist must portray his subject matter as effectively as possible within the allotted pages. What to leave out becomes, at times, as important as what to include. Without such considerations, this volume might have grown to twice or three times its size and become unbalanced, or become so crowded with minutiae as to be dull and boring. In either event, the utility of the book would have been greatly impaired.

As in the preparation of all my previous atlases, my major efforts in this work were again necessarily directed towards gathering, absorbing and digesting the information about each subject so that I might properly portray it. Thus study, learning and analysis of the subject matter became as time consuming, or more so, than the actual painting of the pictures. One cannot intelligently portray a subject unless one understands it. My goal was to picture or diagram the essence of each subject, avoiding the incidental or inconsequential. In some instances I have, however, included topics which, at present, do not seem to have great practical application but which, in the future, may give important clues to pathogenesis, diagnosis or treatment. All this was greatly facilitated, indeed made possible, through the devoted cooperation of the many distinguished consultants who are listed individually on other pages of this volume. I herewith express my appreciation to each and every one of them for the time, effort and guidance which they gave me, and for the knowledge which they imparted to me. I also thank the many others who, although not officially consultants, nevertheless helped me with advice or information or by supplying reference material to me. They are also credited elsewhere in this book. I especially thank Dr. Matthew B. Divertie for his careful and thorough review of both the pictorial and text material and for his many constructive suggestions.

The production of this book involved a tremendous amount of organizational work, such as assembling and compiling the material as it grew in volume, correlating illustrations and text, grammatical checking, reference checking, type specification, page layout, proofreading, and a multitude of mechanical and practical details incidental to publication. I tremendously admire the efficiency with which these matters were handled by Mr. Philip Flagler and his staff at CIBA, including Ms. Gina Dingle, Ms. Barbara Bekiesz, Ms. Kristine Bean and Mr. Pierre Lair. Finally, I once more give praise to the CIBA Pharmaceutical Company and its executives for their vision in sponsoring this project and for the free hand they have given me in executing it. I have tried to do justice to it.

Frank H. Netter, M.D.

Contributors and Consultants

The artist, editors, and publishers express their appreciation to the following authorities for their generous collaboration:

Murray D. Altose, M.D.
Associate Professor of Medicine,
Case Western Reserve University
School of Medicine;
Director, Pulmonary Division,
Cleveland Metropolitan General Hospital,
Cleveland, Ohio

Mary Ellen Avery, M.D.
Thomas Morgan Rotch Professor of Pediatrics,
Harvard Medical School;
Physician-in-Chief,
The Children's Hospital Medical Center,
Boston, Massachusetts

Howard A. Buechner, M.D.
Professor of Medicine and Chief,
Pulmonary Disease Section, Louisiana State
University School of Medicine in New Orleans;
Senior Visiting Physician,
Charity Hospital of Louisiana,
New Orleans, Louisiana

Neil S. Cherniack, M.D.
Professor of Medicine,
Case Western Reserve University
School of Medicine,
Cleveland, Ohio

Hyun Taik Cho, M.D.
Senior Instructor of Surgery,
Mount Sinai School of Medicine of
The City University of New York;
Assistant Attending Surgeon,
Beth Israel Medical Center,
New York, New York

Jacob Churg, M.D.
Professor of Pathology,
Mount Sinai School of Medicine of
The City University of New York;
Chief, Division of Renal Pathology,
The Mount Sinai Hospital,
New York, New York

Robert W. Colman, M.D.
Professor of Medicine and Pathology;
Chief, Coagulation Unit,
The University of Pennsylvania
School of Medicine,
Philadelphia, Pennsylvania

Edmund S. Crelin, Ph.D., D.Sc.
Professor and Chief, Section of Anatomy,
Department of Surgery;
Chairman, Human Growth and
Development Study Unit,
Yale University School of Medicine,
New Haven, Connecticut

Matthew B. Divertie, M.D.
Professor of Medicine, Mayo Medical School;
Consultant, Division of Thoracic Diseases,
Department of Internal Medicine and
Section of Respiratory Care,
Department of Anesthesiology, Mayo Clinic,
Rochester, Minnesota

Paul E. Epstein, M.D.
Cardiovascular-Pulmonary Division,
The University of Pennsylvania
School of Medicine
Philadelphia, Pennsylvania

Alfred P. Fishman, M.D
William Maul Measey Professor of Medicine;
Director, Cardiovascular-Pulmonary Division,
Department of Medicine;
Principal Investigator, Lung Center,
The University of Pennsylvania
School of Medicine,
Philadelphia, Pennsylvania

Albert Haas, M.D.
Professor of Experimental
Rehabilitation Medicine;
Director, Pulmonary Services,
Department of Rehabilitation Medicine,
New York University School of Medicine,
New York, New York

Henry O. Heinemann, M.D.*
Professor of Medicine,
Cornell University Medical College,
New York, New York

John Franklin Huber, M.D., Ph.D.
Professor Emeritus of Anatomy,
Temple University School of Medicine,
Philadelphia, Pennsylvania

Roland H. Ingram, Jr., M.D.
Associate Professor of Medicine,
Harvard Medical School;
Director, Respiratory Disease Division,
Peter Bent Brigham Hospital,
Boston, Massachusetts

*Deceased

Sukahamay Lahiri, Ph.D.
Associate Professor of Physiology,
The University of Pennsylvania
School of Medicine,
Philadelphia, Pennsylvania

Jose F. Landa, M.D.
Associate, Division of Pulmonary Diseases,
Mount Sinai Medical Center,
Miami Beach, Florida;
Instructor, Department of Medicine,
University of Miami School of Medicine,
Miami, Florida

Victor J. Marder, M.D.
Professor of Medicine;
Co-Chief, Hematology Unit,
University of Rochester
School of Medicine and Dentistry,
Rochester, New York

Edward D. Michaelson, M.D.
Associate, Division of Pulmonary Diseases,
Mount Sinai Medical Center,
Miami Beach, Florida

Wallace T. Miller, M.D.
Professor and Vice Chairman,
Department of Radiology,
The University of Pennsylvania
School of Medicine;
Chief, Chest Division,
Hospital of the University of Pennsylvania,
Philadelphia, Pennsylvania

Roger S. Mitchell, M.D.
Professor Emeritus of Medicine,
University of Colorado School of Medicine,
Denver, Colorado

W. Spencer Payne, M.D.
Professor of Surgery, Mayo Medical School;
Consultant in Thoracic and
Cardiovascular Surgery, Mayo Clinic,
Rochester, Minnesota

Giuseppe G. Pietra, M.D.
Professor of Pathology,
The University of Pennsylvania
School of Medicine,
Philadelphia, Pennsylvania

Lynne M. Reid, M.D.
S. Burt Wolbach Professor of Pathology,
Harvard Medical School;
Pathologist-in-Chief,
The Children's Hospital Medical Center,
Boston, Massachusetts

James W. Ryan, M.D., Ph.D.
Associate Professor of Medicine,
University of Miami School of Medicine,
Miami, Florida

Una S. Ryan, Ph.D.
Associate Professor of Medicine,
University of Miami School of Medicine
Miami, Florida

Marvin A. Sackner, M.D.
Director, Medical Services,
Mount Sinai Medical Center,
Miami Beach, Florida;
Professor of Medicine,
University of Miami School of Medicine,
Miami, Florida

Charles V. Sanders, Jr., M.D.
Associate Professor of
Medicine and Microbiology;
Director, Infectious Diseases,
Louisiana State University
Medical Center in New Orleans,
New Orleans, Louisiana

Max L. Som, M.D.
Emeritus Professor of Otolaryngology,
Mount Sinai School of Medicine of
The City University of New York;
Attending Head and Neck Surgeon (off service),
Beth Israel Hospital
New York, New York

D. Eugene Strandness, Jr., M.D.
Professor of Surgery,
Department of Surgery,
University of Washington
School of Medicine,
Seattle, Washington

Morton N. Swartz, M.D.
Professor of Medicine,
Harvard Medical School;
Chief, Infectious Disease Unit,
Massachusetts General Hospital,
Boston, Massachusetts

Alvin S. Teirstein, M.D.
Director, Pulmonary Division;
Florette and Ernst Rosenfeld and
Joseph Solomon Professor of Medicine,
Mount Sinai School of Medicine of
The City University of New York,
New York, New York

Joseph J. Timmes, M.D.
Professor of Surgery, College of
Medicine and Dentistry of New Jersey,
New Jersey Medical School;
Director of Surgery, Medical Center,
Jersey City, New Jersey

Milton H. Uhley, M.D.
Attending Physician,
Department of Medicine,
Cedars-Sinai Medical Center,
Los Angeles, California

Earle B. Weiss, M.D.
Director, Division of Respiratory Diseases,
Saint Vincent Hospital;
Professor of Medicine,
University of Massachusetts Medical School,
Worcester, Massachusetts

William Weiss, M.D.
Professor of Medicine;
Director, Division of Occupational Medicine,
Hahnemann Medical College and Hospital,
Philadelphia, Pennsylvania

William I. Wolff, M.D.
Professor of Clinical Surgery,
Mount Sinai School of Medicine of
The City University of New York;
(Former) Director of Surgery,
Beth Israel Medical Center,
New York, New York

J. Edwin Wood, III, M.D.
Director, Department of Medicine,
Pennsylvania Hospital;
Professor of Medicine,
The University of Pennsylvania
School of Medicine,
Philadelphia, Pennsylvania

Morton M. Ziskind, M.D.
Professor of Medicine;
Director, Pulmonary Diseases Section,
Department of Medicine,
Tulane University School of Medicine,
New Orleans, Louisiana

Acknowledgments

We would like to thank all our contributors and consultants for the hard work and care to detail they have given to Volume 7 of THE CIBA COLLECTION OF MEDICAL ILLUSTRATIONS. Without their help, publication would never have been possible. We especially thank Dr. Matthew B. Divertie, who not only acted as medical consultant for the editorial staff but also edited much of the text.

It is, of course, impossible to give credit to everyone who has, in one way or another, had a hand in preparing this work. There are, however, those whose assistance we particularly acknowledge, namely: Dr. Alfred P. Fishman, for his guidance in the selection of many contributors and in the early organization of the project, in addition to his own contribution as a collaborator; Dr. Edward Coopersmith for help in the preparation of Plates (IV) 97-104; Dr. Edward Hicks, Jr. for help in developing Plates (IV) 122 and (V) 9 and 10; Dr. David Koffler for the demonstration of immunologic tests in the development of Plates (IV) 145 and 147; Dr. Wallace T. Miller for supplying x-ray films for Plates (IV) 54, 55, 57, 59, 61, 63 and 64; Dr. Emil A. Naclerio for the use of his article "Chest Trauma" (CLINICAL SYMPOSIA Vol. 22, No. 3) from which illustrations were modified for Plates (IV) 126 and 133, and (V) 27 and 28; Dr. Louis E. Siltzbach for the loan of material in the development of Plate (IV) 142; Dr.

David C. Stark and Dr. Raymond Miller for the demonstration of the use of the Carlens tube; Dr. Austin J. Sumner for supplying electromyographic tracings; Dr. Wen Lan Wang for supplying two slides used in Plate (IV) 95; and Dr. William Z. Yahr for the extensive demonstrations and descriptions he supplied for preparation of the plates on surgery of the lung.

Within the CIBA organization we must express our special gratitude to Ms. Gina Dingle, who enthusiastically and successfully handled the reins as Production Editor. Likewise to Mr. Pierre Lair, our Production Manager and Art Director, who patiently and with meticulous attention to detail supervised the typography, layout and production of the book from start to finish. Thanks are also due to Ms. Kristine Bean, Ms. Barbara Bekiesz, Mr. Jack Cesareo, Jr. and Ms. Helen Sward, who all helped bring this book to fruition.

Our sincere appreciation is also tendered to Ms. Julia Stair, one of our most experienced editorial consultants, who assisted us with proofreading and copy editing, and did a remarkably expeditious job of indexing. Likewise, we extend our appreciation to Ms. Sylvia Covet who helped us with our early organizational and editorial work.

The production of Volume 7 has been carried out by the CIBA staff and several organizations with whom we have worked closely in the past. Notable among them is Cesareo Studio of Elmsford, New York, whose careful work in preparing the mechanical overlays for

Dr. Netter's plates has been invaluable. Likewise, Case-Hoyt Corporation of Rochester, New York, has not only done its usual fine job of printing the volume, but has also worked with us to solve the many problems encountered in preparing both art and manuscript for press. Mr. Donald McCloskey of Case-Hoyt has distinguished himself in his liaison work on the project and has served both organizations with perseverance, good humor and a very real understanding of the needs of all parties. Also, The Type Group Inc. of New York City has worked with us diligently on the typesetting, and William F. Zahrndt & Son Inc. of Rochester, New York, has done a handsome and expeditious job with the binding. We thank them all for their fine work.

As in the past, we have tried with this book to maintain those attributes of previous volumes of THE CIBA COLLECTION OF MEDICAL ILLUSTRATIONS which have made them so sought after over the years. At the same time, we have adjusted certain aspects of layout and typography in an attempt to enhance the design and readability of the book. We also continue to search for new printing techniques to improve the reproduction of Dr. Netter's plates. We hope these changes will subtly enhance the end result. It has been an exciting and rewarding project from beginning to end, and we thank all who have helped us along the way.

ALISTER BRASS, M.D.
PHILIP B. FLAGLER

Preface to the Second Edition

Although it is a little over one year since the first edition of Respiratory System was published, the demand for copies has been so great that we are reprinting—a record for THE CIBA COLLECTION OF MEDICAL ILLUSTRATIONS and yet a further tribute to the enormous popularity of Dr. Netter's medical paintings.

In preparing the second edition we have corrected all the typographic and other errors we and our diligent readers have detected in the first printing (remarkably few for a volume of this length and complexity), and have made

three important additions to the book. The first is on page 46—a list of the abbreviations and symbols used in Dr. Murray D. Altose's section on respiratory physiology. The second, on page 104, is a new Plate and accompanying text on the use of computerized tomography in the diagnosis of chest diseases, prepared by Dr. Wallace T. Miller. Finally, in response to a request from Dr. Henry J. Heimlich, we have substituted for the original pictures of a woman attempting to save an infant from choking (page 273) two new illustrations by

Dr. Netter demonstrating the correct way of using the Heimlich Maneuver on a choking infant.

Of the many people who have helped to bring this edition of Respiratory System to press it is a pleasure to thank in particular Ms. Gina Dingle, our production editor, and Mr. Pierre Lair who, as production manager, has painstakingly supervised the revised color printing which enhances this volume.

ALISTER BRASS, M.D.

Contents

Section I

Anatomy and Embryology

Frank H. Netter, M.D.

in collaboration with

Edmund S. Crelin, Ph.D., D.Sc.   *Plates 32-41*

John Franklin Huber, M.D., Ph.D.   *Plates 1-19*

Lynne M. Reid, M.D.   *Plates 21-26, 30-31*

Una S. Ryan, Ph.D. and James W. Ryan, M.D., Ph.D.   *Plates 27-29*

Earle B. Weiss, M.D.   *Plate 20*

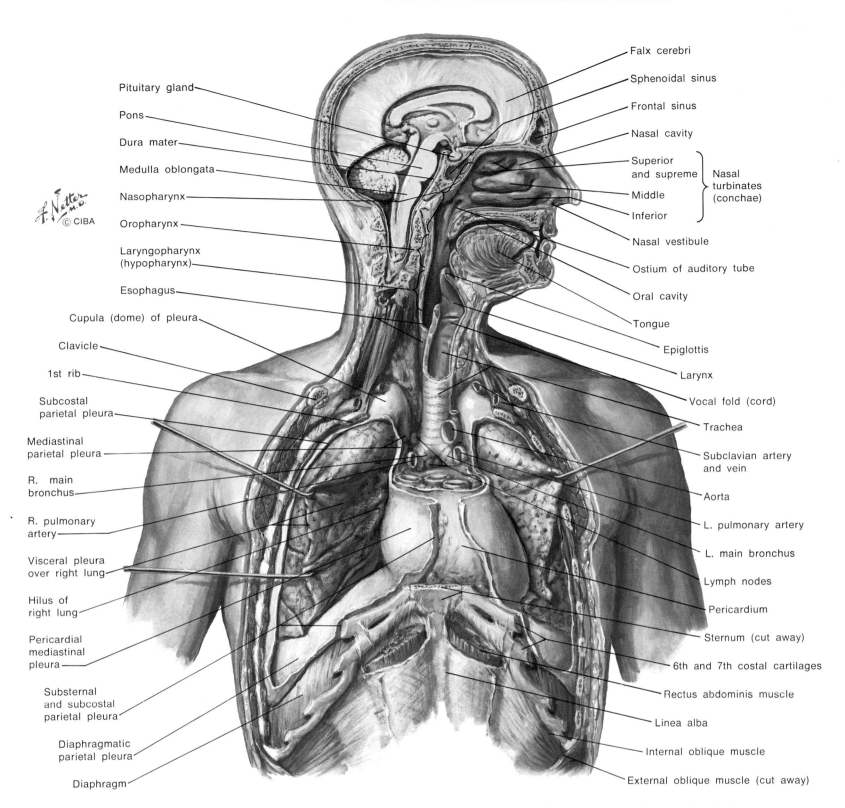

Pituitary gland

Pons

Dura mater

Medulla oblongata

Nasopharynx

Oropharynx

Laryngopharynx (hypopharynx)

Esophagus

Cupula (dome) of pleura

Clavicle

1st rib

Subcostal parietal pleura

Mediastinal parietal pleura

R. main bronchus

R. pulmonary artery

Visceral pleura over right lung

Hilus of right lung

Pericardial mediastinal pleura

Substernal and subcostal parietal pleura

Diaphragmatic parietal pleura

Diaphragm

Falx cerebri

Sphenoidal sinus

Frontal sinus

Nasal cavity

Superior and supreme

Middle

Inferior

Nasal turbinates (conchae)

Nasal vestibule

Ostium of auditory tube

Oral cavity

Tongue

Epiglottis

Larynx

Vocal fold (cord)

Trachea

Subclavian artery and vein

Aorta

L. pulmonary artery

L. main bronchus

Lymph nodes

Pericardium

Sternum (cut away)

6th and 7th costal cartilages

Rectus abdominis muscle

Linea alba

Internal oblique muscle

External oblique muscle (cut away)

SECTION I   PLATE 1

Respiratory System

The respiratory system is made up of the structures involved in exchange of oxygen and carbon dioxide between the blood and the atmosphere, so-called external respiration. The exchange of gases between the blood in the capillaries of the systemic circulation and the tissues in which these capillaries are located is referred to as internal respiration.

The respiratory system consists of the external nose, internal nose and paranasal sinuses; the pharynx, which is the common passage for air and food; the larynx, where the voice is produced; and the trachea, bronchi and lungs. Accessory structures necessary for the operation of the respiratory system are the pleurae, the diaphragm, the

thoracic wall and the muscles which raise and lower the ribs in inspiration and expiration. The muscles of the anterolateral abdominal wall are also accessory to *forceful* expiration (their contraction forces the diaphragm upward by pressing the contents of the abdominal cavity against it from below), and are used in "abdominal" respiration. Certain muscles of the neck can elevate the ribs, thus enlarging the anteroposterior diameter of the thorax, and under some circumstances the muscles attaching the arms to the thoracic wall can also help change the capacity of the thorax.

In the 18 illustrations that follow this one, the anatomy of the respiratory system and significant accessory structures are shown. It is important not only to visualize these structures in isolation, but also to become familiar with their blood supply, nerve supply and relationships with both adjacent structures and the surface of the body. One should keep in mind that these relationships are subject

to the same degree of individual variation that affects all anatomic structures. The illustrations depict the most common situations encountered. No attempt is made to describe all of the many variations which do occur.

One extremely important and clinically valuable concept that is worth emphasizing at this point is the convention of subdividing each lung into lobes and segments on the basis of branching of the bronchial tree. From the standpoint of its embryologic development, as well as of its function as a fully established organ of respiration, the lung is indeed the ultimate branching of the main bronchus which leads into it. The subdivision of the lung on this basis is essential to the anatomist, the physiologist, the pathologist, the radiologist, the surgeon and the chest physician, for without this three-dimensional key there is no exact means of precisely localizing lesions within the respiratory system.

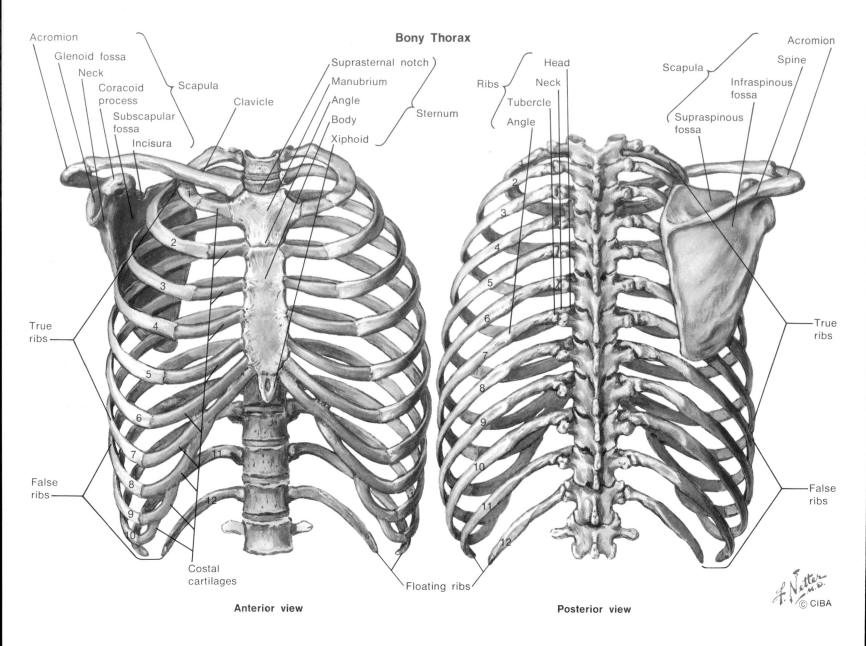

Acromion
Glenoid fossa
Neck
Coracoid process
Subscapular fossa
Incisura
Scapula
Clavicle

Suprasternal notch
Manubrium
Angle
Body
Xiphoid
Sternum

Head
Ribs
Neck
Tubercle
Angle

Scapula
Acromion
Spine
Infraspinous fossa
Supraspinous fossa

True ribs

False ribs

True ribs

False ribs

Costal cartilages

Floating ribs

Anterior view

Posterior view

f. Netter ©CIBA

SECTION I   PLATE 2

Bony Thorax

The skeletal framework of the thorax—the bony thorax—consists of 12 pairs of ribs and their cartilages, 12 thoracic vertebrae and interverte-bral discs, and the sternum. The illustration also includes one clavicle and scapula, since these bones serve as important attachments for some of the muscles involved in respiration.

The sternum is made up of three parts—the manubrium, body and xiphoid process. The manubrium and body are not in quite the same plane and thus form the *sternal angle* at their junc-tion, a significant landmark at which the costal cartilage of the second rib articulates with the sternum. The superior border of the manubrium

is slightly concave, forming what is called the *suprasternal notch*.

The costal cartilages of the first through seventh ribs ordinarily articulate with the ster-num, and are called *true ribs*. The costal cartilages of the eighth through tenth ribs (*false ribs*) are usually attached to the cartilage of the rib above, while the ventral ends of the cartilages of the eleventh and twelfth ribs (*floating ribs*) have no direct skeletal attachment.

All the ribs articulate dorsally with the verte-bral column in such a way that their ventral end (together with the sternum) can be raised slightly, as occurs in inspiration. The articulations of the costal cartilages with the sternum, except for the first rib, are true or synovial joints, which allow more freedom of movement than there would be without this type of articulation.

The deep surface of the scapula (the subscapular fossa) fits against the posterolateral aspect of the thorax over the second to seventh ribs, where, to a great extent, it is held by the muscles which are attached to it. The scapula's only bony articula-tion is between its acromion process and the lateral end of the clavicle; this acts as a strut to hold the lateral angle of the scapula away from the thorax. On the dorsal surface of the scapula a spine protrudes which continues laterally into the acromion process. At its vertebral end the spine flattens into a smooth triangular surface with the

base of the triangle at the vertebral border. The spine separates the supraspinous fossa from the infraspinous fossa. Three borders of the scapula are described—superior, lateral, and medial or vertebral. On the superior border is a notch or incisura, and lateral to this the coracoid process protrudes anteriorly.

The lateral angle of the scapula presents a slight concavity, the glenoid fossa, for articulation with the head of the humerus. At the superior end of the glenoid fossa is the supraglenoid tuberosity, and at its inferior margin is the infraglenoid tuberosity.

The clavicle articulates at its medial end with the superolateral aspect of the manubrium of the sternum, and at its lateral end with the medial edge of the acromion process of the scapula. Its medial two-thirds is curved slightly anteriorly, and its lateral third is curved posteriorly. Muscu-lar attachments to the medial and lateral parts of the clavicle leave its middle portion less protected and thus readily subject to fracture.

The vertebral levels of the bony landmarks on the ventral aspect of the thorax are variable, and differ somewhat with the phase of respiration. In general, the upper border of the manubrium is at the level of the second to third thoracic vertebra, the sternal angle opposite the fourth to fifth thoracic vertebra, and the xiphisternal junction at the level of the ninth thoracic vertebra.

Rib Characteristics and Costovertebral Articulations

1st rib viewed from above

Subclavius muscle

Scalenus anterior muscle

Grooves for subclavian vein and artery

Head

Neck

Tubercle

Red = muscle origins

Blue = muscle insertions

Scalenus medius

Head

Neck

Tubercle

Angle

1st digitation; 2nd digitation of serratus anterior muscle

Scalenus posterior

Tubercle

Head

Neck

2nd rib viewed from above

Angle

Articular facet for transverse process

Superior; inferior

Articular facets for vertebrae

Rib Characteristics and Costovertebral Articulations

A typical rib has a head, a neck and a body. The head articulates with one or two vertebral bodies (see below). A tubercle at the lateral end of the relatively short neck articulates with the transverse process of the lower of the two vertebrae with which the head of the rib articulates. As the body is followed anteriorly, the "angle" of the rib is formed. At the inferior border of the body is the costal or subcostal groove, partially housing the intercostal artery, vein and nerve. Each rib is continued anteriorly by a costal cartilage by which it is attached either directly or indirectly to the sternum, except for the eleventh and twelfth ribs, which have no sternal attachment.

The first and second ribs differ from the typical rib, and therefore need special description. The first rib—shortest and most curved of all the ribs—is quite flat, and its almost horizontal surfaces face roughly superiorly and inferiorly. On its superior surface are grooves for the subclavian artery and subclavian vein, separated by a tubercle for the attachment of the scalenus anterior muscle.

The second rib is a good deal longer than the first, but its curvature is very similar. Its angle, which is close to the tubercle, is not at all marked. Its external surface faces to some extent superiorly but a bit more outward than that of the first rib.

The typical articulation of a rib with the vertebral column involves both the head and tubercle of the rib. The head has two articular facets, the superior facet making contact with the vertebral body above and the inferior one with the vertebral body below. Between these the head of the rib is bound to the intervertebral disc by the intraarticular ligament. The articular facet on the tubercle

Costal groove

A middle rib viewed from behind

Transverse process (cut off)

Radiate ligament

Costotransverse (neck) ligament

Lateral costotransverse (head) ligament

Superior costotransverse (neck) ligament

Intertransverse ligament

Costovertebral ligaments viewed from right posterior

Costovertebral ligaments viewed from above

Radiate ligament

Interarticular ligament

Superior articular facet

Superior costotransverse ligament (cut off)

Synovial cavities

Lateral costotransverse (head) ligament

Costotransverse (neck) ligament

of the rib contacts the transverse process of the lower of the two vertebrae. These are true or synovial joints, with articular cartilages, joint capsules and synovial cavities. The articulations of the first, tenth, eleventh and twelfth ribs are each with only one vertebra, the vertebra of the same number.

The ligaments related to the typical articulation of a rib with the vertebral column are as follows: for articulation of the head of the rib, the intraarticular ligament and the capsular ligament, with a thickening of its anterior part forming the radiate ligament; and, for the costotransverse joint, the thin capsular ligament,

the lateral costotransverse ligament between the lateral part of the tubercle of the rib and the tip of the transverse process, and the superior costotransverse ligament attached to the transverse process of the rib above.

The first and the last two (or three) ribs each has a single articular facet that makes contact with an impression on the side of the thoracic vertebra of the same number. No intraarticular ligament is present, so there is just a single synovial cavity, in contrast to the two synovial cavities present for the typical rib. The lowest ribs do not have synovial joints between their tubercles and the transverse processes of the related vertebrae.

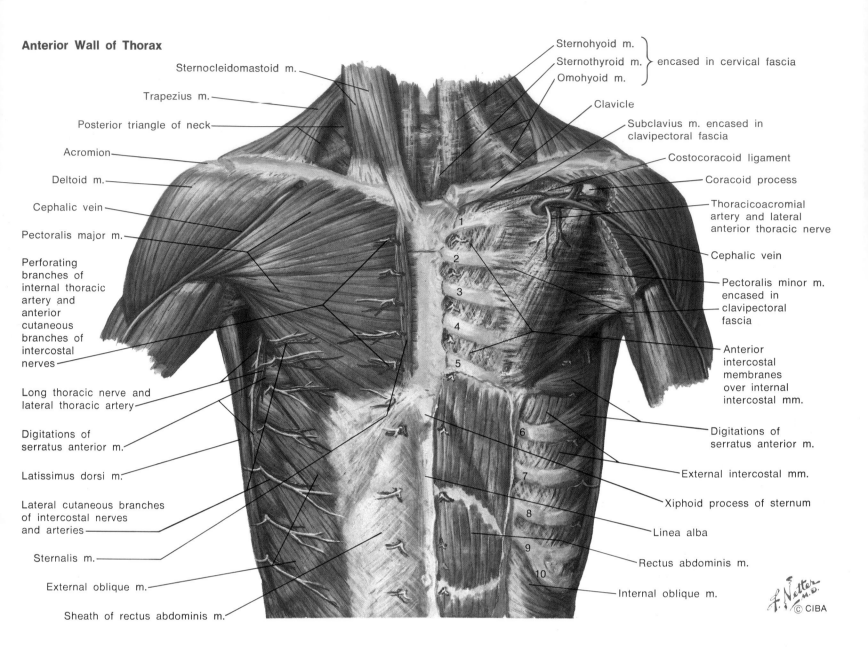

Sternocleidomastoid m.
Trapezius m.
Posterior triangle of neck
Acromion
Deltoid m.
Cephalic vein
Pectoralis major m.
Perforating branches of internal thoracic artery and anterior cutaneous branches of intercostal nerves
Long thoracic nerve and lateral thoracic artery
Digitations of serratus anterior m.
Latissimus dorsi m.
Lateral cutaneous branches of intercostal nerves and arteries
Sternalis m.
External oblique m.
Sheath of rectus abdominis m.

Sternohyoid m.
Sternothyroid m. } encased in cervical fascia
Omohyoid m.
Clavicle
Subclavius m. encased in clavipectoral fascia
Costocoracoid ligament
Coracoid process
Thoracicoacromial artery and lateral anterior thoracic nerve
Cephalic vein
Pectoralis minor m. encased in clavipectoral fascia
Anterior intercostal membranes over internal intercostal mm.
Digitations of serratus anterior m.
External intercostal mm.
Xiphoid process of sternum
Linea alba
Rectus abdominis m.
Internal oblique m.

SECTION I PLATE 4

Anterior Thoracic Wall

The anterior thoracic wall is covered by skin and the superficial fascia, which contains the mammary glands. Its framework is formed by the anterior part of the bony thorax, described and illustrated on page 4.

The muscles here belong to three groups: muscles of the upper extremity, muscles of the anterolateral abdominal wall, and intrinsic muscles of the thorax (Plates 4, 5 and 6).

Muscles of Upper Extremity

These muscles include the pectoralis major, pectoralis minor, serratus anterior, and subclavius.

The *pectoralis major muscle* has three areas of origin: clavicular, sternocostal and abdominal. The clavicular origin is the anterior surface of roughly the medial half of the clavicle. The sternocostal origin is the anterior surface of the

manubrium and body of the sternum, and the costal cartilages of the first six ribs. The small and variable abdominal origin is the aponeurosis of the external abdominal oblique muscle. The pectoralis major inserts onto the crest of the greater tubercle of the humerus.

The *pectoralis minor muscle* arises from the superior margins and external surfaces of the third, fourth and fifth ribs close to their costal cartilages, and from the fascia covering the intervening intercostal muscles. The pectoralis minor inserts onto the coracoid process of the scapula. The pectoralis major and minor muscles are supplied by the medial and lateral anterior thoracic nerves, which are branches of the medial and lateral cords of the brachial plexus.

The *serratus anterior muscle* arises by muscular digitations from the external surfaces and superior borders of the first eight or nine ribs, and from the fascia covering the intervening intercostal muscles. It inserts onto the ventral surface of the vertebral border of the scapula. Its nerve supply is the long thoracic nerve, a branch of the brachial plexus (fifth, sixth and seventh cervical nerves), which courses inferiorly on the external surface of the muscle.

The *subclavius muscle* has a tendinous origin from the area of the junction of the first rib and its costal cartilage, and inserts into a groove toward the lateral end of the lower surface of the clavicle.

It receives its nerve supply from the lateral trunk of the brachial plexus.

Muscles of Anterolateral Abdominal Wall

These muscles, which are partially on the anterior thoracic wall, are the external abdominal oblique and the rectus abdominis.

The *external abdominal oblique muscle* originates by fleshy digitations from the external surfaces and inferior borders of the fifth to twelfth ribs. The fasciculi from the last two ribs insert into the iliac crest, and the remaining fasciculi end in an aponeurosis which inserts in the linea alba.

The superior end of the *rectus abdominis muscle* is attached primarily to the external surfaces of the costal cartilages of the fifth, sixth and seventh ribs. The rectus abdominis muscle is enclosed in a sheath formed by the aponeuroses of the external oblique, the internal oblique and the transverse abdominis muscles.

The muscles of the anterolateral abdominal wall are supplied by the thoracicoabdominal branches of the lower six thoracic nerves.

Intrinsic Muscles of Thorax

These muscles, which help to form the anterior thoracic wall, are the external and internal intercostal muscles and the transversus thoracis muscle.

(Continued)

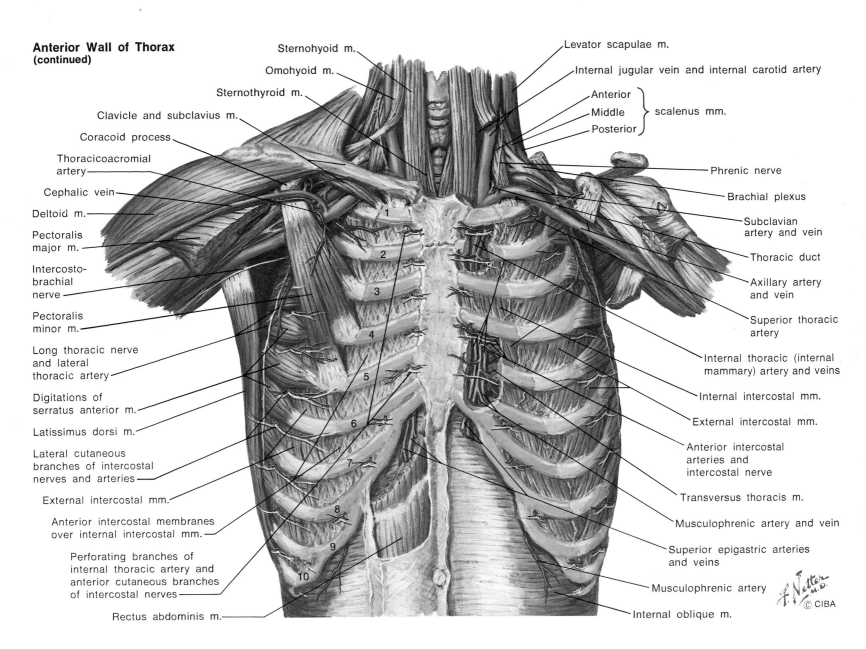

Sternohyoid m.

Omohyoid m.

Sternothyroid m.

Clavicle and subclavius m.

Coracoid process

Thoracicoacromial artery

Cephalic vein

Deltoid m.

Pectoralis major m.

Intercosto-brachial nerve

Pectoralis minor m.

Long thoracic nerve and lateral thoracic artery

Digitations of serratus anterior m.

Latissimus dorsi m.

Lateral cutaneous branches of intercostal nerves and arteries

External intercostal mm.

Anterior intercostal membranes over internal intercostal mm.

Perforating branches of internal thoracic artery and anterior cutaneous branches of intercostal nerves

Rectus abdominis m.

Levator scapulae m.

Internal jugular vein and internal carotid artery

Anterior / Middle / Posterior } scalenus mm.

Phrenic nerve

Brachial plexus

Subclavian artery and vein

Thoracic duct

Axillary artery and vein

Superior thoracic artery

Internal thoracic (internal mammary) artery and veins

Internal intercostal mm.

External intercostal mm.

Anterior intercostal arteries and intercostal nerve

Transversus thoracis m.

Musculophrenic artery and vein

Superior epigastric arteries and veins

Musculophrenic artery

Internal oblique m.

f. Netter © CIBA

Anterior Thoracic Wall
(Continued)

The *external intercostal muscles* each arise from the lower border of the rib above and insert onto the upper border of the rib below. Their fibers are directed downward and medially. They extend from the tubercles of the ribs to the beginnings of the costal cartilages, from which they continue medially as the anterior intercostal membranes. The *internal intercostal muscles* each arise from the inner lip and floor of the costal groove of the rib above and from the related costal cartilage. They insert onto the upper border of the rib below. These muscles extend from the sternum to the angles of the ribs, from which they continue to the vertebral column as the posterior intercostal membranes. The fibers of the internal intercostal muscles are directed downward and laterally.

Some authors describe *innermost intercostal muscles,* which are deep to the internal intercostals, but these are incomplete and variable. The intercostal muscles are supplied by the related intercostal nerves.

A muscle occasionally present, the *sternalis,* lies on the origin of the pectoralis major muscle parallel to the sternum. Its variable attachments are to the costal cartilages, the sternum, the rectus sheath, and the sternocleidomastoid and pectoralis major muscles.

On the inner surface of the anterior thoracic wall lies a thin sheet of muscular and tendinous fibers called the *transversus thoracis muscle.* This muscle arises from the posterior surfaces of the xiphoid process, the lower third of the body of the sternum, and the sternal ends of the related costal cartilages. It is inserted by muscular slips onto the inner surfaces of the second or third to the sixth costal cartilages.

Nerves of Anterior Thoracic Wall

The nerve supply of the skin of the anterior thoracic wall has two sources: the anterior and middle supraclavicular nerves (branches of the cervical plexus made up mostly of fibers from the fourth cervical nerve) cross over the clavicle to supply the skin of the infraclavicular area; the anterior and lateral cutaneous branches of the related intercostal nerves pierce the muscles to supply the skin of the remainder of the anterior thoracic wall.

Arteries of Anterior Thoracic Wall

Arteries supplying the anterior thoracic wall come from several sources. There is typically an artery in the upper part of the intercostal space and one in the lower part of the space. Posteriorly, nine pairs of intercostal arteries come from the back of the aorta and run forward in the lower nine intercostal spaces. Also posteriorly, the first intercostal space receives the highest intercostal branch of the costocervical trunk from the subclavian artery. This same artery anastomoses with the highest aortic intercostal artery, contributing to the supply of the second intercostal space. Near the angle of the rib, each aortic intercostal artery gives off a collateral intercostal branch which descends to run forward along the upper border of the rib below the intercostal space. These arteries anastomose with the intercostal branches of the internal thoracic (internal mammary) artery, of which there are two in each of the upper five or six spaces.

Veins of Anterior Thoracic Wall

Like venous drainage elsewhere, that of the anterior thoracic wall exhibits considerable variation. This account will not attempt to cover it

(Continued)

Anterior Thoracic Wall
(Continued)

Anterior Thoracic Wall from Within

- Manubrium of sternum
- L. sternothyroid m.
- L. sternohyoid m.
- L. internal jugular v.
- Brachiocephalic (innominate) a.
- R. subclavian a. and v.
- L. brachiocephalic (innominate) v.
- L. scalenus anterior m.
- R. internal thoracic (internal mammary) a. and v.
- L. pericardiacophrenic a. and v. and phrenic n.
- Anterior intercostal a. and v. and intercostal n.
- Right clavicle
- Penetrating a. and v. and anterior cutaneous branch of intercostal n.
- Internal intercostal m.
- Innermost intercostal m.
- L. internal thoracic (internal mammary) a. and vv.
- Diaphragm
- Transversus abdominis m.
- Body of sternum
- Xiphoid
- Sternal origin of diaphragm
- R. musculophrenic a. and v.
- R. superior epigastric a. and v.
- Transversus thoracis m.

F. Netter M.D. © CIBA

completely. The most frequent pattern involves the veins accompanying the internal thoracic (internal mammary) arteries and the azygos, hemiazygos and accessory hemiazygos veins. The veins accompanying the internal thoracic arteries receive tributaries corresponding to the arterial branches, and empty into the brachiocephalic (innominate) veins of the same side. The first posterior intercostal vein usually empties into either the brachiocephalic (innominate) or the vertebral vein. The right highest intercostal vein usually drains blood from the second and third intercostal spaces and passes inferiorly to empty into the azygos vein. The left highest intercostal vein also receives the second and third posterior intercostal veins and empties into the lower border of the left brachiocephalic vein.

The fourth to the eleventh posterior intercostal veins on the right side empty into the azygos vein, which is ordinarily formed by the junction of the right ascending lumbar vein and the right subcostal vein. The latter courses superiorly on the right side of the thoracic vertebrae to the level of the fourth posterior intercostal vein, where it passes in front of the root of the lung to empty into the superior vena cava just before this vessel enters the pericardial sac. On the left side, the ascending lumbar vein and the subcostal vein form the hemiazygos vein, which usually receives the lower four

posterior intercostal veins as it runs superiorly to the left of the vertebral column. Here it crosses at about the level of the ninth thoracic vertebra to empty into the azygos vein. The accessory hemiazygos vein receives the fourth to the eighth posterior intercostal veins as it courses inferiorly to the left of the vertebral column before crossing at about the level of the eighth thoracic vertebra, also to empty into the azygos vein.

Lymphatic Drainage of Anterior Thoracic Wall

The lymphatic drainage of the anterior thoracic wall involves three general groups of lymph

nodes: sternal (internal thoracic), phrenic (diaphragmatic) and intercostal. The sternal nodes lie along the superior parts of the internal thoracic arteries. There are several groups of phrenic nodes on the superior surface of the diaphragm, and there is an intercostal node or two at the vertebral end of each intercostal space. The efferents of the sternal nodes usually empty into the bronchomediastinal trunk. The efferents of the phrenic nodes ordinarily go to the sternal nodes. The upper intercostal nodes send their efferents to the thoracic duct, while the lower ones on each side drain into a vessel that courses inferiorly into the cisterna chyli.

Dorsal Aspect of Thorax

External occipital protuberance

Posterior triangle

Sternocleidomastoid m.

Trapezius m.

Spine of scapula

Infraspinatus fascia

Teres major m.

Teres minor m.

Deltoid m.

Splenius capitis m.

Accessory (XI) nerve

Levator scapulae m.

Rhomboideus minor m.

Rhomboideus major m.

Supraspinatus m.

Infraspinatus m.

Teres major m.

Teres minor m.

T1

6

T2

Latissimus dorsi m.

External oblique m.

Lumbar trigone (of Petit) and internal oblique m.

Iliac crest

Cut end of latissimus dorsi m.

Lower digitations of serratus anterior m.

Digitations of external oblique m.

Serratus posterior inferior m.

Lumbodorsal fascia over long muscles of back (sacrospinalis)

Medial } cutaneous branches of posterior
Lateral } rami of thoracic nerves

F. Netter ©CIBA

Dorsal Aspect of Thorax

The dorsal aspect of the thorax is also covered by skin and superficial fascia, with the cutaneous nerves to the skin of the back ramifying in the latter. These cutaneous nerves are branches of the posterior primary divisions (dorsal rami) of the thoracic nerves: for the upper six thoracic levels the medial branch, and for the lower six the lateral branch.

The more superficial muscles on the posterior aspect of the thorax belong to the group connecting the upper extremity to the vertebral column. They are the trapezius, latissimus dorsi, rhomboideus major, rhomboideus minor and levator scapulae.

The *trapezius muscle* arises from about the medial third of the superior nuchal line, the external occipital protuberance and the posterior margin of the ligamentum nuchae, and from the spinous processes of the seventh cervical and all of the thoracic vertebrae, and the related supraspinous ligaments. The lower fibers converge into an aponeurosis which slides over the triangular area at the medial end of the spine of the scapula and is attached at the apex of this triangle. The middle group of fibers is inserted on the medial margin of the acromion and the upper margin of the posterior border of the spine of the scapula. The upper group of fibers ends on the posterior border of the lateral third of the clavicle. The trapezius is supplied by the spinal part of the eleventh cranial nerve and branches from the anterior divisions (ventral rami) of the third and fourth cervical nerves. When contracting, the muscle tends to pull the scapula medially while at the same time rotating it, thus carrying the shoulder superiorly. If the shoulder is fixed, the upper fibers tilt the head so that the face goes upward toward the opposite side.

The *latissimus dorsi muscle* has a broad origin: by a small muscular slip from the outer lip of the iliac crest just lateral to the sacrospinalis muscle, and by an extensive aponeurosis attached to the spinous processes of the lower six thoracic vertebrae, the lumbar and sacral vertebrae, and the related supraspinous ligaments. This muscle is inserted into the depth of the intertubercular groove of the humerus. Its nerve supply comes from the sixth, seventh and eighth cervical nerves by way of the thoracodorsal branch of the brachial plexus. This muscle helps with extension, adduction and medial rotation at the shoulder joint, and helps to depress the raised arm against resistance.

The *rhomboideus major and minor muscles* are often difficult to separate, but the major is described as arising from the tips of the spinous processes and supraspinous ligaments of the second to fifth thoracic vertebrae. Its insertion is into the vertebral border of the scapula via a tendinous arch running from the lower angle of the smooth triangle at the root of the spine to the inferior angle. The rhomboideus minor muscle arises from the spinous processes of the first thoracic and last cervical vertebrae and the lower part of the ligamentum nuchae, and is inserted into the vertebral border of the scapula at the base of the triangle forming the root of the scapular spine. The rhomboideus muscles are supplied by fibers from the *(Continued)*

Dorsal Aspect of Thorax (continued)

Spinous process T1

Splenius capitis and cervicis mm.

Scalenus posterior m.

Serratus posterior superior m.

External intercostal mm.

Lumbodorsal fascia over long muscles of back (sacrospinalis)

Long muscles of back cut away to reveal short vertebrocostal and intervertebral mm.

Serratus posterior inferior m.

Digitations of external oblique m. of abdomen

Internal oblique m.

Tendon of origin of transversus abdominis m.

L2

Dorsal Aspect of Thorax
(*Continued*)

Lateral Aspect of Thorax

Scalenus mm. { Anterior / Middle / Posterior

Accessory (XI) nerve

Levator scapulae m.

Brachial plexus

Subclavian artery and vein

Superior thoracic artery

Anterior intercostal membrane over internal intercostal m.

Perforating branch of internal thoracic artery and anterior cutaneous branch of intercostal nerve

Intercostobrachial nerve

External intercostal m.

Lateral thoracic artery

Lateral cutaneous branches of intercostal nerves and arteries

Serratus anterior m.

Scapula retracted

Teres major m.

Subscapularis m.

Long thoracic nerve

F. Netter M.D. © CIBA

fifth and sixth cervical nerves by way of the dorsoscapular branch of the brachial plexus. The rhomboideus major and minor muscles tend to draw the scapula toward the vertebral column and also slightly superiorly, with the lower fibers of the major helping to rotate the scapula so that the shoulder is depressed.

The *levator scapulae muscle* originates in four tendinous slips attached to the transverse processes of the first four cervical vertebrae. Its insertion is the vertebral border of the scapula from its superior angle to the smooth triangle at the medial end of the spine scapula. Its nerve supply is primarily by cervical plexus branches from the ventral rami of the third and fourth cervical nerves. The levator scapulae, as the name indicates, elevates the scapula, drawing it medially and rotating it so that the tip of the shoulder is depressed.

Just deep to the group of muscles connecting the upper extremity to the vertebral column lie the serratus posterior superior and serratus posterior inferior muscles.

The *serratus posterior superior muscle* has an origin via a thin aponeurosis attached to the lower part of the ligamentum nuchae and to the spinous processes and related supraspinous ligaments of the seventh cervical and upper two or three thoracic vertebrae. It is inserted by fleshy digitations into the upper borders of the second to fifth ribs lateral to their angles. This muscle helps to increase the size of the thoracic cavity by elevating the ribs. The *serratus posterior inferior muscle* arises by means of a thin aponeurosis from the spinous processes and related supraspinous ligaments of the last two thoracic vertebrae and the first two or three lumbar vertebrae. This muscle inserts by fleshy digitations into the lower borders of the last four ribs, just beyond their angles. It tends to pull the last four ribs downward and outward. The serratus

posterior muscles receive branches of the ventral rami of the thoracic nerves at the levels at which they are located.

Just deep to the serratus posterior superior muscle lie the thoracic portions of the splenius cervicis and capitis muscles.

The *splenius cervicis muscle* has a tendinous origin from the spinous processes of the third to sixth thoracic vertebrae, and wraps around the deeper muscles to insert by tendinous fasciculi onto the transverse processes of the upper two or three cervical vertebrae. The *splenius capitis muscle* arises from the inferior half of the ligamentum nuchae and the spinous processes of the seventh cervical

and the first three or four thoracic vertebrae. It is inserted onto the occipital bone just inferior to the lateral third of the superior nuchal line. The splenius muscles tend to pull the head and neck backward and laterally and to turn the face toward the same side. They are supplied by branches of the posterior primary divisions of the middle and lower cervical nerves.

The groove lateral to the spinous processes of the thoracic vertebrae is filled by the *sacrospinalis muscle*, which is covered by the thoracic part of the lumbodorsal fascia. Deep to the sacrospinalis muscle lie the short vertebrocostal and intervertebral muscles; they will not be described here.

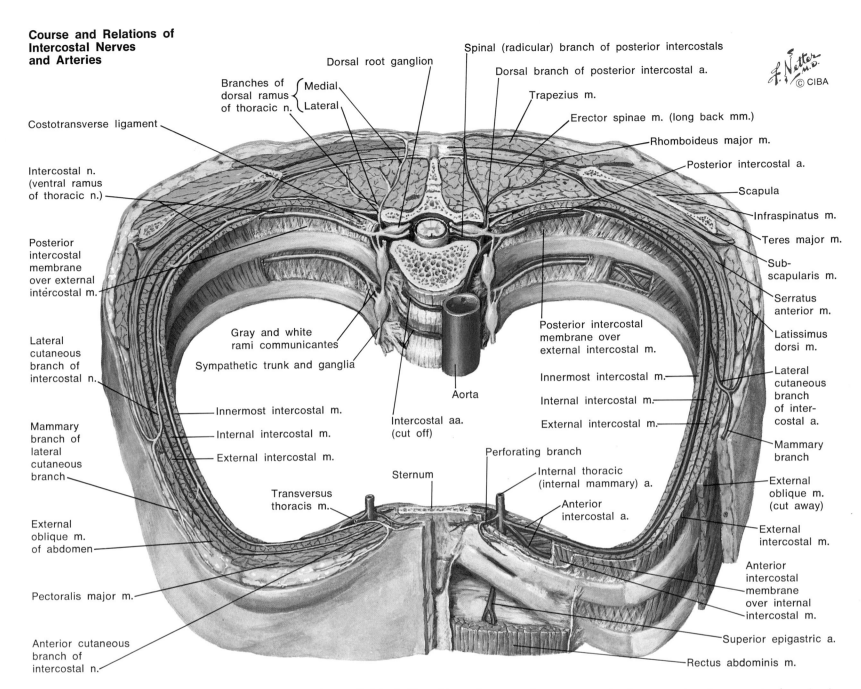

Costotransverse ligament

Branches of dorsal ramus of thoracic n. { Medial / Lateral

Dorsal root ganglion

Spinal (radicular) branch of posterior intercostals

Dorsal branch of posterior intercostal a.

Trapezius m.

Erector spinae m. (long back mm.)

Rhomboideus major m.

Posterior intercostal a.

Scapula

Infraspinatus m.

Teres major m.

Sub-scapularis m.

Serratus anterior m.

Latissimus dorsi m.

Intercostal n. (ventral ramus of thoracic n.)

Posterior intercostal membrane over external intercostal m.

Lateral cutaneous branch of intercostal n.

Mammary branch of lateral cutaneous branch

Gray and white rami communicantes

Sympathetic trunk and ganglia

Innermost intercostal m.

Internal intercostal m.

External intercostal m.

Aorta

Intercostal aa. (cut off)

Posterior intercostal membrane over external intercostal m.

Innermost intercostal m.

Internal intercostal m.

External intercostal m.

Lateral cutaneous branch of intercostal a.

Mammary branch

External intercostal m.

External oblique m. of abdomen

Pectoralis major m.

Transversus thoracis m.

Sternum

Perforating branch

Internal thoracic (internal mammary) a.

Anterior intercostal a.

External oblique m. (cut away)

External intercostal m.

Anterior intercostal membrane over internal intercostal m.

Anterior cutaneous branch of intercostal n.

Superior epigastric a.

Rectus abdominis m.

Course and Relations of Intercostal Nerves and Arteries

The typical thoracic spinal nerve is formed by the junction of a dorsal root and a ventral root near the intervertebral foramen below the vertebra having the same number as the nerve. The *dorsal root* is made up of a series of rootlets which emerge from one segment of the spinal cord between its dorsal and lateral white columns, and contains the nerve cell bodies of the afferent neurons which enter the spinal cord through it. This collection of nerve cell bodies causes a swelling of the root, named the dorsal root ganglion. A series of rootlets composed of axons of ventral horn gray cells leaves the same segment of the cord between the lateral and ventral white columns to form the *ventral root* of the spinal nerve.

The dorsal and ventral roots join near the intervertebral foramen to make up the very short *common trunk* of the spinal nerve, which divides almost immediately into the dorsal ramus (posterior primary division) and the ventral ramus (anterior

primary division). The white and gray rami communicantes, which connect the ganglia of the sympathetic trunk and the thoracic nerves of the same level, join the ventral ramus near its origin.

The *dorsal ramus* of the thoracic nerve, passing posteriorly, pierces the erector spinae muscle (which it supplies), the trapezius muscle and the other superficial muscles of the back (depending on the level) to reach the superficial fascia. Here it divides into a smaller medial branch and a longer lateral cutaneous branch, which supply the skin.

The *ventral ramus* of the thoracic nerve is the intercostal nerve of that particular level (for the twelfth thoracic nerve, the subcostal nerve). From the seventh to the eleventh thoracic levels the ventral rami of the thoracic nerves continue from the intercostal spaces into the anterior abdominal wall. The intercostal nerve runs forward in the thoracic wall between the innermost intercostal muscle and the internal intercostal muscle. It lies inferior to the intercostal vein and intercostal artery, and gives off a collateral branch to the lower part of the space, as do the vein and artery. The intercostal nerve has a lateral cutaneous branch at the lateral aspect of the thorax which pierces the overlying intercostal muscles to reach the subcutaneous tissue. There it divides into an

anterior (mammary) and a posterior branch. At the anterior end of the intercostal space, the intercostal nerve ends by becoming the anterior cutaneous nerve, which divides into a lateral branch and a shorter and smaller medial branch.

The aorta, lying on the anterior aspect of the vertebral bodies, gives off pairs of posterior (aortic) intercostal arteries. They course forward in the upper part of the intercostal spaces between the intercostal vein above and the intercostal nerve below, to anastomose within the anterior intercostal branches of the internal thoracic and musculophrenic arteries. Collateral branches run in the inferior parts of the intercostal space. The right posterior intercostal arteries lie on the anterior aspect and the right side of the vertebral bodies as they travel to reach the intercostal spaces of the right side.

To reach the pleural cavity from the outside at the anterolateral aspect of the thorax, a needle would pass through the following layers: skin, superficial fascia, intercostal muscles and related deep fascial layers, subpleural fascia, and parietal layer of the pleura. If the needle is carefully inserted near the lower part of the intercostal space, *i.e.*, above the rib margin, one is reasonably sure of avoiding the intercostal nerve and vessels.

Diaphragm (viewed from above)

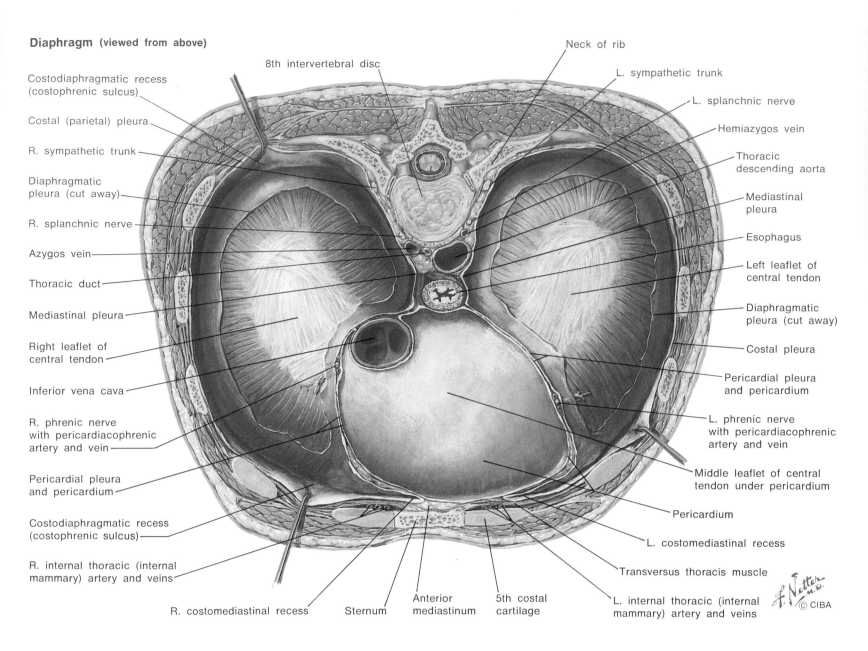

Costodiaphragmatic recess (costophrenic sulcus)

Costal (parietal) pleura

R. sympathetic trunk

Diaphragmatic pleura (cut away)

R. splanchnic nerve

Azygos vein

Thoracic duct

Mediastinal pleura

Right leaflet of central tendon

Inferior vena cava

R. phrenic nerve with pericardiacophrenic artery and vein

Pericardial pleura and pericardium

Costodiaphragmatic recess (costophrenic sulcus)

R. internal thoracic (internal mammary) artery and veins

8th intervertebral disc

Neck of rib

L. sympathetic trunk

L. splanchnic nerve

Hemiazygos vein

Thoracic descending aorta

Mediastinal pleura

Esophagus

Left leaflet of central tendon

Diaphragmatic pleura (cut away)

Costal pleura

Pericardial pleura and pericardium

L. phrenic nerve with pericardiacophrenic artery and vein

Middle leaflet of central tendon under pericardium

Pericardium

L. costomediastinal recess

Transversus thoracis muscle

L. internal thoracic (internal mammary) artery and veins

R. costomediastinal recess

Sternum

Anterior mediastinum

5th costal cartilage

SECTION I   PLATE 10

Diaphragm (Viewed from Above)

The diaphragm is a musculotendinous septum separating the thoracic from the abdominal cavity. Thus it forms the floor of the thoracic cavity.

The origin of the diaphragm is from the outlet of the thorax, and has three parts: sternal, costal and lumbar.

The *sternal origin* is by two fleshy slips from the posterior aspect of the xiphoid process.

The *costal origin* is by fleshy slips which interdigitate with the slips of origin of the transversus abdominis muscle. These arise on the inner surfaces of the costal cartilages and adjacent parts of the last six ribs on both the right and left sides.

The *lumbar portion* of the origin is by a right and a left crus, and right and left medial and lateral lumbocostal arches. The tendinous crura blend with the anterior longitudinal ligament of the vertebral column and are attached to the anterior surfaces of the lumbar vertebral bodies and related intervertebral discs—to the first three on the right and the first two on the left. The medial lumbocostal arch, a thickening of the fascia covering the psoas major muscle, extends from the side of the body of the first or second lumbar vertebra to the front of the transverse process of the first (sometimes also the second) lumbar vertebra. The

lateral lumbocostal arch, passing across the quadratus lumborum muscle, extends from the transverse process of the first lumbar vertebra to the tip and lower border of the twelfth rib.

From the extensive origin just described, the fibers converge to insert in a three-leafed central tendon. Contraction of the muscular portion of the diaphragm pulls the central tendon downward, thus increasing the volume of the thoracic cavity and bringing about inspiration.

The diaphragmatic nerve supply is by way of the right and left phrenic nerves, which are branches of the right and left cervical plexuses and receive their fibers primarily from the fourth cervical nerves, with some contribution from the third and fifth cervical nerves.

Several structures pass between the thoracic and abdominal cavities through apertures in the diaphragm.

The *aortic hiatus* is at the level of the twelfth thoracic vertebra and is actually between the diaphragm and the vertebra. This opening also transmits the azygos vein and the thoracic duct.

The *esophageal hiatus* is at about the level of the tenth thoracic vertebra, in the fleshy part of the diaphragm. It also transmits the right and left vagus nerves and small esophageal arteries and veins.

The foramen for the *inferior vena cava* is situated at about the level of the disc, between the eighth

and ninth thoracic vertebrae, at the junction of the right and middle leaflets of the central tendon. Some branches of the right phrenic nerve also pass through this foramen.

The right crus is pierced by the right greater and lesser splanchnic nerves, and the left crus is pierced by the left greater and lesser splanchnic nerves and the hemiazygos vein. The sympathetic trunks usually do not pierce the diaphragm but pass behind the medial lumbocostal arches.

The base of the fibrous pericardial sac is partially blended with the middle leaflet of the central tendon of the diaphragm. The diaphragmatic portions of the parietal pleura are closely blended with the upper surfaces of the right and left portions of the diaphragm. Where the diaphragmatic pleura reflects at a sharp angle to become the costal pleura, the costodiaphragmatic recess or costophrenic sulcus is formed. Where the costal pleura reflects to become pericardial pleura, the costomediastinal recess is formed.

It should be noted that the dome of the diaphragm on the right side is as high as the fifth costal cartilage (varying with the phase of respiration) and on the left is only slightly lower, so that some of the abdominal viscera are covered by the thoracic cage.

For an illustration of the diaphragm viewed from below, see CIBA COLLECTION, Volume 3/II, page 21.

Topography of Lungs (Anterior View)

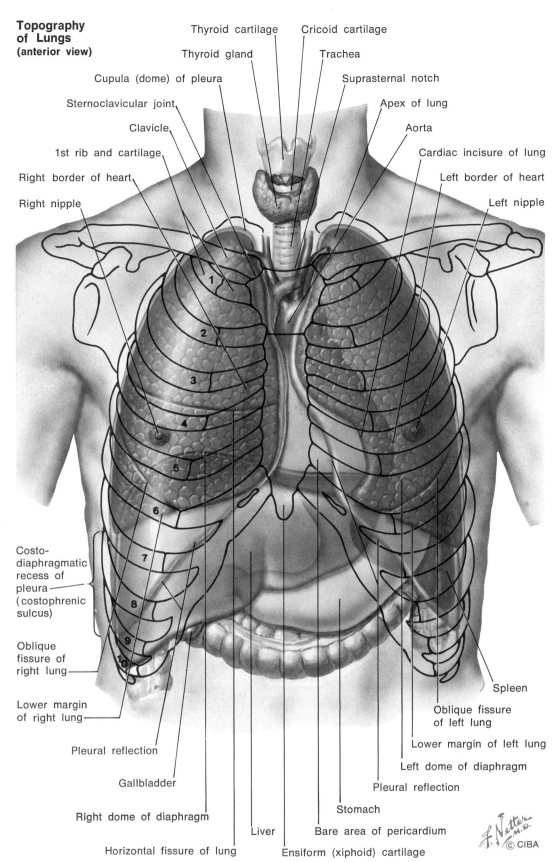

Topography of Lungs (anterior view)

Thyroid cartilage
Cricoid cartilage
Thyroid gland
Trachea
Cupula (dome) of pleura
Suprasternal notch
Sternoclavicular joint
Apex of lung
Clavicle
Aorta
1st rib and cartilage
Cardiac incisure of lung
Right border of heart
Left border of heart
Right nipple
Left nipple

Costo-diaphragmatic recess of pleura (costophrenic sulcus)

Oblique fissure of right lung

Lower margin of right lung

Pleural reflection

Gallbladder

Right dome of diaphragm

Horizontal fissure of lung

Liver

Ensiform (xiphoid) cartilage

Bare area of pericardium

Stomach

Pleural reflection

Left dome of diaphragm

Lower margin of left lung

Oblique fissure of left lung

Spleen

Since the apex of each lung reaches as far superiorly as the vertebral end of the first rib, the lung usually extends about an inch above the medial one-third of the clavicle when viewed from the front. Thus the lung projects into the base of the neck.

The anterior border of the right lung descends behind the sternoclavicular joint and almost reaches the midline at the level of the sternal angle. It continues inferiorly posterior to the sternum to the level of the sixth chondrosternal junction. There the inferior border curves laterally and slightly inferiorly, crossing the sixth rib in the midclavicular line and the eighth rib in the midaxillary line. It then runs posteriorly and medially at the level of the spinous process of the tenth thoracic vertebra. These levels are, of course, variable and apply to the lung in expiration. In inspiration the levels for the inferior border would be roughly two ribs lower.

The anterior border of the left lung is similar in position to that of the right lung. However, at the level of the fourth costal cartilage it deviates laterally because of the heart, causing a cardiac notch in this border of the lung. The inferior border of the left lung is similar in position to that of the right lung except that it extends farther inferiorly, since the right lung is pushed up by the liver below the diaphragm on the right side.

The oblique fissure of the right lung, separating the lower lobe from the upper and middle lobes, ends at the lower border of the lung near the midclavicular line. The horizontal fissure separating the middle from the upper lobe begins at the oblique fissure and runs horizontally forward to the lung's anterior border, which it reaches at about the level of the fourth costal cartilage.

Since the left lung ordinarily has only two lobes, there is usually no horizontal fissure in this lung. The oblique fissure of the left lung is similar in its location to the corresponding fissure of the right side.

It should be remembered that extra fissures may occur in either lung. When such fissures do occur, they are likely to be found between bronchopulmonary segments and, in the left lung, between the superior and inferior divisions of the upper lobe, giving rise to a "three-lobed" left lung.

The lungs seldom extend as far inferiorly as the parietal pleura, so some of the diaphragmatic parietal pleura is usually in contact with costal parietal pleura. This area—which, of course, varies in size with the phase of respiration—is called the costodiaphragmatic recess of the pleura or the costophrenic sulcus. A similar but much less extensive area is present where the anterior border of the lung does not extend to its limits medially—especially in expiration—and the costal and mediastinal parietal pleurae are in contact. This area is called the costomediastinal recess.

The diaphragm separates the liver from the right lung and, depending on the size of the liver, from the left lung. The left lung is also separated by the diaphragm from the stomach and the spleen.

The nipple in the male and in the female (depending on the size and functional state of the breast) usually overlies the fourth intercostal space in approximately the midclavicular line.

Topography of Lungs
(Posterior View)

The apex of the lung extends as far superiorly as the vertebral end of the first rib and therefore as high as the first thoracic vertebra. From there, the lung extends inferiorly as far as the diaphragm, with the base of the lung resting on the diaphragm and fitted to its superior surface. Because of the diaphragm's domed shape, the level of the highest point on the base of the right lung is about at the eighth to ninth thoracic vertebra. The highest point on the base of the left lung is a fraction of an inch lower. From these high points the bases of the two lungs follow the curves of the diaphragm to reach the levels described on page 13 for the inferior borders of the lungs.

The highest point on the oblique fissure of the two lungs is on their posterior aspects, at about the level of the third to fourth thoracic vertebra, a little over an inch from the midline.

If the arm is raised over the head, the vertebral border of the scapula approximates the position of the oblique fissure of the lung. If the shoulder is brought forward as far as possible, the scapula is carried laterally, so that the area in which auscultation can be satisfactorily carried out on the posterior aspect of the chest is significantly widened.

The parietal pleura is separated from the visceral pleura by a potential space (the pleural cavity), which under normal circumstances contains only a minimal amount of serous fluid. Caudal to the inferior margin of the lung the costal parietal pleura is in contact with the diaphragmatic parietal pleura, forming what is called the costodiaphragmatic recess (costophrenic sulcus). This

Topography of Lungs (posterior view)

Labels: Cupula (dome) of pleura; 1st rib; Oblique fissure of right lung; Clavicle; Horizontal fissure of lung; Right margin of parietal pleura; Apex of left lung; 1st rib; Oblique fissure of left lung; Spine of scapula; Left margin of parietal pleura; L. costodiaphragmatic recess of pleura (l. costophrenic sulcus); Spleen; Pleural reflection; Lower margin of left lung; Left kidney; Left dome of diaphragm; L. suprarenal gland; Liver; Lower margin of right lung; Pleural reflection; Right kidney; Right dome of diaphragm; R. suprarenal gland

allows for the caudal movement of the inferior margin of the lung on inspiration.

Under abnormal circumstances the pleural cavity may contain air, increased amounts of serous fluid, blood or pus. The accumulation of a significant amount of any of these in the pleural cavity compresses the lung and causes respiratory difficulties.

The diaphragm separates the base of the left lung from the fundus of the stomach and the spleen. Because of this relationship, if the stomach becomes overfilled with retained food or gas it can push the diaphragm upward and embarrass respiratory activity.

The base of the right lung is separated from the liver by the diaphragm. Because of this relationship, if the liver increases in size it can elevate the diaphragm and push against the lung, possibly limiting its expansion. An abscess on the diaphragmatic surface of the liver can rupture through the diaphragm and involve the related pleural cavity and lung.

It should be remembered that in the illustration the lungs are shown in relation to the bony thorax, scapula and diaphragm, but overlying the structures shown are the deep and superficial muscles of the back, in addition to the superficial fascia and skin.

Medial Surface of Right Lung

Groove for subclavian artery

Apex

Area for trachea

Groove for brachiocephalic (innominate) vein

Area for esophagus

Groove for azygos vein

Groove for 1st rib

R. upper lobe bronchus

Groove for superior vena cava

Upper lobe

Area for thymus and mediastinal fatty tissue

Oblique fissure

Lower lobe

Cut edge of pleura

Anterior (sternal) margin

Pulmonary arteries

Upper lobe

Bronchial arteries

Hilus

Bronchi

Horizontal fissure

Superior pulmonary veins

Cardiac depression

Lymph nodes

Middle lobe

Inferior pulmonary veins

Oblique fissure

Lower lobe

Diaphragmatic surface

Groove for inferior vena cava

Puimonary ligament

Groove for esophagus

Inferior margin

Medial Surface of Left Lung

Area for trachea and esophagus

Apex

Groove for subclavian artery

Groove for arch of aorta

Groove for brachiocephalic (innominate) vein

Upper lobe

Groove for 1st rib

Oblique fissure

Area for thymus and mediastinal fatty tissue

Lower lobe

Anterior (sternal) margin

Upper lobe

Hilus

Cardiac depression

Cardiac notch (incisure)

Oblique fissure

Lingula

Lower lobe

Groove for descending aorta

Lower lobe

Pulmonary ligament

Groove for esophagus

Inferior margin

Diaphragmatic surface

f. Netter M.D. © CIBA

Medial Surface of Lungs

The medial (mediastinal) surfaces of the right and left lungs present concave mirror images of the right and left sides of the mediastinum. In other words, in addition to the structures forming the root of the lung, the medial lung surface presents distinct impressions made by the structures constituting the mediastinum (Plates 18 and 19).

Medial Surface of Right Lung. The oblique and horizontal fissures (if complete) divide the right lung into upper, middle and lower lobes. The pleura reflects directly from the parietal to the

visceral surface around the root of the lung, except where it forms the pulmonary ligament, which extends from the inferior aspect of the root vertically down to the medial border of the base of the lung.

The main structures forming the root of the right lung are: the superior and inferior pulmonary veins, which are situated anterior and inferior; the pulmonary artery; and the bronchus, which is posterior in position. A number of lymph nodes are also present.

Much of the ventral and inferior portion of the mediastinal surface shows the impression caused by the heart. Superior to this is the groove caused by the superior vena cava, with the groove for the right brachiocephalic (innominate) vein above that. Near the apex of the lung is the groove for the right subclavian artery. Arching over the root of the lung is the groove caused by the azygos vein. Superior to this are the areas for the trachea (anteriorly) and the esophagus (posteriorly). The area for the esophagus continues inferiorly posterior to the root of the lung.

Since the inferior margin of the outer, costal surface of the lung extends downward farther than the lower margin of the medial surface, the diaphragmatic surface of the lung can also be seen when the medial aspect of the lung is observed.

Medial Surface of Left Lung. The oblique fissure (if complete) divides the left lung into upper and lower lobes. The relationship of the pleura to

the root of the left lung is similar to that described for the right lung.

Structures forming the root of the left lung are the pulmonary artery superiorly, the bronchus posteriorly, and the superior and inferior pulmonary veins anteriorly and inferiorly. Some lymph nodes are also present.

A large impression caused by the heart is present anterior and inferior to the root of the lung. It is responsible for a rather marked "cardiac notch" in the anterior border of the upper lobe of the left lung. Inferior to this notch is a projection of the upper lobe, the lingula.

Arching over the root of the left lung and continuing inferiorly — posterior to the root — to the base of the lung is a groove for the aortic arch and the descending aorta.

Superior to the groove for the aortic arch are, from behind forward, areas for the esophagus and trachea, the groove for the left subclavian artery, the groove for the left brachiocephalic (innominate) vein, and a groove caused by the first rib.

The portion of the medial surface of the left lung posterior to the areas for the descending aorta and esophagus is in contact with the thoracic vertebral bodies and the vertebral ends of the ribs, except where separated from them by structures lying in the position described above.

As on the right side, the diaphragmatic surface of the left lung can be seen as the medial aspect of the lung is observed.

Bronchopulmonary Segments

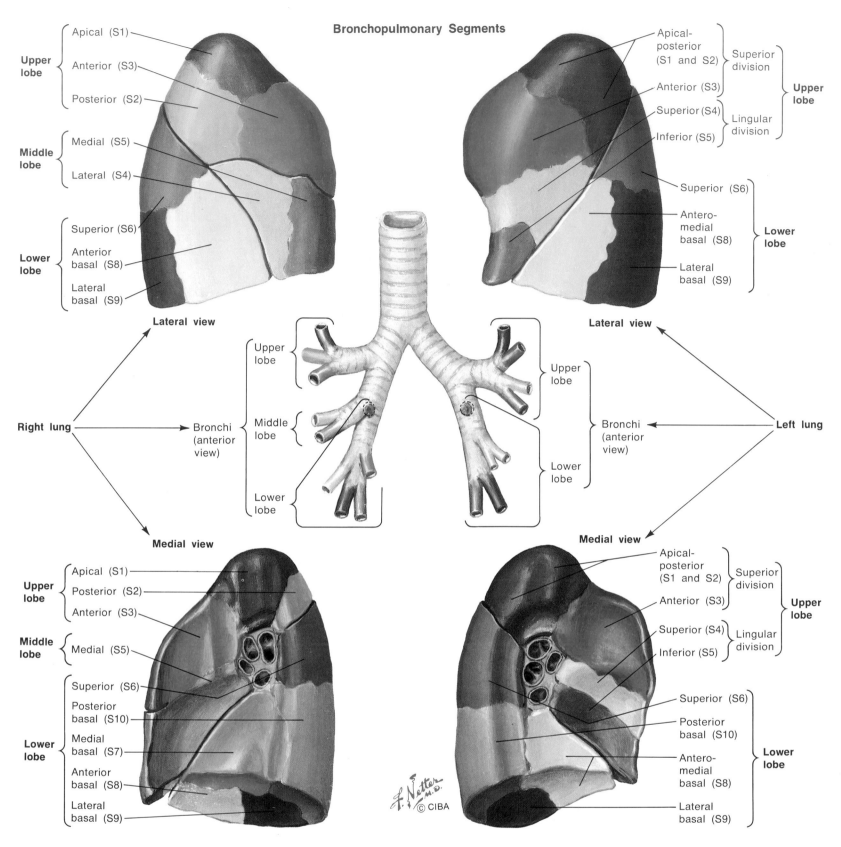

Bronchopulmonary Segments

Upper lobe — Apical (S1), Anterior (S3), Posterior (S2)
Middle lobe — Medial (S5), Lateral (S4)
Lower lobe — Superior (S6), Anterior basal (S8), Lateral basal (S9)

Lateral view

Upper lobe — Apical-posterior (S1 and S2) / Superior division, Anterior (S3), Superior (S4) / Lingular division, Inferior (S5)
Superior (S6), Antero-medial basal (S8), Lateral basal (S9) — **Lower lobe**

Lateral view

Right lung → Bronchi (anterior view)

Upper lobe, Middle lobe, Lower lobe

Upper lobe, Lower lobe

Bronchi (anterior view) ← Left lung

Medial view

Upper lobe — Apical (S1), Posterior (S2), Anterior (S3)
Middle lobe — Medial (S5)
Lower lobe — Superior (S6), Posterior basal (S10), Medial basal (S7), Anterior basal (S8), Lateral basal (S9)

Medial view

Apical-posterior (S1 and S2) / Superior division, Anterior (S3), Superior (S4) / Lingular division, Inferior (S5) — **Upper lobe**
Superior (S6), Posterior basal (S10), Antero-medial basal (S8), Lateral basal (S9) — **Lower lobe**

F. Netter M.D. © CIBA

SECTION I   PLATE 14

Bronchopulmonary Segments

A bronchopulmonary segment can be defined as that portion of the lung which is supplied by the terminal branching of a lobar bronchus. In general, the artery supplying a segment tends to follow the segmental bronchus. The segmental veins are at the periphery of the segment and thus can be helpful in delineating it.

Right Lung

The right main bronchus gives rise to three lobar bronchi: upper, middle and lower. Any two of these may occasionally have a common stem.

Right Upper Lobe. The *apical segment* (S1) of the right upper lobe forms the apex of the right lung. It extends into the root of the neck as high as the vertebral end of the first rib. Toward the lateral aspect of the lung, the apical segment dips downward slightly between the posterior and anterior segments. This boundary line is roughly at the level of the first rib anteriorly and almost down to the second rib posteriorly.

The *posterior segment* (S2) extends from the apical segment down to the lateral portion of the horizontal fissure and the upper part of the oblique fissure.

The *anterior segment* (S3) extends from the apical segment above down to the horizontal fissure at about the level of the fourth rib.

Right Middle Lobe. The middle lobe bronchus branches into two segmental bronchi, the complete branchings of which become the *lateral segment* (S4) and *medial segment* (S5) of the lobe. These segments are separated by a vertical plane extending from the hilus out to the costal surface of the lung and reaching its inferior border just anterior to the lower end of the oblique fissure. The segments are related to the anterior parts of the fourth and fifth ribs and their costal cartilages.

Right Lower Lobe. The lower lobe bronchus gives off a posteriorly directed superior segmental bronchus just below the level of the orifice of the middle lobe bronchus. The *superior segment* (S6) of the lower lobe occupies the entire superior part of

(Continued)

Pulmonary Segments in Relationship to Ribs

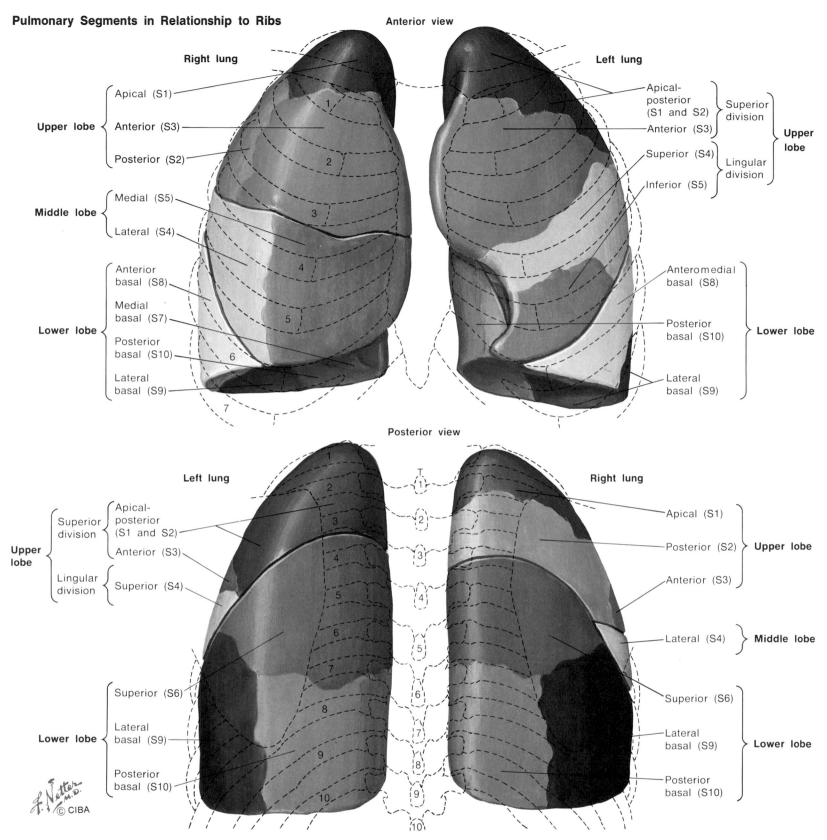

Anterior view

Right lung

Upper lobe
- Apical (S1)
- Anterior (S3)
- Posterior (S2)

Middle lobe
- Medial (S5)
- Lateral (S4)

Lower lobe
- Anterior basal (S8)
- Medial basal (S7)
- Posterior basal (S10)
- Lateral basal (S9)

Left lung

Upper lobe
- Superior division: Apical-posterior (S1 and S2), Anterior (S3)
- Lingular division: Superior (S4), Inferior (S5)

Lower lobe
- Anteromedial basal (S8)
- Posterior basal (S10)
- Lateral basal (S9)

Posterior view

Left lung

Upper lobe
- Superior division: Apical-posterior (S1 and S2), Anterior (S3)
- Lingular division: Superior (S4)

Lower lobe
- Superior (S6)
- Lateral basal (S9)
- Posterior basal (S10)

Right lung

Upper lobe
- Apical (S1)
- Posterior (S2)
- Anterior (S3)

Middle lobe
- Lateral (S4)

Lower lobe
- Superior (S6)
- Lateral basal (S9)
- Posterior basal (S10)

SECTION I PLATE 15

Bronchopulmonary Segments
(Continued)

the lower lobe and extends from the upper part of the oblique fissure at about the level of the vertebral end of the third rib to the level of the vertebral end of the fifth or sixth rib.

Inferior to the level at which the superior segmental bronchus arises, the lower lobe divides into four basal segmental bronchi: *medial* (S7), *anterior* (S8), *lateral* (S9) and *posterior* (S10). The basal segments of the lower lobe form the base of the lung and rest upon the diaphragm. The medial basal segment is sometimes partially sepa-

rated from other basal segments by an extra fissure; in this event it has sometimes been called the *cardiac lobe* of the lung.

Left Lung

The left main bronchus is longer than the right and not in so direct a line with the trachea. Foreign bodies, therefore, are somewhat more likely to enter the right than the left bronchus.

Left Upper Lobe. The upper lobe bronchus subdivides into a superior division bronchus and an inferior or lingular division bronchus. The superior division can be thought of as corresponding to the right upper lobe, with the lingular division corresponding to the right middle lobe, there is usually no fissure separating the two and

their segmental subdivisions are not the same.

Unlike the situation on the right, the superior division of the left upper lobe has only two segments: the *apical-posterior segment* (S1 + S2)—which corresponds to a combination of the right apical and posterior segments—and the *anterior segment* (S3). The inferior or lingular division also has two segments, *superior* (S4) and *inferior* (S5).

Left Lower Lobe. The segments here are similar to those of the right lower lobe, except that the portion corresponding to the right anterior basal and medial basal segments is supplied on the left by two bronchi which have a common stem, and thus forms a single *anteromedial basal* (S8) segment. Other left lower lobe segments are: *superior* (S6), *lateral basal* (S9) and *posterior basal* (S10).

Relations of Trachea and Main Bronchi

The trachea lies on the anterior aspect of the esophagus as it passes through the inlet of the thorax, then courses inferiorly to approximately the level of the upper border of the fifth thoracic vertebra. There it divides into the right and left main bronchi.

As the aorta arches over the root of the left lung, it first lies anterior to the trachea and then on its left side. The major arteries arising from the aortic arch are in close relationship with the trachea. The brachiocephalic (innominate) artery at first is anterior to the trachea and then is on its right side, before dividing into the right common carotid and right subclavian arteries. The left common carotid artery is first anterior to and then on the left lateral aspect of the trachea.

The left brachiocephalic (innominate) vein crosses from left to right, anterior to the trachea and partly separated from it by the major branches of the aortic arch. The right brachiocephalic vein is separated from the trachea by the right brachiocephalic artery.

The beginning of the right main bronchus lies anterior to the esophagus. As it courses inferiorly and laterally to divide into the lobar bronchi, it is posterior to the right pulmonary artery. The bronchus crosses in front of the azygos vein and is separated from the thoracic duct by the esophagus. The relationship to other structures at the root of the lung is shown in Plate 13.

The beginning of the left main bronchus also lies anterior to the esophagus, whence it runs laterally and inferiorly to reach the hilus of the left lung. Since its course is less vertical than that of the right main bronchus (less in a direct line with the trachea), foreign bodies are a little more likely to enter the right bronchus than the left.

The left recurrent laryngeal nerve arises from the left vagus nerve as it crosses the arch of the aorta, and swings posteriorly to loop around the aortic arch just lateral to the ligamentum arteriosum. This nerve then runs cranially in the groove between the trachea and the esophagus to reach the larynx.

The trachea begins at the lower border of the larynx (just below the cricoid cartilage) at about the level of the sixth cervical vertebra and ends at about the level of the upper border of the fifth thoracic vertebra, where it divides into the two main bronchi. The thyroid gland lies on the anterior and both lateral aspects of the highest part of the trachea.

The esophagus starts as a continuation of the pharynx at the lower border of the larynx and continues through the thorax. It then passes through the esophageal hiatus of the diaphragm

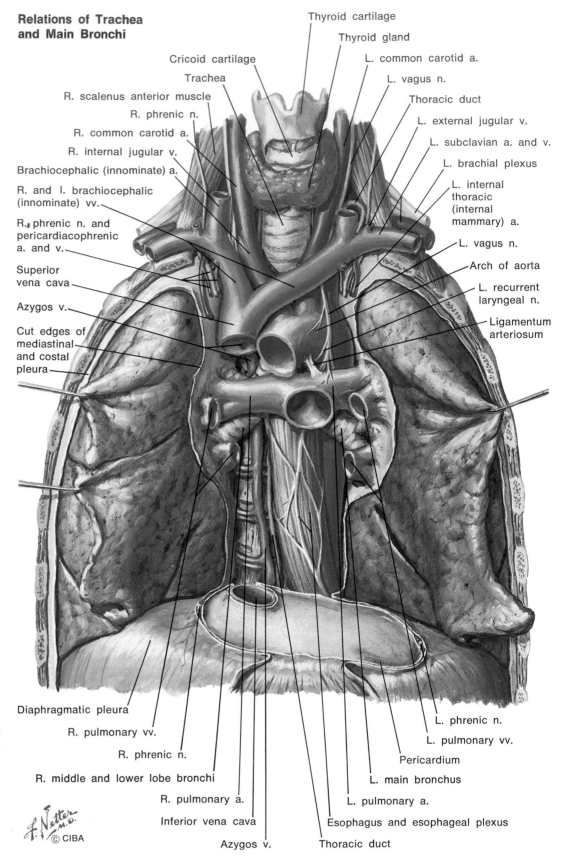

Relations of Trachea and Main Bronchi

Thyroid cartilage
Thyroid gland
Cricoid cartilage
L. common carotid a.
Trachea
L. vagus n.
R. scalenus anterior muscle
Thoracic duct
R. phrenic n.
L. external jugular v.
R. common carotid a.
L. subclavian a. and v.
R. internal jugular v.
L. brachial plexus
Brachiocephalic (innominate) a.
L. internal thoracic (internal mammary) a.
R. and l. brachiocephalic (innominate) vv.
L. vagus n.
R. phrenic n. and pericardiacophrenic a. and v.
Arch of aorta
Superior vena cava
L. recurrent laryngeal n.
Azygos v.
Ligamentum arteriosum
Cut edges of mediastinal and costal pleura
Diaphragmatic pleura
L. phrenic n.
R. pulmonary vv.
L. pulmonary vv.
R. phrenic n.
Pericardium
R. middle and lower lobe bronchi
L. main bronchus
R. pulmonary a.
L. pulmonary a.
Inferior vena cava
Esophagus and esophageal plexus
Azygos v.
Thoracic duct

to enter the abdominal cavity and terminate at the stomach.

The ligamentum arteriosum, the remnant of the ductus arteriosus, runs from the beginning of the left pulmonary artery to the undersurface of the arch of the aorta. In fetal life the ligamentum arteriosum shunts blood from the pulmonary artery to the aorta, so that fetal blood does not pass through the pulmonary circulation.

Some of the many other structures shown in this illustration should be especially noted. One of them is the esophageal plexus, which is made up primarily of the vagus nerves. These nerves split into several bundles below the root of the

lung and form the plexus on the surfaces of the esophagus. Other contributions to the plexus come from the sympathetic trunks and splanchnic nerves. At the lower end of the plexus, two trunks are formed, which pass through the esophageal hiatus of the diaphragm. The anterior trunk is mostly the left vagus, and the posterior trunk mostly the right vagus.

Also worthy of note are: the pulmonary veins, shown cut at the roots of the right and left lungs; the parietal pleura, cut to expose the lungs, each of which is covered by visceral pleura; the cut edge of the pericardium; and the inferior vena cava passing through the diaphragm.

Bronchial Arteries

Bronchial Arteries

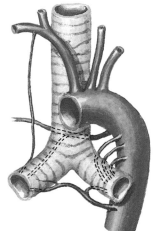

Trachea pulled to left by hook

Esophagus

3rd r. intercostal artery (1st aortic intercostal)

R. bronchial artery

R. main bronchus

L. main bronchus pulled to right by hook

Superior l. bronchial artery

Aorta pulled aside

Inferior l. bronchial artery

Esophageal artery

Variations in bronchial arteries

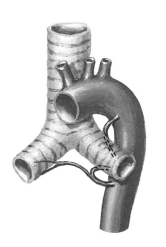

R. and l. bronchial arteries originating from aorta by single stem

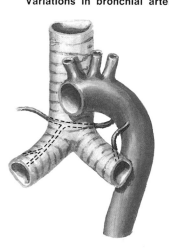

Only a single bronchial artery to each bronchus

Supernumerary bronchial arteries to either or both bronchi. Very rarely a bronchial artery may originate from subclavian artery as shown

Two sets of arteries enter the lungs. In general, the branches of the *pulmonary arteries* follow the bronchi and ramify into capillary networks between the alveoli. Thus the exchange of oxygen and carbon dioxide between the alveolar air and the capillary blood is made possible. The *bronchial arteries* supply the tissues of the lungs, including the walls of the pulmonary vessels.

The origin of the right bronchial artery is quite variable. It often arises from the third right intercostal artery (the first right aortic intercostal artery) and descends to reach the posterior aspects of the right main bronchus. It may also arise from a common stem with the left inferior bronchial artery, which leaves the descending aorta slightly inferior to the spot where the left main bronchus crosses it. Or it may arise from the inferior aspect of the arch of the aorta and course behind the trachea to reach the posterior aspect of the right main bronchus.

On the left side, there is usually a superior bronchial artery and an inferior bronchial artery. The superior artery tends to arise from the inferior

aspect of the aortic arch near the place where it becomes the descending aorta. The inferior artery is likely to come from near the beginning of the descending aorta toward its posterior aspect. The left bronchial arteries come to lie on the posterior surface of the left main bronchus and follow the branching of the bronchial tree.

Some of the more common variations of the bronchial arteries are shown in the lower part of the illustration. The right bronchial artery and the inferior left bronchial artery may come from a common stem arising from the descending aorta. There may be only a single bronchial artery on the left. Supernumerary bronchial arteries may be

present, going to either bronchus or both bronchi.

The majority of those who have studied the blood supply of the lungs seem to agree that there are precapillary anastomoses between the bronchial and pulmonary arteries, which can enlarge when either of these two systems becomes obstructed. Whether these anastomoses are able to maintain full function of the involved area of the lung has not been completely established.

Some branches of the bronchial arteries spread out on the surface of the lung, beneath the pleura, where they form a capillary network that contributes to the blood supply of the visceral layer of the pleura.

Mediastinum

The mediastinum or mediastinal septum is that portion of the thorax which lies between the right and left pleural sacs and is bounded ventrally by the sternum and dorsally by the bodies of the thoracic vertebrae. It extends from the diaphragm inferiorly to the inlet of the thorax superiorly.

For descriptive purposes, the mediastinum is divided into parts related to the pericardial sac. Above a plane extending from the sternal angle to the lower border of the body of the fourth thoracic vertebra is the superior mediastinum. The part below this plane is divided into the anterior mediastinum, which is anterior to the pericardial sac; the middle mediastinum, which contains the pericardial sac and its contents; and the posterior mediastinum, behind the pericardial sac.

The *superior mediastinum* contains the aortic arch; the brachiocephalic (innominate) artery; the beginnings of the left common carotid and left subclavian arteries; the right and left brachiocephalic (innominate) veins as they come together to form the superior vena cava; the right and left vagus, cardiac, phrenic and left recurrent laryngeal nerves, and the trachea; the esophagus and thoracic duct; the remains of the thymus; and a few lymph nodes.

The *anterior mediastinum* contains only a small amount of fascia and a few lymph nodes and vessels.

The *middle mediastinum* contains the pericardium and heart, the beginning of the ascending aorta, the terminal part of the superior vena cava with the azygos vein opening into it, the pulmonary artery dividing into its right and left branches, the terminal parts of the right and left pulmonary veins, and the right and left phrenic nerves.

The *posterior mediastinum* contains the thoracic part of the descending aorta, the bifurcation of the trachea and the right and left main bronchi, the esophagus, the azygos and hemiazygos veins, the right and left vagus nerves, the splanchnic nerves, the thoracic duct, and many lymph nodes.

The interrelationships of the above structures have great clinical significance, since a space-occupying lesion of any one of them can affect any of the other neighboring structures. Attention is therefore directed to a number of these relationships, which can be appreciated by careful scrutiny of Plates 18 and 19.

The esophagus lies near the ventral aspects of the thoracic vertebral bodies, with the right intercostal arteries, thoracic duct and hemiazygos vein

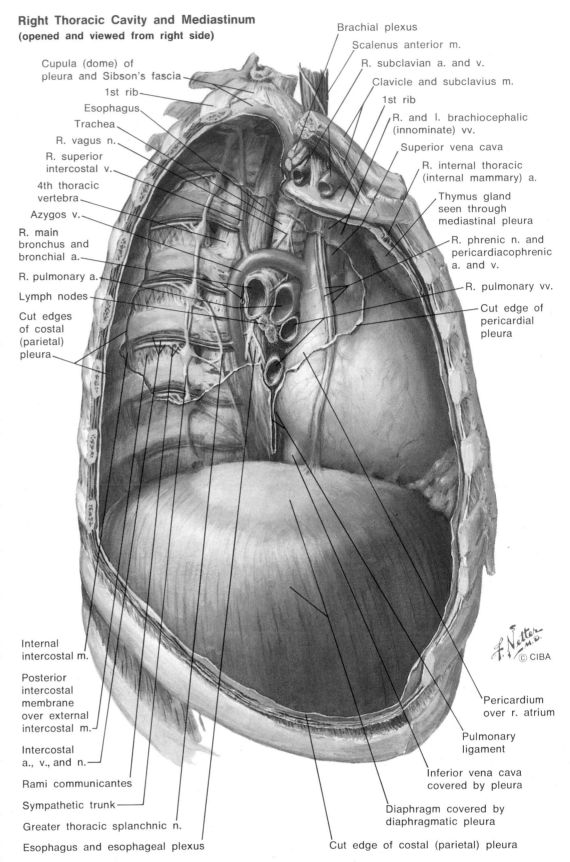

Right Thoracic Cavity and Mediastinum
(opened and viewed from right side)

Cupula (dome) of pleura and Sibson's fascia
1st rib
Esophagus
Trachea
R. vagus n.
R. superior intercostal v.
4th thoracic vertebra
Azygos v.
R. main bronchus and bronchial a.
R. pulmonary a.
Lymph nodes
Cut edges of costal (parietal) pleura

Brachial plexus
Scalenus anterior m.
R. subclavian a. and v.
Clavicle and subclavius m.
1st rib
R. and l. brachiocephalic (innominate) vv.
Superior vena cava
R. internal thoracic (internal mammary) a.
Thymus gland seen through mediastinal pleura
R. phrenic n. and pericardiacophrenic a. and v.
R. pulmonary vv.
Cut edge of pericardial pleura

Internal intercostal m.
Posterior intercostal membrane over external intercostal m.
Intercostal a., v., and n.
Rami communicantes
Sympathetic trunk
Greater thoracic splanchnic n.
Esophagus and esophageal plexus

Pericardium over r. atrium
Pulmonary ligament
Inferior vena cava covered by pleura
Diaphragm covered by diaphragmatic pleura
Cut edge of costal (parietal) pleura

between it and the vertebral bodies. It partially overlaps the azygos vein to its right side. The right and left vagus nerves form a plexus around the esophagus, the left vagus trunk being on its anterior aspect and the right vagus trunk on its posterior aspect.

As the trachea passes through the superior mediastinum, it lies anterior to the esophagus. It continues in this relationship as it passes into the posterior mediastinum to bifurcate.

Anteriorly, in the superior mediastinum, are the remnants of the thymus. The right and left brachiocephalic veins and the superior vena cava are the most anterior of the major structures;

posterior to them are the aortic arch, the brachiocephalic artery and the beginnings of the left common carotid and left subclavian arteries. Posterior to these are the trachea and esophagus.

Right Thoracic Cavity

The structures forming the root of the right lung are the right main bronchus and, posterior and somewhat superior, the right pulmonary artery, with the right pulmonary veins anterior and inferior in position.

The azygos vein arches over the root of the right lung to empty into the superior vena cava. As it

(Continued)

Left Thoracic Cavity and Mediastinum
(opened and viewed from left side)

Labels (clockwise from top):
- Cupula (dome) of pleura and Sibson's fascia
- 1st rib
- Esophagus
- Thoracic duct
- 3rd thoracic vertebra
- L. superior intercostal v.
- L. vagus n.
- L. recurrent laryngeal n.
- Aorta
- Accessory hemiazygos v.
- Cut edges of costal pleura
- Lymph node
- Intercostal v., a., and n.
- Internal intercostal m.
- Posterior intercostal membrane over external intercostal m.
- Rami communicantes
- Sympathetic trunk
- Greater thoracic splanchnic n.
- Esophagus and esophageal plexus under pleura
- Diaphragm covered by diaphragmatic pleura
- Cut edge of costal (parietal) pleura
- Costo-diaphragmatic recess (costophrenic sulcus)
- Pulmonary ligament
- Fat pad
- L. pulmonary vv.
- Cut edge of pericardial pleura
- Pericardium
- L. phrenic n. and pericardiacophrenic a. and v.
- L. main bronchus and bronchial a.
- L. pulmonary a.
- Ligamentum arteriosum
- L. internal thoracic (internal mammary) a.
- Thymus gland under pleura
- Cut edge of mediastinal pleura
- L. brachiocephalic (innominate) v.
- Clavicle and subclavius m.
- L. subclavian a. and v.
- Brachial plexus
- Scalenus anterior m.

F. Netter M.D. © CIBA

Mediastinum
(*Continued*)

begins to arch, it receives the right superior intercostal vein, which accepts blood from the upper three or four intercostal spaces.

Below the root of the lung, the pleura reflects from the parietal to the visceral surface, as it does on the anterior and posterior surfaces of the root of the lung. Since there are no structures between the two layers at this point, they become the pulmonary ligament.

Coursing vertically near the necks of the ribs is the thoracic portion of the right ganglionated sympathetic trunk, which is connected with each intercostal nerve by a gray and a white ramus communicans. Branching from the fifth (or sixth) to the twelfth ganglia are the splanchnic nerves, which course medially and inferiorly to pierce the crus of the diaphragm and enter the abdominal cavity.

The right phrenic nerve and the pericardiacophrenic artery and vein pass vertically between the mediastinal parietal pleura and the fibrous pericardial sac to reach the diaphragm, which they supply.

The medial "wall" of the right thoracic cavity is formed by the thoracic vertebral bodies and the mediastinal septum, of which the most massive part is the pericardial sac containing the heart. The posterior, lateral and anterior walls comprise the thoracic cage, which is limited inferiorly by the diaphragm.

Left Thoracic Cavity

The structures forming the root of the left lung are the left main bronchus, located posteriorly; the left pulmonary artery, in an anterior and superior position; and the left pulmonary veins, which are anterior and inferior in position.

The aorta arches over and descends posterior to the root of the left lung. As it descends, it lies at first to the left of the thoracic vertebral bodies (starting with the lower border of the fourth vertebra); it then approaches the anterior aspect of the vertebral bodies, where it lies as it pierces the diaphragm. The aorta gives off nine pairs of intercostal arteries. They supply the lower nine intercostal spaces.

The ligamentum arteriosum (the remnant of the ductus arteriosus) runs between the left pulmonary artery and the aortic arch.

The thoracic portion of the left ganglionated sympathetic trunk is similar to the portion on the

right side, and does not need special description.

The left phrenic nerve and the left pericardiacophrenic artery and vein cross the aortic arch and descend between the mediastinal parietal pleura and the pericardial sac to pass through the muscular part of the diaphragm.

The left vagus nerve passes in front of the arch of the aorta, giving off its recurrent branch, which passes under the arch to course upward to the larynx. The vagus nerve continues caudally on the posterior aspect of the root of the lung to enter the esophageal plexus, from which the left vagal trunk emerges to follow the esophagus into the abdomen.

The left superior intercostal vein usually drains blood from the upper three or four intercostal spaces. It crosses the aortic arch and the beginnings of the left subclavian and left common carotid arteries and empties into the left brachiocephalic vein. It often anastomoses with the accessory hemiazygos vein.

The medial wall of the left thoracic cavity is formed by the thoracic vertebral bodies and the mediastinal septum, which consists mostly of the pericardial sac and the contained heart. As with the right thoracic cavity, the posterior, lateral and anterior walls form the thoracic cage, which is limited inferiorly by the diaphragm.

Innervation of Tracheobronchial Tree

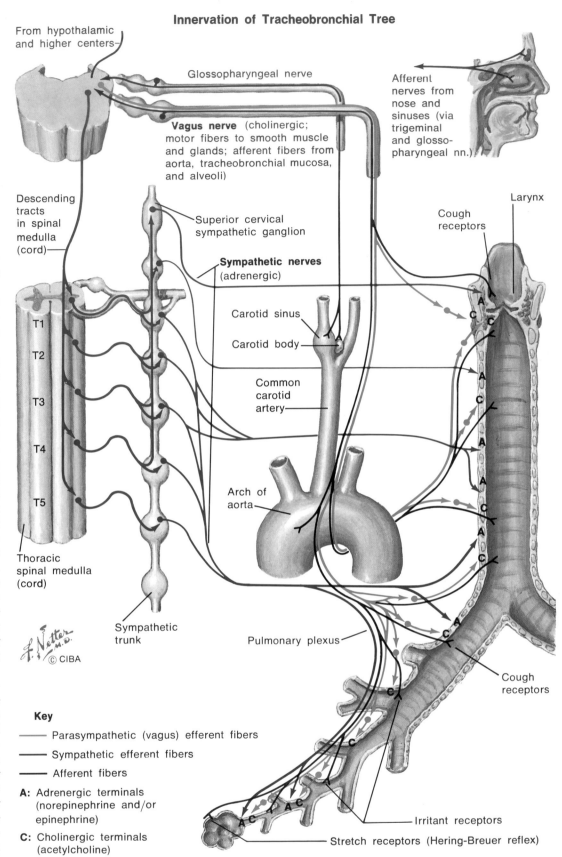

Vagus nerve (cholinergic; motor fibers to smooth muscle and glands; afferent fibers from aorta, tracheobronchial mucosa, and alveoli)

From hypothalamic and higher centers

Glossopharyngeal nerve

Afferent nerves from nose and sinuses (via trigeminal and glossopharyngeal nn.)

Descending tracts in spinal medulla (cord)

Superior cervical sympathetic ganglion

Sympathetic nerves (adrenergic)

Carotid sinus

Carotid body

Common carotid artery

Arch of aorta

Thoracic spinal medulla (cord)

Sympathetic trunk

Pulmonary plexus

Larynx

Cough receptors

Cough receptors

Irritant receptors

Stretch receptors (Hering-Breuer reflex)

T1 T2 T3 T4 T5

Key

— Parasympathetic (vagus) efferent fibers

— Sympathetic efferent fibers

— Afferent fibers

A: Adrenergic terminals (norepinephrine and/or epinephrine)

C: Cholinergic terminals (acetylcholine)

Innervation of Lungs and Tracheobronchial Tree

The tracheobronchial tree and lungs are innervated by the autonomic nervous system. Three types of pathways are involved: *autonomic afferent, parasympathetic efferent* and *sympathetic efferent.* Each type of fiber is discussed here, while the neurochemical control of respiration is covered in the section on physiology (see pages 75 and 76).

Autonomic Afferent Fibers. Afferent fibers from *stretch receptors* in the alveoli as well as fibers from *irritant receptors* in the bronchi and bronchioles travel via the pulmonary plexus (located around the tracheal bifurcation and roots of the lungs) to the vagus nerve. Similarly, fibers from *irritant receptors* in the trachea and from *cough receptors* in the larynx reach the central nervous system via the vagus nerve. *Chemoreceptors* in the carotid and aortic bodies and *pressor receptors* in the carotid sinus and aortic arch also give rise to afferent autonomic fibers. The fibers from the carotid sinus and carotid body travel via the glossopharyngeal nerve, whereas those from the aortic body and aortic arch travel via the vagus nerve. Other receptors in the nose and nasal sinuses give rise to afferent fibers that form parts of the trigeminal and glossopharyngeal nerves. In addition, the respiratory centers are controlled to some extent by impulses from the hypothalamus and higher centers as well as from the reticular activating system.

Parasympathetic Efferent Fibers. All parasympathetic preganglionic efferent fibers to the tracheobronchial tree are contained in the vagus nerve, originating chiefly from cells in the dorsal vagal nuclei that are closely related to the medullary respiratory centers. The fibers relay with short postganglionic fibers in the vicinity of or within the walls of the tracheobronchial tree. This parasympathetic efferent pathway carries motor impulses to the smooth muscle and glands of the tracheobronchial tree. The impulses are cholinergically mediated and produce bronchial smooth muscle contraction, glandular secretion and vasodilation.

Sympathetic Efferent Fibers. The preganglionic efferent fibers emerge from the spinal medulla (cord) at levels T1 or T2 to T5 or T6 and pass to the sympathetic trunks via white rami communicantes. Fibers carrying impulses to the larynx and upper trachea ascend in the sympathetic trunk and synapse in the cervical sympathetic ganglia with postganglionic fibers to those structures. The remainder synapse in the upper thoracic ganglia of the sympathetic trunks, whence the postganglionic fibers pass to the lower trachea, the bronchi and the bronchioles, largely via the pulmonary plexus. The postganglionic

nerve endings are adrenergic. Sympathetic stimulation relaxes bronchial and bronchiolar smooth muscle, inhibits glandular secretion and causes vasoconstriction.

Pharmacologic studies indicate that there are two types of adrenergic receptors, alpha and beta. The alpha receptors are located primarily in smooth muscle and exocrine glands. Beta receptors have been differentiated pharmacologically into beta$_1$, located in the heart, and beta$_2$, located in smooth muscle throughout the body, including bronchial and vascular smooth muscle. Generally, alpha stimulation is excitatory. Beta stimulation may be inhibitory (relaxation of bronchial smooth

muscle) or excitatory (increase in both heart rate and force of contraction). Beta stimulation also tends to mobilize energy by glycogenolysis and lipolysis. For further discussion of this topic, see pages 122 and 123.

Certain tissues contain both alpha and beta receptors. The result of stimulation depends on the nature of the stimulating catecholamine and the relative proportion of the two types of receptors. In the lungs, beta$_2$ stimulation (there are no beta$_1$ receptors here) causes bronchodilatation and possibly decreased secretion of mucus; alpha adrenergic stimulation by pharmacologic agents causes bronchoconstriction.

Structure of Trachea and Major Bronchi

Thyroid cartilage
Cricothyroid ligament
Cricoid cartilage

Connective tissue sheath
Cartilage
Elastic fibers
Gland
Small artery
Lymph vessels
Nerve
Epithelium

Connective tissue sheath (cut away)

Intercartilaginous ligaments

Tracheal cartilages

Anterior wall

Cross section through trachea

Mucosa showing longitudinal folds formed by dense collections of elastic fibers

Posterior wall

Nerve
Small arteries
Gland
Elastic fibers

Trachealis muscle
Esophageal muscle
Epithelium
Lymph vessels

Eparterial bronchus

To upper lobe

To upper lobe

To lingula

To middle lobe

R. main bronchus

L. main bronchus

To lower lobe

To lower lobe

Intrapulmonary | Extrapulmonary | Intrapulmonary

The trachea or windpipe passes from the larynx to the level of the fourth thoracic vertebra where it divides into the two main bronchi that enter the right and left lungs. About 20 C-shaped plates of cartilage support the anterior and lateral walls of the trachea and main bronchi. The posterior wall—or membranous trachea—is free of cartilage, but interlacing bundles of muscle fibers lie in this region and insert into the posterior ends of the cartilage plates.

Mucous glands are particularly numerous posteriorly. Some lie between the cartilage plates, and some are external to the muscle layer with ducts that penetrate this layer to open on the mucosal surface. Posteriorly, elastic fibers are grouped in longitudinal bundles immediately beneath the basement membrane of the tracheal epithelium, and these appear to the naked eye as broad flat bands that give a ridged effect to the inner lining of the trachea; they are not so obvious anteriorly. The bands of elastic fibers are thinner and surround the entire circumference of the lower airways.

Just above the point at which the main bronchus enters the lung, the cartilage plates come together to completely encircle the airway. Posteriorly, the ends of the plates meet and the membranous region disappears. The plates are no longer C-shaped but are smaller, more irregular and arranged around the wall. Where the main bronchus divides into lobar bronchi—at the hilus of the lung—the plates of cartilage are large and saddle-shaped to support this region of bifurcation.

At the level where cartilage completely surrounds the circumference of the airway, the muscle coat undergoes a striking rearrangement. It no longer inserts into the cartilage—as in the trachea—but forms a separate layer of interlacing bundles internal to it. The airway lumen can now be occluded by contraction of the muscle; but the

trachea is never subjected to such sphincteric action.

The right main bronchus is shorter than the left, and angles away from the trachea less sharply than the left. Foreign bodies lodge more often in the right main bronchus than in the left bronchus.

Lobes and Segments. The right lung has three lobes and the left has two, although the lingula of the left lung is analogous to the right middle lobe.

The bronchopulmonary segments are the topographic units of the lung, and are a means of identifying regions of the lung either radiologically or surgically; there are eight bronchopulmonary segments in the left lung but 10 in the right lung

(Plate 14). A segment is not a functional end unit because it is not isolated by connective tissue. Neighboring segments share common venous and lymphatic drainage, and, by collateral ventilation, air passes across segmental boundaries. The pleura isolates one lobe from another, but since the main or oblique fissure is complete in only about 50% of subjects, even a lobe is not always an end unit.

For counting orders or generations of airways, it is sometimes appropriate to count the trachea as the first generation, the main bronchi as the second generation, and so on. To compare features within a segment, it is better to count the segmental bronchi as the first generation.

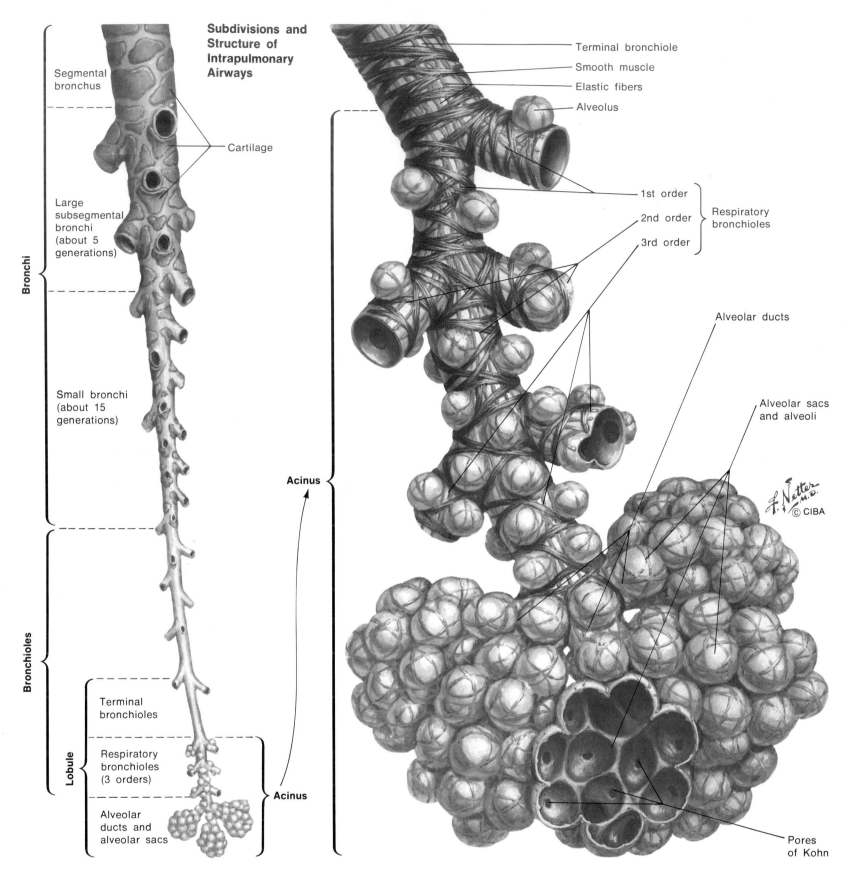

Subdivisions and Structure of Intrapulmonary Airways

Bronchi
- Segmental bronchus
- Cartilage
- Large subsegmental bronchi (about 5 generations)
- Small bronchi (about 15 generations)

Bronchioles

Lobule
- Terminal bronchioles
- Respiratory bronchioles (3 orders)
- Alveolar ducts and alveolar sacs

Acinus

Terminal bronchiole
Smooth muscle
Elastic fibers
Alveolus

Respiratory bronchioles
- 1st order
- 2nd order
- 3rd order

Alveolar ducts

Alveolar sacs and alveoli

Acinus

Pores of Kohn

Intrapulmonary Airways

According to the distribution of cartilage, airways are divided into bronchi and bronchioles. *Bronchi* lie proximal to the last plate of cartilage found along an airway. *Bronchioles* are distal to the bronchi, beyond the last plate of cartilage and proximal to the alveolar region. Cartilage plates become sparser toward the periphery and in the last generations of bronchi are found only at the points of branching. The large bronchi have enough inherent rigidity to sustain patency in massive lung collapse; the small bronchi collapse like the bronchioles and alveoli. Small and large bronchi have submucosal mucous glands in their walls.

When any airway is pursued to its limit, the *terminal bronchiole* is reached. Three to five terminal bronchioles make up a *lobule*. The *acinus* or respiratory unit of the lung is defined as the lung supplied by a terminal bronchiole. Acini vary in size and shape. In the adult the acinus may be up to 1 cm in diameter. Within the acinus three to eight generations of *respiratory bronchioles* may be found, which have the structure of bronchioles in part of their walls, but with alveoli opening directly to their lumina as well. Beyond these lie the alveolar ducts and sacs, before the alveoli proper are reached.

None of these units is isolated from its neighbor by connective tissue septa. Collateral air passage occurs between acinus and acinus, and between lobule and lobule through the pores of Kohn in the alveolar wall, and through accessory communications between the distal bronchioles and adjacent alveoli.

Connective tissue forms a sheath around airways and blood vessels. It also forms septa that are relatively numerous in some parts of the edges of the lingula and middle lobe and parts of the costodiaphragmatic and costovertebral edges. These septa impede collateral ventilation but, since in man they never completely isolate one unit from its neighbor, do not prevent collateral air drift.

Structure of Bronchi and Bronchioles—Light Microscopy

Section of large bronchus

Higher magnification of epithelium

- Ciliated columnar epithelium with many goblet cells
- Basal cells
- Basement membrane
- Blood vessel
- Lamina propria with elastic fibers
- Lymph vessel
- Smooth muscle
- Blood vessels
- Submucosal glands
- Nerve fiber
- Stroma with elastic fibers and lymphocyte collections
- Perichondrium
- Cartilage
- Lymph vessels

Section of medium-sized bronchus

- Ciliated columnar epithelium with many goblet cells
- Basement membrane
- Blood vessels
- Lamina propria with elastic fibers
- Smooth muscle
- Submucosal glands
- Nerve fiber
- Lymph vessels
- Cartilage
- Alveoli

Section of bronchiole

Ciliated cuboidal epithelium with few goblet cells, smooth muscle ring, blood vessels, and nerve fibers; stroma contains many elastic fibers. Cartilaginous plates, glands, and lymph vessels absent

The airways are the hollow tubes that conduct air to the respiratory region of the lung. They are lined throughout their length by pseudostratified, ciliated, columnar epithelium supported by a basement membrane. (See page 26 for details of cell types and their arrangement.) The remainder of the wall includes a muscle coat and accessory structures such as submucosal glands, together with connective tissue. In the bronchi, cartilage provides additional support.

In an adult the diameter of the main bronchus is about 2 cm and the diameter of a terminal bronchiole is about 1 mm. These measurements vary with age and the size of the individual, and with the functional state of the airway, so it is helpful to designate airways by their order or generation along an axial pathway. The epithelium is higher in the large airways and gradually thins toward the periphery.

Immediately beneath the basement membrane elastic fibers are collected into fine bands that form longitudinal ridges. In cross section, the fiber bundles are at the apices of the bronchial folds. The rest of the wall is made up of loose connective tissue in which lie blood vessels, nerves, capillaries and lymphatics.

Blood Supply. The bronchial arteries supply the capillary bed in the airway wall, forming one plexus internal and another external to the muscle layer. (See also Plate 26.)

Venous Drainage. The capillary bed of the bronchi and bronchioles drains to the pulmonary veins. At each point of airway bifurcation two venous tributaries join. Only at that hilus is there some drainage to the azygos system through veins called the true bronchial veins.

Lymphatics. Lymph glands lie internal to and between the plates of cartilage, and internal and external to the muscle layer. Lymphatics are numerous in airway walls. They are not found in the alveolar walls, but start in the region of respiratory and terminal bronchioles.

Nerve Supply. Large nerves—both myelinated and nonmyelinated—are seen in the wall of the airway. Motor nerves supply the lymph glands and the muscles. Intraepithelial nerve endings that are almost certainly sensory fibers have also been described, but whether there are also motor nerve endings at the epithelial level is not certain.

As the lumen tapers toward the periphery and the airway wall becomes thinner, the small airways are more intimately related to the surrounding alveoli. Functional interaction between the two is probably very important at this level, and inflammation spreads easily through the walls of small airways.

Ultrastructure of Tracheal, Bronchial and Bronchiolar Epithelium

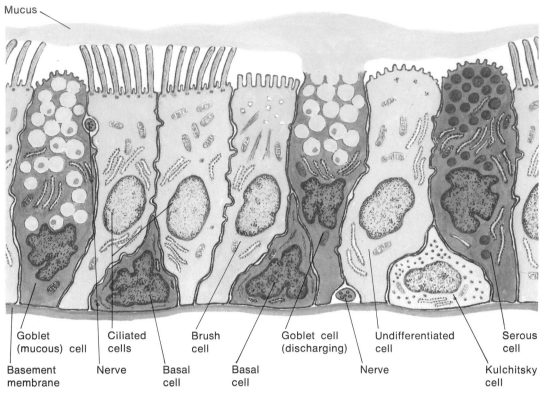

Trachea and large bronchi. Ciliated and goblet cells predominant, with some serous cells and occasional brush cells, undifferentiated (intermediate) cells, and Clara cells. Numerous basal cells and occasional Kulchitsky cells present

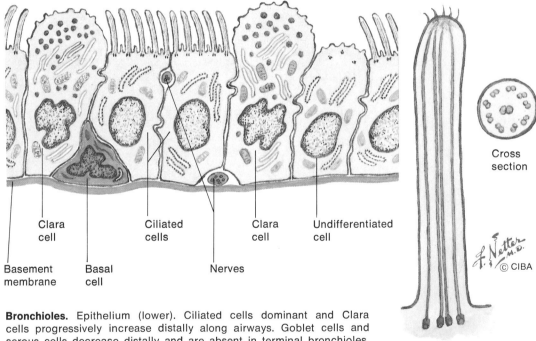

Bronchioles. Epithelium (lower). Ciliated cells dominant and Clara cells progressively increase distally along airways. Goblet cells and serous cells decrease distally and are absent in terminal bronchioles. Occasional undifferentiated and brush cells may be present. Basal cells and especially Kulchitsky cells are uncommon in distal airways

The lining of the respiratory airways is predominantly a pseudostratified, ciliated, columnar epithelium in which all cells are attached to the basement membrane but not all reach the lumen. In the smaller peripheral airways the epithelium may be only a single layer thick and cuboidal rather than columnar, since basal cells are absent.

Ciliated cells are present in even the smallest airways and respiratory bronchioles, where they are adjacent to alveolar lining cells. The "ciliary escalator" starts at the most distal point of the airway epithelium. In smaller airways, the cilia are not as tall as in central airways. Eight epithelial cell types can be identified in man, although ultrastructural features and cell kinetics have been studied mainly in animals. The following classification is based on studies in the rat: the (1) basal and (2) Kulchitsky cells are attached to the basement membrane but do not reach the lumen, (3) the intermediate cell is probably the precursor that differentiates into (4) the ciliated cell, (5) the brush cell, or one of the secretory cells, (6) the mucous (goblet) cell, (7) the serous cell or (8) the Clara cell.

The *basal cell* divides, and daughter cells pass to the superficial layer.

The *Kulchitsky cell* contains numerous neurosecretory granules and is part of the APUD (amine precursor uptake and decarboxylation) system making active peptides. Kulchitsky cells are more numerous before birth.

The *intermediate cell* is columnar. It has electron-lucent cytoplasm and no special features. It is probably the cell that differentiates into the others.

The *ciliated cell* carries the cilia. The cilium is now known to have nine double pairs of axonemes and a special axoneme in the center. The arrangement is modified at the base and at the apex, where a coronet of small claws has recently been identified. The feet of the axonemes are arranged so that a cilium "plugs" into the cytoplasm. The axonemes are attached to each other by "arms" of dynein, a contractile protein, and these provide the mechanism for ciliary motion.

The *brush cell* resembles a similar cell type found in the gut and in the nasal sinuses. Its function in the respiratory tract is not known.

The *mucous (goblet) cell* is a secretory cell containing numerous large and confluent secretory granules. Recently it has been shown by electron microscopy that confluence represents fusion of the

two trilaminar membranes of adjacent granules to produce a pentalaminar layer.

The *serous cell* resembles the serous cell of the submucosal gland and contains small, discrete, electron-dense secretory granules. Its cytoplasm is also more electron-dense than that of the Clara cell.

The *Clara cell* also contains small, discrete, electron-dense granules but in comparison with the serous cell, the cytoplasm is electron-lucent and there is relatively more smooth than rough endoplasmic reticulum.

The serous cell is mainly found centrally, the Clara cell only distally. These are the more common secretory cells of the airways, but irritation, drugs

or infection may lead to an increase in the number of secretory cells; the serous and Clara cells then develop into mucous cells. Differentiated cells are seen in mitosis, but this is probably not the main way in which cell numbers increase.

The basement membrane is well defined and becomes thinner in small airways. In certain diseases—notably asthma—it increases in thickness, although its structure remains normal.

Nerve fibers are seen within the epithelium. They are nonmyelinated and without a Schwann cell sheath. Their vesicle content suggests that the fibers are sensory or motor and either cholinergic or adrenergic in type.

Bronchial Submucosal Glands

Bronchial Submucosal Glands

Bronchial lumen

Ciliated duct

Collecting duct

Mucous tubules

Serous tubules

Tall cells packed with mito-chondria. M = myoepithelial cell; BM = basement membrane

Electron-lucent granules within cells and in lumen. N = nerve

Branch from and at ends of mucous tubules. Small, discrete electron-dense granules

M   BM   M   N   BM   M   N   BM

The submucosal glands of the human airway are of the branched tubuloacinar type: *tubulo* refers to the main part of the secretory tubule and *acinar* to the blind end of such a tubule.

Three-dimensional reconstruction of the gland reveals its various zones:

1. To form the *ciliated duct* bronchial epithelium with its mixed population of cells dips into the mouth of a gland—seen on naked-eye examination as a hole of pinpoint size in the surface epithelium of the bronchus.

2. This part of the duct expands into the *collecting duct,* which may be up to 0.25 mm in diameter and 1 mm long. It is lined by a columnar epithelium in which the cells are eosinophilic after hematoxylin and eosin staining; on electron microscopy, they are seen to be packed with mitochondria. These cells resemble the cells of the striated duct of the salivary gland, except that the formed cells lack the folds of membrane responsible for the appearance of striation. The collecting duct passes obliquely from the lumen, but since the airway wall is generally cut for examination at right angles to the lumen, the usual macroscopic section does not include the full length of the duct. It is usually seen as a rather large "acinus" comprised of cells without secretory granules.

3 and 4. Of the order of 13 tubules arise from one collecting duct. They may branch several times and are closely intertwined. The secretory cells lining these tubules are of two types: *mucous* and *serous.* Mucous cells line the central or proximal part of a tubule; serous cells line the distal part. Outpouchings or short-sided tubules may arise from the sides of the mucous tubules, and these are lined by serous cells. The peripheral part of a tubule usually

branches several times, and each of the final blind endings is lined with serous cells.

The gland tissue is internal to a basement membrane. In addition to the cell types described above, the following are found: (1) myoepithelial cells, (2) "clear" cells (probably immunoblasts) and (3) nerve fibers, including motor fibers. Outside the basement membrane are rich vascular and lymphatic networks and the nerve plexus.

In cross section the submucosal gland is seen to be compact, and in a main bronchus of an adult is of the order of 0.2 mm thick, or less than one-third the thickness of the airway wall between the surface and the cartilage layer. This ratio is similar in both

children and adults, and in airways at various positions in the pattern of branching. This gland-to-wall ratio is a useful way of measuring gland size, since gland hypertrophy is a hallmark of many human diseases.

In man, the secretory tubules of the mucous and serous cells contain mainly an acid glycoprotein, either sialic acid or its sulfate ester.

The concentration of bronchial submucosal gland openings in the trachea is of the order of one gland opening per mm². The glands become sparser toward the periphery, their fall in concentration being parallel to the diminution in the amount of cartilage.

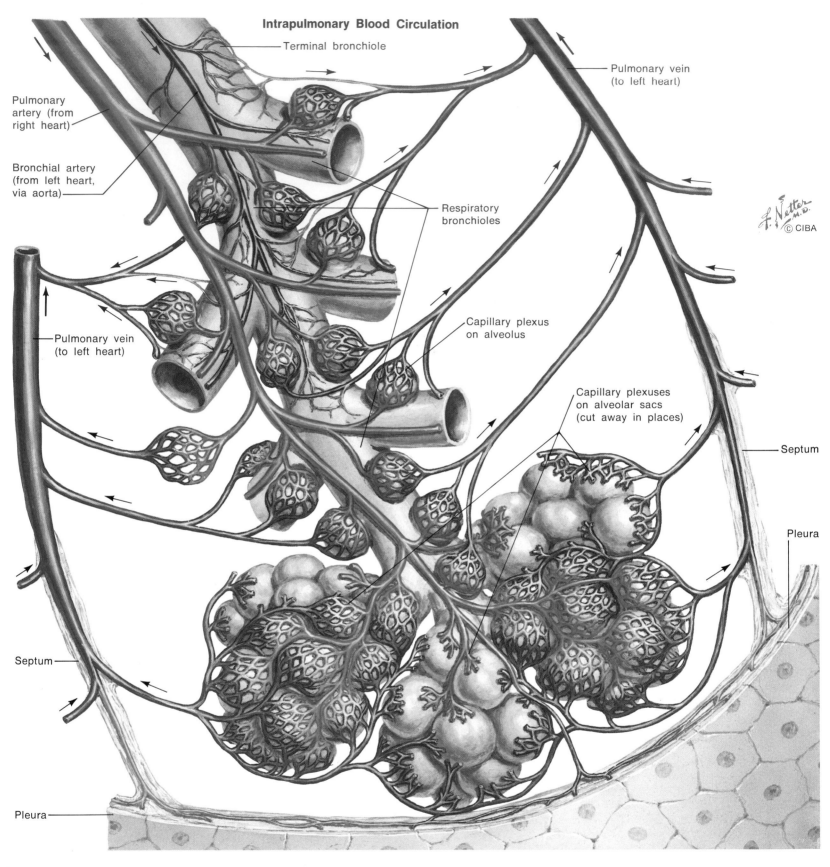

Intrapulmonary Blood Circulation

Terminal bronchiole

Pulmonary artery (from right heart)

Bronchial artery (from left heart, via aorta)

Respiratory bronchioles

Pulmonary vein (to left heart)

Capillary plexus on alveolus

Capillary plexuses on alveolar sacs (cut away in places)

Pulmonary vein (to left heart)

Septum

Pleura

Septum

Pleura

Intrapulmonary Blood Circulation

The human lung is supplied by two arterial systems, *pulmonary* and *bronchial*—one from each side of the heart—and is drained by two venous systems, *pulmonary* and *true bronchial*. The pulmonary veins drain the regions supplied by the pulmonary artery and also the airways within the lung that are supplied by the bronchial artery. The true bronchial veins serve only the perihilar region

that is supplied mainly by the bronchial artery, and drain to the azygos system and right atrium.

Arteries. The *bronchial arteries* arise from the aorta and supply the capillary plexus in the full length of the airway wall from the hilus to the respiratory bronchiole.

The *pulmonary artery* branches run with airways and their accompanying bronchial arteries in a single connective tissue sheath, the *bronchoarterial bundle*. The pulmonary artery breaks up into a capillary bed only when it reaches the alveoli of the respiratory bronchiole. It supplies all capillaries in the alveolar walls, which constitute the respiratory surface of the lung.

Veins. All intrapulmonary drainage is to pulmonary veins. The veins lie at the periphery of any unit—acinus, lobule or segment. Veins receive tributaries from (1) the alveolar capillary network, (2) the pleura and (3) the airways.

Precapillary Anastomoses. Pulmonary and bronchial arteries, and hence the right and left sides of the heart, communicate through the capillary bed in the region of the respiratory bronchiole and through the intrapulmonary venous bed. Pulmonary-to-bronchial artery anastomoses are present in the walls of the larger airways, but normally are closed. They open if blood flow is interrupted in either system and in certain diseases.

Fine Structure of Alveolar Capillary Unit

The cellular nature of the alveolar capillary unit was not recognized until the lungs were examined by electron microscopy. Indeed, it was thought that a simple membrane separated blood and air at the level of the terminal airspace. However, even at its narrowest, the boundary between blood and air is composed of at least two cell types (the type I alveolar epithelial cell and the endothelial cell) and extracellular material, namely, the surfactant-lining layer, the basement membranes and the so-called endothelial fuzz, a surface coating thought to be composed of mucopolysaccharides. Plate 27 shows part of a terminal airspace and cross sections of surrounding capillaries. In man, the diameter of the alveoli varies from 100 to 300 microns. The capillary segments are much smaller in diameter (10 to 14 microns), and may be separated from one another by even smaller distances. Each alveolus (there are 300 million alveoli in human lungs) may be associated with as many as 1000 capillary segments.

The thinness of the cellular boundary between blood and air suggests, correctly, that the two major cell types are remarkably flat, and have a paucity of intracellular organelles; however, they present enormous surface areas to air on one side and blood on the other (approximately 70 m²). A *priori*, these cells can play no more than a passive role in all physical and metabolic events involving airborne or bloodborne substrates.

The airspace is lined by epithelial type I cells, interspersed with larger polygonal type II cells. Together, all the alveolar epithelial cells form a complete epithelial layer sealed by tight junctions. The cellular layer lining the alveoli is remarkably impermeable to salt-containing solutions, but little is known about specific metabolic activities of type I alveolar cells. On the

other hand, the type II alveolar and endothelial cells play an active role in the metabolic functioning of the lung, respectively producing surfactant, and processing circulating vasoactive substances.

Alveolar Cells and Surface-Active Layer

As illustrated in Plate 28, in addition to being large, the type II alveolar cell is distinguished from the type I alveolar cell by having short, blunt projections on the free alveolar surface and lamellar inclusion bodies. There is now considerable evidence indicating that the lamellar bodies of type II cells are the source of the surfactant-lining

layer. Freeze-fractured* replicas of lung tissue show a striking array of ribs and particles on the lamellar bodies, with the same measurements as the lattice of tubular myelin, a component of the lining layer of the terminal airspace. In addition, electron microscopic studies of thin sections have

(Continued)

*Freeze-fracturing is a process which can expose the internal faces of cell membranes. Material (either fixed or fresh) is frozen and fractured under vacuum; the plane of fracture frequently passes through the hydrophobic terminals of the fatty acids in the membrane, thus exposing two complementary internal faces of the membrane: the "protoplasmic" half (P, inner fracture face) and the "exoplasmic" half (E, outer fracture face), as illustrated in Plate 28.

Fine Structure of Alveolar Capillary Unit
(Continued)

Type II Alveolar Cell and Surface-Active Layer
Electron microscopic features

Plasma membrane of type II cell
Cytoplasm
Lamellar body extruding contents
Multivesicular body
Lamellar bodies
Mitochondria
Surface phase
Subphase
Tubular myelin
Surface-active layer

Freeze-fracture preparation of a lamellar body with closely apposed, fractured lamellae. Series of parallel ribs, each ca. 80 Å in width evident on lamellae A and B, the series angled to each other. Particles or knobs, ca. 100 Å in diameter, prominent on lamella C but also apparent between ribs

shown lamellar bodies that appear to be released from the type II cells by a process similar to exocytosis. After release into the airspace, the contents of the lamellar bodies seem to unravel to yield tubular myelin. Besides lamellar bodies, type II cells are rich in mitochondria and multivesicular bodies. The intracellular origins of the lamellar bodies are not known with certainty. However, they do not appear much before birth and may require hormones such as cortisol and thyroxine for full maturation.

Alveolar macrophages are migratory cells and, after fixation for microscopy, they are usually seen free in the alveolar space or closely applied to the surface of type I cells. Alveolar macrophages are characterized by irregular cytoplasmic projections and large numbers of lysosomes. Alveolar macrophages are important in the defense mechanisms of the lungs.

The cellular components of the blood-air barrier frequently consist only of the extremely flattened extensions of endothelial cells and type I alveolar cells. In other regions the wall contains such cell types as smooth muscle cells, pericytes, fibroblasts and occasional plasma cells. Smooth muscle cells are found around the mouth of each alveolus in man. Pericytes occur around pulmonary alveolar capillaries, but less frequently than on systemic capillaries. In lung capillaries they have recently been noted to have a close association with the capillary basement membrane within which they are ensheathed. The pericytes are also characterized by having finely branched cytoplasmic processes that approach the endothelial cells and a web of cytoplasmic filaments that run along the membrane close to the endothelium. They also are the exclusive or predominant source of the vesicles that lie along the outer cell membrane. Lysosomal elements are rare. Pericytes can be distinguished from fibroblasts

in that the latter are free of a basement membrane sheath.

Endothelial Cell Structure

Details of the fine structure of pulmonary capillary endothelial cells are shown in Plate 29. The endothelium is of the continuous type (not fenestrated), and the cells are frequently linked by tight junctions. Around the nucleus, endothelial cells contain mitochondria, Golgi apparatus, rough endoplasmic reticulum, multivesicular bodies, microtubules, microfilaments and Weibel-Palade bodies. However, the slender extensions of the cells are practically devoid of

organelles, and in some regions may be as thin as 0.1 micron.

Recent evidence indicating that endothelium has a role in processing circulating vasoactive substances by the lungs has prompted reexamination of the fine structure of pulmonary endothelial cells. The most striking feature of these cells is the large number of caveolae intracellulares, many of which directly face the vascular lumen but which are also found on the abluminal surface as vesicles. These caveolae vastly increase the surface area of the endothelium, and their position in direct communication with the blood makes them
(Continued)

Fine Structure of Alveolar Capillary Unit
(Continued)

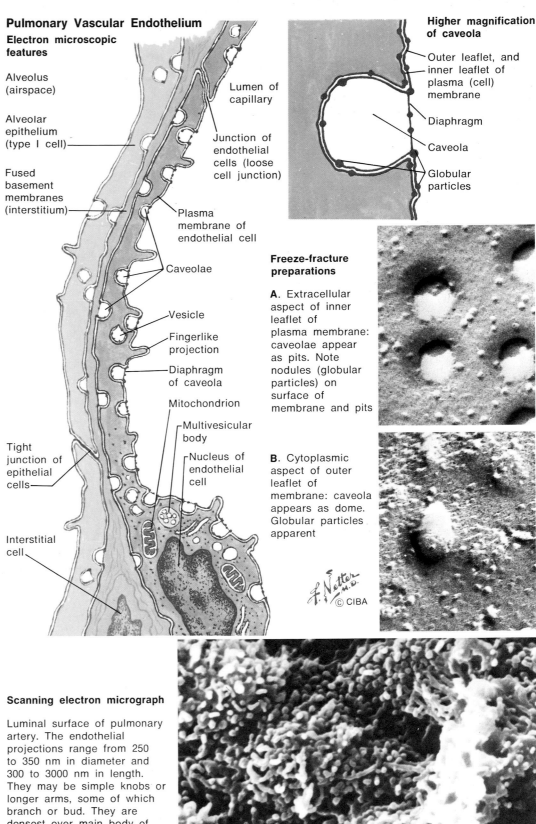

Pulmonary Vascular Endothelium

Electron microscopic features

Alveolus (airspace)

Alveolar epithelium (type I cell)

Fused basement membranes (interstitium)

Tight junction of epithelial cells

Interstitial cell

Lumen of capillary

Junction of endothelial cells (loose cell junction)

Plasma membrane of endothelial cell

Caveolae

Vesicle

Fingerlike projection

Diaphragm of caveola

Mitochondrion

Multivesicular body

Nucleus of endothelial cell

Higher magnification of caveola

Outer leaflet, and inner leaflet of plasma (cell) membrane

Diaphragm

Caveola

Globular particles

Freeze-fracture preparations

A. Extracellular aspect of inner leaflet of plasma membrane: caveolae appear as pits. Note nodules (globular particles) on surface of membrane and pits

B. Cytoplasmic aspect of outer leaflet of membrane: caveola appears as dome. Globular particles apparent

F. Netter M.D.

© CIBA

Scanning electron micrograph

Luminal surface of pulmonary artery. The endothelial projections range from 250 to 350 nm in diameter and 300 to 3000 nm in length. They may be simple knobs or longer arms, some of which branch or bud. They are densest over main body of cells but extend laterally to overlap adjacent cells

ideally suited for processing circulating vasoactive substances. In addition, they possess fine structural features that may be important in the metabolic functions of the lungs.

The luminal stoma of the caveola is spanned by a delicate diaphragm composed of a single lamella (by contrast with the unit membrane construction of the endothelial plasma membrane and caveola membrane). This diaphragm may well create a specialized microenvironment within the caveola. The diaphragm is well placed as an ultrafilter, but whether it functions in this way is not known. Moreover a rim or ring of beads (seen in transverse sections as dense knobs) encircles the stoma of the caveola and may help to maintain the patency of the stoma and the integrity of the diaphragm. The caveola membrane also contains irregularly spaced globular structures, some of which are thought to be enzymes or binding sites. The former interpretation is supported by findings obtained by cytochemical and immunocytochemical enzyme localization techniques. 5'-Nucleotidase and angiotensin-converting enzyme occur in spatial arrangements like those of the globular structures seen on the caveola membrane.

When the pulmonary capillary endothelial cell membrane is freeze-fractured, the caveolae appear as pits on the P face and as domes on the E face. Intramembranous particles, about 80 to 100 Å in diameter, are randomly scattered on both faces, except in association with caveolae, where they occur in rings or plaques. These rings correspond to the skeletal rim seen in thin sections. The intramembranous particles also occur on the curved faces of the caveola membrane. It is not known whether the particles are enzymes, but their size and position make them ideally suited for processing circulating substances, especially those likely to be insoluble in lipid membranes.

The endothelial surface is greatly amplified by numerous fingerlike projections. In addition to the caveolae, these projections can be seen in sections of vessels of all sizes. However, the array of endothelial projections is most strikingly demonstrated in scanning electron micrographs. The size (250 to 350 nm in diameter and 300 to at least 3000 nm long) and density of the projections are such that they may prevent the formed elements of blood from approaching the endothelial surface and have the effect of directing an eddy flow of plasma along the cells. Their function is not known, but they may aid in the exchange of nutrients and in the processing of circulating hormones.

As described above, the relationships of capillaries to alveoli are very nearly perfect for the bulk exchange of oxygen and carbon dioxide. Although the ability of the lungs to process circulating vasoactive hormones is not known to be related to gas exchange, the structure and situation of the lungs within the circulatory system, which make them well suited for gas exchange, may explain how the lungs are also so efficient in processing some hormones. The narrow caliber and vast surface area of the lung capillaries ensure that the layer of hormone-carrying plasma on the endothelial cells is very thin, an ideal situation for facilitating interactions between plasma solutes (*e.g.*, hormones) and the surface structures of the endothelial cells (*e.g.*, enzymes).

Routes of Lymphatic Drainage of Lungs

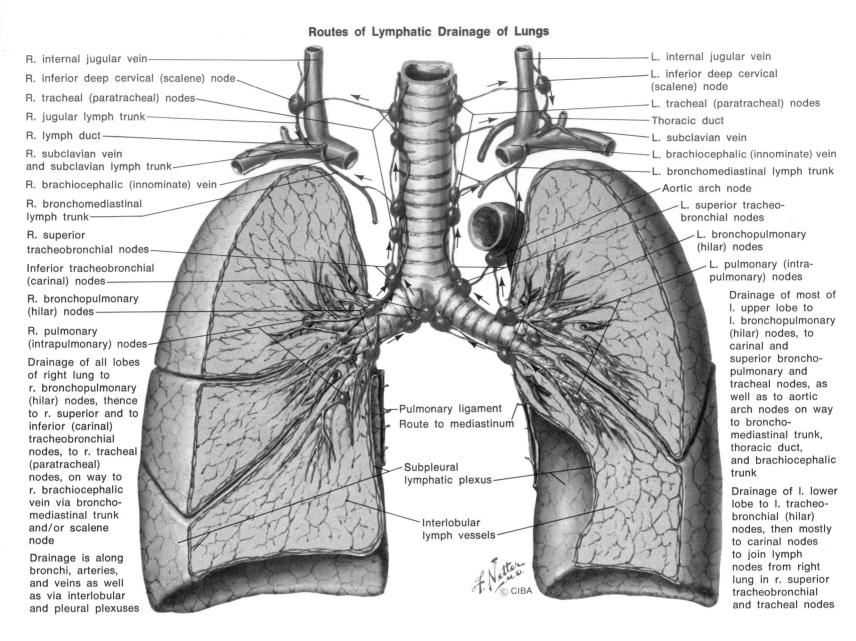

R. internal jugular vein
R. inferior deep cervical (scalene) node
R. tracheal (paratracheal) nodes
R. jugular lymph trunk
R. lymph duct
R. subclavian vein and subclavian lymph trunk
R. brachiocephalic (innominate) vein
R. bronchomediastinal lymph trunk
R. superior tracheobronchial nodes
Inferior tracheobronchial (carinal) nodes
R. bronchopulmonary (hilar) nodes
R. pulmonary (intrapulmonary) nodes

Drainage of all lobes of right lung to r. bronchopulmonary (hilar) nodes, thence to r. superior and to inferior (carinal) tracheobronchial nodes, to r. tracheal (paratracheal) nodes, on way to r. brachiocephalic vein via bronchomediastinal trunk and/or scalene node

Drainage is along bronchi, arteries, and veins as well as via interlobular and pleural plexuses

L. internal jugular vein
L. inferior deep cervical (scalene) node
L. tracheal (paratracheal) nodes
Thoracic duct
L. subclavian vein
L. brachiocephalic (innominate) vein
L. bronchomediastinal lymph trunk
Aortic arch node
L. superior tracheobronchial nodes
L. bronchopulmonary (hilar) nodes
L. pulmonary (intrapulmonary) nodes

Drainage of most of l. upper lobe to l. bronchopulmonary (hilar) nodes, to carinal and superior bronchopulmonary and tracheal nodes, as well as to aortic arch nodes on way to bronchomediastinal trunk, thoracic duct, and brachiocephalic trunk

Drainage of l. lower lobe to l. tracheobronchial (hilar) nodes, then mostly to carinal nodes to join lymph nodes from right lung in r. superior tracheobronchial and tracheal nodes

Pulmonary ligament
Route to mediastinum

Subpleural lymphatic plexus

Interlobular lymph vessels

Lymphatic Drainage of Lungs and Pleura

Considerable inconsistency exists in the terminology as well as the descriptions of the lymphatic channels and distribution of the lymph vessels of the lung. There are discrepancies between the terminology of the *Nomina Anatomica* adopted by anatomists and the terms commonly and conveniently used by clinicians, surgeons and radiologists. For this reason, in the illustrations the terms in common usage are included in parentheses after the official *Nomina Anatomica* designations.

The groups of lymph nodes involved in drainage of the lungs are as follows:

1. The pulmonary (intrapulmonary) nodes within the lung, located chiefly at bifurcations of the larger bronchi.

2. The bronchopulmonary (hilar) nodes situated in the pulmonary hilus at the site of entry of the main bronchi and vessels.

3. The tracheobronchial nodes, which anatomists subdivide into two groups: a *superior* group situated in the obtuse angles between the trachea and bronchi, and an *inferior* (carinal) group situated below or at the carina, *i.e.,* at the junction of the two main bronchi.

4. The tracheal (paratracheal) group situated alongside and to some extent in front of the trachea throughout its course. These are sometimes subdivided into *lower* tracheal (paratracheal) nodes and an *upper* group in accordance with their relative positions.

5. The inferior deep cervical (scalene) nodes situated in relation to the lower part of the internal jugular vein, usually under cover of the scalenus anterior muscle.

6. The aortic arch nodes situated under the arch of the aorta.

The major lymph channels on the *right* side are (1) the bronchomediastinal lymph trunk, which collects lymph from the mediastinum, and (2) the

jugular lymph trunk. The latter commonly unites with (3) the subclavian trunk to form a right lymphatic duct, which in turn joins the origin of the right brachiocephalic vein. In some cases, however, these three major lymphatic channels join the brachiocephalic vein independently. On the *left* side the thoracic duct curves behind the internal jugular vein to enter the right brachiocephalic vein at the junction of the subclavian and internal jugular veins. There may or may not be a separate right bronchomediastinal lymph trunk; if present, it may join the thoracic duct or enter the brachiocephalic vein independently.

Within the lung, lymphatic plexuses course along the bronchi, the pulmonary arteries and the pulmonary veins. There are similar plexuses in the interlobular planes, connective tissue septa and the pleural lining. In the bronchi there are fine lymph channels in the submucosa that communicate with much larger vessels in the adventitia. The bronchial lymph plexuses extend only to the terminal bronchioli, or possibly as far as respiratory bronchioli. Beyond this point, the lymph is collected by the interlobular lymphatics. The bronchial pathways communicate with the lymph vessels along the accompanying pulmonary arteries. The pulmonary veins that lie at the edge of the respiratory units—whether acinus, lobule or

(Continued)

Distribution of Lymphatics in Lungs and Pleura

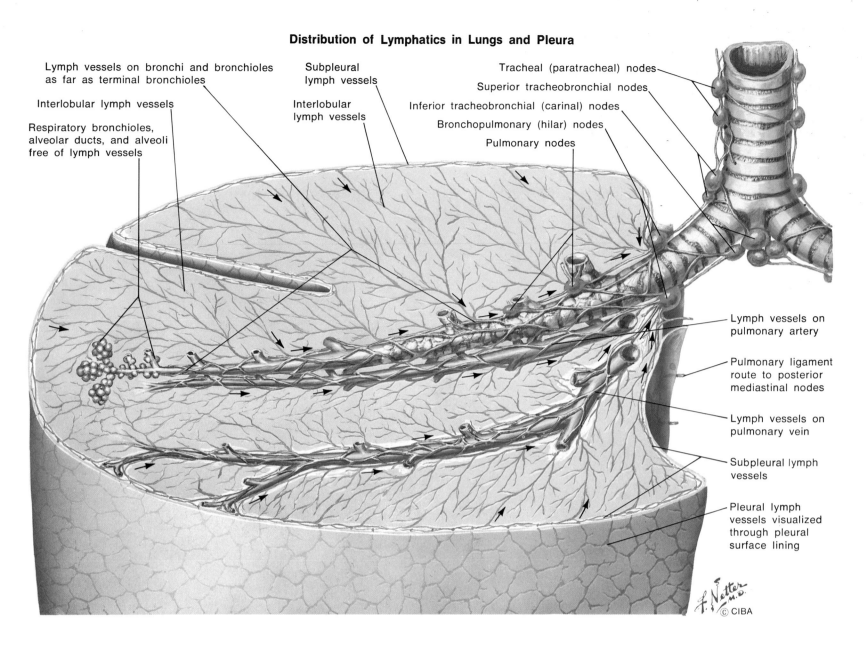

Lymph vessels on bronchi and bronchioles as far as terminal bronchioles

Interlobular lymph vessels

Respiratory bronchioles, alveolar ducts, and alveoli free of lymph vessels

Subpleural lymph vessels

Interlobular lymph vessels

Tracheal (paratracheal) nodes

Superior tracheobronchial nodes

Inferior tracheobronchial (carinal) nodes

Bronchopulmonary (hilar) nodes

Pulmonary nodes

Lymph vessels on pulmonary artery

Pulmonary ligament route to posterior mediastinal nodes

Lymph vessels on pulmonary vein

Subpleural lymph vessels

Pleural lymph vessels visualized through pleural surface lining

Lymphatic Drainage of Lungs and Pleura

(Continued)

segment—are surrounded by connective tissue, and also have lymphatic plexuses in their walls. They are separated from the bronchi and arteries, but, at least centrally, communicating channels connect the various lymphatic systems which form a fine network beneath the pleural surface over the surface of the lungs and the interlobar fissures. When injected, distended (see page 113) or infiltrated by carcinoma (see page 165) the network may be visualized as such. It was former-

ly thought to drain, in its entirety, to the hilar nodes, but it has now been shown to communicate not only with the arterial and venous channels but with the interlobular plexuses as well. Only the portion of the pleural drainage close to the hilus supplies the nodes there. The interlobular vessels pass to the bronchial, arterial and venous pulmonary plexuses and to the pulmonary and bronchopulmonary nodes.

Almost all the lymph from the lungs eventually reaches the bronchopulmonary (hilar) lymph glands, with or without passing through pulmonary nodes on its way. Some lymph may bypass the hilus and go directly to the tracheobronchial nodes. From the *right* lung, drainage from the bronchopulmonary (hilar) group is to the superior and inferior (carinal) tracheobronchial and the right tracheal (paratracheal) nodes. Thence it goes either by way of the bronchomediastinal trunk to the right brachiocephalic vein, or via the inferior deep cervical (scalene) nodes to the same vein, or through both these channels. On the *left* side, the course is somewhat different. Here, most or all of the drainage from the *upper* lobe, after passing through the bronchopulmonary (hilar) nodes, moves either by way of the tracheobronchial and tracheal (paratracheal) nodes, bronchomediastinal trunk, scalene nodes and thoracic duct to the brachiocephalic vein, or by way of the aortic arch

nodes to the same termination. From the *left lower* lobe and usually from the lingula, lymph flows to the right after passing through the bronchopulmonary (hilar) nodes, and goes mostly to the lower tracheobronchial (carinal) lymph nodes. It then follows the same course as lymph from the right lung by way of the right tracheal (paratracheal) nodes—an important point in disease, especially tumors of the left lower lobe.

A number of factors may cause deviation from these major pathways of lymph drainage. The pulmonary lymphatic vessels contain many valves that normally direct the flow centripetally, *i.e.*, toward the hilus. Obstruction in parts of the system, however, may cause a "backing-up" effect, with incompetence of the valves, reversal of flow and opening of collateral channels. It is noteworthy that in pulmonary edema, the pulmonary lymph vessels have been found to be greatly distended (see page 236). Some lymph may leave the lungs through vessels that emerge in the pulmonary ligaments, and pass to posterior mediastinal nodes. Nagaishi states that some of the pulmonary drainage may even reach intraabdominal lymph nodes, although he does not describe the transit route. Finally, there are probably crossconnections between the right and left tracheal (paratracheal) nodes, a situation that may further alter the drainage pathways.

Development of Lower Respiratory System

Developing Respiratory Tract at 4 to 5 Weeks

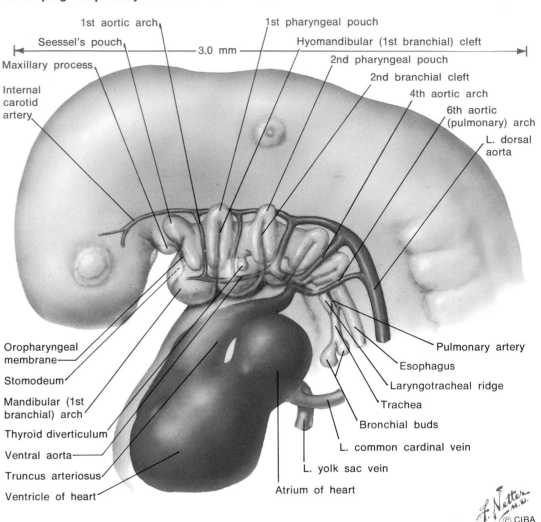

1st aortic arch
Seessel's pouch
Maxillary process
Internal carotid artery
1st pharyngeal pouch
Hyomandibular (1st branchial) cleft
2nd pharyngeal pouch
2nd branchial cleft
4th aortic arch
6th aortic (pulmonary) arch
L. dorsal aorta
3.0 mm
Oropharyngeal membrane
Stomodeum
Mandibular (1st branchial) arch
Thyroid diverticulum
Ventral aorta
Truncus arteriosus
Ventricle of heart
Pulmonary artery
Esophagus
Laryngotracheal ridge
Trachea
Bronchial buds
L. common cardinal vein
L. yolk sac vein
Atrium of heart

Pharynx at 4 to 5 Weeks
(ventral view)

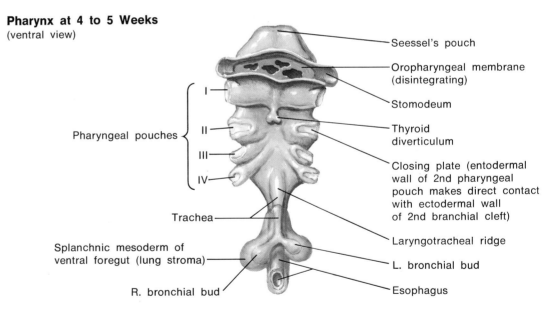

Pharyngeal pouches { I, II, III, IV }
Trachea
Splanchnic mesoderm of ventral foregut (lung stroma)
R. bronchial bud
Seessel's pouch
Oropharyngeal membrane (disintegrating)
Stomodeum
Thyroid diverticulum
Closing plate (entodermal wall of 2nd pharyngeal pouch makes direct contact with ectodermal wall of 2nd branchial cleft)
Laryngotracheal ridge
L. bronchial bud
Esophagus

The development of the respiratory system in man is an interesting demonstration of ontogeny recapitulating phylogeny. The embryology of the system goes through the fish, amphibian, reptilian and mammalian evolutionary stages of man's ancestry. In the change from an aqueous to an aerobic environment, many basic structures were modified but retained as parts of the respiratory system, whereas others became nonrespiratory structures. At the same time entirely new respiratory structures evolved. The olfactory organ of aqueous forms was incorporated into the respiratory system of terrestrial forms, and the simple sphincter mechanism of the swim bladder of fish became the larynx of air-breathers, which also took on the function of phonation. In contrast, that part of the respiratory system involved in the gas exchange vital to life has essentially not changed throughout vertebrate evolution. Exchange of oxygen and carbon dioxide between the external environment and the circulating blood stream occurs through a wet epithelium in both gills and lungs.

The respiratory system in man differs from the other major body systems in that it is not operational until birth. Therefore, development of the antenatal respiratory system is genetically determined independently of the functional demands of the growing embryo and fetus. The system's physiologic development is mainly one of preparation for instant action at birth, a feat unmatched by any other system. When the fetus passes from the uterine aquatic environment, the partially collapsed, fluid-filled lungs immediately function efficiently to sustain life. The chief cause of perinatal death of human infants is failure of the respiratory system to work properly. In the majority of perinatal deaths all other body systems are functioning normally.

Primitive Respiratory Tube

During the fourth week the first indication of the future respiratory tree is a groove that runs lengthwise in the floor of the pharynx, just caudal to the pharyngeal pouches. From the outside this laryngotracheal groove appears as a ridge. The ridge grows caudally to become a tube, the lung bud, and the cranial or upper part of the tube becomes the larynx. The caudal part becomes the future trachea, which soon develops two knob-like enlargements at its distal end, the bronchial buds (Plate 32).

Trachea

As the trachea lengthens, anterior to and parallel with the esophagus, the bronchial buds are carried progressively more caudal in the body until they reach their definitive position in the thorax. During this growth period mesenchymal cells from the splanchnic mesoderm surround the tracheal tube of entoderm and give rise to the connective tissue, smooth muscle and cartilage of the tracheal wall. By and during the eighth week, the rudiments of the 16 to 20 C-shaped tracheal cartilages appear (Plate 35). These mesenchymal rudiments transform into cartilage in a cranial to caudal direction up to the tenth week. Only the epithelial lining and glands of the trachea are derived from entoderm. The lining starts to become ciliated at 10 weeks, with the cilia beating *(Continued)*

Development of Lower Respiratory System
(Continued)

Sagittal Section at 5 to 6 Weeks

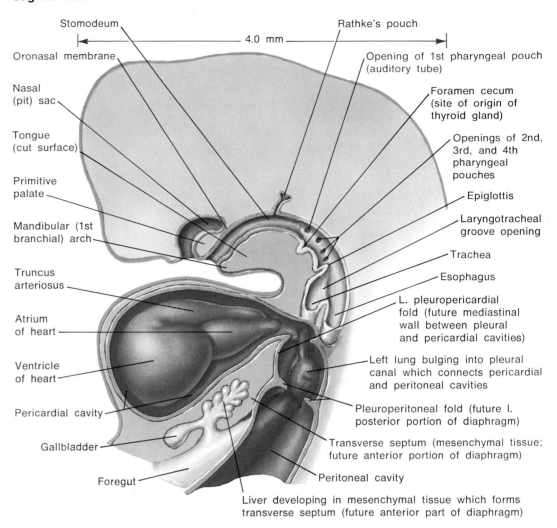

Stomodeum
Oronasal membrane
Nasal (pit) sac
Tongue (cut surface)
Primitive palate
Mandibular (1st branchial) arch
Truncus arteriosus
Atrium of heart
Ventricle of heart
Pericardial cavity
Gallbladder
Foregut

4.0 mm

Rathke's pouch
Opening of 1st pharyngeal pouch (auditory tube)
Foramen cecum (site of origin of thyroid gland)
Openings of 2nd, 3rd, and 4th pharyngeal pouches
Epiglottis
Laryngotracheal groove opening
Trachea
Esophagus
L. pleuropericardial fold (future mediastinal wall between pleural and pericardial cavities)
Left lung bulging into pleural canal which connects pericardial and peritoneal cavities
Pleuroperitoneal fold (future l. posterior portion of diaphragm)
Transverse septum (mesenchymal tissue; future anterior portion of diaphragm)
Peritoneal cavity
Liver developing in mesenchymal tissue which forms transverse septum (future anterior part of diaphragm)

toward the larynx. By 12 weeks the mucosal glands begin to appear in a cranial to caudal direction. All major microscopic features are recognizable by the end of the fifth month. However, the infantile trachea differs grossly from the adult form because it is short and narrow compared with a relatively very large larynx. This size difference continues for several months after birth.

Bronchi

The bronchial buds of the trachea become the two main bronchi. As soon as the right bronchus appears, it is a little larger than the left one and tends to be more vertically oriented (Plates 32 and 35). These differences become more pronounced up to and after the time the bronchi mature, and this fact accounts for the fact that foreign bodies enter the right main bronchus much more often than the left.

During the fifth week each main bronchus gives rise to two bronchial buds. These buds develop secondary branches to the future lobes: the upper, middle and lower lobes on the right side and the upper and lower lobes on the left (Plate 33). By the seventh week tertiary branches appear (Plate 34), 10 in the right lung and 8 in the left. These tertiary branches will supply the clinically important bronchopulmonary segments, which become separated from one another by tenuous connective-tissue septa (Plate 35). The tenuous connective tissue surrounding each segment delineates a separate respiratory unit of the lung, but some collateral ventilation does occur between segments. A branch of the pulmonary artery accompanies each segmental bronchus to serve as

Bronchi and Lungs at 5 to 6 Weeks

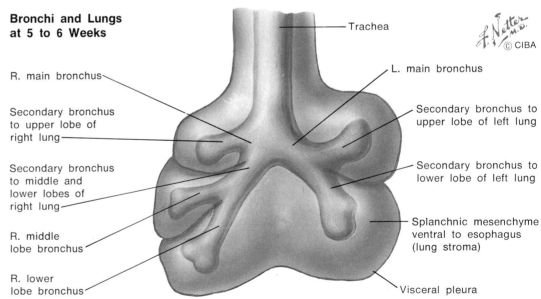

R. main bronchus
Secondary bronchus to upper lobe of right lung
Secondary bronchus to middle and lower lobes of right lung
R. middle lobe bronchus
R. lower lobe bronchus

Trachea
L. main bronchus
Secondary bronchus to upper lobe of left lung
Secondary bronchus to lower lobe of left lung
Splanchnic mesenchyme ventral to esophagus (lung stroma)
Visceral pleura

the independent blood supply to a bronchopulmonary segment. Again, some collateral circulation occurs across segments. The pulmonary veins do not accompany the segmental bronchi and arteries but run chiefly through the substance of the lung between the segments, as do the lymphatic vessels.

Branching of the segmental bronchi continues until, by the sixth month, about 17 orders of branching have been formed. Additional branching continues postnatally and until puberty, when about 24 orders of branches have been established. Once the full complement of branches has appeared, no new ones will form to replace any lost

through trauma or disease. The mature lung makes up for any branches lost by enlarging the remaining functional segments, which then do more work (compensatory hyperinflation).

Cartilage, Smooth Muscle and Connective Tissue

By the tenth week cartilage is present in the main bronchi and by the twelfth week in the segmental bronchi. Cilia appear in the lining of the main bronchi at 12 weeks and in the segmental bronchi at 13 weeks. At birth the ciliated epithelium extends to the terminal bronchioles.

(Continued)

Respiratory System at 6 to 7 Weeks

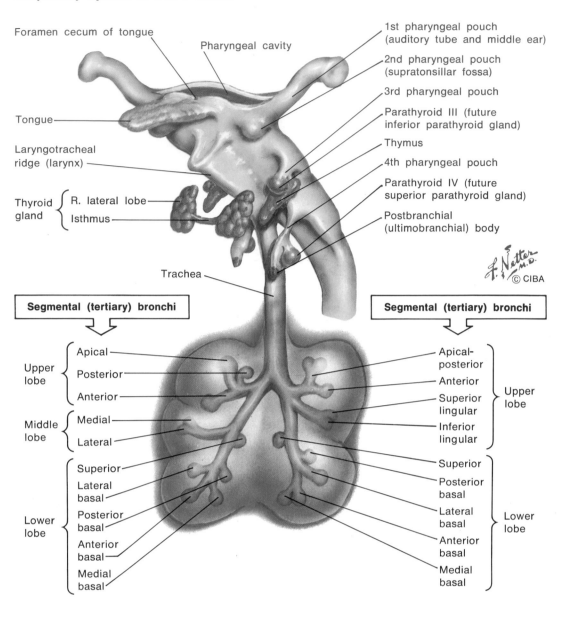

Foramen cecum of tongue

Pharyngeal cavity

Tongue

Laryngotracheal ridge (larynx)

Thyroid gland { R. lateral lobe / Isthmus }

Trachea

1st pharyngeal pouch (auditory tube and middle ear)

2nd pharyngeal pouch (supratonsillar fossa)

3rd pharyngeal pouch

Parathyroid III (future inferior parathyroid gland)

Thymus

4th pharyngeal pouch

Parathyroid IV (future superior parathyroid gland)

Postbranchial (ultimobranchial) body

Segmental (tertiary) bronchi

Upper lobe { Apical / Posterior / Anterior }

Middle lobe { Medial / Lateral }

Lower lobe { Superior / Lateral basal / Posterior basal / Anterior basal / Medial basal }

Segmental (tertiary) bronchi

Apical-posterior / Anterior / Superior lingular / Inferior lingular } Upper lobe

Superior / Posterior basal / Lateral basal / Anterior basal / Medial basal } Lower lobe

Although the l. anterior basal and the l. medial basal bronchi are sometimes considered together as the l. anteromedial basal bronchus, they are usually separate structures and are so designated

Development of Lower Respiratory System
(Continued)

Mucous glands appear in the bronchi at 13 weeks and actively produce mucus by 14 weeks. At 28 weeks, seven-eighths of the potential adult number of mucous glands are present in the respiratory tubes.

By the third month smooth muscle cells differentiate to form the posterior wall of the trachea and extrapulmonary main bronchi, which permanently lack cartilage. Smooth muscle cells form bundles arranged obliquely and circularly around the bronchioles, including the terminal bronchioles, whose entire walls have no cartilage. The smooth muscle that extends to the alveolar ducts acts as a sphincter. In an allergic reaction, such as bronchial asthma, smooth muscle spasm greatly increases airway resistance. High surface tension in the terminal airways containing a large accumulation of mucus then further reduces the smaller than normal bronchiolar diameter during expiration. Since inspiration is effected by contraction of powerful muscles and is associated with widening and lengthening of the bronchial tree muscles, an asthmatic can usually inspire adequately. He has great difficulty exhaling, however, because expiration normally results from passive recoil of the stretched thoracic wall and lungs. To overcome the increased airway resistance of an asthmatic attack, muscles of the anterior abdominal wall must be contracted and stabilized, thus allowing the diaphragm to push with greater force and drive air out of the lungs with maximum effort.

Autonomic innervation of the lungs is not extensive; all effects of both sympathetic and parasympathetic innervation are mild. Parasym-

pathetic stimulation can cause moderate contraction of smooth muscle of the respiratory tubes and perhaps some dilation of the blood vessels. In contrast, sympathetic stimulation can mildly dilate the tubes and mildly constrict the vessels. Therefore, sympathomimetic drugs can be helpful in inhibiting the spasmodic contraction of the respiratory tube smooth muscle during an asthmatic attack.

Pleural Cavities

The pericardial, pleural and peritoneal cavities develop as subdivisions of two primitive coelomic cavities that extend along the length of the embryo. Normally each is only a potential space with serous lining which produces a slimy secretion. This reduces friction as the ordinarily apposed surfaces rub against each other. Following trauma or other forms of pathology the cavities may become actual spaces containing proteinaceous exudate, air or blood.

During the second week of life the two coelomic cavities in the region of the developing heart fuse into a single pericardial coelom. While

the pericardial cavity is becoming established, it is in open communication caudally on each side with the still paired primitive coeloms in the embryo's future abdominal region. Partitioning of the pericardial coelom from these primitive coeloms starts by the establishment of a shelf of mesenchyme, the transverse septum, into which the liver becomes incorporated as it is developing (Plate 33). This transverse septum grows in from the anterior body wall toward the dorsal or posterior body wall, but never reaches it and finally becomes part of the diaphragm. Therefore, the two channels of communication between the pericardial coelom and the two primitive coelomic cavities persist to become the pleural canals.

Pleural Canals. In the fish stage of vertebrate evolution the transverse septum completely separates the pericardial and peritoneal cavities. In lungfish, the air bladder projects directly into a common pleuroperitoneal space, while in amphibians and reptiles the lungs are found in a similar space caudal to the pericardial cavity. In man, the amphibian and reptilian evolutionary stage of
(Continued)

Development of Lower Respiratory System
(Continued)

Larynx, Tracheobronchial Tree, and Lungs at 7 to 10 Weeks

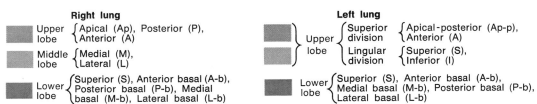

Thyrohyoid membrane

Greater cornu
Lesser cornu — Hyoid cartilage (later develops into bone)
Body

Thyroid cartilage

Position of cricoid lamina

Thyrocricoid membrane

Arch of cricoid cartilage

Trachea

Tracheal cartilages

L. main bronchus

R. main bronchus

L. pulmonary artery

R. pulmonary artery

Upper lobe of right lung

Superior division of upper lobe of left lung

Ap

Ap-p

P

A

A

S

S

S

L

I

L-b

M

Middle lobe of right lung

Lingular division of upper lobe of left lung

M-b

L-b

M-b

P-b

A-b

Lower lobe of right lung

Lower lobe of left lung

L-b

A-b

P-b

Tertiary branches of bronchi to bronchopulmonary segments

Right lung

Upper lobe	Apical (Ap), Posterior (P), Anterior (A)
Middle lobe	Medial (M), Lateral (L)
Lower lobe	Superior (S), Anterior basal (A-b), Posterior basal (P-b), Medial basal (M-b), Lateral basal (L-b)

Left lung

Upper lobe	Superior division	Apical-posterior (Ap-p), Anterior (A)
	Lingular division	Superior (S), Inferior (I)
Lower lobe	Superior (S), Anterior basal (A-b), Medial basal (M-b), Posterior basal (P-b), Lateral basal (L-b)

lung development occurs when the growing lungs project into the pleural canals. Each pleural cavity then becomes isolated by the growth of the pleuropericardial and pleuroperitoneal folds. These in turn become associated with the transverse septum (see below).

Pleuropericardial and Pleuroperitoneal Folds. The vertically oriented pleuropericardial folds arise on each side from the body walls where the common cardinal veins swing around to enter the sinus venosus, which subsequently becomes the right atrium. These body-wall folds bulge into the pleural canals between the lungs and the heart (Plates 33 and 37). When the free borders of the pleuropericardial folds fuse with midline mesenchymal tissue at the base of the heart, they completely separate what is now the pericardial cavity from the pleuroperitoneal coelom (Plate 37). At this time the latter space contains the lungs as well as the abdominal and pelvic viscera.

The pleuroperitoneal folds are actually two horizontally oriented ridges of the dorsolateral body wall where the common cardinal veins are located (Plate 33). Each fold grows anteriorly and medially to fuse with the transverse septum and mesenchymal tissue surrounding the aorta, esophagus and inferior vena cava. The two pleural canals are then walled off from the newly formed peritoneal cavity, and the formation of the pleural cavities and diaphragm is completed (Plates 36 and 38).

Diaphragm

A diaphragm is lacking in fish, amphibians, reptiles and birds. In mammals, it is the principal respiratory muscle. Although there are numerous accessory respiratory muscles, they cannot support life to a normal degree without a functioning diaphragm. Reptiles have a dual muscular respiratory mechanism: the action of the trunk muscles creates negative pressure, and the floor of the mouth pushes air into the lungs under positive pressure. The reptilian action of the muscles of the floor of the mouth is also the chief respiratory muscular mechanism in amphibians ("frog-breathing"). In birds, which like mammals evolved from reptiles, respiration is accomplished chiefly by the intercostal trunk muscles that move the ribs, to which the lungs are attached.

In the evolutionary transition from gill-breathing to lung-breathing, original muscles from the mandibular arch gave rise to the musculature of the floor of the mouth, especially the mylohyoid muscle. In amphibians and reptiles, air brought in through the nares is forced into the lungs by the musculatory action of the floor of the mouth. In mammals, a new respiratory muscle — the diaphragm — evolved from structures lacking muscle in certain reptiles: specifically, the transverse septum and two unfused coelomic folds that are the pleuroperitoneal folds in mammalian development.

(Continued)

Sagittal Section at 6 to 7 Weeks

Rathke's pouch

Foramen cecum of tongue

Opening of 1st pharyngeal pouch (auditory tube)

Openings of 2nd, 3rd, and 4th pharyngeal pouches

Lateral palatine process (portion of future palate)

Oronasal membrane

Median palatine process

Epiglottis

R. nasal sac

Maxillary fold

Oral cavity

Arytenoid swelling which borders laryngeal opening (glottis)

Ethmoid fold

Trachea

Esophagus

— 7.0 mm —

Development of Lower Respiratory System
(Continued)

Mandibular (1st branchial) arch

Tongue (cut surface)

Pericardial cavity

Ventricle of heart

Transverse septum contribution to diaphragm

Falciform ligament

Liver (cut surface)

Left atrium of heart

L. common cardinal vein

Lesser omentum

Left lung bulging into l. pleural cavity which has developed from pleural canal

Pleuroperitoneal fold contribution to diaphragm

Greater omentum

Stomach bulging into left side of peritoneal cavity

Pleuropericardial fold which separates l. pleural cavity from pericardial cavity

Diaphragmatic musculature in mammals develops from a common mass of mesoderm at the posterior region of the branchial arches from which the tongue and infrahyoid muscles are also derived (Plate 38). The transverse septum, the largest single contribution to the diaphragm, develops in the neck or cervical region of the embryo (Plates 33 and 38). The diaphragmatic striated musculature migrates to the transverse septum, along with branches of the third, fourth and fifth cervical spinal nerves, which become its exclusive motor nerve through the phrenic nerve. By differential growth, especially an increase in size of the thoracic region, there is a so-called migration and descent of the diaphragm to a much more caudal position. At the end of the eighth week the diaphragm is attached to the dorsal body wall at the level of the first lumbar segment. The phrenic nerves, which are located in the body wall where the pleuropericardial folds develop, lengthen as the diaphragm descends. They are, therefore, relocated to a position between the pericardium and the pleurae as the pleural cavities increase in size (Plate 37).

Once the transverse septum, the two pleuroperitoneal folds and the numerous other minor folds unite to complete the diaphragm at or during the seventh week, the diaphragmatic musculature becomes peripherally positioned (Plate 38), while its domelike central area remains tendinous. As soon as the diaphragm is completely developed, it begins to contract at irregular intervals. Near term, these contractions, which are essentially hiccups, become more vigorous and

more frequent. They exercise the muscles for the time when air-breathing begins at birth.

During inhalation, the diaphragm flattens as it contracts. This action reduces the intrathoracic pressure by enlarging the thoracic cavity, and with it the intrapulmonary space. The vocal folds are separated, and thus air rushes into the lungs at atmospheric pressure. Normal inspiration is caused chiefly by the contraction of the diaphragm. Other powerful striated muscles that assist the diaphragm are in the neck and chest region, and are attached to the skull, clavicle, ribs, vertebral column and upper limbs. Therefore, inspiration is effected by the contraction of

powerful muscles, whereas expiration is largely a passive action caused by recoil of the stretched tissues of the thoracic wall and lungs.

The diaphragm is subject to developmental defects that permit herniation of abdominal viscera into the thorax. The most common diaphragmatic congenital hernia is related to defective development of the left pleuroperitoneal fold (Plate 38).

Pleura and Mediastinum

The lungs develop much later than the heart, as was the case throughout their evolutionary history. The small lungs, posterior to a relatively very
(Continued)

Development of Lower Respiratory System
(Continued)

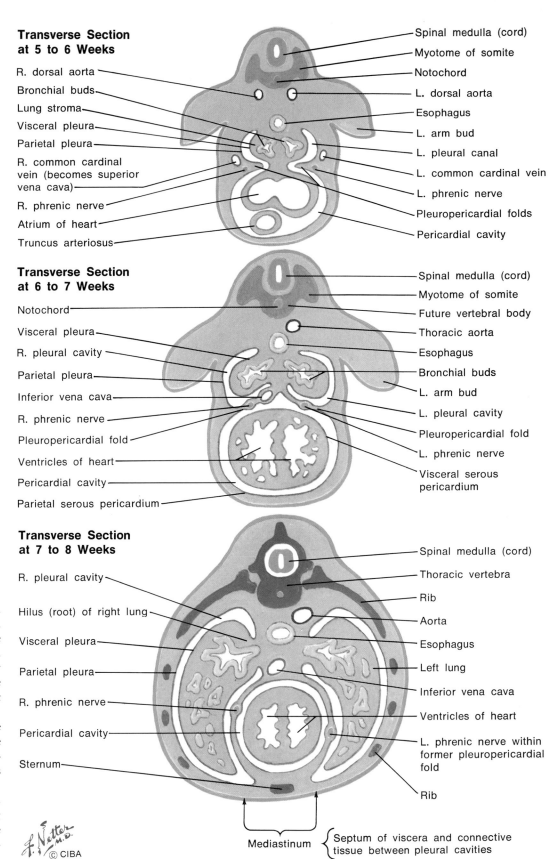

Transverse Section at 5 to 6 Weeks

- R. dorsal aorta
- Bronchial buds
- Lung stroma
- Visceral pleura
- Parietal pleura
- R. common cardinal vein (becomes superior vena cava)
- R. phrenic nerve
- Atrium of heart
- Truncus arteriosus
- Spinal medulla (cord)
- Myotome of somite
- Notochord
- L. dorsal aorta
- Esophagus
- L. arm bud
- L. pleural canal
- L. common cardinal vein
- L. phrenic nerve
- Pleuropericardial folds
- Pericardial cavity

Transverse Section at 6 to 7 Weeks

- Notochord
- Visceral pleura
- R. pleural cavity
- Parietal pleura
- Inferior vena cava
- R. phrenic nerve
- Pleuropericardial fold
- Ventricles of heart
- Pericardial cavity
- Parietal serous pericardium
- Spinal medulla (cord)
- Myotome of somite
- Future vertebral body
- Thoracic aorta
- Esophagus
- Bronchial buds
- L. arm bud
- L. pleural cavity
- Pleuropericardial fold
- L. phrenic nerve
- Visceral serous pericardium

Transverse Section at 7 to 8 Weeks

- R. pleural cavity
- Hilus (root) of right lung
- Visceral pleura
- Parietal pleura
- R. phrenic nerve
- Pericardial cavity
- Sternum
- Spinal medulla (cord)
- Thoracic vertebra
- Rib
- Aorta
- Esophagus
- Left lung
- Inferior vena cava
- Ventricles of heart
- L. phrenic nerve within former pleuropericardial fold
- Rib

Mediastinum { Septum of viscera and connective tissue between pleural cavities

large heart, grow in an anterior direction on each side of it (Plate 37). The pleural cavities open in advance of the growing lungs so that they are already prepared to receive them. By the eighth week the lungs are larger than the heart and nearly surround it. The pleural cavities now occupy the two sides of the thoracic cavity. All other thoracic viscera, including the heart, great vessels, esophagus and associated connective tissue, are now between the two pleural cavities, from the vertebral column to the sternum. This broad medial septum of viscera and connective tissue is known as the mediastinum.

As the lungs protrude into the pleural canals (Plate 33), they are invested by the lining mesothelium of these spaces which becomes the visceral pleura (Plate 37). Before the pleuro-pericardial folds wall off the pleural canals from the pericardial coelom, the mesothelium lining the walls of these thoracic subdivisions is continuous (Plates 33 and 37). As soon as the pleural canals become the pleural cavities, the lining of the walls of the canals becomes the parietal pleura. The region where the visceral pleura reflects off the lungs and becomes continuous with the parietal pleura shifts medially and becomes smaller to envelop the structures that constitute the root of the lung.

Throughout human development the right lung is larger than the left, as is the case with the right and left pleural cavities. This size differential is related to the shift of the heart to the left side of the thorax. In adult mammals and reptiles,

the right lung also tends to be larger than the left. In adult man, the space occupied by the heart produces the cardiac notch of the left lung.

Terminal Respiratory Tubes

The amphibian stage of development of portions of the respiratory tubes occurs at 4 to 5 weeks when the bronchial buds are present (Plate 32). Amphibian lungs are essentially two air sacs, each with a large single lumen. In reptilians, segmental bronchi are present at 7 to 8 weeks (Plate 35). The reptilian lung has branching respiratory tubes ending in terminal sacs that are much like mammalian primitive alveoli. They

add greatly to the surface area where gas exchange occurs; in contrast, the amphibian lung has only rudimentary alveoli.

Alveolar development does not begin in the human fetus until airway development is complete at 16 weeks. Between the fourth and sixth months the last airway is transformed to a terminal or respiratory bronchiole. Generally, each respiratory bronchiole divides into three to six alveolar ducts (Plate 39). Each alveolar duct first ends in a bulging terminal sac lined by cuboidal or columnar epithelium that ultimately evolves into definitive alveoli. Capillaries multiply so that the

(Continued)

Development of Lower Respiratory System
(Continued)

Innervation of Muscle Masses of Tongue, Neck, and Diaphragm at 5 to 6 Weeks

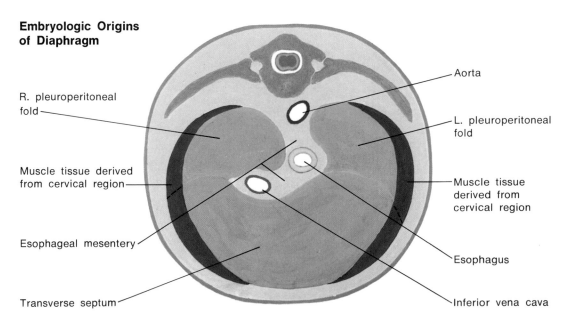

— 4.0 mm —

Hypoglossal (XII) nerve

Myelencephalon (future medulla oblongata)

Myotome of 1st cervical somite

Spinal medulla (cord)

Sensory ganglion of 1st cervical nerve

Superior ramus of ansa cervicalis

Inferior ramus of ansa cervicalis

Ansa cervicalis

Lingual muscle mass (future tongue)

Infrahyoid muscle mass (future so-called strap muscle)

Diaphragmatic muscle mass

Transverse septum (future anterior portion of diaphragm)

4th cervical nerve

Phrenic nerve

© CIBA

Embryologic Origins of Diaphragm

R. pleuroperitoneal fold

Muscle tissue derived from cervical region

Esophageal mesentery

Transverse septum

Aorta

L. pleuroperitoneal fold

Muscle tissue derived from cervical region

Esophagus

Inferior vena cava

region of terminal airspaces becomes highly vascularized.

During the sixth month the epithelium of the terminal sacs thins where it is in contact with a capillary (Plate 39). The epithelial cells become so thin when the alveoli fill with air that, before the advent of electron microscopy, there seemed to be breaks in the lining where only capillary endothelium separated the blood from the alveolar air (Plate 40). The capillaries, covered by the thin epithelial cells, line the alveolar spaces (Plate 40). These very thin cells, constituting the major part of the alveolar surface, are known as type I pneumocytes. Other cells, scattered along the lining of the alveoli, are cuboidal, have microvilli on their luminal surfaces, and contain osmiophilic inclusions of surfactant or its precursors. These cells are known as type II pneumocytes, and they also appear during the sixth month.

The original mesenchyme that gives rise to the pulmonary capillaries and lymphatics is also the source of the fibrocytes that produce an abundance of elastic fibers in the lungs (Plate 39). Once the lungs become inflated with air, the elastic fibers are constantly stretched and, by attempting to contract, contribute to the normal recoil or collapsing tendency of the lungs. On the other hand, the natural tendency of the chest wall is to expand. The resulting negative pressure in the pleural cavities helps to keep the lungs expanded. The visceral pleura continually absorbs fluid so that only a small amount of it remains in the potential intrapleural space at all times. Since the elastic fibers of the lungs are stretched even more during inspiration, they are the chief structures responsi-

ble for returning the enlarged alveoli and bronchioles to their more contracted resting dimensions during normal passive expiration.

Alveolar-Capillary (Respiratory) Membrane. By the 28th week the lung has lost its glandular appearance. The respiratory airways end in a cluster of large thin-walled sacs separated from one another by a matrix of loose connective tissue. At this stage respiration can be supported because gas exchange can occur at the terminal sacs, and surfactant is present to maintain alveolar stability. The primitive alveoli do not become definitive as true alveoli until after birth, at which time they are only shallow bulges of the walls of the terminal

sacs and respiratory bronchioles. Even so, the thickness of the blood-air barrier, which is also known as the *respiratory* or *alveolar-capillary membrane,* is about 0.4 micron. This is within the range found in the adult: that is, 2.5 microns to less than 0.1 micron (a micron is 0.001 mm). In the lungs of the newborn infant there are 24 million primitive alveoli (Plate 40).

During the first three years of life the increase in lung size is due to alveolar multiplication rather than to greater alveolar size. From the third to the eighth year the alveoli increase in size as well as in number until there are 300 million in the two

(Continued)

Development of Lower Respiratory System
(Continued)

Terminal Air Tube at 20 Weeks

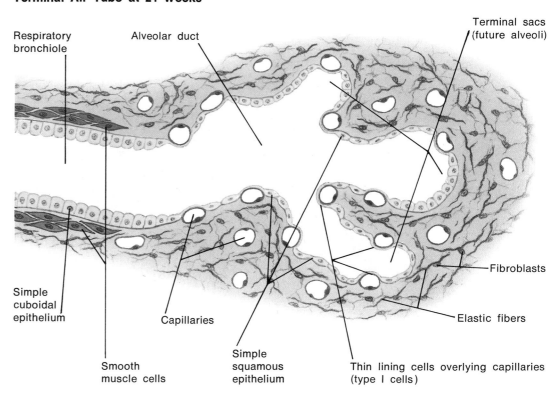

Terminal Air Tube at 24 Weeks

lungs. After the eighth year alveoli become larger only until the chest wall stops growing. At age 8 the diameter of the mature alveolus is 100 to 300 microns. Physical diffusion of oxygen from the alveolus into the red blood cell or erythrocyte and of carbon dioxide in the opposite direction occurs through the respiratory membrane, which consists of an alveolar type I pneumocyte and a capillary endothelial cell and their respective basement membranes. Consequently, oxygen and carbon dioxide do not have to pass across a great distance between the erythrocyte and the alveolus and gas diffusion can be accomplished very rapidly. The total surface area of the respiratory membrane of both lungs is about 70 m², which is vast when compared to the 1.7 m² of total body surface of an adult. The average diameter of a pulmonary capillary is only about 7 microns (Plate 40). The extensive alveolar and associated capillary endothelial surface is also responsible for a large water vapor loss during respiration; adult lungs eliminate about 800 ml of water a day in expired air.

Surfactant

No matter how complete the development of the respiratory system at birth, one factor that determines whether or not it will support life is the presence of a substance known as pulmonary surfactant. Therefore, because of its functional implications, the most important morphologic event is the appearance at about the 23rd week of lamellar inclusion bodies in the type II pneumocytes of the lining of the terminal sacs. These bodies are precursors of surfactant, a lipoprotein mixture rich in phospholipids, especially dipalmitoyl lecithin. Surfactant has a "detergent"

property of lowering surface tension in the fluid layer which lines the primitive alveoli once air enters the lungs, and it acts as an antiatelectasis factor to maintain patency of terminal airspaces (Plate 40).

Surface tension of a fluid is measured in dynes/cm. A drop of water on a sheet of glass tends to round up into a compact mass because of its surface tension of about 72 dynes/cm at the air-water interface. If household detergent is added to the drop of water, its surface tension is reduced to about 20 dynes/cm and it spreads into a very thin film on the glass (Plate 41). In a similar manner surfactant reduces surface tension of the fluid layer

lining the alveolus to about 5 dynes/cm. Its ability to form a monomolecular layer at the interface between air and the alveolar lining fluid (Plate 40) allows some air to be retained within the alveolus at all times.

Although surfactant is present in the lungs as early as the 23rd week, the lungs at this stage are unable to retain air after inflation, and they collapse completely before 28 to 32 weeks. The quantity of surfactant within the lungs increases markedly toward term — one of the most important reasons why older fetuses have a better chance of survival as air-breathers. Surfactant must be

(Continued)

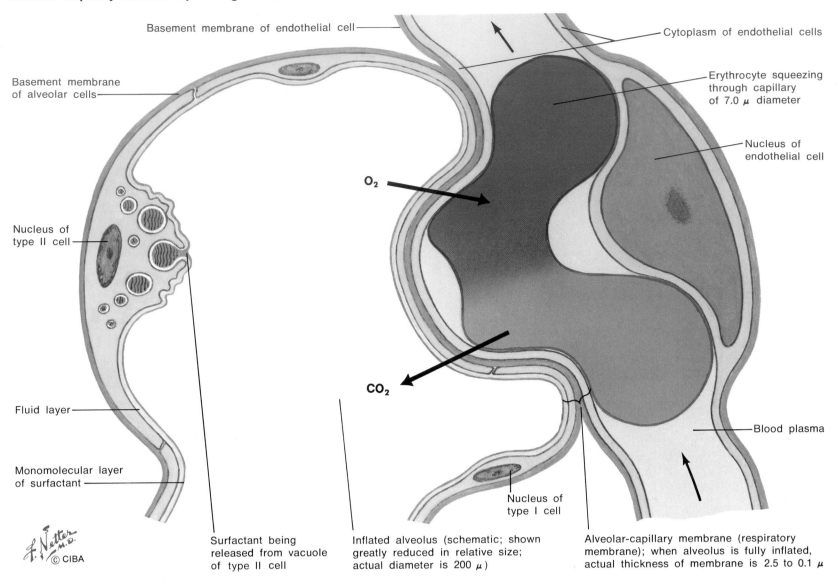

Basement membrane of endothelial cell

Cytoplasm of endothelial cells

Basement membrane of alveolar cells

Erythrocyte squeezing through capillary of 7.0 μ diameter

Nucleus of endothelial cell

O₂

Nucleus of type II cell

CO₂

Blood plasma

Fluid layer

Monomolecular layer of surfactant

Nucleus of type I cell

Surfactant being released from vacuole of type II cell

Inflated alveolus (schematic; shown greatly reduced in relative size; actual diameter is 200 μ)

Alveolar-capillary membrane (respiratory membrane); when alveolus is fully inflated, actual thickness of membrane is 2.5 to 0.1 μ

SECTION I   PLATE 40

Development of Lower Respiratory System
(Continued)

produced continually, because it has a half-life of from 14 to 24 hours. A deficiency of surfactant is associated with the infant respiratory distress syndrome (RDS), also known as hyaline membrane disease (see pages 250 to 252). This is due to the relative instability of the immature lung because of failure to produce surfactant in amounts sufficient for neonatal respiration. Death from the disease occurs within a few hours to a few days after birth. The alveoli of the dead infants are filled with a proteinaceous fluid that resembles a glassy or hyaline membrane.

The high incidence of RDS in premature infants is due to their low initial concentrations of surfactant. Prematurity, cesarean section and perinatal asphyxia are recognized predisposing factors. Surface tension of lung extracts of newborn infants with a birth weight of 1200 g or more

is only about 5 dynes/cm. In extracts from infants with a birth weight less than 1200 g who have hyaline membrane disease, it may be four times that value.

Before birth the respiratory tubes are filled with fluid, some of it amniotic fluid brought in by "practice" inspiratory movements. However, most of the fluid is produced by the lining of the respiratory tubes, as much as 120 ml/hour near term. This pulmonary fluid passes through the oral and nasal cavities to mix with the amniotic fluid. Amniotic fluid contains phospholipids, and amniocentesis before the 35th week usually shows that the ratio of lecithin to sphingomyelin is less than or equal to one, since the latter remains constant as gestation advances. Such a ratio indicates that the fetus is immature in regard to surfactant production. A ratio of more than 2:1 indicates that the fetal lungs are sufficiently mature to prevent the development of RDS.

The role of thyroxine and adrenal corticosteroids in stimulating lung maturation and surfactant production has not yet been settled and is still under investigation. Surfactant is present in the lungs of all vertebrate air-breathers. The amount of surfactant correlates well with alveolar surface area and with the amount of certain saturated phospholipids in the lung tissue in a stepwise fashion up the phylogenetic scale from amphibians through reptiles to mammals.

First Breath

Before the first breath, the lungs are filled with fluid. Therefore, the lungs of a stillborn infant who has not taken a breath of air differ from those of an infant who has. They are firm, do not crepitate when handled and, since they contain no air, sink in water. Some of the fluid normally within the lungs at birth is extruded from the mouth; most of it is removed through the lymphatic vessels in the region of the primitive alveoli. The pleural lymphatic vessels are relatively larger and more numerous in the fetus and newborn infant than in the adult, and lymph flow is high during the first few hours after birth. The flow is less two days later but is still higher than in the adult.

A certain amount of fluid must of necessity always remain in the alveoli, but in the partially atelectatic (collapsed) primitive alveoli, the surface tension of the viscid fluid tends to hold the walls of the alveoli together. Therefore, the first breath of some 30 to 40 ml in volume requires a tremendous physical effort, and a negative intrathoracic pressure — as much as 40 to 100 cm of water — is needed for expansion. This is about 14 times the pressure required to produce breaths of a similar volume subsequently (Plate 41).

Contraction of the diaphragm is mainly responsible for the first breath that is often associated
(Continued)

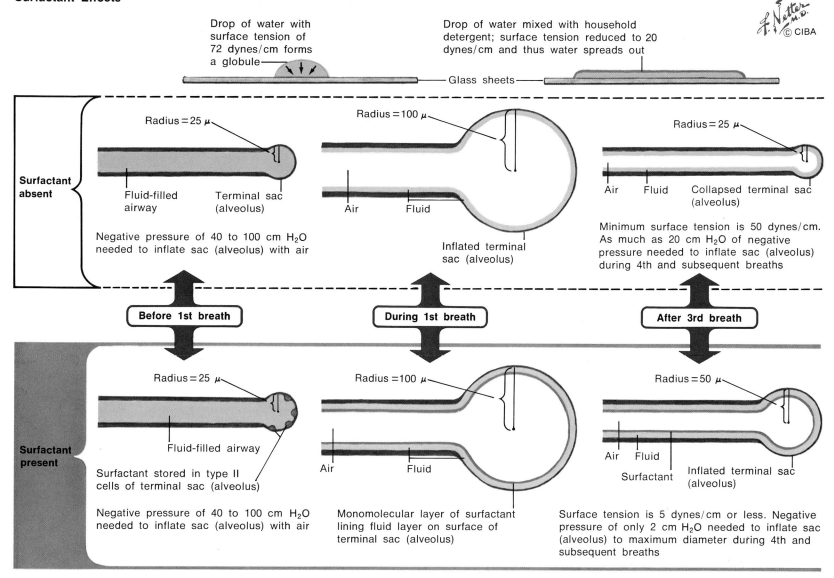

Drop of water with surface tension of 72 dynes/cm forms a globule

Drop of water mixed with household detergent; surface tension reduced to 20 dynes/cm and thus water spreads out

Glass sheets

Surfactant absent

Radius = 25 μ

Fluid-filled airway — Terminal sac (alveolus)

Negative pressure of 40 to 100 cm H₂O needed to inflate sac (alveolus) with air

Radius = 100 μ

Air — Fluid

Inflated terminal sac (alveolus)

Radius = 25 μ

Air Fluid Collapsed terminal sac (alveolus)

Minimum surface tension is 50 dynes/cm. As much as 20 cm H₂O of negative pressure needed to inflate sac (alveolus) during 4th and subsequent breaths

Before 1st breath   **During 1st breath**   **After 3rd breath**

Surfactant present

Radius = 25 μ

Fluid-filled airway

Surfactant stored in type II cells of terminal sac (alveolus)

Negative pressure of 40 to 100 cm H₂O needed to inflate sac (alveolus) with air

Radius = 100 μ

Air — Fluid

Monomolecular layer of surfactant lining fluid layer on surface of terminal sac (alveolus)

Radius = 50 μ

Air Fluid

Surfactant Inflated terminal sac (alveolus)

Surface tension is 5 dynes/cm or less. Negative pressure of only 2 cm H₂O needed to inflate sac (alveolus) to maximum diameter during 4th and subsequent breaths

Development of Lower Respiratory System
(Continued)

with the first good cry, but the accessory muscles of respiration offer little assistance at this time. Expansion of the chest wall is slight in the days just after birth. In fact, the thoracic skeleton contains so much flexible cartilage that the chest wall tends to collapse with each inspiration, especially in the premature infant.

When air expands the primitive alveolus during the first breath, surfactant (or its precursors stored in type II pneumocytes) is rapidly discharged into the alveolar space (Plate 41). This monomolecular layer prevents the development of an air-water interface that otherwise would have 7 to 14 times as much surface tension as does the air-surfactant interface.

According to the Laplace equation, the pressure required to prevent collapse of a bubble due to surface tension is inversely proportional to the bubble's radius. Since the radii of primitive alveoli are very small, the collapsing forces are correspondingly high. Therefore, as the lungs deflate,

the alveolar radii are further reduced and the collapsing forces are proportionately increased. Alveoli lacking surfactant thus cannot retain air after expiration, and collapse (Plate 41); infants in whom hyaline membrane disease develops have so little air in their nonexpanded alveoli that at autopsy the lungs immediately sink when placed in water. Surfactant has the fortunate property of increasing its activity as its surface area is reduced. Therefore, on expiration the surfactant effectively lowers the alveolar surface tension so that air can be retained.

Without sufficient surfactant, all breaths after the first would require great physical effort. A negative pressure as great as 20 cm of water is required to reinflate a collapsed primitive alveolus with a radius of 25 microns and a minimal surface tension of 50 dynes/cm. By contrast, with surfactant present the alveolus of a deflated lung would have a radius of 50 microns and its minimal surface tension would be only 5 dynes/cm or less. Thus, a negative pressure of only 2 cm of water is all that would be needed to maximally reinflate it under these conditions (Plate 41). The physical effort a premature infant lacking surfactant requires to breathe is so great that exhaustion of the infant will soon result unless mechanical support is provided.

Although the second breath is much easier for a normal full-term infant, breathing is usually not

completely normal until about 40 minutes after birth. The entire lung does not become fully inflated as soon as respiration begins, and for the first week to 10 days after birth small parts of the lungs may still remain underinflated.

The onset of breathing at birth is accompanied by important and immediate circulatory system readjustments that allow adequate blood flow through the lungs. During fetal life only about 12% of the cardiac output goes to the lungs because most of the flow from the right ventricle is shunted away from the pulmonary artery to the aorta through the large ductus arteriosus. The fluid-filled atelectatic lungs create a high resistance in the pulmonary circulation by compressing the blood vessels. Expansion of the lungs induces vasodilation of the pulmonary vessels and results in a sudden increase in blood flow — up to 200% or more. This increased pulmonary blood flow, coupled with the cutting off of the large placental circulation when the umbilical cord is tied, actually means that a smaller quantity of blood is propelled a shorter distance within the infant. Therefore, the most crucial event at birth is the expansion of the lungs with the first breath of air, rather than the alterations occurring in the vascular system. Once respiration is established, the normal vascular system is well prepared to meet the functional demands imposed on it after birth.

Section II

Physiology

Frank H. Netter, M.D.

in collaboration with

Murray D. Altose, M.D. *Plates 1-21*

Neil S. Cherniack, M.D. and Sukahamay Lahiri, Ph.D. *Plates 25-31*

Henry O. Heinemann, M.D. *Plates 22-24*

List of Abbreviations and Symbols

V_T	tidal volume		P_{CO_2}	partial pressure of carbon dioxide
FRC	functional residual capacity		P_{N_2}	partial pressure of nitrogen
ERV	expiratory reserve volume		Pa_{O_2}	partial pressure of oxygen in arterial blood
RV	residual volume		Pa_{CO_2}	partial pressure of carbon dioxide in arterial blood
IC	inspiratory capacity			
IRV	inspiratory reserve volume		PA_{O_2}	partial pressure of oxygen in alveolar gas
TLC	total lung capacity		PA_{CO_2}	partial pressure of carbon dioxide in alveolar gas
VC	vital capacity			
Raw	resistance of tracheobronchial tree to flow of air into the lung		PA_{H_2O}	partial pressure of water in alveolar gas
P_L	recoil pressure of lung		$P\bar{A}_{O_2}$	mean partial pressure of oxygen in alveolar gas
P_W	recoil pressure of the chest wall			
P_{RS}	recoil pressure of the total respiratory system		$P\bar{A}_{CO_2}$	mean partial pressure of carbon dioxide in alveolar gas
P_B	atmospheric pressure		$P\bar{A}_{CO}$	mean partial pressure of carbon monoxide in alveolar gas
Pbs	pressure at the external surface of the chest		$P\bar{E}_{CO_2}$	mean partial pressure of carbon dioxide in mixed expired air
Palv	alveolar pressure			
Ppl	pleural pressure		$P\bar{c}_{O_2}$	mean partial pressure of oxygen in capillary blood
Pao	pressure at the airway opening			
Re	Reynolds number		$\dot{V}_I$	inspired volume of ventilation per minute
ρ	density of gas		$\dot{V}_E$	expired volume of ventilation per minute
μ	viscosity of gas		FI_{O_2}	fraction of oxygen in inspired air
$\dot{V}$	gas volume per minute		FI_{N_2}	fraction of nitrogen in inspired air
$\dot{V}_{max}$	maximal rate of airflow during forced expiration		FE_{O_2}	fraction of oxygen in expired air
			FE_{CO_2}	fraction of carbon dioxide in expired air
$\dot{V}_{max.\ 50}$	rate of airflow at 50% of VC		FE_{N_2}	fraction of nitrogen in expired air
Rus	resistance of the upstream segment of tracheobronchial tree		RQ	respiratory quotient
			$\dot{V}_{CO_2}$	amount of carbon dioxide eliminated per minute
FEV_1	forced expiratory volume in 1 second			
FEV_3	forced expiratory volume in the first 3 seconds		V_D	volume of dead space gas
			V_A	volume of alveolar gas
$FEF_{25-75\%}$	forced midexpiratory flow (between 25 and 75% of the FVC)		R	respiratory exchange ratio
			$\dot{V}_A/\dot{Q}_C$	ratio of alveolar ventilation to pulmonary capillary blood flow
V iso $\dot{V}$	volume of isoflow			
MVV	maximal voluntary ventilation		$\dot{Q}_S$	shunt flow
Vc	volume of blood in pulmonary capillary bed		$\dot{Q}_t$	total cardiac output
			Cc_{O_2}	concentration of oxygen in end-capillary blood
θ	amount of oxygen taken up by 1 ml of blood/mm Hg pressure gradient		Ca_{O_2}	concentration of oxygen in arterial blood
			$C\bar{v}_{O_2}$	concentration of oxygen in mixed venous blood
$D_{L_{O_2}}$	diffusing capacity of the lung for oxygen			
$D_{L_{CO}}$	diffusing capacity of the lung for carbon monoxide		S_{O_2}	percentage saturation of hemoglobin with oxygen
$\dot{V}_{O_2}$	rate of oxygen uptake per minute		Sa_{O_2}	percentage saturation of hemoglobin with oxygen in arterial blood
$\dot{V}_{CO}$	rate of carbon monoxide uptake per minute		$S\bar{v}_{O_2}$	percentage saturation of hemoglobin with oxygen in mixed venous blood
P_{O_2}	partial pressure of oxygen			

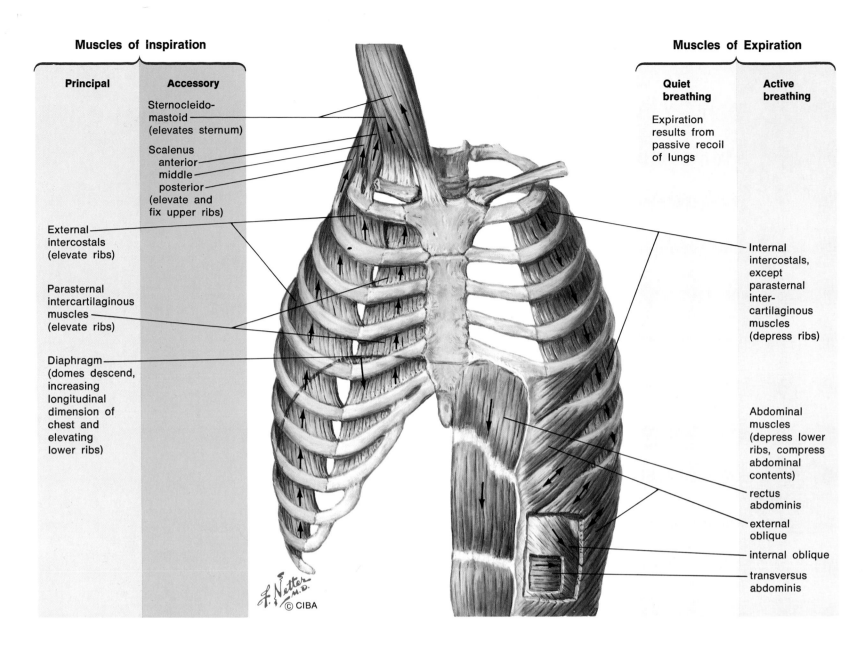

Muscles of Inspiration

Principal	Accessory

Sternocleidomastoid (elevates sternum)

Scalenus
anterior
middle
posterior
(elevate and
fix upper ribs)

External intercostals (elevate ribs)

Parasternal intercartilaginous muscles (elevate ribs)

Diaphragm (domes descend, increasing longitudinal dimension of chest and elevating lower ribs)

Muscles of Expiration

Quiet breathing	Active breathing

Expiration results from passive recoil of lungs

Internal intercostals, except parasternal intercartilaginous muscles (depress ribs)

Abdominal muscles (depress lower ribs, compress abdominal contents)

rectus abdominis

external oblique

internal oblique

transversus abdominis

Pulmonary Mechanics and Gas Exchange

The major responsibility of the lung is to add oxygen to and remove carbon dioxide from the blood passing through the pulmonary capillary bed. This function is achieved through a series of complex processes. Contraction of the inspiratory muscles provides the force to overcome the resistance of the lung and chest wall, and results in passage of air along the tracheobronchial tree into the alveoli of the lung. There, alveolar air and pulmonary capillary blood, although separated by the ultrathin alveolar-capillary membrane, come into intimate contact. Oxygen diffuses across the alveolar-capillary membrane into the blood while carbon dioxide passes in the opposite direction, and the adequacy of gas exchange can be determined from the tensions of oxygen and carbon dioxide in the blood leaving the lungs.

Assessment of the mechanical properties of the lung and chest wall and evaluation of the efficiency of gas exchange in the lungs may prove useful in a number of ways. Abnormalities can be revealed early when the impairment may still be reversible. Pulmonary function testing is also helpful in elucidating the basis for breathlessness, a common pulmonary symptom, and is important in characterizing the pathophysiology and providing a measure of the severity of various pulmonary diseases. The range of pulmonary function tests, their accepted symbols, techniques of performance and interpretation are summarized on pages 267 and 268.

Respiratory Muscles

The chest expands and the lungs are filled with air by the contraction of the inspiratory muscles (Plate 1). The diaphragm is the principal muscle of inspiration and provides for the movement of more than two-thirds of the air that enters the lungs during quiet breathing. Contraction of the diaphragm causes its domes to descend and the chest to expand longitudinally. At the same time, because of the vertically oriented attachments of the diaphragm to the costal margins, its contractions also elevate the lower ribs.

Contraction of the intercostal muscles (external intercostals and parasternal intercartilaginous muscles) also raises the ribs during inspiration. As the ribs are elevated, the anteroposterior and transverse dimensions of the chest enlarge because of the pattern of movement of the ribs around the axis of their necks. Upward displacement of the upper ribs is accompanied by an increase in the anteroposterior dimension, while elevation of the lower ribs is associated with an increase in the transverse dimension of the chest.

In addition to the diaphragm and intercostal muscles, other accessory inspiratory muscles may contribute to the movement of the chest. The scalene muscles make their major contribution during high levels of ventilation when the upper parts of the chest must be enlarged. These muscles arise from the transverse processes of the lower five cervical vertebrae and insert into the upper aspect of the first and second ribs. Contraction of these muscles elevates and fixes the uppermost part of the rib cage.

Another accessory muscle, the sternomastoid (sternocleidomastoid), normally becomes active only at high levels of ventilation. Contraction of the sternomastoid muscle is frequently apparent during severe asthma and with other disorders that obstruct the movement of air into the lungs. The sternomastoid muscle elevates the sternum and slightly enlarges the anteroposterior and longitudinal dimensions of the chest.

In contrast to inspiration, expiration during quiet breathing occurs passively as a result of recoil of the lung. However, expiration does become active at higher levels of ventilation and

(Continued)

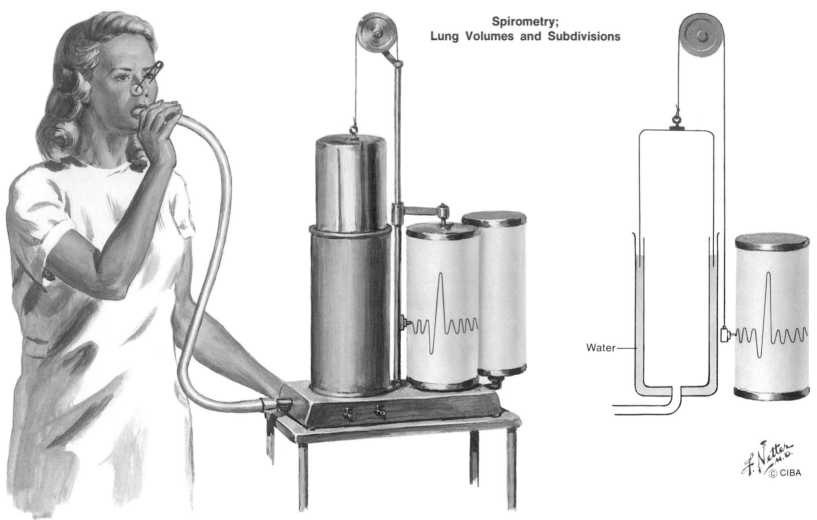

Water

© CIBA

SECTION II PLATE 2

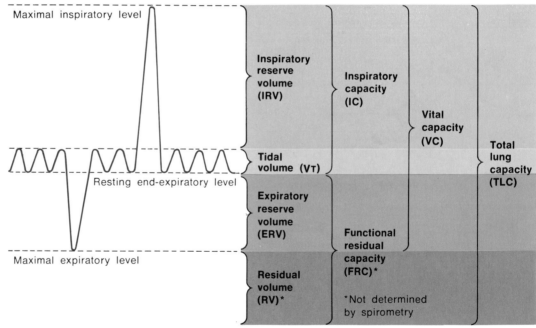

Maximal inspiratory level

Inspiratory reserve volume (IRV)

Inspiratory capacity (IC)

Vital capacity (VC)

Tidal volume (VT)

Resting end-expiratory level

Total lung capacity (TLC)

Expiratory reserve volume (ERV)

Functional residual capacity (FRC)*

Maximal expiratory level

Residual volume (RV)*

*Not determined by spirometry

Pulmonary Mechanics and Gas Exchange
(Continued)

when movement of air out of the lungs is impeded. Muscles involved in active expiration include the internal intercostal muscles which depress the ribs, the external and internal oblique abdominal muscles, and the transversus and rectus abdominis muscles which compress the abdominal contents, depress the lower ribs and pull down the anterior part of the lower chest. These expiratory muscles also play important roles in regulating breathing during talking, singing, coughing, defecation and parturition.

The strength of the respiratory muscles can be determined from maximal static respiratory pressures—i.e., maximal pressure generated during a forced inspiratory or expiratory maneuver against a manometer or pressure gauge. Pressure developed during an isometric contraction of the respiratory muscles depends on the length of those muscles and is therefore related to the lung volume at which the maneuver is performed. Maxi-

mal static inspiratory pressure is measured when the inspiratory muscles are optimally lengthened following a complete expiration to residual volume. Similarly, maximal static expiratory pressure is determined after a full inspiration to total lung capacity, when the expiratory muscles are in their most mechanically advantageous position.

Measurement of maximal static respiratory pressures is clinically useful in the evaluation of patients with neuromuscular disorders, since respiratory muscle weakness, when severe, can reduce the ventilatory capacity and can result in breathlessness, even when lung function is otherwise normal.

Lung Volumes and Subdivisions

Tidal volume (VT) is the volume of air that enters the lungs during inspiration and leaves the lungs during expiration in normal breathing.

The volume of air in the lungs at the end of expiration during normal breathing is referred to as the *functional residual capacity* (FRC). This volume is maintained by the opposing recoil forces of the lung and chest wall while the respiratory muscles are at rest.

FRC is composed of two volumes: *expiratory reserve volume* (ERV) is the maximal additional
(Continued)

Determination of Functional Residual Capacity (FRC)

Closed-Circuit Helium Dilution Method

A. Start of determination

B. After rebreathing

Body Plethysmograph Method

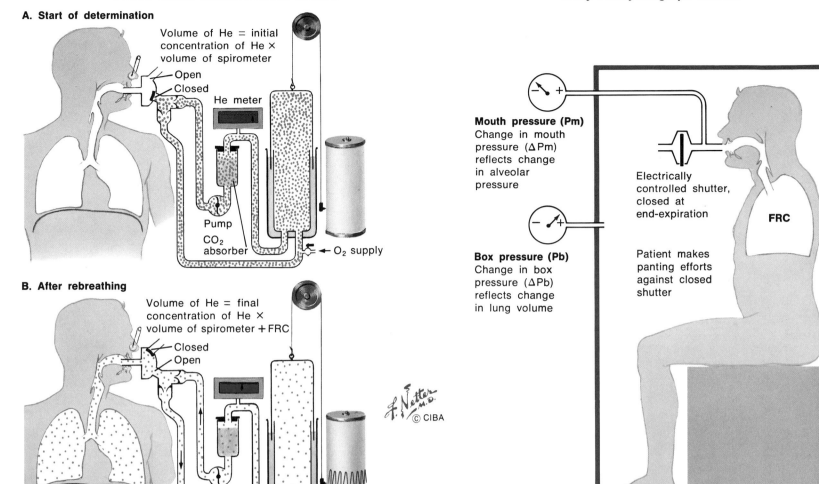

Volume of He = initial concentration of He × volume of spirometer

Open
Closed
He meter

Pump
CO_2 absorber
← O_2 supply

Volume of He = final concentration of He × volume of spirometer + FRC

Closed
Open

Mouth pressure (Pm) Change in mouth pressure (ΔPm) reflects change in alveolar pressure

Electrically controlled shutter, closed at end-expiration

FRC

Box pressure (Pb) Change in box pressure (ΔPb) reflects change in lung volume

Patient makes panting efforts against closed shutter

$$\text{Volume of gas in thorax} = \text{atmospheric pressure} \times \frac{\Delta Pb}{\Delta Pm}$$

Pulmonary Mechanics and Gas Exchange
(Continued)

volume of air that can be exhaled following a normal expiration to FRC, and *residual volume* (RV) is the volume of air remaining in the lungs at the end of a maximal exhalation.

Inspiratory capacity (IC) is the maximal volume of air that can be inhaled from FRC and is made up of two subdivisions: VT and *inspiratory reserve volume* (IRV).

Total lung capacity (TLC) is the volume of air in the lungs following a maximal inspiration, and *vital capacity* (VC) is the maximal volume of air that can be exhaled from the lungs following a maximal inspiration.

Subdivisions of lung volume can be determined by means of a spirometer (Plate 2), a simple gas volume recorder. The commonly used water-filled spirometer consists of a double-walled drum into which a bell is fitted. The bell is attached by a pulley to a pen that writes on a second rotating drum. As air enters the spirometer, the drum rises and, because of the pulley, the pen is lowered.

In order to determine lung volumes and capacities, the patient is seated and breathes quietly

from the spirometer. After several breaths to establish the resting end-expiratory level, a maximal inspiration is taken followed by a slow complete expiration.

By convention, all lung volumes are expressed in terms of body temperature, ambient pressure and saturation with water vapor (BTPS). Since gas volumes measured in a spirometer are at ambient temperature (ATPS) rather than body temperature, appropriate corrections must be made.

RV consists of the air remaining in the lung following a maximal expiration, and consequently this volume cannot be determined directly by spirometry. In practice, FRC is measured by indirect means and RV is ascertained by subtracting ERV from FRC. Three techniques are available to determine FRC (Plate 3): closed-circuit helium dilution, open-circuit nitrogen washout and body plethysmography.

The *closed-circuit helium dilution* method involves dilution of helium, an inert, insoluble gas, as it mixes with the air in the lungs. A spirometer is filled with a mixture of 10% helium in air. Starting precisely at the end-expiratory position, the patient begins to breathe from the closed spirometer system. The carbon dioxide is absorbed by soda lime, and the oxygen consumed is replaced by adding oxygen to the spirometer. As the helium in the spirometer mixes with the air in the lung, the concentration of helium in the circuit falls to a new level. Since helium does not cross the

alveolar-capillary membrane, the volume of helium in the system does not change during the test period. Consequently, the initial concentration of helium ($He_{initial}$) multiplied by the volume of gas in the spirometer at the start of the test ($V_{spirometer}$) equals the final concentration of helium (He_{final}) multiplied by the volume of gas in the spirometer at the end of the test plus the volume of air in the lung: *i.e.*, FRC. The equation can be written as follows:

$$He_{initial} \times V_{spirometer} = He_{final} \times (V_{spirometer} + FRC)$$

Solving for FRC, the equation becomes

$$FRC = \frac{V_{spirometer} \times (He_{initial} - He_{final})}{He_{final}}$$

In the *open-circuit nitrogen washout* technique, nitrogen is completely displaced from the lungs during a period of 100% oxygen-breathing. All expired air is collected, and the volume and nitrogen concentration of the sample are measured. Since the total volume of nitrogen in the expired air equals the volume of nitrogen in the lung before the start of the test, the volume of expired air multiplied by the nitrogen concentration of the expired air equals the volume of air in the lung (FRC) multiplied by the initial concentration of nitrogen in the lung.

The volume of gas in the thorax can also be measured by means of a *body plethysmograph*, a
(Continued)

Pulmonary Mechanics and Gas Exchange
(Continued)

closed chamber within which the patient is seated. In a constant-volume, variable-pressure plethysmograph, the patient breathes in and out gently against a closed shutter. During an inspiratory effort against the closed shutter following a normal expiration, the pressure in the airways and alveoli falls below atmospheric levels, and the gas in the lung undergoes decompression. Because the plethysmograph is sealed, the resulting increase in lung volume is reflected by an increase in the pressure within the plethysmograph. An obstructed expiratory effort produces the opposite effect.

Thoracic gas volume is determined by applying Boyle's law, which states that, for a gas at a constant temperature, the product of pressure and volume is constant. Boyle's law can also be expressed as follows:

$$P \times V = (P + \Delta P) \times (V + \Delta V)$$

where P = initial pressure; V = initial volume; ΔP is a change in pressure; and ΔV, a corresponding change in volume. This expression can be simplified, solving for V:

$$V = (P + \Delta P) \times \frac{\Delta V}{\Delta P}$$

With respect to the respiratory system, V represents the initial volume of gas in the thorax, *i.e.*, FRC; P represents the pressure in the alveoli at the end of a normal expiration, *i.e.*, atmospheric pressure; ΔP represents the change in alveolar pressure during breathing efforts against a closed shutter; and ΔV represents the change in thoracic gas volume resulting from gas expansion or compression during obstructed breathing. Changes in alveolar pressure are determined from changes in mouth pressure (ΔPm), and changes in the volume of thoracic gas are reflected by changes in the pressure within the plethysmograph (ΔPb). Since changes in alveolar pressure during the gentle breathing maneuver against a closed shutter are extremely small as compared to atmospheric pressure, FRC can be calculated from the following further simplified equation:

$$FRC = \text{atmospheric pressure} \times \frac{\Delta Pb}{\Delta Pm}$$

Mechanics of Ventilatory Apparatus

The ventilatory apparatus consists of the lungs and surrounding chest wall. The chest wall includes not only the rib cage but also the diaphragm and abdominal wall. The lungs fill the
(Continued)

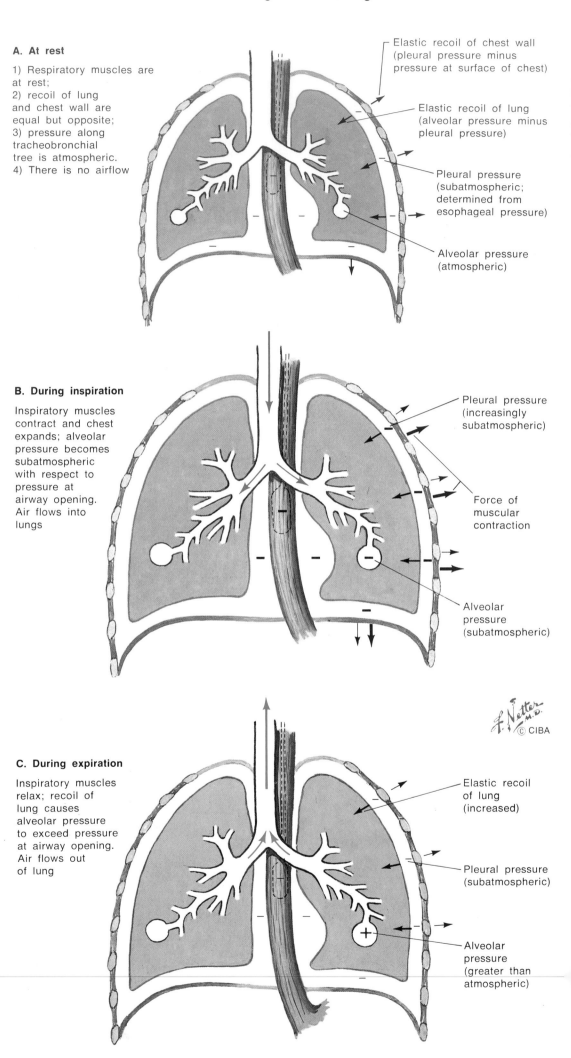

A. At rest

1) Respiratory muscles are at rest;
2) recoil of lung and chest wall are equal but opposite;
3) pressure along tracheobronchial tree is atmospheric.
4) There is no airflow

- Elastic recoil of chest wall (pleural pressure minus pressure at surface of chest)
- Elastic recoil of lung (alveolar pressure minus pleural pressure)
- Pleural pressure (subatmospheric; determined from esophageal pressure)
- Alveolar pressure (atmospheric)

B. During inspiration

Inspiratory muscles contract and chest expands; alveolar pressure becomes subatmospheric with respect to pressure at airway opening. Air flows into lungs

- Pleural pressure (increasingly subatmospheric)
- Force of muscular contraction
- Alveolar pressure (subatmospheric)

C. During expiration

Inspiratory muscles relax; recoil of lung causes alveolar pressure to exceed pressure at airway opening. Air flows out of lung

- Elastic recoil of lung (increased)
- Pleural pressure (subatmospheric)
- Alveolar pressure (greater than atmospheric)

Measurement of Elastic Properties of Lung

Pulmonary Mechanics and Gas Exchange
(Continued)

chest so that the visceral pleura is in contact with the parietal pleura of the chest cage. Consequently, the lungs and chest wall act in unison, and from a mechanical point of view may be regarded as a pump that can be characterized by its elastic, flow-resistive and inertial properties (Plates 4 and 5).

At the end of a normal expiration the respiratory muscles are at rest. The elastic recoil of the lung, directed centripetally, is balanced by the elastic recoil of the chest, directed centrifugally, and these opposing forces generate a subatmospheric pressure of approximately 5 cm H_2O in the potential space between the visceral and parietal pleurae. Provided there is no movement of air into or out of the lungs, the pressure along the entire airway from the mouth to the alveoli is at atmospheric level. The difference between alveolar and pleural pressure, the pressure difference across the lung, is the transpulmonary pressure.

As the inspiratory muscles contract during inspiration and the chest expands, the pleural pressure becomes increasingly subatmospheric. Because of the resistance offered by the tracheobronchial tree to the flow of air into the lung (Raw), the alveolar pressure also becomes subatmospheric. At a given rate of airflow, the difference between alveolar pressure and the pressure at the airway opening, which remains at atmospheric level, is a measure of the flow-resistance of the airways:

$$\text{Airway resistance} = \frac{\text{alveolar pressure} - \text{airway opening pressure}}{\text{rate of airflow}}$$

Movement of air into the lungs continues until the alveolar pressure again reaches atmospheric level, so that the pressure difference between the alveoli and the airway opening no longer exists.

At the end of inspiration, the volume of air in the lungs is greater and the pleural pressure is more subatmospheric than at the end of the preceding expiration. Since alveolar pressure has returned to atmospheric level, the difference between alveolar and pleural pressure—the transpulmonary pressure—is increased. The change in transpulmonary pressure required to effect a given change in the volume of air in the lungs is a measure of the elastic resistance of the lungs:

$$\text{Lung elastic resistance} = \frac{\text{change in transpulmonary pressure}}{\text{change in lung volume}}$$

The forces required to overcome elastic resistance are stored during inspiration; expiration

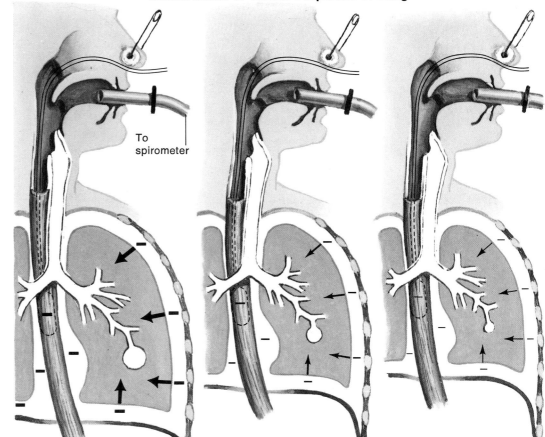

During a slow expiration from TLC, flow is periodically interrupted and measurements are made of lung volume and of transpulmonary pressure. Transpulmonary pressure is difference between alveolar and pleural pressures. Pleural pressure is determined from pressure in esophagus. Since there is no airflow, alveolar pressure is same as pressure at airway opening

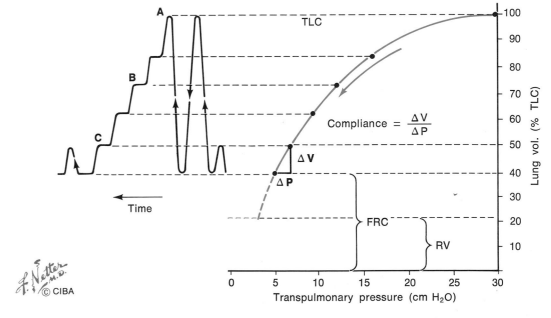

occurs when these forces are released. The recoil of the lung causes the alveolar pressure to exceed the pressure at the mouth, and consequently air flows out of the lung.

Elastic Properties of the Lung. The compliance or distensibility of the lungs is determined from the relationship between changes in lung volume and changes in transpulmonary pressure. The elastic properties of the lungs (Plate 5) are determined when airflow is stopped. Under these conditions, alveolar pressure equals the pressure at the mouth; pleural pressure is determined indirectly from the pressure in the esophagus by means of a balloon catheter. In practice, during a

slow exhalation following a full inspiration to total lung capacity, airflow is interrupted and measurements are made of lung volume and transpulmonary pressure.

Pressure-volume characteristics of the lung are nonlinear. Thus, compliance of the lung is least at high volumes and greatest as residual volume is approached. Forces favoring further collapse of the lung can be demonstrated throughout the range of vital capacity, even at low lung volumes. If the opposing forces of the chest wall on the lung are eliminated by removing the lung from the thorax or by opening the chest, the lung will
(Continued)

Pulmonary Mechanics and Gas Exchange
(*Continued*)

collapse to a virtually airless state to reach its equilibrium position.

Lung tissue elasticity arises from the fibers of elastin and collagen that are present in the alveolar walls and surround the bronchioles and pulmonary capillaries. The elastin fibers can approximately double their resting length and are probably the chief determinant of lung tissue elasticity. In contrast, the collagen fibers are poorly extensible and act primarily to limit expansion at high lung volumes. Lung expansion probably occurs through an unfolding and geometric rearrangement of the fibers analogous to the way a nylon stocking is easily stretched even though the individual fibers are elongated very little.

The distensibility of the lungs increases with advancing age as a result of alterations in the elastin and collagen fibers in the lung. Pulmonary emphysema, which destroys alveolar walls and enlarges alveolar spaces, similarly increases lung compliance. In contrast, compliance of the lung is reduced by disorders such as pulmonary fibrosis, which affect the interstitial tissues of the lung, and by diffuse alveolar consolidation and edema, which also interfere with expansion of the lung.

Surface Tension (Plate 6). Particularly at small lung volumes, the elastic behavior of the lung depends on the surface tension of the film lining the alveoli. The attractive forces between

molecules of the liquid film are stronger than those between the film and the gas in the alveoli. Consequently, the area of the surface film shrinks. The behavior of the surface film has been examined in experimental animals by comparing pressure-volume relationships of air-filled lungs with those of saline-filled lungs. Since saline eliminates the liquid-air interface without affecting tissue elasticity, lungs distended with liquid require a lower transpulmonary pressure to maintain a given lung volume than do lungs inflated with air.

This observation is explained by Laplace's law, which states that the pressure inside a spherical structure such as an alveolus is directly proportional to the tension in the wall and inversely proportional to the radius of curvature. When the liquid-air interface and surface tension forces are abolished by instillation of saline into the alveolar spaces, the pressure required to maintain a given lung volume is reduced. Thus, surface forces make a major contribution to the retractive forces of the lung.

The surface tension of the film lining the alveolar walls depends on lung volume: surface tension is high when the lungs are inflated and low at small lung volumes. These variations in surface tension with changes in lung volume require that the surface film contain a special type of surface-active material. The surface-active material lining the alveoli, *surfactant,* is considered a product of the type II granular pneumocyte and has dipalmitoyl lecithin as an important constituent. Surfactant serves a number of important functions. Its low surface tension, particularly at low lung volumes, increases the compliance of the lung and facilitates expansion during the subsequent breath. Furthermore, the stability of alveoli at low lung volumes is maintained. If the surface tension remained constant instead of changing with lung volume, a greater pressure would be required to keep an alveolus open as its radius of curvature diminished with decreasing lung volume. Small alveoli would consequently empty into communicating larger ones, and atelectasis would regularly occur.

Elastic Properties of the Chest Wall and Total Respiratory System (Plate 7). The elastic recoil of the chest wall is such that, if the chest were unopposed by the lungs, it would enlarge to approximately 70% of the total lung capacity. This represents the equilibrium or resting position of the chest wall, where the pressure across the chest wall (the difference between pleural pressure and the pressure at the surface of the chest when the respiratory muscles are completely at rest) is zero. If the volume of gas in the lungs is increased to further expand the thorax, the chest wall, like the lung, will recoil inward, resisting expansion and favoring a return to the equilibrium position. Conversely, at volumes less than 70% of total lung capacity, the recoil of the chest is opposite to that of the lung and is directly outward.

Elastic recoil properties of the chest wall, which play an important role in determining the subdivisions of lung volume, may be rendered abnormal by disorders such as marked obesity, kyphoscoliosis and ankylosing spondylitis.

The lung and chest wall are considered to be in series with each other, so that the algebraic sum of the pressures exerted by the recoil of the lung (P_L) and the recoil of the chest wall (P_W) makes up the

recoil pressure of the total respiratory system (P_{RS}):

$$P_{RS} = P_L + P_W$$

The recoil of the lung is determined from the difference between alveolar pressure ($Palv$) and pleural pressure (Ppl). The recoil of the chest wall when the respiratory muscles are at rest is determined from the difference between pleural pressure (Ppl) and the pressure at the external surface of the chest (Pbs). Thus, the recoil of the entire respiratory system can be expressed as follows:

$$P_{RS} = (Palv - Ppl) + (Ppl - Pbs)$$

When the respiratory muscles are completely at rest and the pressure at the surface of the chest is at atmospheric levels,

$$P_{RS} = Palv$$

The elastic properties of the total respiratory system can be evaluated in a number of ways. Each method requires that a given lung volume be maintained during complete relaxation of all the respiratory muscles. This function is generally accomplished by application of external forces such as positive pressure to the airways or negative pressure around the chest, or through voluntary relaxation of the respiratory muscles while the airway opening is occluded. Since there is no airflow, the alveolar pressure is the same as the pressure at the mouth.

Functional residual capacity represents the equilibrium or resting position of the lung–chest wall system where the recoil pressure is zero. At any volume above functional residual capacity, the recoil pressure exceeds atmospheric levels, favoring a decrease in lung volume; at volumes below functional residual capacity, the recoil pressure is less than atmospheric pressure and the respiratory system tends to retract outward in an attempt to increase lung volume.

Flow-Resistive Properties of the Lung. Total pulmonary nonelastic resistance is made up of the flow-resistance of the airways (*airway resistance*) and the frictional resistance to the displacement of lung tissue during breathing (*tissue resistance*) (Plates 8 and 9). Tissue resistance normally comprises only 10 to 20% of the total pulmonary nonelastic resistance, but may increase significantly in certain lung diseases affecting parenchymal tissues.

A large proportion of the resistance to airflow is offered by the upper respiratory tract. Resistance to airflow through the nasal passages is so high that during nose breathing nasal resistance may comprise 50% of the total airway resistance. The mouth, pharynx, larynx and trachea account for 20 to 30% of airway resistance during quiet mouth breathing, but as much as 50% of total airway resistance when minute ventilation is increased. The major sites of the remaining airway resistance are in the medium-sized lobar, segmental and subsegmental bronchi, up to about the seventh generation of airways. With additional branching distally, the number of airways in any generation as well as the total cross-sectional area of the tracheobronchial tree increase progressively. Consequently, the small peripheral airways, particularly those less than 2 mm in diameter, contribute only about 10 to 20% to the total airway resistance of the normal lung.

(Continued)

Surface Forces in Lung

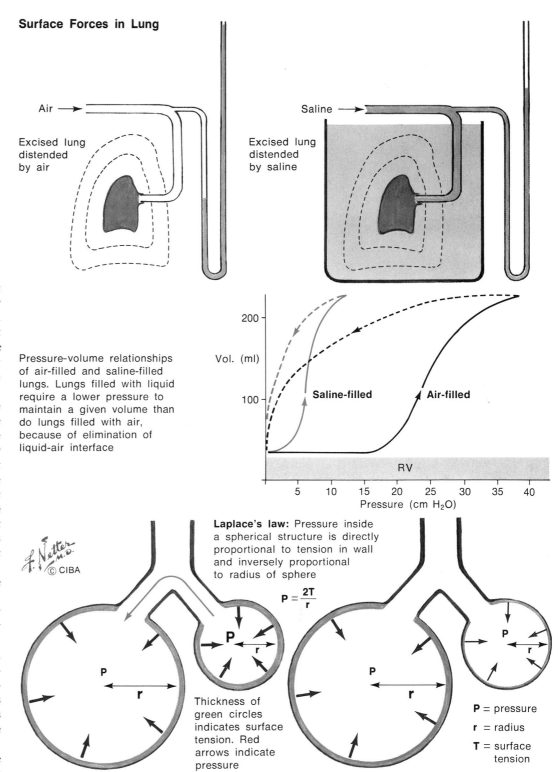

Pressure-volume relationships of air-filled and saline-filled lungs. Lungs filled with liquid require a lower pressure to maintain a given volume than do lungs filled with air, because of elimination of liquid-air interface

Laplace's law: Pressure inside a spherical structure is directly proportional to tension in wall and inversely proportional to radius of sphere

$$P = \frac{2T}{r}$$

Thickness of green circles indicates surface tension. Red arrows indicate pressure

P = pressure
r = radius
T = surface tension

Without surfactant. Surface tension in both alveoli is the same. A greater pressure is required to keep small alveolus open. Small alveolus tends to empty into larger one

With surfactant. Surface tension reduced in small alveolus. Pressure distending both alveoli is approximately the same. Alveoli are stabilized, and tendency for small alveolus to empty into larger one is reduced

Pulmonary Mechanics and Gas Exchange
(Continued)

The airways, like the lung parenchyma, exhibit elasticity and are capable of being compressed or distended. Thus the diameter of any airway will vary with the transmural pressure applied to that airway—*i.e.,* the difference between the pressure within the airway and the pressure surrounding the airway. The pressure surrounding the intrathoracic airways approximates pleural pressure, since these airways are in a sense tethered to the parenchymal tissue and exposed to the expansive forces required to overcome the elastic recoil of the lung. Airway caliber depends on the volume of air in the lung. As lung volume enlarges, elastic recoil forces of the lung will increase, and the traction applied to the walls of the intrathoracic airways will become greater. The airways therefore widen, and airway resistance falls. Conversely, at low lung volumes, transmural airway pressure is lower, and airway resistance increases. If elastic recoil of the lung is reduced—for example, through destruction of alveolar walls (the pathologic process in pulmonary emphysema)— at any given lung volume the transmural airway pressure is less, airways are narrower, and airway resistance is greater.

Effects of a change in transmural pressure on airway caliber depend on compliance of the airway; this, in turn, depends on the structural support of that airway. The trachea, for instance, is almost completely surrounded by cartilaginous rings which tend to prevent complete collapse even when the transmural pressure is negative. The bronchi are less well supported by incomplete cartilaginous rings and plates, while bronchioles have no cartilaginous support but can be made stiffer by contraction of the smooth muscle in their walls.

Airway caliber may also be compromised and airway resistance increased in patients with lung disease because of mucosal edema, hypertrophy and hyperplasia of mucous glands; increased elaboration of mucus; and hypertrophy of bronchial smooth muscle.

The driving pressure producing airflow along the tracheobronchial tree is the difference between alveolar pressure (Palv) and the pressure at the airway opening (Pao). Airway resistance (Raw) is defined as the ratio of driving pressure and the rate of airflow ($\dot{V}$) according to the equation:

$$Raw = \frac{Palv - Pao}{\dot{V}}$$

Airway resistance is readily determined by a body plethysmograph. The patient, seated in the plethysmograph chamber, pants at a frequency of two to three breaths per second, and airflow is measured with a pneumotachograph. While these efforts are continuing, a shutter at the airway opening is closed, and alveolar pressure is ascertained from the change in mouth pressure using the technique employed in determination of functional residual capacity (Plate 3).

Since airway resistance varies inversely with the volume of air in the lungs, it is important to take lung volume into account when assessing the significance of the measurement of airway resistance. To do so, one calculates *specific conductance* (SGaw), the inverse of airway resistance divided by the lung volume at which the measurement was made.

Pressure-Flow Relationships. The relationship between driving pressure and the resulting rate of airflow along the tracheobronchial tree is extremely complicated because the airways comprise a system of irregular branching tubes which are neither rigid nor perfectly circular. For purposes of simplification, the pressure-flow relationship in rigid tubes may be considered a model for those in the lung.

The driving pressure required to overcome friction depends on the rate and the pattern of airflow.

(Continued)

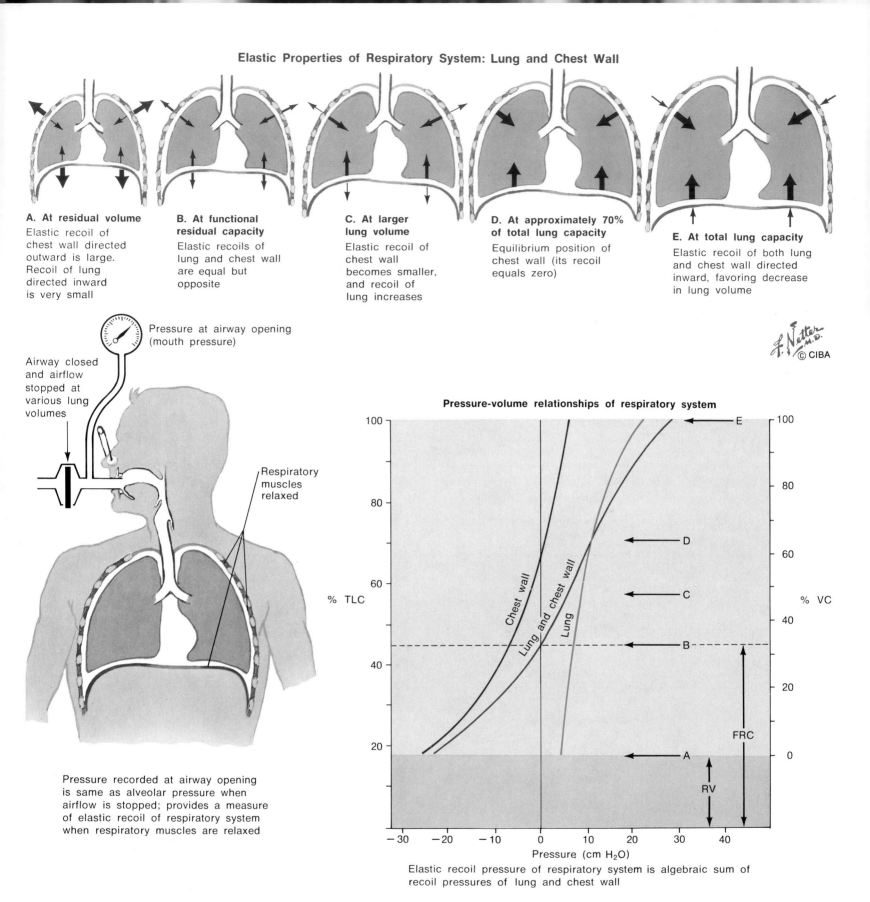

Elastic Properties of Respiratory System: Lung and Chest Wall

A. At residual volume
Elastic recoil of chest wall directed outward is large. Recoil of lung directed inward is very small

B. At functional residual capacity
Elastic recoils of lung and chest wall are equal but opposite

C. At larger lung volume
Elastic recoil of chest wall becomes smaller, and recoil of lung increases

D. At approximately 70% of total lung capacity
Equilibrium position of chest wall (its recoil equals zero)

E. At total lung capacity
Elastic recoil of both lung and chest wall directed inward, favoring decrease in lung volume

Pressure at airway opening (mouth pressure)

Airway closed and airflow stopped at various lung volumes

Respiratory muscles relaxed

Pressure recorded at airway opening is same as alveolar pressure when airflow is stopped; provides a measure of elastic recoil of respiratory system when respiratory muscles are relaxed

Pressure-volume relationships of respiratory system

Elastic recoil pressure of respiratory system is algebraic sum of recoil pressures of lung and chest wall

Pulmonary Mechanics and Gas Exchange
(Continued)

There are two major patterns of airflow (Plate 9). *Laminar flow* is characterized by streamlines that are parallel to the sides of the tube and capable of sliding over one another. The streamlines at the center of the tube move faster than those closest to the walls, so that the flow profile is parabolic. The pressure-flow characteristics of laminar flow depend on the length (l) and radius (r) of the tube and the viscosity of the gas (μ) according to the equation of Poiseuille

$$\frac{P}{\dot{V}} = \frac{8\mu\, l}{\pi\, r^4}$$

where P is the driving pressure and $\dot{V}$ is the flow rate. The critical importance of the tube radius in determining the driving pressure for a given flow is apparent from the equation. If the radius of the tube is halved, the pressure required to maintain a given flow rate must be increased 16-fold.

Turbulent flow occurs at high flow rates and is characterized by a complete disorganization of streamlines. The molecules of gas may then move laterally, collide with one another, and change their velocities. Under these circumstances pressure-flow relationships change. The rate of airflow is no longer directly proportional to the driving pressure as during laminar flow; rather,

(Continued)

Pulmonary Mechanics and Gas Exchange
(Continued)

the driving pressure to produce a given rate of airflow is proportional to the square of flow. Also, the driving pressure is dependent on gas density but is little affected by the viscosity of the gas.

At lower flow rates during expiration, particularly at branches in the tracheobronchial tree where flow in two separate tubes comes together into a single channel, the parabolic profile of laminar flow may become blunted, the streamlines may separate from the walls of the tube, and minor eddy formation may develop. This is referred to as a mixed or *transitional flow* pattern. With a mixed flow pattern the driving pressure to produce a given flow is dependent on both the viscosity and the density of the gas.

Whether the pattern of flow is laminar or turbulent is determined from the Reynolds number (Re), a dimensionless number which depends upon the rate of airflow ($\dot{V}$), the density of the gas (ρ), the viscosity of the gas (μ), and the radius of the tube (r), according to the equation:

$$\text{Re} = \frac{2\,\dot{V}\,\rho}{\pi\,\text{r}\,\mu}$$

In straight, smooth, rigid tubes, turbulence results when the Reynolds number exceeds 2000. It is apparent that turbulence is most likely to occur when the rate of airflow and the gas density are high, the viscosity is low, and the tube radius is small.

In a normal lung, laminar flow patterns occur only in the very small peripheral airways where the flow through any given airway is extremely slow. In the remainder of the tracheobronchial tree, flow is transitional, and in the trachea turbulence regularly occurs.

Flow-Volume Relationships. An assessment of the flow-resistive properties of the airways is obtained from the flow-volume curve, which illustrates the relationship between airflow and lung volume during a maximal expiratory maneuver (Plate 10). An individual inhales maximally to total lung capacity and then exhales to residual volume as forcefully, rapidly and completely as possible. During the forced expiration, the rate of airflow rises quickly to a maximal value at a lung volume close to total lung capacity. As the lung volume decreases, intrathoracic airways narrow, airway resistance increases and rate of airflow progressively falls.

A family of flow-volume curves is produced by repeating full expiratory maneuvers over the entire vital capacity at different levels of effort. At

Distribution of Airway Resistance

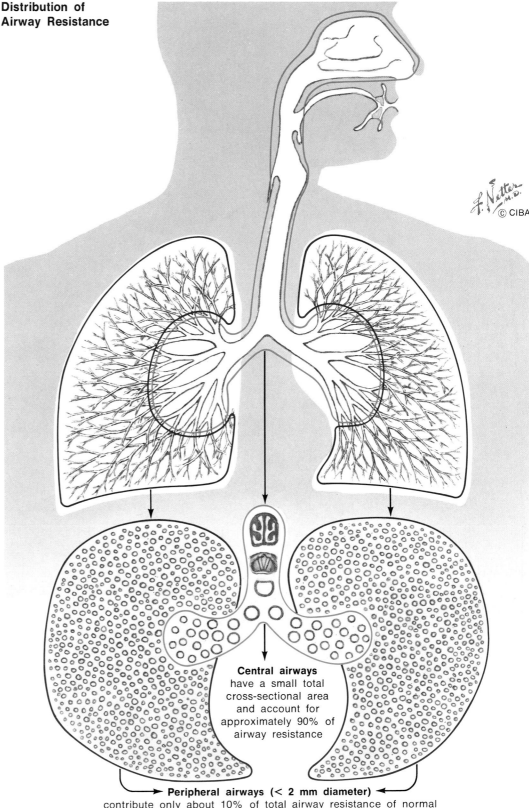

Central airways have a small total cross-sectional area and account for approximately 90% of airway resistance

→ **Peripheral airways (< 2 mm diameter)** ← contribute only about 10% of total airway resistance of normal lung since number of airways and total cross-sectional area in any generation are very large

large lung volumes close to total lung capacity, rate of airflow increases progressively with increasing effort. However, at intermediate and low lung volumes, expiratory flow reaches maximal levels after only moderate effort is exerted and thereafter increases no further despite increasing efforts.

The rate of airflow during expiration is influenced by both lung volume and effort expended. The relationship between effort alone and expiratory airflow is illustrated by *isovolume pressure-flow curves* (Plate 10). During repeated expiratory maneuvers performed with various degrees of effort, simultaneous measurements are made of airflow,

pleural pressure and lung volume. At given lung volumes, airflow is plotted against pleural pressure, providing a measure of the degree of effort.

At all lung volumes, pleural pressure becomes less subatmospheric and subsequently exceeds atmospheric pressure as the expiratory effort is progressively increased. Correspondingly, the rate of airflow increases. At lung volumes greater than 75% of vital capacity, airflow increases progressively with rising pleural pressure; airflow is thus considered to be effort-dependent. In contrast, at volumes below 75% of vital capacity, flow levels off as the pleural pressure exceeds atmospheric

(Continued)

Patterns of Airflow

Pulmonary Mechanics and Gas Exchange
(Continued)

pressure and becomes fixed at a maximal level. Thereafter, further increases in effort and in pleural pressure effect no further rise in flow, and airflow is considered to be effort-independent. Since airflow remains constant despite an increasing driving pressure, it follows that resistance to airflow must also be increasing proportionally with pleural pressure, probably because of compression and narrowing of intrathoracic airways.

Factors that determine airflow during a maximal expiratory maneuver are illustrated by means of a model of the lung (Plate 10). The alveoli are represented by an elastic sac and the intrathoracic airways by a compressible tube, both enclosed within a pleural space.

At a given lung volume, when airflow is arrested, pleural pressure is subatmospheric and counterbalances the elastic recoil pressure of the lung. The alveolar pressure (Palv), the sum of the elastic recoil pressure of the lung (PL) and pleural pressure (Ppl), is zero. Since airflow has ceased, pressures along the entire airway are also at atmospheric levels.

During a forced expiration pleural pressure rises above atmospheric levels and increases alveolar pressure (Plate 11). Airway pressure falls progressively from the alveolus toward the airway opening in overcoming resistance. At a point along the airway, referred to as the *equal pressure point,* the drop in airway pressure from that in the alveolus equals the recoil pressure of the lung. At the equal pressure point, the intraluminal pressure and the pressure surrounding the airways are equal and are the same as pleural pressure. Downstream, toward the airway opening, the transmural pressure becomes negative as the intramural airway pressure falls below pleural pressure. Consequently, the airways are subjected to dynamic compression.

The equal pressure point divides the airways into two components arranged in series: an upstream segment, from the alveoli to the equal pressure point, and a downstream segment, from the equal pressure point to the airway opening. Once maximal expiratory flow is achieved, the position of the equal pressure point becomes fixed. Further increases in pleural pressure with increasing expiratory force simply produce more compression of the downstream segment but do not affect airflow through the upstream segment.

The driving pressure of the upstream segment—*i.e.,* the pressure drop along the airways of that segment—equals the elastic recoil pressure of the lung. Consequently, the maximal rate of airflow during forced expiration ($\dot{V}_{max}$) can

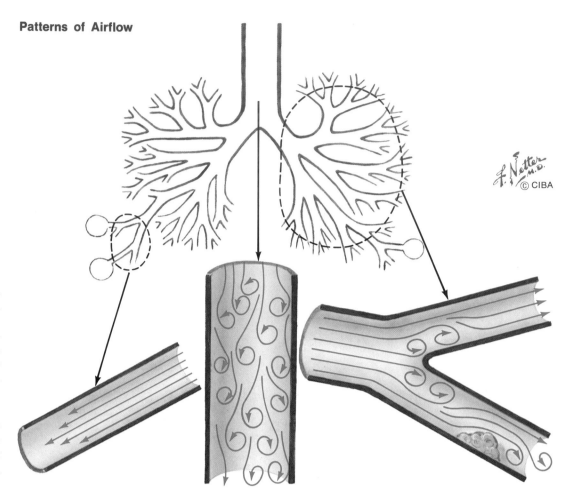

Laminar flow occurs mainly in small peripheral airways where rate of airflow through any airway is low. Driving pressure is proportional to gas viscosity

Turbulent flow occurs at high flow rates in trachea and larger airways. Driving pressure is proportional to square of flow and is dependent on gas density

Transitional flow occurs in larger airways, particularly at branches and at sites of narrowing. Driving pressure is proportional to both gas density and gas viscosity

Poiseuille's law. Resistance to laminar flow is inversely proportional to tube radius to the 4th power and directly proportional to length of tube. When radius is halved, resistance is increased 16-fold. If driving pressure is constant, flow will fall to one-sixteenth. Doubling length only doubles resistance. If driving pressure is constant, flow will fall to one-half

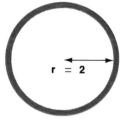

r = 2

Resistance ~1

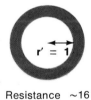

r′ = 1

Resistance ~16

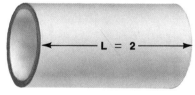

L = 2

Resistance ~2

L′ = 4

Resistance ~4

be expressed in terms of the elastic recoil pressure of the lung (PL) and the resistance of the upstream segment (Rus), according to the equation:

$$\dot{V}_{max} = \frac{P_L}{Rus}$$

Measurements of the rate of airflow during forced expiration form the basis of many of the tests used in assessment of flow-resistive properties of the lung. It is apparent, however, that the maximal rate of expiratory airflow depends on numerous factors, including: lung volumes at which airflow is determined; force of expiration (particularly at high lung volumes); elastic recoil

pressure of the lung as well as resistance of small peripheral airways; and the cross-sectional area of larger central airways.

Dynamic Compliance and Work of Breathing. Changes in lung volume and pleural pressure during a normal breathing cycle, displayed as a *pressure-volume loop* (Plate 12), describe the elastic and flow-resistive properties of the lung as well as the work performed by the respiratory muscles on the lung.

Airflow momentarily ceases at the end of both expiration and inspiration; the change in pleural pressure between these two points reflects the
(Continued)

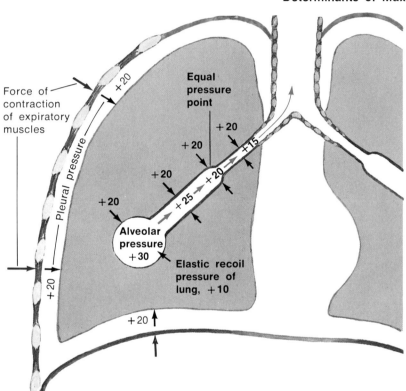

Expiratory Flow-Volume Curves Performed with Progressively Increasing Levels of Effort from A to D

At high lung volumes, rate of airflow during expiration increases progressively with increasing effort. At intermediate and low lung volumes, airflow reaches maximal levels after only modest effort is exerted and thereafter increases no further despite increasing effort

Isovolume Pressure-Flow Curves

At lung volumes greater than 75% of VC, airflow increases progressively with increasing pleural pressure. Airflow is effort-dependent. At volumes below 75% of VC, airflow levels off as pleural pressure exceeds atmospheric pressure. Thereafter airflow is effort-independent, since further increases in pleural pressure result in no further rise in rate of airflow

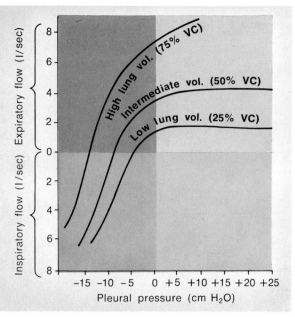

Determinants of Maximal Expiratory Flow

At onset of maximal airflow, contraction of expiratory muscles at a given lung volume raises pleural pressure above atmospheric level (+20 cm H₂O). Alveolar pressure (sum of pleural pressure and lung recoil pressure) is yet higher (+30 cm H₂O). Airway pressure falls progressively from alveolus to airway opening in overcoming resistance. At equal pressure point of airway, pressure within airway equals pressure surrounding it (pleural pressure). Beyond this point, as intraluminal pressure drops further, below pleural pressure, airway will be compressed

With further increases in expiratory effort, at same lung volume, pleural pressure is greater and alveolar pressure is correspondingly higher. Fall in airway pressure and location of equal pressure point are unchanged, but beyond equal pressure point, intrathoracic airways will be compressed to a greater degree by higher pleural pressure. Once maximal airflow is achieved, further increases in pleural pressure produce proportional increases in resistance of segment downstream from equal pressure point, so rate of airflow does not change

SECTION II   PLATE 10

Pulmonary Mechanics and Gas Exchange
(Continued)

increasing elastic recoil of the lungs as the lung volume enlarges. The slope of the line connecting the end-expiratory and end-inspiratory points on the pressure-volume loop provides a measure of the dynamic compliance of the lung. In addition, during inspiration, while air is flowing into the lungs, the change in pleural pressure at any given lung volume from that at the end-expiratory posi-

tion reflects not only increasing lung elastic recoil but also the pressure required to overcome the frictional resistance of the airways and the nonelastic resistance of lung tissues.

In normal individuals, *dynamic compliance* closely approximates static lung compliance and remains essentially unchanged when breathing frequency is increased up to 60 breaths per minute. Thus lung units in parallel with one another normally fill and empty evenly and synchronously, even when airflow is high and the change in lung volume is rapid. For the distribution of ventilation to parallel lung units to be independent of the rate of airflow, the resistance and

compliance of these units must be distributed so that the time constants (*i.e.,* the product of resistance and compliance of individual units) are approximately the same. Time constants of lung units distal to airways 2 mm in diameter are in the order of 0.01 second, and fourfold differences in time constants are necessary to cause dynamic compliance to fall progressively with increasing respiratory frequency.

Patchy narrowing of small peripheral airways produces regional differences in time constants. At low breathing frequencies, when rate of airflow is low, ventilation is evenly distributed. But as

(Continued)

Pulmonary Mechanics and Gas Exchange
(Continued)

breathing frequency increases, ventilation tends to be distributed to areas that offer the least resistance to airflow. Therefore, lung units fed by narrowed airways receive proportionally less ventilation than do areas of the lung where the airways remain normal. A given change in pleural pressure thus produces a smaller overall change in lung volume and, as a result, dynamic compliance falls.

Measurement of the frequency dependence of dynamic compliance is time-consuming and technically difficult, but this test has proved useful in the diagnosis of obstruction in small peripheral airways when other conventional tests of lung mechanics show results that are still within normal limits.

The mechanical *work of breathing* (Plate 12) performed by the respiratory muscles in overcoming the forces of the lung alone can be readily evaluated during spontaneous breathing from the pleural pressure and the change in volume of air in the lung.

The product of pressure (P) and volume (V) has the dimension of work (W), according to the equation

$$W = \int P dV$$

and the work of breathing done on the lungs can be determined from the area of a dynamic pressure-volume loop.

During inspiration, work to overcome the elastic forces of the lung is determined from the area of the trapezoid EABCD. The area of the loop AB'CBA is the work in overcoming nonelastic forces during inspiration, and the area of the loop EAB'CD is the total work of breathing during inspiration.

Because of the elastic recoil of the lung, expiration is passive during quiet breathing; the elastic recoil of the lung is sufficient to overcome nonelastic forces during expiration. At high levels of ventilation and when airway resistance is increased, additional mechanical work during expiration may be required to overcome nonelastic forces. Under these circumstances pleural pressure exceeds atmospheric pressure, and the expiratory portion of the loop extends beyond the confines of the trapezoid EABCD.

The work of breathing at any given level of ventilation depends on the pattern of breathing. Large tidal volumes increase the elastic work of breathing whereas high breathing frequencies increase the work against flow-resistive forces.
(Continued)

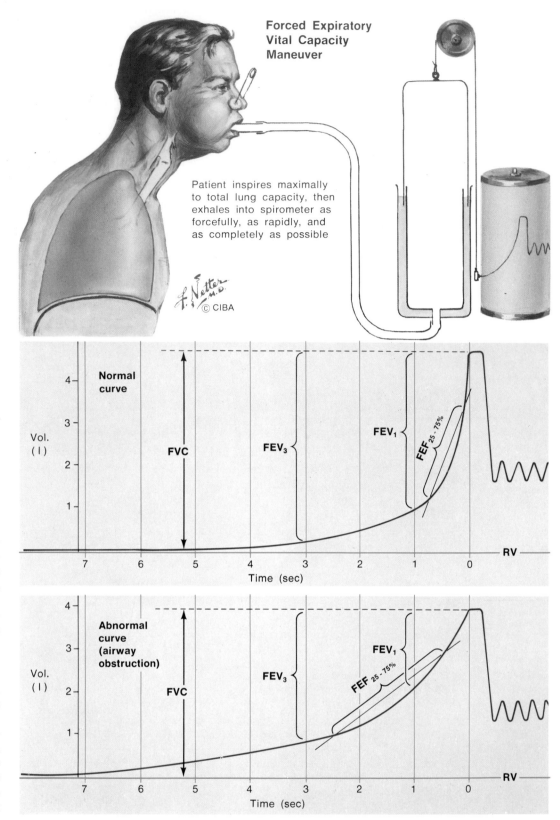

Forced Expiratory Vital Capacity Maneuver

Patient inspires maximally to total lung capacity, then exhales into spirometer as forcefully, as rapidly, and as completely as possible

Maximal Expiratory Flow-Volume Curve

Airway obstruction increases residual volume. Vital capacity is slightly reduced, and total lung capacity is elevated. Despite larger volumes of air in lungs, expiratory airflow is markedly reduced

In restrictive pulmonary disorders, all lung volumes are reduced. Low levels of expiratory airflow are consequent to reduced lung volumes and do not reflect airway obstruction

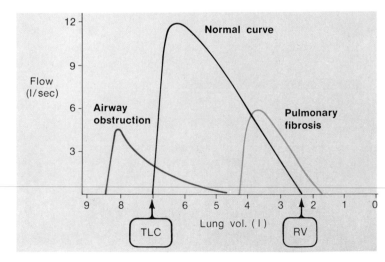

Pulmonary Mechanics and Gas Exchange
(Continued)

During quiet breathing and during exercise, individuals tend to adjust tidal volume and breathing frequency at values that minimize muscle force and work of breathing. Similar adjustments are seen in patients with pulmonary disorders. Individuals with pulmonary fibrosis and increased elastic work of breathing are likely to breathe shallowly and rapidly, while patients with airway obstruction and increased nonelastic work of breathing usually breathe more deeply and slowly.

In order to perform their work on the lung and chest wall during breathing, the respiratory muscles require oxygen. The work of breathing, therefore, can also be considered from the point of view of the energy required, determined from the oxygen cost of breathing. Total oxygen consumption is determined at rest and at an increased level of ventilation produced by voluntary hyperventilation, or breathing carbon dioxide. If no other factors act to increase oxygen consumption, the added oxygen uptake at the higher level of ventilation is attributed to the metabolism of the respiratory muscles.

The oxygen cost of breathing in normal individuals is approximately 1 ml/liter of ventilation, and is less than 5% of total oxygen consumption. At higher levels of ventilation, however, the oxygen cost of breathing progressively increases. Patients with pulmonary disorders demonstrate a higher oxygen cost of quiet breathing as well as a disproportionate increase at elevated levels of ventilation.

Assessment of Dynamic Lung Function

The rate of airflow out of the lungs during a rapid, forceful and complete expiration from total lung capacity to residual volume provides an indirect measure of the flow-resistive properties of the lung (Plate 11). This forced vital capacity maneuver is usually traced on a spirogram, which records the volume exhaled over time. Rates of airflow are determined by calculating the volume exhaled during particular time intervals. In practice, measurements are made of the volume exhaled during the first second (*i.e.,* forced expiratory volume in one second, FEV_1) and over the first three seconds (FEV_3). FEV_1 and FEV_3 are generally expressed as a percentage of the forced vital capacity (FVC): $FEV_1/FVC\%$ and $FEV_3/FVC\%$. An additional common measurement is that of the mean rate of airflow over the middle half of the FVC—*i.e.,* between 25 and 75% of the FVC. This value, previously called the maximal midexpiratory flow rate (MMFR), is now referred to as the forced midexpiratory flow ($FEF_{25-75\%}$).

At large lung volumes close to total lung capacity, maximal expiratory flow is effort-dependent and consequently varies with the degree of force exerted by the patient. In contrast, a maximal effort is not required to achieve maximal rates of airflow at intermediate and low lung volumes. The $FEF_{25-75\%}$, which does not take the first portion of expiration into account, and the FEV_1 and FEV_3, measured over large ranges of lung volume, are little affected by suboptimal efforts and are good indexes of airway resistance.

Asthma, bronchitis and emphysema, which produce airway obstruction, decrease expiratory flow rates, and the extent of reduction is proportional to the severity of the obstruction (Plate 12). Mild airway obstruction may decrease only the $FEF_{25-75\%}$ or the $FEV_3/FVC\%$ without affecting the FEV_1; with increasing airway obstruction all expiratory flow rates fall below predicted values.

Restrictive disorders (such as pulmonary fibrosis), which increase the elasticity of the lung but generally do not produce airway obstruction, primarily decrease the vital capacity (Plate 12). Correspondingly, the FEV_1, FEV_3 and $FEF_{25-75\%}$ may be small also. However, when the FEV_1 and FEV_3 are expressed as percentages of FVC, the values are normal and may even exceed predicted values.

A forced expiratory vital capacity maneuver can also be recorded by directly displaying the rate of airflow against the volume of air expelled from the lung. The resulting plot is called a maximal expiratory flow-volume curve. Conventionally, measurements are made of maximal rates of expiratory airflow ($\dot{V}_{max}$) at 75, 50 and 25% of vital capacity.

When airflow is plotted against the absolute volume of air in the lungs, a number of effects of obstructive and restrictive lung disorders become evident.

Airway obstruction increases the residual volume because of actual closure of narrowed and poorly supported airways. The vital capacity is often normal or only slightly reduced, so that the total lung capacity is usually elevated. The increased lung volume is important in preserving the rate of expiratory airflow: airways are widened, elastic recoil pressure of the lung is increased, and expiratory muscles are shorter and in a mechanically more efficient position. Nonetheless, at any given lung volume, expiratory airflow remains markedly reduced.

Comparing maximal expiratory flow-volume curves obtained during the breathing of air and during the breathing of a mixture of 80% helium and 20% oxygen is useful in locating the major sites of airway obstruction. Normally, resistance to airflow is primarily located in large central airways, and during a forced expiratory vital capacity maneuver airflow is turbulent. Since turbulent airflow is density-dependent, breathing a helium-oxygen mixture 64% less dense than air increases the rate of airflow during a forced expiratory vital capacity maneuver at all but the very lowest lung volumes. At low lung volumes approaching residual volume, flow falls to low levels and becomes laminar, so that airflow while breathing air and when breathing a helium-oxygen mixture is the same. This point is called the volume of isoflow (V iso $\dot{V}$).

Disorders of peripheral airways less than 2 mm in diameter may increase airway resistance, so that a greater proportion of the overall airway resistance is now located in small airways where flow remains laminar. Since laminar flow is independent of gas density, breathing a helium-oxygen mixture would result in smaller increases in airflow. Response to helium-oxygen can be assessed from V iso $\dot{V}$ and from the increase in the rate of airflow at 50% of the vital capacity ($\Delta\dot{V}_{max\ 50}$).

Restrictive disorders characteristically reduce all lung volumes. The residual volume is low, and, because of increased lung elasticity, which acts to resist complete expansion, vital capacity and total lung capacity are also decreased. Throughout expiration, airflow remains at low levels. However, with respect to the actual lung volume, flow rates are in fact normal and often greater than expected.

Another commonly employed test of dynamic lung function is the *maximal voluntary ventilation* (MVV). For this test the patient is instructed to breathe as hard and as fast as possible for 12 seconds, and the minute ventilation is calculated. The MVV is dependent on achievement of high rates of airflow, and consequently is affected by changes in airway resistance. A good correlation exists between the MVV and the FEV_1, and the MVV is usually reduced in patients with obstructive airway disorders. The test can also be influenced by changes in the elastic properties of the lung as well as by poor strength, motivation and coordination. Although an abnormal test does not point toward any specific defect, a normal MVV usually indicates that there is no gross impairment of lung function.

Distribution of Ventilation

In the upright position, pleural pressure is more negative with respect to atmospheric pressure at the apex of the lung than at the base (Plate 13). Pleural pressure increases by approximately 0.25 cm H_2O per centimeter of vertical distance from the top to the bottom of the lung because of the weight of the lung and the effects of gravity.

(Continued)

Work of Breathing

Normal

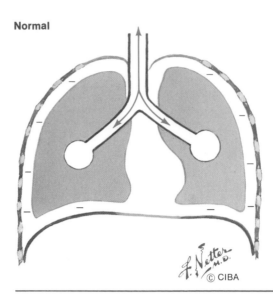

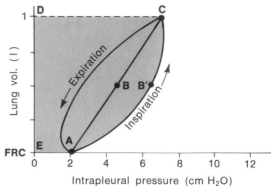

Work performed on lung during breathing can be determined from dynamic pressure-volume loop. Work to overcome elastic forces is represented by area of trapezoid EABCD. Additional work required to overcome flow-resistance during inspiration is represented by area of right half of loop AB'CBA

Pulmonary Mechanics and Gas Exchange
(Continued)

Because of these differences in pleural pressure, the transpulmonary pressure is greater at the top than at the bottom of the lung, so that at most lung volumes the alveoli at the lung apices are more expanded than those at the lung bases.

At low lung volumes approaching residual volume, the pleural pressure at the bottom of the lung actually exceeds intraluminal airway pressure and leads to closure of peripheral airways. The first portion of a breath taken from residual volume enters alveoli at the lung apex. However, in the tidal volume range and above, because of regional variations in lung compliance, ventilation per alveolus is greater at the bottom than at the top of the lung.

The distribution of ventilation and volume at which airways at the lung bases begin to close can be assessed by the *single-breath nitrogen washout and closing volume test* (Plate 13). The concentration of nitrogen at the mouth is measured and plotted against expired lung volume following a single full inspiration of 100% oxygen from residual volume to total lung capacity. The initial portion of the inspiration, which consists of dead-space gas rich in nitrogen, goes to the upper lung zones, while the remainder of the breath, containing only oxygen, is distributed preferentially to the lower lung zones. The result is that the concentration of oxygen in the alveoli of the lung bases is greater than in those of the lung apices.

During the subsequent expiration the initial portion of the washout consists of dead space and contains no nitrogen *(phase I)*. Then, as alveolar gas containing nitrogen begins to be washed out, the concentration of nitrogen in the expired air rises to reach a plateau. The portion of the curve where the concentration of nitrogen rises steeply is called *phase II*, while the plateau is referred to as *phase III*. Provided gas enters and leaves all regions of lung synchronously and equally, phase III will be flat. When the distribution of ventilation is nonuniform, gas coming from different alveoli will have different nitrogen concentrations, producing a rising nitrogen concentration during phase III.

At low lung volumes, when the airways at the lung bases close, only the alveoli at the top of the lung continue to empty. Since the concentration of nitrogen in the alveoli of the upper lung zones is higher, there will be an abrupt increase in slope of the nitrogen-volume curve *(phase IV)*. The volume at which this increase in slope occurs is referred to as the *closing volume*.

The earliest pathologic changes produced by chronic bronchitis and emphysema include inflammation, fibrosis and increased elaboration of

Obstructive disease

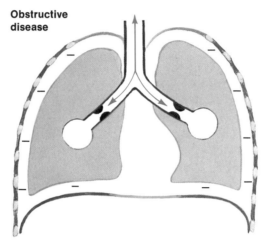

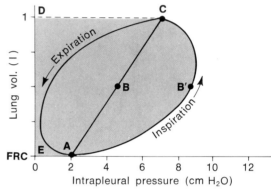

In disorders characterized by airway obstruction, work to overcome flow-resistance is increased; elastic work of breathing remains unchanged

Restrictive disease

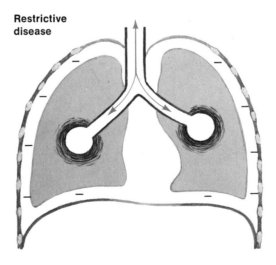

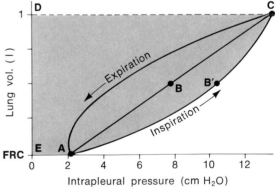

Restrictive lung diseases result in increase of elastic work of breathing; work to overcome flow-resistance is normal

mucus in the peripheral bronchioles less than 2 to 3 mm in diameter. These changes promote premature airway closure at larger than normal lung volumes even before other tests of dynamic lung function become abnormal, so that the closing volume test can be applied in the early diagnosis of small airway disease.

The closing volume test, however, is nonspecific, since loss of lung elasticity alone will increase the closing volume. This feature accounts for the progressive increase in closing volume seen with advancing age in normal individuals and may in part explain the increased closing volume regularly noted in those who smoke cigarettes.

Pulmonary Circulation

Mixed venous blood from the entire systemic circulation is collected in the right atrium and passes to the right ventricle (Plate 14). Contraction of the right ventricle delivers its entire output along the pulmonary arteries to the capillary bed, where gas exchange takes place. The pulmonary capillaries consist of a fine network of thin-walled vessels, but since the surface area of the capillary bed is approximately 70 m², it may be regarded as a sheet of flowing blood rather than as individual channels. At any one moment, the
(Continued)

Pulmonary Mechanics and Gas Exchange
(Continued)

pulmonary capillary bed holds only about 100 ml of blood; most of the remainder of the blood in the pulmonary circulation is contained in the compliant pulmonary venules and veins which, along with the left atrium, serve as a reservoir for the left ventricle.

Intravascular Pressure. Whereas the systemic circulation regulates the blood supply, redistributing blood flow to various organs such as the muscles, kidneys and gastrointestinal tract in response to their specific requirements, the pulmonary circulation is concerned only with blood flow to the lungs. Pulmonary vascular pressures are very low compared with those in the systemic circulation. Systolic pulmonary artery pressure is approximately 25 mm Hg, diastolic pressure is 8 mm Hg, and mean arterial pressure is about 14 mm Hg. Pressure in the left atrium is 5 mm Hg, only slightly less than the pressure in the large pulmonary veins; left atrial pressure is accurately reflected in *pulmonary wedge pressure.* Pulmonary capillary pressure cannot be measured directly but lies somewhere between arteriolar and venular pressures. The pressure drop across the entire pulmonary circulation—the difference between mean pulmonary artery pressure and mean left atrial pressure—constitutes the driving pressure which produces blood flow through the lungs.

Blood Flow. Pulmonary blood flow can be determined in a number of ways. The Fick method makes use of the principle that the amount of oxygen taken up by the blood passing through the lungs is reflected by the difference in oxygen content between arterial and mixed venous blood. Pulmonary blood flow can be calculated with the following equation:

$$\text{Pulmonary blood flow} = \frac{\text{oxygen uptake}}{\text{arterial-venous oxygen content difference}}$$

Blood flow can also be measured by the thermodilution and indicator dilution techniques, in which a tracer substance is injected into the venous system and the concentration and time of appearance of the substance in the arterial blood are recorded. These three methods measure average blood flow only. Instantaneous pulmonary blood flow can be determined by means of a body plethysmograph, with the patient seated and inhaling a mixture of 80% nitrous oxide and 20% oxygen. Nitrous oxide is a particularly soluble gas, and its rate of uptake by the capillary blood and removal from the lung are limited by the rate of pulmonary blood flow. The instantaneous

(Continued)

Pleural Pressure Gradient. Pleural pressure in upright position is more subatmospheric at top of lung and increases down lung consequent to weight of lung and force of gravity

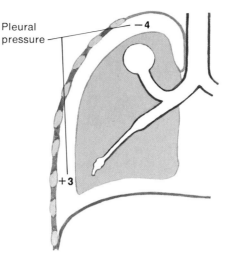
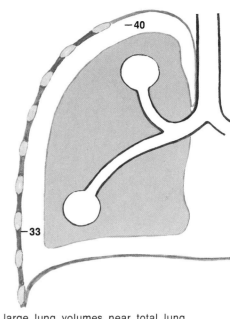

At low lung volumes, alveoli at top of lung are larger than those at bottom. When pleural pressure at lung bases exceeds atmospheric pressure, airways are compressed and tend to close

At large lung volumes near total lung capacity, alveoli at top and bottom of lung are about same size. During normal breathing, alveoli at bottom of lung expand more than those at top

Closing Volume. A single full breath of 100% O_2 is inhaled from residual volume to total lung capacity. Initial portion of breath (dead-space air, rich in N_2) enters alveoli in upper lung zones. Remainder of breath (O_2 only) preferentially goes to lower lung zones, so concentration of N_2 is lower in alveoli of lung bases. During subsequent expiration, concentration of N_2 at mouth is plotted against expired lung volume

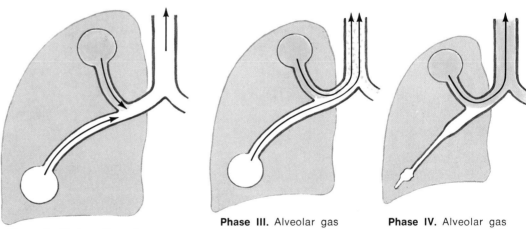

Phase I. First portion of breath exhaled is free of N_2 and contains only O_2 remaining in dead space

Phase II. Mixture of dead-space and alveolar gas

Phase III. Alveolar gas from both upper and lower lung zones

Phase IV. Alveolar gas primarily from upper lung zones containing a relatively high concentration of N_2

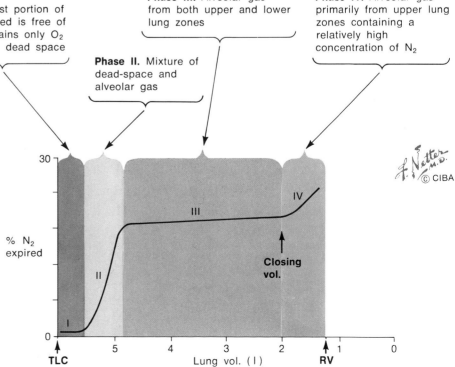

Pulmonary Mechanics and Gas Exchange
(Continued)

measurements possible with this technique have demonstrated that blood flow through the pulmonary capillary bed is, in fact, pulsatile.

Pulmonary Vascular Resistance. Pulmonary vascular resistance (Plate 15) is calculated from the driving pressure across the pulmonary circulation—*i.e.,* mean pulmonary artery pressure minus mean left atrial pressure—and pulmonary blood flow according to the following equation:

$$\text{Pulmonary vascular resistance} = \frac{\text{driving pressure}}{\text{pulmonary blood flow}}$$

Since blood flow through the systemic and pulmonary circulations is essentially the same, while the pressure drop across the pulmonary circulation is only one-tenth that across the systemic circulation, it follows that pulmonary vascular resistance is one-tenth of the systemic resistance. Major sites of pulmonary vascular resistance are the arterioles and capillaries.

The pulmonary circulation has the capacity to accommodate twofold to threefold increases in cardiac output with only small changes in pulmonary artery pressure. This state commonly exists during exercise. The increase in blood flow with little change in driving pressure indicates that, as pulmonary blood flow increases, pulmonary vascular resistance actually falls. This fall in vascular resistance results from an increasing cross-sectional area of the vascular bed. Blood vessels already conducting blood may increase their caliber. Also, vessels previously closed may open and begin to conduct blood as the cardiac output rises.

Pulmonary blood vessels are extremely thin-walled and compliant. Their caliber depends on the transmural pressure—*i.e.,* the difference between the pressure inside the blood vessel and that surrounding the vessel. The smallest pulmonary capillaries are surrounded by alveoli and are subjected to alveolar pressure. Increase in alveolar pressure produced by positive pressure breathing, for example, can result in compression and closure of these alveolar vessels. The influence exerted on larger arteries and veins is different. Larger blood vessels are tethered to the lung parenchyma, which acts as a spring to hold the vessels open. The pressure surrounding these extraalveolar blood vessels more closely approximates pleural pressure. As lung volume and elastic recoil of the lung increase, the pull on the extraalveolar vessels is greater, the vessels dilate, and their resistance falls. In contrast, alveolar vessels become stretched and compressed as the alveoli enlarge

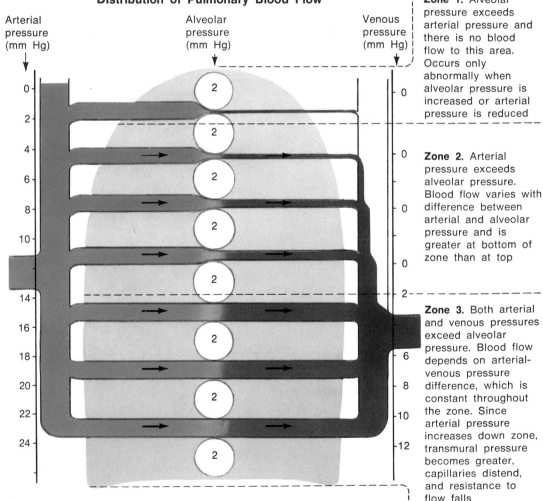

Vascular Pressure in Systemic and Pulmonary Circulations (mm Hg)

(Bar above figures = mean)

with increasing lung volume so that their resistance rises. Overall pulmonary vascular resistance is probably lowest at functional residual capacity, and deviations in lung volume in either direction from the usual end-expiratory position tend to increase vascular resistance.

Distribution of Pulmonary Blood Flow (Plate 14). The pulmonary arterial system can be regarded as a continuous vertical column of blood. The intravascular hydrostatic pressure is affected

by gravity, so that in the upright position the pulmonary artery pressure is greater at the bottom than at the top of the lung. Similarly, venous pressure is different at various levels of the lung. Consequently, blood flow is not distributed evenly throughout the lung but progressively decreases from the base to the apex. In the supine position, as the direction of gravitational forces changes, blood flow to the lung apices increases,

(Continued)

Pulmonary Vascular Resistance

Effects of increases in pulmonary blood flow and vascular pressures

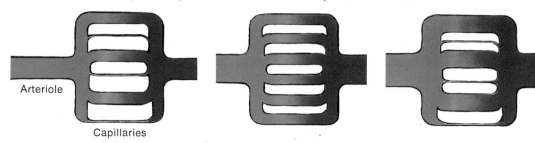

Normally some pulmonary capillaries are closed and conduct no blood

Recruitment: More capillaries open as pulmonary vascular pressure or blood flow increases

Distention: At high vascular pressures individual capillaries widen and acquire a larger cross-sectional area

Pulmonary Mechanics and Gas Exchange
(Continued)

and pulmonary blood flow becomes more uniformly distributed. Exercise, by increasing blood flow to all areas of the lung, also lessens regional differences in pulmonary blood flow.

Normally, pulmonary artery pressure is just sufficient to deliver blood to the lung apices. A drop in hydrostatic pressure produced by hemorrhage or shock may lower the intravascular pressure at the lung apex below alveolar pressure. Since the extraluminal pressure exceeds the intraluminal pressure, the highly compliant blood vessels will then be compressed and become occluded. This area at the apex of the lung is called zone 1. Farther down the lung, pulmonary artery pressure increases and exceeds alveolar pressure. If, however, alveolar pressure is greater than venous pressure (zone 2), blood flow will be regulated by the difference between arterial and alveolar pressures rather than by the arterial-venous pressure difference. This arrangement, analogous to a waterfall in which flow over the fall is independent of the height of the fall, can be simulated by a Starling resistor, a compressible tube passing through a compression chamber. Because of the effects of gravity, pulmonary artery pressure increases down zone 2, but since alveolar pressure remains unchanged, the driving pressure producing flow becomes greater. Still farther down the lung (zone 3), venous pressure exceeds alveolar pressure, and flow is determined as usual from the difference between arterial and venous pressures. Throughout zone 3, despite increase in pulmonary artery pressure, the arterial-venous pressure difference remains unchanged. However, the transmural distending pressure across the capillary wall does become greater. As a result of distention of blood vessels and/or recruitment of new capillaries, blood flow does increase. At the very bottom of the lung, blood flow falls. Because the elastic recoil pressure is less in the lower lung zones, the action of the alveolar walls on the extraalveolar blood vessels is smaller. The vessels are, therefore, poorly distended, and the pulmonary vascular resistance is greater.

Factors Affecting the Pulmonary Vascular Bed. A variety of neural stimuli as well as chemical and humoral substances can affect the pulmonary vascular bed (Plate 15). Pulmonary blood vessels are innervated by both sympathetic and parasympathetic nerves, but under normal circumstances in man, the autonomic nervous system has virtually no role in determining pulmonary vascular resistance. Hypoxemia is a potent stimulus affecting the pulmonary vascular bed; it constricts both precapillary and postcapillary

Effects of lung volume

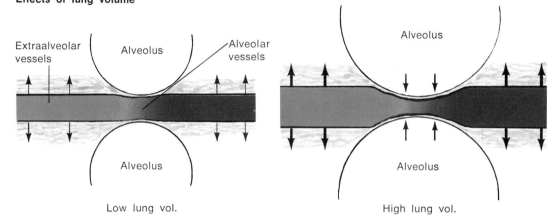

As lung volume increases, increasing elastic recoil of lung dilates extraalveolar capillaries and their resistance falls. Alveolar vessels, in contrast, are compressed by enlarging alveoli and their resistance increases

Effects of chemical and humoral substances

vessels. This effect is independent of neural and humoral mechanisms, since it can be demonstrated even in the isolated lung. The effects of hypercapnia *per se* on the pulmonary vasculature are variable. They appear to depend on changes in hydrogen ion concentration. Acidosis, whether respiratory or metabolic, increases pulmonary vascular tone, and acidosis and hypoxemia are considered to act synergistically in constricting pulmonary vessels and increasing pulmonary vascular resistance. Chemical and humoral agents that act on the pulmonary vascular bed include epinephrine, norepinephrine, histamine and angiotensin, all of which produce

pulmonary vasoconstriction, and bradykinin and acetylcholine, which result in vasodilatation. While prostaglandins appear to have a role in pulmonary vasoconstriction, their exact place has not been determined.

Pulmonary vascular resistance may be increased by various cardiopulmonary disorders. Pulmonary fibrosis, characterized by a diffuse increase in fibrous tissue in the lung, obliterates and compresses pulmonary capillaries. Pulmonary emboli directly obstruct pulmonary arteries and arterioles and may produce secondary vasoconstriction through the release of vasoactive

(Continued)

Pulmonary Mechanics and Gas Exchange
(Continued)

substances. Primary pulmonary hypertension is presumed to result from pulmonary arteriolar sclerosis, which thickens the walls and decreases the caliber of the vessels. These disorders require a greater force of contraction of the right ventricle to overcome the added resistance and to maintain blood flow, and may lead to hypertrophy, strain and ultimately failure of the right ventricle.

Diffusion

Oxygen and carbon dioxide pass between the alveoli and the pulmonary capillary blood by *diffusion,* the passive tendency of molecules to move from a region of higher to one of lower concentration (Plate 16).

Gas Phase Diffusion. Different steps in the pathway of gas transfer involve diffusion. Because of the rapidly increasing cross-sectional area of the bronchial tree, inspired air is carried by bulk movement only as far as the alveolar ducts. At that point airflow effectively stops, and thereafter movement of gas molecules and mixing of gas in the alveoli take place by diffusion. The diffusion rate of a gas in a gaseous medium is inversely proportional to the molecular weight of the gas. Light molecules move faster and collide more frequently than heavy molecules and thus diffuse more rapidly. Gaseous diffusion of oxygen (molecular weight 32) is faster than that of carbon dioxide (molecular weight 44).

The distance for gaseous diffusion is small in normal alveoli, and complete mixing of newly

inspired air with gas already present in alveoli occurs within a fraction of a second. However, in emphysema, in which the alveolar spaces are enlarged, this time may be considerably prolonged and may be a limiting factor in gas transfer.

Membrane Diffusion. Gas transfer across the alveolar-capillary membrane involves diffusion between a gas phase and a liquid phase. Diffusion in liquids depends on the solubility of the gas in the liquid. Consequently, despite its greater molecular weight, carbon dioxide is considerably more soluble than oxygen and diffuses approximately 20 times more rapidly than does oxygen.

Barriers to Diffusion. The effective barriers across which gas must pass include the surface lining of the alveoli, alveolar epithelium, basement membranes, capillary endothelium, a layer of plasma in the capillary blood and red blood cell membrane. The diffusion rate of a gas across these barriers also depends on the difference in partial pressure of the gas between the alveoli and pulmonary capillary blood. This pressure gradient is the driving pressure, which results in the transfer of gas across the alveolar-capillary membrane.

Alveolar-Capillary Partial Pressure Gradients. The difference in partial pressures of oxygen between alveolar air and capillary blood is greatest at the beginning of the capillary where venous blood with a P_{O_2} of 40 mm Hg enters. Oxygen moves rapidly along its concentration gradient from alveolus to capillary blood. Although the transit time of blood through the pulmonary capillaries is only 0.75 second, diffusion is so rapid that the P_{O_2} of air and that of blood reach equilibrium before the blood has passed even halfway along the capillary. When the alveolar-capillary membrane is thickened and diffusion is moderately impaired, oxygen transfer is slowed, but the P_{O_2} of capillary blood may still come into equilibrium with that of alveolar air within the available time.

During exercise, pulmonary blood flow is increased, and the transit time of blood through pulmonary capillaries is shortened. Normally, the diffusion reserve of the lung is so great that the alveolar air and capillary blood reach equilibrium with respect to P_{O_2} even in the reduced time available for gas transfer. If, however, the alveolar-capillary membrane is abnormal, even though equilibrium is achieved at rest, the P_{O_2} of capillary blood may not reach equilibrium with the levels in alveolar air before blood leaves the capillary during exercise.

Although the diffusion rate of carbon dioxide greatly exceeds that of oxygen, the time required for equilibrium between alveolar air and capillary blood is approximately the same for the two gases. Even when diffusion is considerably impaired, any alveolar–end-capillary gradient for carbon dioxide remains extremely small and virtually never poses a significant clinical problem.

Blood Phase Diffusion. After reaching the plasma of capillary blood, oxygen must pass into the red blood cell and combine chemically with hemoglobin (Plate 20). The time required for the chemical combination of oxygen and hemoglobin significantly delays the diffusion process. This time is determined by the volume of blood in the pulmonary capillary bed (Vc) and the amount of oxygen taken up by 1 ml of blood/mm Hg pressure gradient (θ).

Diffusing Capacity and Its Components. The diffusing capacity of the lung is simply a measure of the lung's ability to conduct a gas from the alveoli to the capillary blood. It is defined as the amount of gas transferred from alveoli to capillary blood per unit time as a function of the mean partial pressure gradient. The diffusing capacity of the lung for oxygen ($D_{L_{O_2}}$) is determined from the equation

$$D_{L_{O_2}} = \frac{\dot{V}_{O_2}}{P_{\bar{A}_{O_2}} - P_{\bar{c}_{O_2}}}$$

where $\dot{V}_{O_2}$ is the oxygen uptake per minute, $P_{\bar{A}_{O_2}}$ is the mean alveolar oxygen tension, and $P_{\bar{c}_{O_2}}$ is the mean capillary oxygen tension. This flow-pressure ratio has the dimensions of conductance, and its reciprocal ($1/D_L$) is an expression of the resistance to diffusion. The resistance to diffusion has two components: membrane component and intravascular component.

The *membrane component* of the resistance to diffusion is determined from the thickness of the blood-gas barrier and from the area available for diffusion. When the alveoli are destroyed or their walls disrupted, and when the pulmonary capillaries are obliterated or blood flow is obstructed, the effective area for diffusion is reduced. The thickness of the barrier is increased by interstitial pulmonary edema and fibrosis and by intraalveolar edema and consolidation. Furthermore, the distance oxygen must travel to reach the hemoglobin molecules in the red blood cells is increased if the pulmonary capillaries are dilated and if there is hemodilution with an increase in the quantity of plasma within the capillaries. The *intravascular component* of the resistance to diffusion results from the finite reaction time of oxygen with hemoglobin and depends on the number of red blood cells in the pulmonary capillaries and their hemoglobin concentration.

Measurements of Diffusing Capacity of Lung for Carbon Monoxide. The diffusing capacity of the lung for oxygen is not routinely determined because the mean capillary P_{O_2} cannot be readily ascertained. The gas most suitable for measuring the lung's diffusing capacity is carbon monoxide, which has diffusing characteristics similar to those of oxygen. Because of the great affinity of carbon monoxide for hemoglobin, virtually all the carbon monoxide that passes from the alveoli into the capillary blood is taken up by the hemoglobin. Hence the partial pressure of carbon monoxide in the plasma remains so low that for practical purposes it can be ignored, and the diffusing capacity of the lung for carbon monoxide ($D_{L_{CO}}$) can be determined from the simplified equation

$$D_{L_{CO}} = \frac{\dot{V}_{CO}}{P_{\bar{A}_{CO}}}$$

where $\dot{V}_{CO}$ is the amount of carbon monoxide taken up per minute and $P_{\bar{A}_{CO}}$ is the mean alveolar carbon monoxide tension.

There are a number of techniques for measuring the diffusing capacity of the lung for carbon monoxide. The single-breath test involves a single full inspiration of a very low concentration of carbon monoxide followed by a 10 second period of breath-holding. Inspired and expired concentrations of carbon monoxide are measured; volume of gas in the lung is determined; and rate of carbon *(Continued)*

Pathways of O₂ and CO₂ Diffusion

Alveolus
Surface-lining fluid
Alveolar epithelium
Basement membranes (fused)
Capillary endothelium
Plasma

Red blood cell { membrane
intracellular fluid
hemoglobin molecules

O₂   CO₂

$P_{O_2} = 150$ mm Hg
$P_{CO_2} = 0$ mm Hg } Atmospheric air at airway opening

Pulmonary Mechanics and Gas Exchange
(*Continued*)

monoxide uptake from the lung is calculated. This method is relatively simple and requires no blood samples. However, breath-holding is an artificial condition and may be difficult for patients with lung disease who are short of breath. In steady state methods, a very dilute mixture of carbon monoxide is breathed until the rate of uptake of carbon monoxide from the lung is constant. The adequacy of the procedure depends on the accuracy with which the alveolar carbon monoxide concentration is determined. The diffusing capacity during exercise increases the accuracy of the test and is most readily determined by steady state techniques.

Gas Exchange

Properties of Gases. A gas consists of molecules in a state of random motion. The molecules fill any container in which they are enclosed, and as they collide with one another and with the walls of the enclosing container, a pressure is exerted.

The respiratory gases, which include oxygen, carbon dioxide and nitrogen, follow the laws of perfect gases, expressed as

$$PV = nrT$$

where P is pressure, V is volume, n is the number of gas molecules, r is the gas constant, and T is the absolute temperature. This expression indicates that if temperature is kept constant, the volume occupied by an aliquot of gas varies inversely with the pressure to which it is subjected (Boyle's law). Also, at a constant pressure, the volume of a gas is proportional to the absolute temperature (Charles' law). Similarly, at a constant volume, the pressure exerted by a gas varies directly with the absolute temperature (Gay-Lussac's law).

At sea level the total pressure of atmospheric air is 760 mm Hg. Constituents of air include nitrogen, oxygen, carbon dioxide, water vapor, and inert gases such as argon and neon. Each gas exerts a partial pressure proportional to its concentration. The partial pressure is the same as it would be if that gas alone occupied the entire volume. The sum of the partial pressures of the gases in the mixture equals the total atmospheric pressure.

Inspired atmospheric air is warmed and humidified as it passes through the nasopharynx and tracheobronchial tree. The latter takes part in respiratory heat exchange but by the time air reaches the alveoli, it has been heated to body temperature and fully saturated with water vapor. The water vapor pressure of a saturated gas varies with temperature; at body temperature, regard-

Transfer of O₂ and CO₂ Between Alveolar Air and Capillary Blood

$P_{O_2} = 40$ mm Hg
$P_{CO_2} = 46$ mm Hg

Pulmonary artery
(mixed venous blood)

Alveolus
$P_{O_2} = 100$ mm Hg
$P_{CO_2} = 40$ mm Hg

O₂
CO₂

$P_{O_2} = 100$ mm Hg
$P_{CO_2} = 40$ mm Hg

Pulmonary vein
(arterial blood)

Capillaries

Transit time during exercise

Transit time (sec)

less of barometric pressure, water vapor pressure is 47 mm Hg. Consequently, the total pressure of dry gases in tracheal air is equal to the barometric pressure (760 mm Hg) minus water vapor pressure (47 mm Hg), or 713 mm Hg. The approximate partial pressures of the gases in inspired tracheal air are proportional to their concentrations and are: partial pressure of oxygen (P_{O_2}), 150 mm Hg; of carbon dioxide (P_{CO_2}), less than 1 mm Hg; of nitrogen (P_{N_2}), 563 mm Hg.

Ventilation, Oxygen Uptake and Carbon Dioxide Output. In the alveoli of the respiratory bronchioles, alveolar ducts and alveolar sacs, gas comes into intimate contact with pulmonary

capillary blood, and transfer of oxygen and carbon dioxide occurs (Plate 17). Pulmonary capillary blood continuously removes oxygen from and adds carbon dioxide to alveolar gas. Ventilation, on the other hand, serves to maintain alveolar gas composition by replenishing oxygen and eliminating carbon dioxide to the atmosphere. The composition of alveolar gas depends on the balance between alveolar ventilation and pulmonary capillary blood flow. Both alveolar P_{O_2} and P_{CO_2} vary during the breathing cycle, but the mean alveolar P_{O_2} is approximately 100 mm Hg and the mean alveolar P_{CO_2} is 40 mm Hg.

(*Continued*)

Pulmonary Mechanics and Gas Exchange
(Continued)

Capillary blood generally takes up more oxygen than the amount of carbon dioxide the blood adds to the alveolar gas. As a result, the expired tidal volume is somewhat less than the corresponding inspired volume. Since nitrogen is not exchanged in the lung, any difference between carbon dioxide output and oxygen uptake will be reflected by an increase in the concentration of nitrogen in the expired air as compared to the inspired air. These changes in nitrogen concentration allow the inspired volume of ventilation to be calculated once the expired ventilation is known. The inspired volume of ventilation per minute ($\dot{V}_I$) is determined according to the equation

$$\dot{V}_I = \dot{V}_E \left(\frac{F_{E_{N_2}}}{F_{I_{N_2}}} \right)$$

where $\dot{V}_E$ is the expired volume of ventilation per minute; $F_{E_{N_2}}$ and $F_{I_{N_2}}$ respectively are the concentrations of nitrogen in inspired air.

The ratio of carbon dioxide output to oxygen uptake, the *respiratory exchange ratio,* is normally 0.8. The respiratory exchange ratio is distinct from the *respiratory quotient* (RQ), which is determined by cellular metabolism, but the two are identical under steady state conditions when oxygen and carbon dioxide stores of the body are constant.

Since the quantity of carbon dioxide in inspired air is considered to be negligible, the amount of carbon dioxide eliminated per minute ($\dot{V}_{CO_2}$) can be calculated from $\dot{V}_E$ and the concentration of carbon dioxide in the expired air ($F_{E_{CO_2}}$), according to the equation

$$\dot{V}_{CO_2} = \dot{V}_E \times F_{E_{CO_2}}$$

In contrast, significant quantities of oxygen are present in both inspired and expired air, so that oxygen uptake must be calculated from the difference in the amount of oxygen in inspired and expired air by means of the equation

$$\dot{V}_{O_2} = (\dot{V}_I \times F_{I_{O_2}}) - (\dot{V}_E \times F_{E_{O_2}})$$

where $\dot{V}_{O_2}$ is the oxygen uptake per minute, $F_{I_{O_2}}$ is the concentration of oxygen in inspired air, and $F_{E_{O_2}}$ is the concentration of oxygen in expired air.

Dead Space. The minute volume of ventilation, *i.e.,* total air breathed each minute, is the product of the tidal volume and the breathing frequency. The entire minute volume of ventilation, however, does not participate in gas exchange. A portion of each breath fills the mouth, nose, pharynx, larynx, trachea, bronchi and bronchioles. This volume is called the *anatomic dead space* and numerically equals approximately an individual's ideal

body weight in pounds (about 150 ml in a typical adult). In addition, some inspired air reaches alveoli which are not in contact with pulmonary capillary blood and so does not participate in gas exchange. The total volume of anatomic and alveolar dead space not involved in gas exchange is termed the *physiologic dead space.* Normally, the anatomic and physiologic dead spaces are practically the same, and equal about one-third of the tidal volume. The remaining two-thirds of the tidal volume, the alveolar component, ventilates alveoli perfused by pulmonary capillary blood, participates directly in gas exchange and contributes to maintaining alveolar gas composition.

Each expired tidal volume (V_T) can thus be considered to consist of a volume corresponding to the physiologic dead space (V_D) plus the alveolar component (V_A):

$$V_T = V_D + V_A$$

The concentration of partial pressure of carbon dioxide in the dead space gas is the same as that in inspired air, and is virtually zero. Dead space gas dilutes alveolar gas, so that the partial pressure of carbon dioxide in mixed expired air is lower than in alveolar gas. The volume of dead space can be readily calculated, if one knows the mean partial

(Continued)

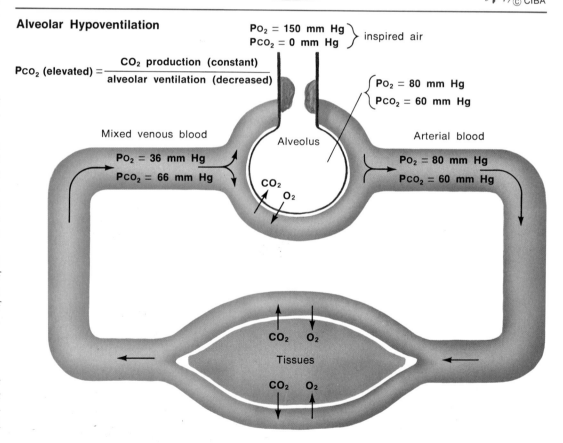

Normal Ventilation

$$P_{CO_2} = \frac{CO_2 \text{ production}}{\text{alveolar ventilation}}$$

$P_{O_2} = 150$ mm Hg
$P_{CO_2} = 0$ mm Hg } inspired air

$P_{O_2} = 100$ mm Hg
$P_{CO_2} = 40$ mm Hg

Mixed venous blood

Alveolus

Arterial blood

$P_{O_2} = 40$ mm Hg
$P_{CO_2} = 46$ mm Hg

CO_2
O_2

$P_{O_2} = 100$ mm Hg
$P_{CO_2} = 40$ mm Hg

CO_2 O_2
Tissues
CO_2 O_2

Alveolar Hypoventilation

$$P_{CO_2} \text{ (elevated)} = \frac{CO_2 \text{ production (constant)}}{\text{alveolar ventilation (decreased)}}$$

$P_{O_2} = 150$ mm Hg
$P_{CO_2} = 0$ mm Hg } inspired air

$P_{O_2} = 80$ mm Hg
$P_{CO_2} = 60$ mm Hg

Mixed venous blood

Alveolus

Arterial blood

$P_{O_2} = 36$ mm Hg
$P_{CO_2} = 66$ mm Hg

CO_2
O_2

$P_{O_2} = 80$ mm Hg
$P_{CO_2} = 60$ mm Hg

CO_2 O_2
Tissues
CO_2 O_2

Ventilation-Perfusion ($\dot{V}A/\dot{Q}C$) Relationships

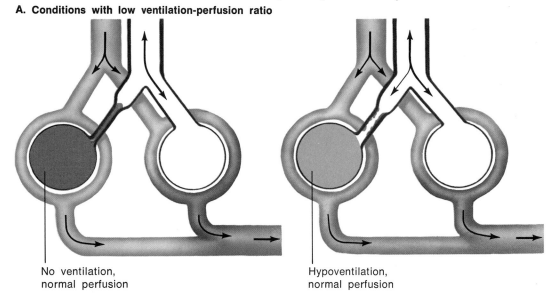

A. Conditions with low ventilation-perfusion ratio

No ventilation,
normal perfusion

Hypoventilation,
normal perfusion

B. Conditions with high ventilation-perfusion ratio

Normal ventilation,
no perfusion (physiologic dead space)

Normal ventilation,
hypoperfusion

Pulmonary Mechanics and Gas Exchange
(Continued)

pressure of carbon dioxide in mixed expired air ($P\bar{E}_{CO_2}$) and in alveolar gas ($P\bar{A}_{CO_2}$), by using a modification of the Bohr equation:

$$V_D = V_T \left(\frac{P\bar{A}_{CO_2} - P\bar{E}_{CO_2}}{P\bar{A}_{CO_2}} \right)$$

Since dead space gas contains no carbon dioxide, $\dot{V}_{CO_2}$ can be expressed in terms of alveolar ventilation ($\dot{V}\bar{A}$), *i.e.,* the product of the alveolar component of the tidal volume and breathing frequency, and the $P\bar{A}_{CO_2}$:

$$\dot{V}_{CO_2} = \dot{V}\bar{A} \times P\bar{A}_{CO_2} \times \text{a constant}$$

Since partial pressure of carbon dioxide in alveolar gas is essentially the same as that in arterial blood (Pa_{CO_2}), the relationship can also be expressed:

$$\dot{V}_{CO_2} = \dot{V}\bar{A} \times Pa_{CO_2} \times \text{a constant}$$

This equation indicates that in a steady state the arterial P_{CO_2} is regulated by the balance between metabolic activity and alveolar ventilation.

Alveolar Hypoventilation. A fall in the overall level of ventilation can reduce alveolar ventilation below that required by the metabolic activity of the body. Under this condition of alveolar hypoventilation (Plate 17), the rate at which oxygen is added to alveolar gas and carbon dioxide is eliminated to the atmosphere is lowered so that the alveolar P_{O_2} falls and the alveolar P_{CO_2} rises. As a result of this derangement, pulmonary capillary blood is less well oxygenated, and the arterial P_{O_2} falls below normal values. Similarly, less carbon dioxide is removed from pulmonary capillary blood than is produced by tissue metabolism, so that arterial P_{CO_2} rises above the normal range.

Alveolar hypoventilation can occur during severe disorders of the lung and following injury to the chest cage. It can also result when the central nervous system is depressed by the administration of narcotics, sedatives and anesthetics, and consequent to disorders of the brain such as stroke, meningitis and increased intracranial pressure. Even when central respiratory activity is normal, neuromuscular disorders that affect the respiratory muscles such as polyneuritis, myasthenia gravis and polymyositis can reduce the level of ventilation and cause alveolar hypoventilation.

Alveolar Gas Composition. The adequacy of gas exchange in the lung is determined from the arterial P_{O_2} and P_{CO_2}. If ventilation and pulmonary blood flow were evenly and uniformly distributed to all the gas exchange units in the lung and there were no barriers to diffusion across the alveolar-capillary membrane, partial pressures of oxygen and carbon dioxide in arterial blood and alveolar gas would be identical. Because of regional variations in distribution of both ventilation and

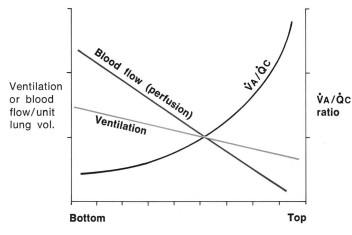

Ventilation or blood flow/unit lung vol.

Blood flow (perfusion)

Ventilation

$\dot{V}A/\dot{Q}C$

$\dot{V}A/\dot{Q}C$ ratio

Bottom **Top**

Both ventilation and blood flow are gravity-dependent and decrease from bottom to top of lung. Gradient of blood flow is steeper than that of ventilation so that ventilation-perfusion ratio increases up lung

blood flow in the lung, however, this ideal condition is not encountered. Differences in partial pressures between alveolar gas and arterial blood, which reflect the degree of inefficiency of gas exchange, are found normally and are exaggerated by diseases of the lungs. Thus, a thorough evaluation of gas exchange necessitates the determination of both alveolar and arterial gas tensions.

During quiet breathing, the end-tidal portion of an exhaled breath is considered to consist of alveolar gas. In normal individuals, particularly at rest, P_{O_2} and P_{CO_2} in an end-tidal sample approximate the mean alveolar values. But in the presence of lung disease, when ventilation and

blood flow in the lung are not evenly matched, alveolar gas composition will vary markedly among gas-exchanging units. Since well-ventilated alveoli empty early while poorly-ventilated lung units empty late, significant changes in expired P_{O_2} and P_{CO_2} continue throughout expiration, and a single sample of end-tidal gas may not reflect the mean alveolar gas composition.

Mean alveolar P_{O_2} and P_{CO_2} can be determined indirectly. Because of the great solubility of carbon dioxide, it is assumed that arterial P_{CO_2} approximates ideal alveolar P_{CO_2}. Alveolar P_{O_2}

(Continued)

Pulmonary Mechanics and Gas Exchange
(*Continued*)

($P_{A_{O_2}}$) can be calculated according to the alveolar air equation

$$P_{A_{O_2}} = F_{I_{O_2}} (P_B - P_{A_{H_2O}}) - P_{A_{CO_2}} \left[F_{I_{O_2}} + \frac{1 - F_{I_{O_2}}}{R} \right]$$

where $F_{I_{O_2}}$ is the inspired oxygen fraction, P_B is the atmospheric pressure, and $P_{A_{H_2O}}$ is the alveolar water tension, both expressed in mm Hg. The equation simply states that the alveolar P_{O_2} is determined from the difference between the inspired P_{O_2} and the alveolar P_{CO_2}, with a correction when the respiratory exchange ratio (R) is different from unity.

Ventilation-Perfusion Relationships (Plate 18). Efficient gas exchange requires that both ventilation and blood flow be distributed uniformly and in appropriate proportions to each of the numerous gas-exchanging units in the lung. Overall, the ratio of alveolar ventilation to pulmonary capillary blood flow ($\dot{V}_A/\dot{Q}_C$) is about 0.8. Under these circumstances the $P_{A_{O_2}}$ is approximately 100 mm Hg and the $P_{A_{CO_2}}$ is 40 mm Hg.

When an individual is in the upright position, ventilation decreases from the bottom to the top of the lung. Pulmonary blood flow also decreases from the bottom to the top of the lung, but the change in blood flow is greater than the change in ventilation. Consequently, the ratio of alveolar ventilation to pulmonary blood flow progressively increases from the base to the apex of the lung.

Alveolar ventilation to the apical alveoli at the top of the lung is three times greater than blood flow; *i.e.*, ($\dot{V}_A/\dot{Q}_C$) is 3. Oxygen uptake by the capillary blood becomes limited by the rate of pulmonary blood flow and is reduced. Carbon dioxide output, however, is increased as more carbon dioxide is extracted from each unit of blood flow. As a result, the local respiratory exchange ratio at the top of the lung exceeds 1, the alveolar P_{CO_2} is less, and the alveolar P_{O_2} is greater than the ideal values.

At the base of the lungs, alveolar ventilation is less than pulmonary capillary blood flow, and $\dot{V}_A/\dot{Q}_C$ is approximately 0.6. The relative hypoventilation reduces the local carbon dioxide output more than oxygen uptake, and the respiratory exchange ratio falls. Consequently, at the bottom of the lung the $P_{A_{CO_2}}$ rises and the $P_{A_{O_2}}$ falls as compared to ideal levels.

The normal differences in regional $\dot{V}_A/\dot{Q}_C$ throughout the lung are relatively small and cause only minor derangements in gas exchange. Diseases of the ventilatory system, however, produce more extreme variations in $\dot{V}_A/\dot{Q}_C$ because of abnormalities in airway resistance, lung compliance and blood vessel caliber. In disease, $\dot{V}_A/\dot{Q}_C$ in the lung may range from zero to infinity, markedly reducing the efficiency of gas exchange and causing hypoxemia.

There are hundreds of thousands of gas-exchanging units, but for the purposes of simplification it is convenient to use a two-compartment model of the lung to illustrate the effects of alterations of the $\dot{V}_A/\dot{Q}_C$ relationship on gas exchange.

Abnormalities in the distribution of ventilation can result from bronchial narrowing that causes one lung unit to receive only a fraction of the ventilation of the other unit. When pulmonary blood flow is evenly distributed, the $\dot{V}_A/\dot{Q}_C$ of the poorly ventilated but well-perfused lung unit is low as compared to the normal lung unit. The poorly ventilated compartment will have a lower alveolar and end-capillary P_{O_2} and a higher P_{CO_2} than the unit with a normal $\dot{V}_A/\dot{Q}_C$. If the level of ventilation to the abnormal lung unit were to fall to zero, the end-capillary P_{O_2} and P_{CO_2} would approximate that in mixed venous blood. The mean alveolar gas composition is determined algebraically from the amount of ventilation and the alveolar P_{O_2} and P_{CO_2} of each compartment. If the poorly ventilated lung unit has an alveolar P_{O_2} of 60 mm Hg and receives only one-third of the ventilation of the normal lung unit with a $P_{A_{O_2}}$ of 100 mm Hg, the mean alveolar P_{O_2} will be $\frac{(3 \times 100) + 60}{4}$, or 90 mm Hg. Similarly, a normal lung unit with a $P_{A_{CO_2}}$ of 40 mm Hg and a poorly ventilated unit receiving only one-third as much ventilation and having a $P_{A_{CO_2}}$ of 44 mm Hg will produce a mean alveolar P_{CO_2} $\frac{(3 \times 40) + 44}{4}$, or 41 mm Hg.

Because of the alinear characteristics of the oxyhemoglobin dissociation curve, the overall arterial P_{O_2} cannot be determined directly from the mean end-capillary P_{O_2} of the two lung units. It is necessary first to ascertain the average oxygen content or saturation of the end-capillary blood of the two compartments. The oxygen saturation of the end-capillary blood from the poorly ventilated unit with a P_{O_2} of 60 mm Hg is approximately 90%. End-capillary blood from the normal unit with a P_{O_2} of 100 mm Hg is 98% saturated with oxygen. The mixed arterial blood thus will have an oxygen saturation of $\frac{90 + 98}{2}$, or 94%. According to the oxyhemoglobin dissociation curve, this represents a $P_{a_{O_2}}$ of approximately 70 mm Hg at normal pH and temperature.

Although the carbon dioxide dissociation curve is also curvilinear throughout its entire range—between P_{CO_2} of 40 mm Hg, the arterial value, and P_{CO_2} of 46 mm Hg, the mixed venous value—it is essentially linear. Therefore, mixed arterial P_{CO_2} can be determined directly from the average P_{CO_2} of the two compartments.

Disorders of the lungs characterized by gas-exchanging units with low $\dot{V}_A/\dot{Q}_C$ produce large alveolar-arterial P_{O_2} differences, but alveolar-arterial P_{CO_2} differences remain relatively small.

The distribution of pulmonary blood flow can be affected by disorders that constrict, obstruct or obliterate pulmonary blood vessels. Lung units with markedly reduced blood flow contribute little to overall gas exchange, and alveolar gas in those poorly perfused units has a relatively high P_{O_2} and a low P_{CO_2}. When blood flow is zero, the alveolar P_{O_2} and P_{CO_2} approximate that in the conducting airways. Ventilation to poorly perfused or nonperfused alveoli is wasted insofar as it contributes little or nothing to the arterialization of mixed venous blood; therefore, that portion of ventilation is included in the physiologic dead space. The presence of high $\dot{V}_A/\dot{Q}_C$ does not directly produce arterial hypoxemia, but since the dead space is enlarged, the overall level of ventilation must be increased to maintain alveolar ventilation. High $\dot{V}_A/\dot{Q}_C$, however, results in large alveolar-arterial P_{CO_2} differences.

Shunts (Plate 19). Blood flowing through bronchial veins, which empty directly into pulmonary veins, and through thebesian veins of the ventricular myocardium, which drain into the left ventricle, constitute right-to-left shunts carrying up to 5% of the cardiac output. Right-to-left shunting of blood is increased in the presence of abnormal anatomic pathways such as intracardiac septal defects and pulmonary arteriovenous fistulas. Moreover, blood flowing through regions of the lung with $\dot{V}_A/\dot{Q}_C$ of zero is also considered a right-to-left shunt. This particular condition occurs when gas-exchanging units perfused by pulmonary capillary blood receive absolutely no ventilation because of bronchial obstruction or atelectasis, or because the alveoli are filled with fluid or inflammatory secretions.

Right-to-left shunting of blood results in the admixture of venous blood (P_{O_2} 40 mm Hg, P_{CO_2} 46 mm Hg) with properly arterialized end-capillary blood (P_{O_2} 100 mm Hg, P_{CO_2} 40 mm Hg). The major consequence is a fall in the overall arterial P_{O_2}. Changes in arterial P_{CO_2} tend to be insignificant because the difference between mixed venous and arterialized end-capillary P_{CO_2} is small. Furthermore, any increase in arterial P_{CO_2} stimulates respiratory chemoreceptors to increase the level of ventilation and to restore the $P_{a_{CO_2}}$ to normal values.

True right-to-left shunting can be distinguished from $\dot{V}_A/\dot{Q}_C$ abnormalities, and the magnitude of the shunt can be determined from the alveolar-arterial P_{O_2} difference during 100% oxygen-breathing. After a sufficient period of oxygen-breathing, nitrogen is removed from even

(Continued)

Pulmonary Mechanics and Gas Exchange
(Continued)

the most poorly ventilated regions of the lung and replaced with oxygen. The alveoli thus contain only oxygen ($P_{A_{O_2}}$ about 673 mm Hg) and carbon dioxide ($P_{A_{CO_2}}$ about 40 mm Hg). Pulmonary capillary blood perfusing both normal and poorly ventilated gas-exchanging units becomes oxygenated and achieves a P_{O_2} virtually the same as that in alveolar gas. Mixed venous blood passing through shunt channels and pulmonary capillary blood which fails entirely to come into contact with alveolar gas enter the arterial system and lower the overall arterial P_{O_2}, producing an alveolar-arterial P_{O_2} difference.

The fraction of the cardiac output that constitutes the right-to-left shunt can be calculated from the shunt equation

$$\dot{Q}s/\dot{Q}t = \frac{Cc_{O_2} - Ca_{O_2}}{Cc_{O_2} - C\bar{v}_{O_2}}$$

where $\dot{Q}s$ is shunt flow, $\dot{Q}t$ is total cardiac output, and Cc_{O_2}, Ca_{O_2} and $C\bar{v}_{O_2}$ are the oxygen content of end-capillary blood, arterial blood and mixed venous blood, respectively. In general, the oxygen content of blood can be calculated from the P_{O_2}. The end-capillary P_{O_2} is considered equal to the alveolar P_{O_2}. Mixed venous P_{O_2} can be measured directly or determined by assuming an arterial-venous oxygen content of 5 ml/100 ml.

Oxygen Transport

Oxygen diffuses from the alveoli of the lungs into the plasma of pulmonary capillary blood and then enters the red blood cells. Oxygen is carried in the blood in two ways: in physical solution in plasma and in chemical combination with hemoglobin in the red blood cell (Plate 20).

Physical Solution. The amount of oxygen dissolved in plasma is determined by its solubility and is directly proportional to the partial pressure of oxygen in the plasma. Arterial blood with a P_{O_2} of 100 mm Hg contains 0.30 ml of oxygen in solution in each 100 ml of plasma, while mixed venous blood with a P_{O_2} of 40 mm Hg contains only 0.12 ml of dissolved oxygen per 100 ml of plasma. The difference in the amounts of oxygen dissolved in arterial and mixed venous blood reflects the quantity of oxygen given up to the peripheral tissues by the plasma. This volume is clearly inadequate to meet the metabolic needs of the peripheral tissues.

Chemical Combination with Hemoglobin. Over 60 times more oxygen is carried in the blood in chemical combination with hemoglobin. The amount of oxygen combined with hemoglobin varies with the partial pressure of oxygen in a

Shunts

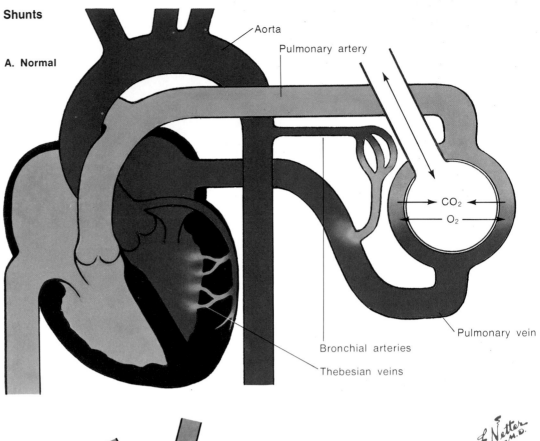

A. Normal

Aorta
Pulmonary artery
CO_2
O_2
Pulmonary vein
Bronchial arteries
Thebesian veins

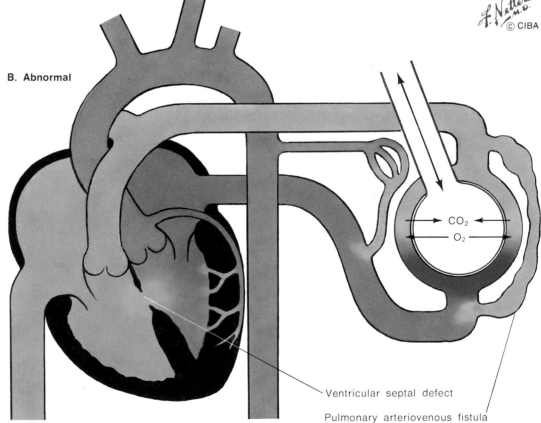

B. Abnormal

CO_2
O_2
Ventricular septal defect
Pulmonary arteriovenous fistula

nonlinear fashion. The relationship between the amount of oxygen combined with hemoglobin and the partial pressure of oxygen in the blood is described by the sigmoid-shaped oxyhemoglobin dissociation curve. The maximal amount of oxygen that can combine with 1 g hemoglobin is 1.34 ml. Assuming a hemoglobin concentration of 15 g Hb/100 ml of blood, the total amount of oxygen in combination with hemoglobin would be 15×1.34, or 20.1 ml O_2/100 ml blood. This represents the oxygen capacity of hemoglobin. The actual amount of oxygen in chemical combination with hemoglobin in relation to the maximal amount of oxygen the hemoglobin can carry is

referred to as the percentage saturation ($S_{O_2}\%$), and can be expressed according to the equation:

$$\text{Oxygen saturation}(\%) = \frac{\text{oxygen combined with hemoglobin}}{\text{oxygen capacity}} \times 100$$

The oxygen saturation of arterial blood with a P_{O_2} of 100 mm Hg is approximately 98%, while that of venous blood with a P_{O_2} of 40 mm Hg is 75%.

Oxyhemoglobin Dissociation Curve. The physiologic advantages of the affinity of hemoglobin for oxygen are illustrated by the oxyhemoglobin dissociation curve. The upper, flat portion
(Continued)

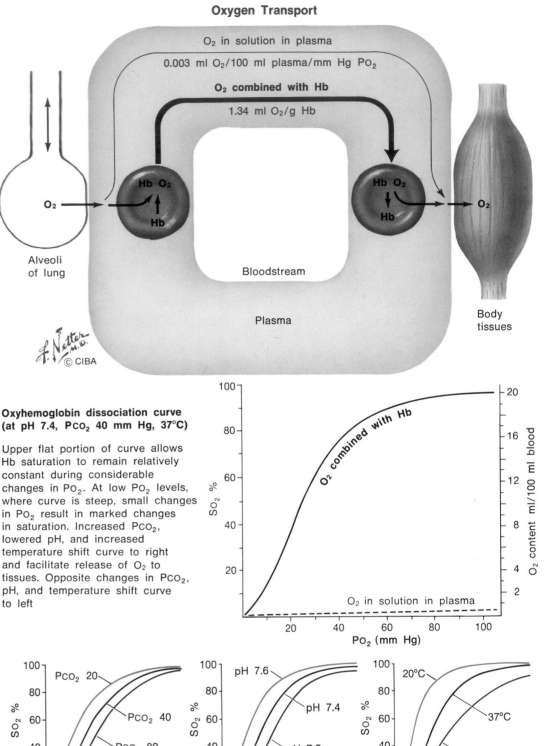

Oxygen Transport

Pulmonary Mechanics and Gas Exchange
(Continued)

of the curve ensures that the arterial oxygen content remains high and relatively constant despite considerable reductions in the oxygen tension of the blood that may result from cardiopulmonary disorders or travel at high altitude. In the periphery, as oxygen in solution leaves the systemic capillary blood and enters the tissues, the P_{O_2} of the blood falls. The middle, steep portion of the oxyhemoglobin dissociation curve allows the release of large quantities of oxygen from hemoglobin at the lowered oxygen tension in the capillary blood to meet the metabolic requirements of the tissues.

Any alteration in the ability of hemoglobin to bind oxygen is reflected in a change in position of the oxyhemoglobin dissociation curve. A decrease in the affinity of hemoglobin for oxygen results in a shift of the curve to the right. This effect is produced by increases in temperature, intracellular hydrogen ion concentration and P_{CO_2}. In the systemic capillaries, where carbon dioxide is added to the blood, the ensuing rise in hydrogen ion concentration and in carbamino compounds decreases oxygen affinity and facilitates the release of oxygen to the peripheral tissues.

An increase in the affinity of hemoglobin for oxygen is seen when temperature is reduced and when the intracellular hydrogen ion concentration and P_{CO_2} are lowered. The result is a shift of the oxyhemoglobin dissociation curve to the left. This is the condition existing in the lung, where the hydrogen ion concentration in the blood falls as carbon dioxide passes into the alveoli; the resulting increase in affinity for oxygen enhances its uptake by hemoglobin in the pulmonary capillaries. The position of the dissociation curve can be determined by measuring the arterial oxygen tension corresponding to 50% saturation of hemoglobin. This normally occurs at about 26 mm Hg, and is known as the P 50 value.

The affinity of hemoglobin for oxygen is also influenced by the presence in the red blood cell of 2,3-diphosphoglycerate (DPG). This organic phosphate, an intermediate product of anaerobic glycolysis, decreases the affinity of hemoglobin for oxygen and promotes the increased release of oxygen that takes place in the peripheral tissues. The amount of DPG in red blood cells is increased when tissue oxygen delivery is compromised by anemia or hypoxemia, and thus serves an important adaptive function in maintaining tissue oxygenation.

Acid-Base Regulation

Since metabolically produced acid is largely eliminated from the body via the lungs in the form

Oxyhemoglobin dissociation curve (at pH 7.4, P_{CO_2} 40 mm Hg, 37°C)

Upper flat portion of curve allows Hb saturation to remain relatively constant during considerable changes in P_{O_2}. At low P_{O_2} levels, where curve is steep, small changes in P_{O_2} result in marked changes in saturation. Increased P_{CO_2}, lowered pH, and increased temperature shift curve to right and facilitate release of O_2 to tissues. Opposite changes in P_{CO_2}, pH, and temperature shift curve to left

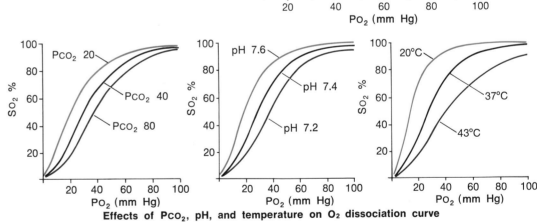

Effects of P_{CO_2}, pH, and temperature on O_2 dissociation curve

of carbon dioxide, the respiratory system is of great importance in acid-base regulation (Plate 21).

Carbon dioxide is carried in the blood in a number of ways. In both plasma and red cells some carbon dioxide is physically dissolved in an amount dependent on the partial pressure. Dissolved carbon dioxide is hydrated to form carbonic acid:

$$CO_2 + H_2O \rightleftharpoons H_2CO_3$$

The equilibrium of this reaction in the plasma is such that the concentration of carbon dioxide remains about 1000 times greater than that of carbonic acid. The red blood cells, however, contain

carbonic anhydrase, which catalyzes the hydration reaction in the red blood cell so that carbonic acid is formed at a much higher rate. Carbonic acid dissociates to form hydrogen ion (H^+) and bicarbonate ion (HCO_3^-). Since large quantities of bicarbonate are formed in the red blood cell and relatively little in the plasma, a concentration gradient is established, and bicarbonate diffuses out of the cells into the plasma. In addition, carbon dioxide is carried in the red blood cell bound to hemoglobin as carbamino-hemoglobin.

The hydrogen ion concentration in the blood is determined by the relationship between dissolved

(Continued)

Role of Lungs and Kidneys in Regulation of Acid-Base Balance

Acid-base balance

Lung   Tissues   Kidney

CO_2 HCO_3^-

Acidosis

Respiratory
Lung disease
Sedatives
Neuromuscular disorders
Brain damage

CO_2 HCO_3^-

CO_2 HCO_3^-

Metabolic
Adds acid:
Diabetes
Uremia
Lactic acidosis
Loses base:
Diarrhea

Alkalosis

Respiratory
Hyperventilation
Fever
Anxiety
Brain disorders

CO_2 HCO_3^-

CO_2 HCO_3^-

Metabolic
Adds base:
Alkali ingestion
Loses acid:
Diuretics
Vomiting
Gastric suction

Pulmonary Mechanics and Gas Exchange
(*Continued*)

carbon dioxide, which is dependent on the P_{CO_2}, and the bicarbonate ion concentration $\left([HCO_3^-]\right)$. This relationship is illustrated by the Henderson-Hasselbalch equation:

$$pH = pK + \log \frac{[HCO_3^-]}{0.03\ P_{CO_2}}$$

Variations in the ratio of $[HCO_3^-]$ and P_{CO_2} produced by either metabolic or respiratory disturbances result in changes in pH from the normal value of 7.4, leading to *acidemia* (*i.e.,* low pH and high hydrogen ion concentration) or to *alkalemia* (*i.e.,* high pH and low hydrogen ion concentration). The arterial P_{CO_2} is a measure of the *respiratory* component while $[HCO_3^-]$ defines the *metabolic* or nonrespiratory contribution to the acid-base status. It is also possible to measure hydrogen ion concentration directly. The normal value in blood is 35 to 45 nm/liter.

Respiratory Disturbances. Respiratory acidosis is seen with alveolar hypoventilation and is characterized by an elevated P_{CO_2} and a low pH. Alveolar hypoventilation can occur when central nervous system function is depressed by sedatives, narcotics and anesthetic agents; as a consequence of disorders of the brain; and when diseases affect the respiratory neuromuscular apparatus. Patients with severe lung disease, in whom the physiologic dead space is markedly increased, may also develop alveolar hypoventilation even though the overall level of ventilation remains normal.

Persistent carbon dioxide retention and acidosis alters the renal threshold and promotes the renal retention of bicarbonate. This compensatory action, which reaches maximal levels in five to seven days, increases the bicarbonate ion concentration and tends to restore the pH toward normal values, even though the P_{CO_2} remains unchanged.

Respiratory alkalosis results from alveolar hyperventilation. The excessive output of carbon dioxide leads to hypocapnia, which elevates the pH. Hyperventilation is seen in excessively anxious or apprehensive individuals, and also occurs secondary to fever and following the ingestion of drugs such as aspirin which act as respiratory stimulants. Certain disorders of the central nervous system that interfere with respiratory control mechanisms produce hyperventilation. In early stages of cardiopulmonary disorders, stimulation of pulmonary mechanoreceptors as well as hypoxemia can stimulate ventilation and induce respiratory alkalosis.

Renal adjustments to chronic respiratory alkalosis involve the excretion of bicarbonate ions by the kidney. Within several days, the bicarbonate ion concentration falls, and despite the persistence of hypocapnia the pH is restored to virtually normal values.

Metabolic Disturbances. Metabolic acidosis is due to an accumulation of nonvolatile acids or to a loss of bicarbonate. Levels of nonvolatile acids are increased in diabetes, uremia and shock, while loss of bicarbonate occurs in chronic renal insufficiency and with diarrhea. The resultant increase in hydrogen ion concentration is a strong respiratory stimulant. As the level of ventilation rises, the arterial P_{CO_2} falls and the change in pH is minimized.

Excessive loss of nonvolatile acids or increases in bicarbonate levels produce *metabolic alkalosis*. Circumstances under which this occurs include prolonged vomiting or gastric suction, ingestion of alkali or administration of thiazide diuretics; these elevate the bicarbonate ion concentration and raise the pH. Since respiratory drive is diminished as the bicarbonate concentration rises and hydrogen ion accumulation falls, ventilation is reduced and the P_{CO_2} increases. These respiratory compensatory mechanisms, although relatively weak, lessen the change in pH. Accelerated renal excretion of bicarbonate also serves to restore acid-base balance toward normal.

Response to Oxidant Injury

Pulmonary Defenses Against Oxidant and Other Noxious Injuries

Inhaled
High O$_2$
Ozone (O$_3$)
NO$_2$
Phosgene

Bloodborne
Busulfan
Thiourea
Oleic acid

Type I cells
Damaged or destroyed (more susceptible to injury)

Type II cells
Proliferated (resistance increased to high oxidant exposure)

Proliferation

May form new type I cells

F. Netter
© CIBA

Glycolysis

Glucose → Glucose-6-P

G-6-PD

Pentose shunt
6-P-gluconate

6-P-GD → CO$_2$

Ribulose-5-P

Activation

Oxidant injury

Lactate ↔ Pyruvate

Oxalacetate

Malate → H$^+$

H$^+$ → NADPH → NADP

Oxidized glutathione → Reduced glutathione

Hydroxy fatty acid

Fatty acid peroxide

Poly-unsaturated fatty acid

α-Tocopherol (vit. E); may protect against peroxidation

The lung is primarily designed for gas exchange between circulating blood and inhaled air. The delicate alveolar-capillary boundary where gas exchange takes place can be injured by inhaled or bloodborne noxious agents. The inhaled substances are either volatile chemicals such as phosgene, oxidants—especially oxygen at partial pressures above atmospheric—or ozone. Chemicals and a growing list of drugs reaching the lungs via the bloodstream can cause injury as well. Among the tissue components of the lung, the type I or membranous pneumocyte, the predominant cell type lining the alveoli, is most susceptible to injury. The type II cell, or granular pneumocyte, proliferates in response to injury in an apparent effort to repair the damage and replace the nonviable type I cell. A lung populated with a larger number of type II cells is more "tolerant" of continued exposure to the harmful effects of, for example, persistently high oxygen tensions.

An example of the response to injury of the lung by noxious agents is what happens after the inhalation of oxidants. Exposure to these compounds leads to the peroxidation of unsaturated lipids in membranes, which can eventually produce visible tissue damage. The organism defends itself against the harmful effects of oxidant injury by mobilization of antioxidants such as alpha tocopherol, or by the conversion of lipid peroxides to hydroxy compounds, a reaction that is promoted by reduced glutathione.

Animals can be made tolerant to oxygen at high partial pressures by exposure to graded increments in the oxygen content of inspired air. This acquired tolerance for oxygen may be a consequence of an increased capacity to maintain glutathione in the reduced state, an interpretation supported by the fact that the activities of enzymes necessary to maintain glutathione in the reduced state (glutathione peroxidase, glutathione reductase) and to generate the needed NADPH (nicotinamide-adenine dinucleotide phosphate) via the pentose phosphate shunt are increased in lung tissue following exposure to oxidant injury. It appears, therefore, that reduced glutathione, which is known to be important as an antioxidant in other tissues such as erythrocytes and phagocytic cells (polymorphonuclear leukocytes, alveolar macrophages), plays a similar role in the tissue components (type II cell) of the lung.

The biochemical sequelae to toxic lung damage are often not as easily defined as in the example cited in the previous paragraphs. The biochemical defects caused by agents such as paraquat, beryllium and diethylnitrosamine, which all affect the lung adversely, have not been identified.

Manifestations of toxic lung damage are frequently not immediately apparent. They may be obscured by rapid repair with proliferation of tissue components, lack of easily detectable biochemical sequelae and the remarkable "reserve" capacity of the lung for gas exchange.

Serotonin Metabolism

A. Normal

R. heart / L. heart

In lung, remaining circulating serotonin is taken up

In liver, most of unbound serotonin is removed

Portal vein

Serotonin from mast cells and other tissue components enters portal blood

Remainder of circulation; relatively free of unbound serotonin

B. Carcinoid tumor

R. heart / L. heart

Lung; incapable of removing excess serotonin

Liver; metastatic carcinoid tumor adds to serotonin production

Portal vein

Gut; carcinoid tumor produces large amount of serotonin

Remainder of circulation; pharmacologically active amounts of serotonin present

Serotonin, if in excess, affects endothelium of right side of heart and pulmonary artery causing pulmonary stenosis and tricuspid insufficiency

In presence of atrial septal defect, similar lesions appear in left heart

Inactivation of Circulating Vasoactive Substances

In 1924 Starling and Verney first noted in an isolated, perfused kidney preparation that vasoconstriction could be prevented if the lung was included in the perfusion system. They concluded that a vasoactive substance was removed during passage of the perfusate through the lung. The substance affecting the renal vasculature was later found to be *serotonin,* which was either removed or inactivated during its journey through the pulmonary circulation. It is now well established, in part because of the pioneering work of Vane, that the lung is intimately concerned with the inactivation and activation of circulating vasoactive substances. These intrapulmonary reactions contribute to the control of peripheral vascular resistance and the "reconditioning" of blood before reentry into the arterial system. The structure of the lung and its location within the circulatory system are eminently suited to fulfilling this role. Here, the entire blood volume has to pass through a single vascular bed and, although the intrapulmonary blood volume at any given moment is small (± 60 ml), it is exposed to a large vascular surface area (± 70 m^2), allowing intimate contact between substances within the blood and the endothelial cells.

The fate of serotonin in the lung is one example of the interaction between circulating vasoactive substances and the endothelium of the pulmonary vasculature. Serotonin (5-hydroxytryptamine) is a potent neurotransmitter which affects the microcirculation in various areas of the body. It is generated in many tissues, with mast cells having the highest production rate. Only a small fraction normally circulates free in the blood, most of the serotonin being bound by thrombocytes. The pharmacologic action of this amine varies from tissue to tissue. In the lung it causes bronchoconstriction.

Serotonin produced in the gastrointestinal tract reaches the liver via the portal circulation. In the liver it is converted by means of a reaction that involves monoamine oxidase to 5-hydroxyindoleacetic acid, a freely diffusible and water-

soluble substance that does not have any known pharmacologic actions. Trace amounts of "free" serotonin in blood reaching the lung are effectively removed by uptake into endothelial cells. This process is apparently dependent on a carrier mechanism which is saturable and requires sodium to be maximally effective. Following its uptake by tissue components of the lung, serotonin is oxidized to 5-hydroxyindoleacetic acid.

Excessive production of serotonin, or the appearance of serotonin-releasing tumor tissue (carcinoid) beyond the liver, will lead to "overflow" of the amine into the hepatic veins and inferior vena cava. The amount of serotonin reaching the lung

under these circumstances may exceed the capacity of the intrapulmonary removal system. Prolonged exposure of the endothelium of the pulmonary vasculature to excess serotonin leads to structural changes in the right side of the heart and large pulmonary vessels. The mechanism underlying these structural changes remains unknown. That the changes are caused by serotonin and not by its metabolites is suggested by the intriguing observation that in the presence of an atrial septal defect with a right-to-left shunt, when larger quantities of serotonin can "overflow" into the systemic circulation, structural changes also develop in the left side of the heart.

Activation of Circulating Precursors of Vasoactive Substances

Renin-Angiotensin System

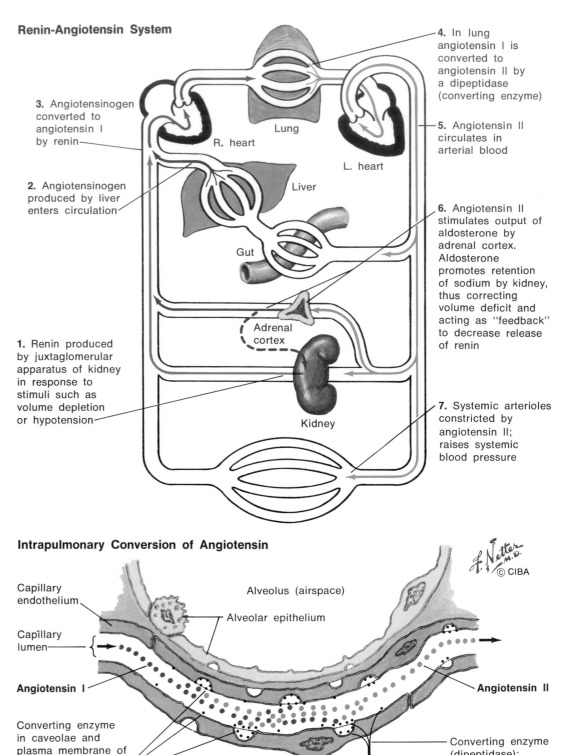

3. Angiotensinogen converted to angiotensin I by renin

2. Angiotensinogen produced by liver enters circulation

Lung

R. heart

L. heart

Liver

Gut

Adrenal cortex

Kidney

1. Renin produced by juxtaglomerular apparatus of kidney in response to stimuli such as volume depletion or hypotension

4. In lung angiotensin I is converted to angiotensin II by a dipeptidase (converting enzyme)

5. Angiotensin II circulates in arterial blood

6. Angiotensin II stimulates output of aldosterone by adrenal cortex. Aldosterone promotes retention of sodium by kidney, thus correcting volume deficit and acting as "feedback" to decrease release of renin

7. Systemic arterioles constricted by angiotensin II; raises systemic blood pressure

Intrapulmonary Conversion of Angiotensin

Capillary endothelium

Alveolus (airspace)

Alveolar epithelium

Capillary lumen

Angiotensin I

Angiotensin II

Converting enzyme in caveolae and plasma membrane of pulmonary vascular endothelium

Converting enzyme (dipeptidase); acts on angiotensin I and other polypeptides (bradykinin) at the phenylalanine-histidine bond

Angiotensin I

| Asp. | Arg. | Val. | Tyr. | Ileu. | His. | Pro. | Phe. | His. | Leu. |

Angiotensin II

| Asp. | Arg. | Val. | Tyr. | Ileu. | His. | Pro. | Phe. |

The fate of angiotensin in the lung is a paradigm for the conversion of an inactive precursor into a vasoactive substance. Angiotensin II, the most potent vasoconstrictor known, is derived from angiotensin I. This conversion is part of a more complex feedback loop originating in the kidneys where, in response to stimuli such as volume depletion or hypotension, renin is released into the bloodstream. Renin is a protease that acts on angiotensinogen (renin substrate), a globulin produced by the liver. The product of the interaction is a decapeptide, angiotensin I. This polypeptide, in turn, is exposed to a dipeptidase (converting enzyme, kininase II) at the endothelial surface of the pulmonary vessels. Kininase II cleaves off two amino acids by acting on a phenyl-alanine-histidine bond, a reaction that requires the presence of chloride ions. The resultant octapeptide, angiotensin II, acts on systemic arterioles to raise peripheral vascular resistance. In addition, the polypeptide promotes the release of aldosterone from the adrenal cortex. The hormone is carried via the bloodstream to the kidneys, where it promotes the retention of sodium for correction of the original intravascular volume deficit. This action completes the feedback loop initiated by volume depletion or hypotension.

Angiotensin II has a short half-life and is inactivated by angiotensinases, which have been identified in many tissues, by cleavage of additional amino acids.

The converting enzyme, which is located within or adjacent to the so-called caveolae (small indentations on the endothelial surface layer of pulmonary capillaries), has been isolated and purified. The enzyme also acts on another circulating vasoactive polypeptide, bradykinin, a nonapeptide that tends to lower systemic blood pressure. However, in contrast to the situation with angiotensin I, cleavage of amino acids from bradykinin abolishes its vasoactive properties.

Converting enzyme has been identified by means of fluorescein-labeled antibodies in the endothelium of blood vessels in many organs other than the lung (liver, spleen, kidneys, pancreas). Thus the presence of converting enzyme is not unique to the lung, although the structural arrangement in the lung does allow maximal conversion of angiotensin I to angiotensin II. The unique feature of the process in the lung is the efficiency of the enzymatic reaction due to the strategic location of the enzyme within the pulmonary vasculature, where a small volume of blood is exposed to a large surface area prior to reentry into the high-pressure arterial system.

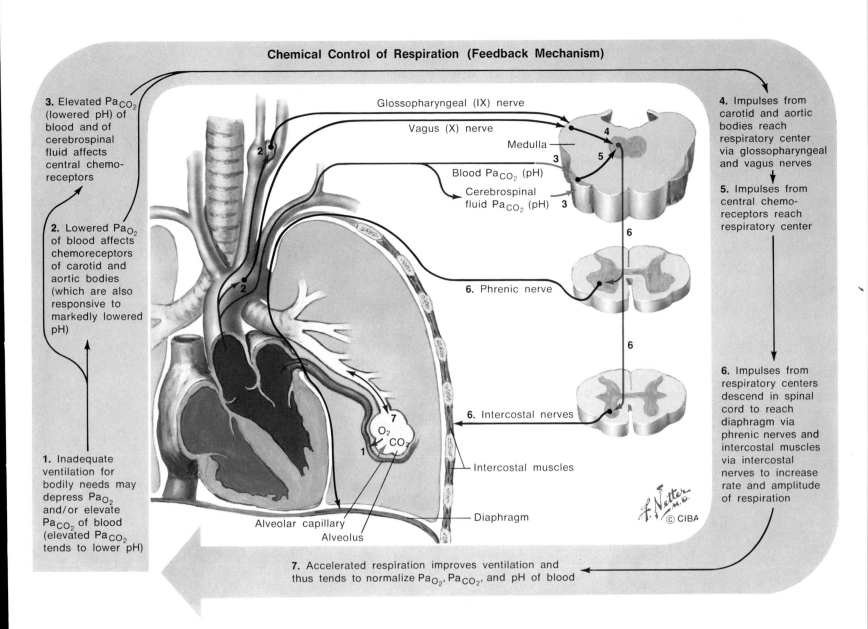

Chemical Control of Respiration (Feedback Mechanism)

3. Elevated Pa_{CO_2} (lowered pH) of blood and of cerebrospinal fluid affects central chemo-receptors

2. Lowered Pa_{O_2} of blood affects chemoreceptors of carotid and aortic bodies (which are also responsive to markedly lowered pH)

1. Inadequate ventilation for bodily needs may depress Pa_{O_2} and/or elevate Pa_{CO_2} of blood (elevated Pa_{CO_2} tends to lower pH)

Glossopharyngeal (IX) nerve

Vagus (X) nerve

Medulla

Blood Pa_{CO_2} (pH)

Cerebrospinal fluid Pa_{CO_2} (pH)

6. Phrenic nerve

6. Intercostal nerves

O_2 CO_2

Intercostal muscles

Alveolar capillary

Alveolus

Diaphragm

4. Impulses from carotid and aortic bodies reach respiratory center via glossopharyngeal and vagus nerves

5. Impulses from central chemo-receptors reach respiratory center

6. Impulses from respiratory centers descend in spinal cord to reach diaphragm via phrenic nerves and intercostal muscles via intercostal nerves to increase rate and amplitude of respiration

7. Accelerated respiration improves ventilation and thus tends to normalize Pa_{O_2}, Pa_{CO_2}, and pH of blood

Control and Disorders of Respiration

Chemical Control of Respiration

Changes in arterial blood gas tension or pH or in the interstitial fluid of the brain cause changes in ventilation that tend to restore gas tension and pH to their usual levels. These compensatory variations in ventilation depend on the normal operation of a negative feedback control system. This system continually samples the pH and Po_2 of the arterial blood and the pH of the interstitial fluid of the brain and adjusts nervous output and ventilation appropriately to maintain blood and body tensions of Pco_2 and Po_2.

Two types of receptors sample changes in arterial blood: (1) those in the vicinity of the bifurcation of the carotid artery into its internal and external branches, which send signals to the brain via the ninth cranial nerve, and (2) those in the aortic arch, which signal the brain through the tenth nerve. The receptors seem to respond directly to changes in arterial Po_2. If the receptors are removed, hypoxia exerts a depressant effect on central neurons and decreases ventilation.

Changes in ventilation caused by hypercapnia seem to depend largely on alterations in cerebrospinal fluid (CSF) and brain interstitial fluid hydrogen ion concentration. Receptors located in the ventrolateral surface of the medulla account for approximately 80% of the increase in ventilation produced when carbon dioxide is inhaled; the carotid artery and possibly the aortic bodies are responsible for the remaining 20%.

The carbon dioxide and oxygen receptors, together with the respiratory neurons themselves, make up the respiratory controller, which regulates ventilation by determining the movement of the thoracic chest bellows—*i.e.,* the lungs, rib cage and inspiratory and expiratory muscles. The respiratory controller also seems to interconnect with other neurons involved in circulatory regulation, and thus allows for coordinated changes in oxygen delivery and carbon dioxide removal from tissues in the face of changing metabolic or environmental conditions. The thoracic bellows and the tissue stores of oxygen and carbon dioxide in physical solution and chemical combination make up the controlled portion of the respiratory regulation system.

If the chest bellows are operating normally, the adequacy of the respiratory controller function can be tested by measuring variations in ventilation produced by different inspired gas concentrations of carbon dioxide and oxygen and relating these changes to alterations in arterial Po_2 and Pco_2. Ventilation increases linearly with a rise in arterial Pco_2, and the slope of the line relating ventilation to arterial carbon dioxide tension is considered to be a measure of respiratory sensitivity to the carbon dioxide stimulus. The slope varies widely in men and women. The usual range is 2 to 5 liters per minute for 1 mm Hg change in arterial Pco_2.

Metabolic acidosis increases ventilation whereas metabolic alkalosis decreases it. Changes in CSF and brain interstitial fluid pH and bicarbonate concentration in steady state metabolic acidosis and alkalosis are less than the changes in plasma pH and bicarbonate concentration.

Ventilation increases hyperbolically as arterial Po_2 declines. Hypoxic ventilatory sensitivity is usually expressed as a change in ventilation for a given change in hypoxic stimulus after linearizing the stimulus–response relationship. A linear relationship is obtained by plotting ventilation against arterial oxygen saturation or against the reciprocal of Pa_{O_2} minus a constant. There is a wide variation in hypoxic sensitivity between the sexes.

Acute hypoxia stimulates ventilation, the increase being approximately hyperbolic as the intensity of hypoxia rises from a Pa_{O_2} of 100 to 40 mm Hg. Since increased ventilation lowers Pa_{CO_2}, the CO_2^--H^+ drive to ventilation is diminished during this stage. This lessened drive can be demonstrated by maintaining Pa_{CO_2} constant during hypoxia. The effect of normocapnic hypoxia is greater than the effect of hypoxia alone. The

(Continued)

Neural Control of Breathing

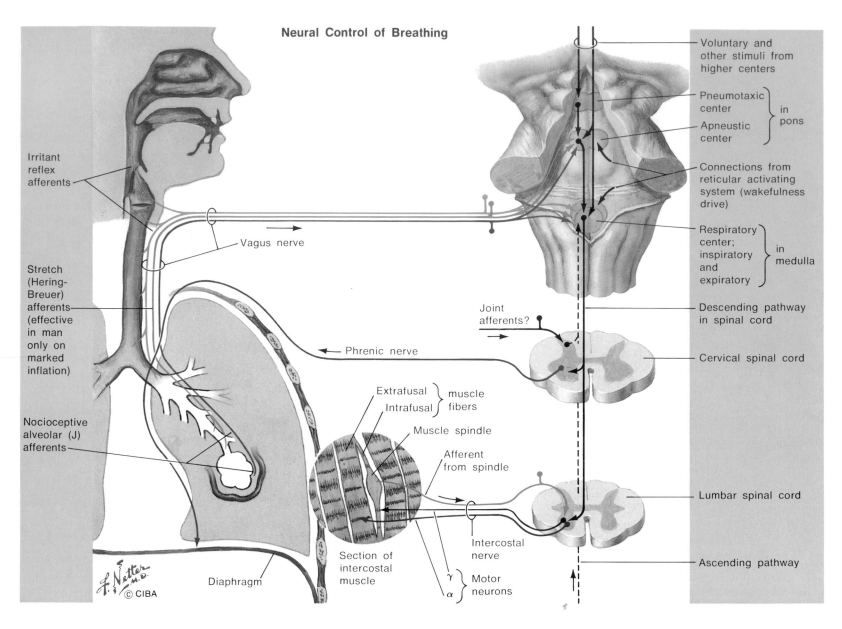

Labels in figure:

Irritant reflex afferents

Stretch (Hering-Breuer) afferents (effective in man only on marked inflation)

Nocioceptive alveolar (J) afferents

Vagus nerve

Diaphragm

Section of intercostal muscle

Extrafusal / Intrafusal muscle fibers

Muscle spindle

Afferent from spindle

Joint afferents?

Phrenic nerve

Intercostal nerve

γ / α Motor neurons

Voluntary and other stimuli from higher centers

Pneumotaxic center / Apneustic center } in pons

Connections from reticular activating system (wakefulness drive)

Respiratory center; inspiratory and expiratory } in medulla

Descending pathway in spinal cord

Cervical spinal cord

Lumbar spinal cord

Ascending pathway

SECTION II   PLATE 26

Control and Disorders of Respiration
(Continued)

carotid chemoreflex is primarily responsible for the hypoxic effect on ventilation. The response of carotid chemoreceptors to hypoxia appears similar to that seen in the central controller. The ventilatory stimulation of hypoxia is abolished by a surgical denervation of the peripheral chemoreceptors.

At sea level or at high altitudes the function of ventilation is to maintain arterial blood gases at an appropriate normal level. Thus a study of arterial blood gases provides indexes for pulmonary insufficiency. The latter can arise from the lungs or from poor ventilation. At sea level hypoxemia and hypercapnia may result from poor ventilation or from mismatching of pulmonary blood flow and airflow. Hypoxemia alone can develop from problems of diffusion or as a result of anatomic or physiologic shunt. However, hypercapnia alone cannot occur unless extra oxygen is inhaled.

Some patients who experience chronic hypoxia develop a blunted ventilatory response to a fall in arterial P_{O_2}. Patients with cyanotic heart disease and adults dwelling at high altitudes exhibit this phenomenon, but it is reversible. Carbon dioxide retention and an increase in arterial P_{CO_2} are seen

when hypoventilation occurs with respect to metabolism or if physiologic dead space is enlarged. Hypoventilation may result from a loss of function of the central $CO_2^--H^+$ sensor, from disorders of medullary respiratory neurons, or from neuromuscular causes. Hyperventilation as a disease entity is rare.

Neural Control of Breathing

Breathing is mediated by the cyclic contraction and relaxation of respiratory muscles primarily controlled by groups of neurons in the pons and medulla. These respiratory neurons are operationally divided into medullary (inspiratory and expiratory), apneustic and pneumotaxic centers.

The respiratory muscles are also under voluntary control of the motor and premotor cortices, which have descending pathways in the corticospinal tract separate from the course of the involuntary control system. The two control systems converge at the segmental levels in the spinal cord for final integration. The respiratory muscles (diaphragm, intercostal and abdominal) receive efferents from the spinal neurons.

Medullary Centers. Recent investigation has established three groups of rhythmic respiratory neurons in the medulla: (1) in the region of the nucleus ambiguus (NA), (2) in the nucleus of the tractus solitarius (NTS) and (3) in the nucleus retroambiguus (NRA) in the lateral medulla at the level of the obex.

The neurons associated with the NTS belong to the dorsal respiratory group (DRG). They are mostly inspiratory cells and are divided into two subgroups: one inhibited (I alpha) and the other excited (I beta) by lung inflation. It has been suggested but not proved that the DRG is the initial intracranial integration and relay site for a number of respiratory reflexes. The afferent inputs include peripheral chemoreceptors, stretch receptors from the lungs and airways, irritant receptors and other afferents.

NA and NRA belong to the ventral respiratory groups (VRG). Both inspiratory and expiratory neurons are present in these nuclei.

VRG and DRG cells project to the contralateral spinal motor neurons. The major function of the VRG is to drive intercostal and abdominal respiratory motor neurons. DRG cells drive the phrenic motor neurons and also VRG cells. Thus it appears that DRG cells are closer in function to the rhythm generator for respiration.

Central Rhythm Generator. In mammals, no pacemaker cells whose output is independent of interaction with other cells have so far been found in the medullary center. Recent findings have not substantiated the belief that an interacting neuronal network is responsible for generating rhythmic activity of the medullary neurons. Merril showed that early-burst VRG inspiratory neurons inhibit VRG expiratory neurons.
(Continued)

76

Control and Disorders
of Respiration
(Continued)

Mitchell and Berger found inhibitory postsynaptic potential in the expiratory group but not in the VRG inspiratory cells. Although inspiratory cells seem to be the source of rhythm generation, a reciprocal active hyperpolarization of some of these cells has also been reported. Clearly, there is much uncertainty regarding the cellular basis of rhythmic breathing.

Descending Pathways. Descending fibers from the cortex fall into two categories: corticobulbar fibers to the reticular formation and corticospinal fibers to the spinal cord. These cortical pathways are located in the dorsolateral columns.

Axons from the dorsal medullary neurons descend in the contralateral ventral and lateral columns and extend to phrenic motor neurons. Descending fibers from the VRG pass primarily to contralateral intercostal spinal motor neurons. Thus, most axons from the rhythmic respiratory neurons decussate at the medullary level and travel to the contralateral motor neurons. The fibers from the inspiratory cells decussate above the obex, and those from the expiratory cells decussate below it, making a clear separation of the two pathways. This anatomic separation provides an opportunity for experimentation and often for localizing lesions leading to respiratory diseases.

Axons from the nonrhythmic respiratory neurons involved with coughing and hiccups presumably descend ipsilaterally.

Vagal Afferents. Pulmonary stretch receptors (PSR) from the respiratory bronchioles synapse with inspiratory cells of NTS. Discharge of these fibers stimulates I beta cells and inhibits I alpha cells. This seems to be the basic mechanism for terminating inspiration, although there may be other pathways. Experimentally induced stretch during expiration prolongs the expiratory phase. Although prolongation of expiration is clearly not simply a lack of inspiration, the mechanism of the expiratory effect of PSR is not known. These two effects of pulmonary stretch receptors are known as the Hering-Breuer reflex.

The strength of PSR activity needed to terminate the inspiratory phase is diminished with the progress of inspiration in a roughly all-or-nothing fashion. It is postulated that this decrease in vagal threshold is due to a matching increase in central generator activity. Vagal expiratory effect, on the other hand, is found during the first 80% of the expiratory period, and the effect is graded; *i.e.,* a stronger stretch produces a longer expiration.

Vagal threshold for both inspiration and expiration alters with the change of respiratory stimulation. Thus, during hypercapnic stimulation of tidal volume the duration of each breath is diminished rather than increased.

Thoracicoabdominal Afferents. The thoracic intercostal muscles contain numerous spindles, pacinian corpuscles and tendon end-organs, whereas the diaphragm is endowed with fewer receptors. Connections between these organs and the spinal motor neurons, which also receive descending fibers from the brain stem and cortex,

provide the basis for monitoring tidal volume or for load detection, principally through the gamma loop system. In man and animals with a strong thoracic cage, this is an appropriate reflex. The Hering-Breuer vagal reflex serves a similar purpose, although subservient to the spinal reflex in man. There is also an intersegmental reflex influence from one stimulated intercostal nerve to another in adjacent segments.

Spinal Integration. Spinal cord segments provide mechanisms for independent integration of information from the descending fibers as well as from the intrasegmental and intersegmental fibers of the spinal cord. Intracellular recording from inspiratory and expiratory motor neurons shows a reciprocal fluctuation of membrane potentials representing the summation of excitatory and inhibitory synaptic input. These are of central origin (central respiratory drive potential), but are modified considerably by local spinal reflexes. Reciprocal active depolarization and hyperpolarization preclude simultaneous contraction of both inspiratory and expiratory muscles.

Other Afferents. Vagus nerves carry a host of information from both the pulmonary and the cardiovascular systems that influences the breathing pattern. Irritant receptors in the upper airways mediate the cough reflex; aortic chemoreceptors stimulate breathing; aortic and cardiac mechanoreceptors cause feeble inhibition; J receptors from the lung parenchyma may influence breathing during pulmonary congestion. Sinus nerves convey stimulatory carotid chemoreflex and inhibitory baroreflex impulses through the glossopharyngeal nerves. Sensory endings in the fifth cranial nerve and olfactory nerves cause sneezing. Pain afferents stimulate breathing, as do joint afferents. Muscular exercise, the most potent stimulus to breathing, in part presumably involves joint afferents.

Medullary Respiratory Neurons and Arterial P_{CO_2} *and* P_{O_2}. Central chemosensitivity for CO_2-H^+ for respiration is well known, but the site and mechanism of excitatory respiratory neurons are not clear. However, hypercapnia has been found to hyperpolarize the respiratory neurons in the NA and NRA. This direct hyperpolarizing effect should increase the carbon dioxide threshold for excitation and decrease neural output as its level is raised. Thus the direct effect of hypercapnia on respiratory neurons does not explain stimulation by carbon dioxide. The electrophysiologic evidence and observations on the chemosensitivity of the superficial medullary surface strongly suggest that the respiratory neurons receive synaptic input from carbon dioxide-excitable elements in another site. In particular, a moderate acute hypoxia seems to decrease excitability of inspiratory neurons directly.

Pneumotaxic Center. A transection through the upper pons increases tidal volume and duration of inspiration and expiration just as a bilateral section of vagus nerves does. Some cells in the upper pons—located in the region of the nucleus parabrachialis medialis (NPBM)—terminate inspiration when electrically stimulated. The threshold stimulus strength for the effect decreases as inspiration progresses. These cells, known as the pneumotaxic center, modulate respiratory rhythm, but they are not the rhythm generator.

Lesions in the region of NPBM in man result in apneustic breathing.

Apneustic Center. Inspiratory apneusis produced by an upper pontine lesion is terminated by a caudal section of the lower pons. Some yet unidentified cells in the region of the lower pons are believed responsible for the apneusis.

Respiratory Response to Exercise

On exercise there is an immediate increase in both depth and rate of breathing. In steady states of moderate exercise, the increment in breathing is such that the alveolar and arterial blood gases remain at nearly normal levels. There is no retention of carbon dioxide, nor does any oxygen debt occur. How this remarkable regulation of breathing is achieved is not known.

Both at rest and during exercise, hypoxia and hypercapnia (CO_2-H^+) stimulate breathing. A combination of hypoxic and hypercapnic stimulation is synergistic. The respiratory response occurs in concert with such other changes as cardiovascular, thermal and proprioceptive compensations and is clearly geared to homeostasis. During intense exercise, however, the oxygen supply may not cope with the demand of the working muscles, resulting in an accumulation of acid and other metabolites. Also, the catecholamine level in blood rises. As a consequence, breathing is stimulated beyond metabolic need, lowering $P_{A_{CO_2}}$, $P_{a_{CO_2}}$ and $[H^+]$ and raising P_{O_2}.

The mean level of chemical stimuli related to respiratory gases obviously cannot explain the response. An associated temperature increase might account for some of the effects, but a rise in blood and body temperatures occurs only slowly and does not explain the rapid augmentation of ventilation at the onset of exercise.

Logical candidates for other sources were the exercising and moving parts of the body and venous blood returning from *active* muscles. Venous blood is depleted of oxygen and enriched with carbon dioxide. Thus, a sensor in the right heart and pulmonary artery was suspected, but its presence still remains to be confirmed in spite of a large amount of investigative work.

The *neural theory* for control of ventilation with afferents from the periphery remains attractive. However, increased metabolism resulting from administration of such drugs as triiodothyronine, dinitrophenol and salicylate increases breathing. But these drugs raise body temperature and are expected to stimulate peripheral chemoreceptors. The mechanism for stimulating breathing in the two instances would then be entirely different.

The dynamic responses to changes in stimuli often provide more insight. Thus, the responses occurring at the start of exercise and during recovery have been considered. It is well known that ventilation at the onset of exercise is suddenly increased, and this is usually attributed to proprioceptive afferent impulses from the joints reaching the respiratory neurons. Since an increased blood flow through the lungs occurs promptly with the onset of exercise, possibly the fast component is related to a resulting increase in chemical stimuli to the lungs. However, the fast component can be shown to be present even without an increase in blood flow. It can also be explained by a delayed neural phenomenon in the central nervous system during the onset of exercise. Termination of exercise is followed by similar fast and slow changes in ventilation.

(Continued)

Control and Disorders of Respiration
(Continued)

The ventilatory effect of hypoxia is augmented by exercise and is very evident in subjects sojourning at high altitudes. Since the mean activity of peripheral chemoreceptors is not increased during exercise, perhaps the augmentation of hypoxic ventilation is due to a multiplication of the impact from the peripheral chemoreceptors by one or more central neuronal factors. However, oscillations of chemoreceptor activity, which are partly due to rapid fluctuations in arterial blood gas levels, are potentially capable of augmenting the ventilation effect, and it is known that these oscillations produce a greater volume of inspiration if they coincide with the peak inspiratory flow. If peak activity of oscillating signals occurred at this time, the tidal volume would be augmented. Since breathing frequency is increased during hypoxic exercise, the minute ventilation would then be increased.

Respiratory Response and Adaptation to Hypoxia

The immediate effect of acute hypoxia is an increase in ventilation, which leads to respiratory alkalosis. The alkalosis decreases the response of arterial peripheral chemoreceptors as well as that of the central chemosensitive mechanism. If the exposure to hypoxia continues—*e.g.,* by residence at high altitude—ventilation increases further after the first few days. In subjects acclimatized to high altitude, carbon dioxide sensitivity is increased, but the mechanism of the secondary increase in ventilation is not clear. One explanation is that a partial compensation of central alkalosis restores the central stimulus for ventilation. However, recent measurements of cerebrospinal fluid (CSF) pH have not supported this explanation. Thus, it has been proposed that chronic hypoxia causes excitation of central respiratory neurons. This central activity is presumably also responsible for the increased respiratory sensitivity to carbon dioxide. Natives of high-altitude areas show a normal acid-base status in arterial blood and CSF.

Respiratory sensitivity to hypoxia does not seem to change even after months of acclimatization to high altitude. However, adult natives at high altitudes show a blunted ventilatory response to hypoxia. At 3,850 meters in the Andes, children up to 12 years of age have a normal sensitivity. Thereafter, their response begins to decline, and by the age of 20 years or so, it is definitely blunted. The phenomenon has been seen regardless of genetic background.

The blunted hypoxic response in adult highlanders is restored to normal after several years of residence at sea level. The development of reduced ventilatory drive at high altitude, then, is an environmental rather than a genetic effect.

These findings are in conformity with observations in subjects with congenital cyanotic heart disease at sea level; corrective cardiac surgery restores their natural response. The mechanism of the development and disappearance of the phenomenon is not known, although peripheral chemoreceptors have been implicated. It is of

Respiratory Response to Exercise

Factors which may account for initial abrupt rise and sharp terminal drop in ventilation

Collaterals to respiratory centers from motor pathways for muscle activation

Proprioceptive afferents from joint receptors to respiratory centers

Other unknown factors

Factors which may play a part in continued elevation of ventilation during continuing exercise

Rise in body temperature accounts for a small part of elevation

Respiratory neurons seem to be more responsive to changes in chemoreceptor activity. Centers may be more sensitive to fluctuation than to absolute values of Pa_{O_2}, Pa_{CO_2}, or pH

Lactic acid production due to anaerobic metabolism in muscle may increase H^+ concentration of blood and CSF, thus affecting chemoreceptors

Possible metabolic receptors in exercising muscle

Other unknown factors

interest that the carotid body of many animals and of man shows enlargement and hyperplasia at high altitude, and the changes are reversible. Any disease or state leading to a decrease in sensitivity to carbon dioxide may result in a worsening of hypoxemia, but this in itself would increase response to carbon dioxide. That is, in the absence of hypoxemia breathing would decrease. However, hypoxia also has a central depressant effect, although the mechanism of this effect is not clear. Be that as it may, without the oxygen and carbon dioxide drive, it is difficult to maintain normal respiration; in the awake state, it is somewhat depressed; during sleep, breathing may cease,

thus manifesting the primary alveolar hypoventilation syndrome, or "Ondine's curse."

Other Effects of Chronic Hypoxia. Of many other effects of chronic hypoxia, increased concentration of red blood cells is most striking. Usually the increment is such that the oxygen content of arterial blood is maintained similar to that at sea level. Occasionally, however, an excessive increase in red blood cells may occur, leading to cardiac failure and pulmonary congestion. In addition, the red blood cells show a diminished hemoglobin affinity for oxygen due to an increase in organic phosphate (2,3-diphosphoglycerate in

(Continued)

Control and Disorders
of Respiration
(Continued)

man) related to respiratory alkalosis and hemoglobin deoxygenation. The latter response may not be beneficial, particularly during exercise at high altitude when loading of blood with oxygen in the lungs is compromised.

The usual cardiovascular response to acute hypoxia is an increased heart rate and cardiac output, which subside with the development of chronic hypoxia. In high-altitude natives, pulmonary hypertension and systemic hypotension are common but reversible features whose mechanisms are not understood.

Hypoxia also elicits a number of adaptive responses which tend to compensate for the loss of alveolar and arterial P_{O_2}. Hypoxia stimulates lung growth, and high-altitude natives possess a greater lung volume than sea-level natives of the same body size; this is associated with an increase in oxygen-diffusing capacity. The difference seems to occur after birth at high altitude and consists of increases in lung parenchyma rather than airways that form completely in fetal life.

Abnormal Breathing Patterns

Alveolar hyperventilation or hypoventilation usually results from multiple rather than single causes. Hyperventilation occurring in pulmonary edema is caused by hypoxemia and probably by stimulation of irritant and J receptors in the lung. Both receptors receive their sensory innervation through the vagi. Stimulation of irritant receptors located in the epithelium of the airways produces coughing, but when the stimulus is not severe enough to do that, hyperventilation results. When J receptors—so called because of their juxtacapillary position—are stimulated by interstitial edema or fibrosis, tachypnea occurs.

The obesity-hypoventilation syndrome is associated with carbon dioxide retention and somnolence. At least three factors contribute to the carbon dioxide retention: (1) the increased weight of the chest wall adds to the work of breathing; (2) the work that the respiratory muscles will do for a given level of chemical drive is limited, and when respiratory work is increased, ventilation tends to decrease; and (3) in obese patients, upper airway obstruction occurs during rapid-eye-movement (REM) sleep when jaw muscles relax. In some patients, the obstruction may be severe and cause increasing respiratory efforts, until the patient awakens and the obstruction is relieved. This produces a pattern of waxing and waning respiratory efforts reminiscent of Cheyne-Stokes breathing. Because the effect of the upper airway obstruction is to reduce ventilation, arterial P_{CO_2} ultimately rises and bicarbonate is retained, further depressing ventilatory responses to hypercapnia.

In some obese patients, the output of respiratory neurons has been measured by electromyography of the diaphragm; it has been shown that when function of the chest bellows is abnormal, diaphragmatic electric activity more faithfully indicates respiratory neuron stimulation than does ventilation. Recordings are made with electrodes

passed down the esophagus and positioned near the diaphragm. Obese patients who maintain normal blood gas tensions and pH seem to have a higher output from respiratory neurons, but this does not seem to be true of similar individuals who retain carbon dioxide. It has therefore been postulated that defective function of the respiratory neurons may contribute to carbon dioxide retention in the obesity-hypoventilation syndrome. Similarly, in myxedema, abnormalities in lung function and respiratory muscle weakness in the presence of impaired respiratory neuron chemosensitivity seem to predispose to carbon dioxide retention.

Factors Affecting Stability of Feedback Control Systems. Cheyne-Stokes breathing is an example of instability in a physiologic feedback control system. It is analogous to instabilities that occur in physical control systems, for which the explanation is the same. Although feedback enhances the accuracy of the control system, it also introduces the possibility that the corrective action taken by the controller may be inappropriate because of the delay required for the controller to receive and process data from sensors.

When the delays are sufficiently great, controller action to correct the effects of a disturbance

(Continued)

Effects of High Altitude on Respiratory Mechanism

Response to hypercapnia persists, thus maintaining normal blood gas tensions; but CO_2 response may be lost under anesthesia, resulting in dangerous hypoxemia

CO_2

Respiratory response to hypoxemia is blunted or lost

O_2

O_2

O_2

in persons born at and living for many years at high altitude

Some physiologic alteration persists for some time after moving to sea level

In children with congenital cyanotic heart disease, similar phenomena occur and persist into later life. Normal response is restored after corrective surgery

Some manifestations of adaptation to chronic hypoxemia

Polycythemia due to increased renal erythropoietic factor

O_2

Facilitation of O_2 dissociation due to elevated diphosphoglycerate

Pulmonary arteriolar constriction and pulmonary hypertension with r. heart hypertrophy

Decreased bicarbonate concentration in blood and in CSF

Pulmonary Edema Hyperventilation

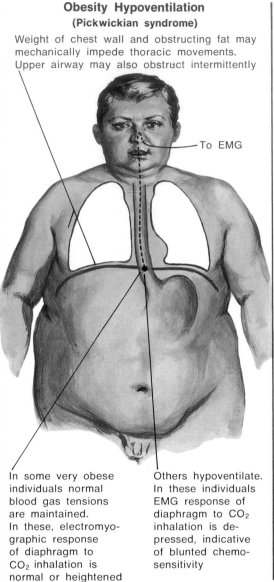

Vagal J (juxtacapillary) receptor or irritant receptor stimulation may cause reflex hyperventilation

Obesity Hypoventilation
(Pickwickian syndrome)

Weight of chest wall and obstructing fat may mechanically impede thoracic movements. Upper airway may also obstruct intermittently

To EMG

In some very obese individuals normal blood gas tensions are maintained. In these, electromyographic response of diaphragm to CO_2 inhalation is normal or heightened

Others hypoventilate. In these individuals EMG response of diaphragm to CO_2 inhalation is depressed, indicative of blunted chemosensitivity

Myxedema Hypoventilation

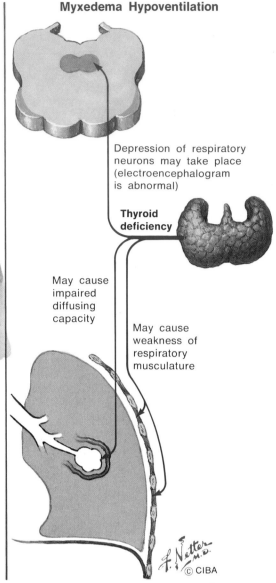

Depression of respiratory neurons may take place (electroencephalogram is abnormal)

Thyroid deficiency

May cause impaired diffusing capacity

May cause weakness of respiratory musculature

Control and Disorders of Respiration
(Continued)

may be postponed too long, causing the output to swing past the desired level. When the controller ultimately is informed of this overshoot, it takes excessive action—now in the opposite direction—causing the output to undershoot the level desired. It is even possible for the output to swing about endlessly, never reaching a steady state.

The output of physical or physiologic systems can oscillate even in the absence of delays. All components of physiologic systems—like physical components with properties of friction and elasticity—cannot instantaneously attain a steady state after being disturbed. The ventilatory system has such properties, and the terms *compliance* (a measure of elasticity), *resistance* (a measure of friction) and *inertia* (a measure of the mass of an object) are used commonly to describe the behavior of the lung. Whether or not oscillations occur depends on the system's damping ratio. When feedback is employed to reduce steady state errors in output, the control system will behave as though it had a reduced damping ratio, and the tendency of the output to oscillate is increased.

Factors Influencing Stability of Ventilatory Control. Some insights into the causes of instability in the ventilatory control system can be obtained by considering oxygen and carbon dioxide control separately. Over a wide range of carbon dioxide tensions at constant oxygen tension, ventilation increases linearly with P_{CO_2}, indicating a constant carbon dioxide controller gain (at least above 30 mm Hg P_{CO_2}). On the other hand, the hyperbolic increase in arterial chemoreceptor discharge and ventilation as arterial P_{O_2} decreases results in an increasing oxygen controller gain during hypoxia.

Differences in the oxygen and carbon dioxide stores also contribute to the difference in the stability of the two systems. The ratio between the volume of carbon dioxide or oxygen stored in the body for a given change in gas tension is a measure of the compliance of the stores. The more gas stored, the greater the compliance (the inverse of elasticity), and the greater the damping. Although both carbon dioxide and oxygen are stored in blood and lung air, large amounts of carbon dioxide but only minute amounts of oxygen are stored in the tissues. Accordingly, the damping or buffering effect of the carbon dioxide stores of the brain stem and the relative linearity of the response of carbon dioxide receptors make its effects on ventilation more stable than those of P_{O_2} via peripheral chemoreceptors. Carbon dioxide control is further stabilized by the increase

in cerebral blood flow that takes place during hypercapnia. The reverse change occurs during hypocapnia, so that the rate and level of change of P_{CO_2} are slowed in the vicinity of the cerebral chemoreceptors during disturbances in the level of metabolism or environmental carbon dioxide concentration. In contrast, the oxygen control system tends to be much more unstable than that for carbon dioxide because of its extremely low damping. This is due to the small size of the carotid and aortic bodies, high blood flow and oxygen consumption, and the alinear characteristics of the oxygen controller. Although the usual stability of ventilatory responses to hypoxia is explained by the multiple physiologic connections between the oxygen and carbon dioxide systems through ventilation, metabolism and the circulation, these same interconnections decrease the stability of carbon dioxide control.

Since both oxygen and carbon dioxide receptors receive information concerning the response of the organism (for example, ventilation) directly or indirectly through the blood, it is apparent that reductions in the speed of the circulation will increase the transportation or transmission lag in both control systems and will promote instability. The time required for the blood to traverse the vessels between the lung and the chemoreceptors is also responsible for the peculiar relationship between alveolar and arterial gas tensions that *(Continued)*

Control and Disorders
of Respiration
(Continued)

occurs during Cheyne-Stokes breathing. Arterial carbon dioxide tension tends to be highest and oxygen tension lowest during hyperpnea; the reverse is true of alveolar gas levels. During Cheyne-Stokes breathing, then, the arterial gas tensions reflect the input to the receptors—the respiratory drive—whereas the alveolar gas tensions reflect the changing ventilatory output. In addition, the duration of the cycle of hyperpnea and apnea tends to vary directly with circulation time, and cycles are usually shorter when Cheyne-Stokes breathing occurs in normal individuals at high altitude than in patients with cardiac disease and slowed circulation times.

Variations of arterial blood gases resulting in oscillations of peripheral chemoreceptor activity are well known. Similarly, blood pressure waves (Mayer waves) generate oscillations of peripheral chemoreceptor discharge. The effect of these receptor activity oscillations is dependent on the timing of input with respect to the phase of respiratory neuronal discharge. The phasic relationship has an important bearing on control of breathing in normal and abnormal situations.

Causes of Cheyne-Stokes Breathing in Clinical Situations. In patients with cardiac disease, pulmonary congestion is a destabilizing force that reduces lung volume and the ability to store carbon dioxide and oxygen, and it may produce reflex hyperpnea. This tends to increase sensitivity to hypoxia and hypercapnia. Arterial hypoxemia may produce reflex hyperpnea, which also tends to augment the ventilatory response to hypoxia and hypercapnia. A fall in arterial oxygen tension may also complicate pulmonary congestion and increase ventilatory sensitivity to carbon dioxide. However, the major factor causing instability in cardiac patients is the prolonged circulation time resulting from heart failure.

In patients with disease of the central nervous system (CNS), gasping respirations can result from severe damage to the respiratory neurons *per se.* However, these kinds of irregular breathing patterns should be distinguished from the regular cycles of Cheyne-Stokes breathing due to control system instability. CNS disease can predispose to instability in several ways. Frequently, patients with CNS disease have an increased carbon dioxide threshold and become apneic in response to slight reductions in carbon dioxide tension. Moreover, the sensitivity of the carbon dioxide receptors may be increased, presumably by removal of inhibiting cortical influences. On the other hand, in some patients with CNS disease, carbon dioxide response is depressed rather than increased, possibly because of lesions in the medulla rather than in the cortex or forebrain. Cheyne-Stokes breathing in patients with depressed carbon dioxide response may be explained by the fact that ventilation is now being controlled by the inherently more unstable oxygen control system. Greater reliance on the oxygen system probably also explains the Cheyne-Stokes breathing that occurs in subjects arriving at high altitude. This is also seen in patients who are given

morphine, which depresses the ventilatory responses to carbon dioxide more than the responses to hypoxia. Finally, in patients with cerebrovascular disease, the reduction in the level of cerebral blood flow and the inability of the cerebral vasculature to respond to changes in arterial P_{CO_2} eliminate this stabilizing factor.

Disturbances in Normal Control of Breathing

A variety of disturbances and disorders can interfere with the function of either the respiratory controller or the chest bellows and produce hyperventilation or hypoventilation.

Disease of the lung itself (parenchyma, airways or circulation) can lower resting arterial oxygen tensions, an event sometimes associated with a rise in arterial P_{CO_2}. The most common cause of inadequate ventilation (alveolar hypoventilation), producing a rise in arterial P_{CO_2} above its usual level of 35 to 45 mm Hg, is *chronic airway obstruction.* The inadequate ventilation has been attributed to the increase in work needed to overcome the elevated airway resistance, and to abnormalities of gas exchange in the lung itself. Hypercapnia does not usually occur in this condition until alveolar ventilation actually decreases.

(Continued)

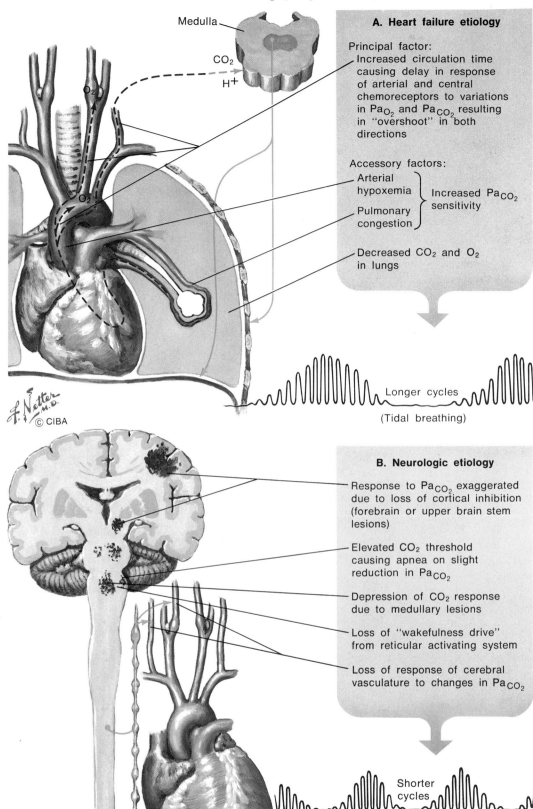

Periodic Breathing (Cheyne-Stokes)

A. Heart failure etiology

Principal factor:
Increased circulation time causing delay in response of arterial and central chemoreceptors to variations in Pa_{O_2} and Pa_{CO_2} resulting in "overshoot" in both directions

Accessory factors:
Arterial hypoxemia
Pulmonary congestion
} Increased Pa_{CO_2} sensitivity

Decreased CO_2 and O_2 in lungs

Longer cycles
(Tidal breathing)

B. Neurologic etiology

Response to Pa_{CO_2} exaggerated due to loss of cortical inhibition (forebrain or upper brain stem lesions)

Elevated CO_2 threshold causing apnea on slight reduction in Pa_{CO_2}

Depression of CO_2 response due to medullary lesions

Loss of "wakefulness drive" from reticular activating system

Loss of response of cerebral vasculature to changes in Pa_{CO_2}

Shorter cycles
(Tidal breathing)

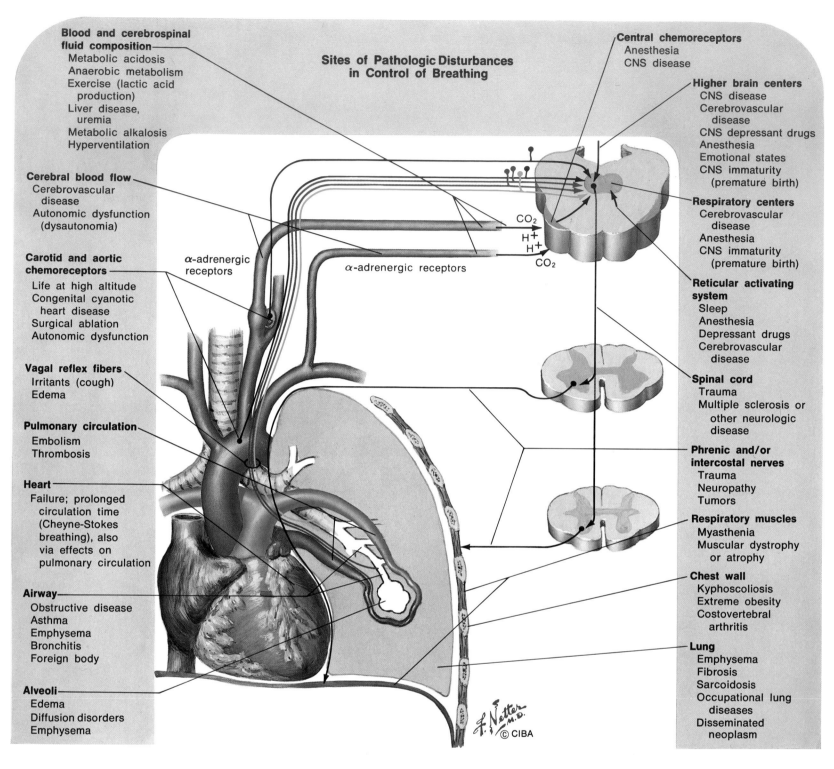

Sites of Pathologic Disturbances in Control of Breathing

Blood and cerebrospinal fluid composition
Metabolic acidosis
Anaerobic metabolism
Exercise (lactic acid production)
Liver disease, uremia
Metabolic alkalosis
Hyperventilation

Cerebral blood flow
Cerebrovascular disease
Autonomic dysfunction (dysautonomia)

Carotid and aortic chemoreceptors
Life at high altitude
Congenital cyanotic heart disease
Surgical ablation
Autonomic dysfunction

Vagal reflex fibers
Irritants (cough)
Edema

Pulmonary circulation
Embolism
Thrombosis

Heart
Failure; prolonged circulation time (Cheyne-Stokes breathing), also via effects on pulmonary circulation

Airway
Obstructive disease
Asthma
Emphysema
Bronchitis
Foreign body

Alveoli
Edema
Diffusion disorders
Emphysema

α-adrenergic receptors

α-adrenergic receptors

CO_2
H^+
H^+
CO_2

Central chemoreceptors
Anesthesia
CNS disease

Higher brain centers
CNS disease
Cerebrovascular disease
CNS depressant drugs
Anesthesia
Emotional states
CNS immaturity (premature birth)

Respiratory centers
Cerebrovascular disease
Anesthesia
CNS immaturity (premature birth)

Reticular activating system
Sleep
Anesthesia
Depressant drugs
Cerebrovascular disease

Spinal cord
Trauma
Multiple sclerosis or other neurologic disease

Phrenic and/or intercostal nerves
Trauma
Neuropathy
Tumors

Respiratory muscles
Myasthenia
Muscular dystrophy or atrophy

Chest wall
Kyphoscoliosis
Extreme obesity
Costovertebral arthritis

Lung
Emphysema
Fibrosis
Sarcoidosis
Occupational lung diseases
Disseminated neoplasm

F. Netter M.D.
© CIBA

Control and Disorders of Respiration
(Continued)

Lung fibrosis and other restrictive lung diseases are usually associated with subnormal levels of arterial P_{CO_2} at rest. In part this is caused by stimulation of ventilation by lung receptors through the vagi relative to the metabolic rate.

Encephalitis and *meningitis* interfere with the function of central nervous system (CNS) hydrogen ion receptors. Maintenance of normal acidity of the interstitial fluid of the brain depends on the cerebral blood flow as well as on ventilation. Usually, cerebral blood flow increases with hypercapnia and hypoxia, while the opposite occurs with hypocapnia or with elevations of P_{O_2}. Even when cerebrovascular disease does not produce ischemia of the respiratory neurons themselves, it can inter-

fere with the control of brain interstitial fluid hydrogen ion levels.

In *familial dysautonomia,* the sympathetic nervous system is ineffective, hypoxia fails to elicit the usual vasoconstriction, blood pressure decreases, and the brain is hypoperfused. Thus, hypoxia can depress ventilation. If the carbon dioxide response is blunted by sleep or anesthesia, apnea may occur.

Prolonged exposure to hypoxia because of *residence at high altitude or cyanotic congenital heart disease* causes depressed ventilatory responses. Whether this inhibition is due to an effect of long-term continuous hypoxia on peripheral chemoreceptors or to CNS neuronal function is unknown.

Prolonged exposure to carbon dioxide causes a compensatory increase in blood and brain interstitial fluid bicarbonate levels which can decrease the change in hydrogen ion concentration produced by P_{CO_2}. This decreases the stimulus (change) at CNS receptors and depresses ventilatory responses

to carbon dioxide. In practice, however, hypercapnia results from respiratory failure, and respiratory acidosis is partly compensated. Metabolic alkalosis has the same effect, and the reverse changes in ventilatory responses are produced by metabolic acidosis. Changes in brain interstitial fluid bicarbonate levels lag behind changes in plasma bicarbonate levels because of the slow transport of bicarbonate between blood and brain extracellular fluid compartments. Accordingly, acute changes in plasma bicarbonate level may not be immediately reflected in the brain, causing the hyperventilation that persists for a time in uremia after plasma acidosis is corrected by dialysis.

An increase in levels of catecholamines and thyroid hormones can increase ventilation. The hyperventilation seen in *liver failure* is intriguing. It may relate to shunting of venous to arterial blood, further complicated by unusual circulating metabolites due to malfunction of the liver.

Section III

Radiology

Frank H. Netter, M.D.

in collaboration with

Wallace T. Miller, M.D. *Plates 1-18*

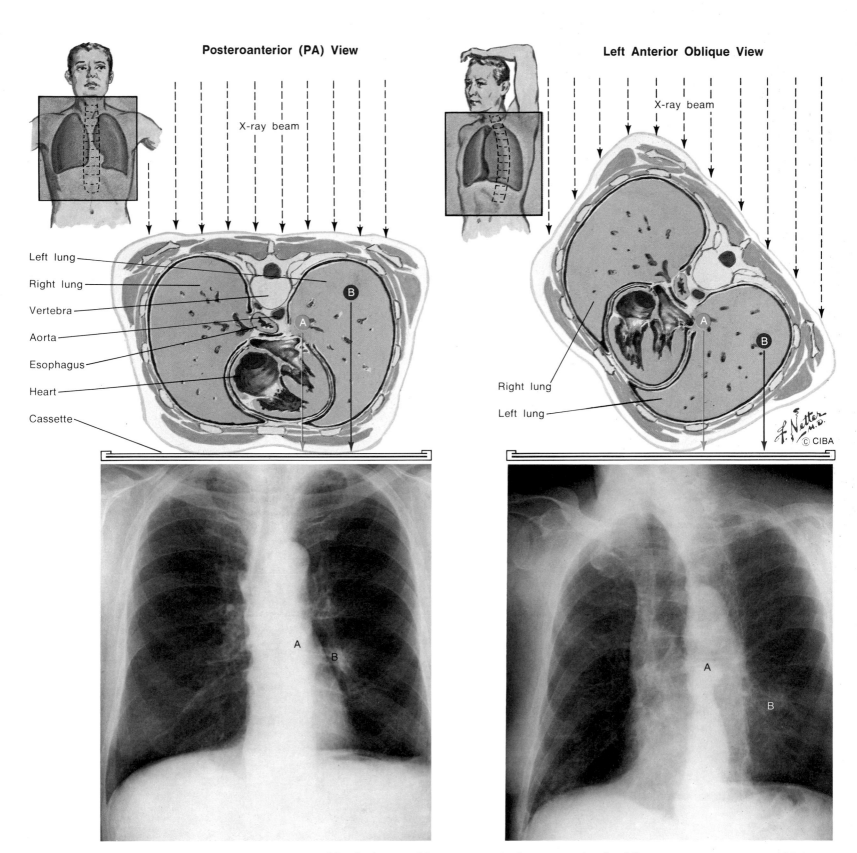

Posteroanterior (PA) View

X-ray beam

Left lung
Right lung
Vertebra
Aorta
Esophagus
Heart
Cassette

Left Anterior Oblique View

X-ray beam

Right lung
Left lung

Roentgenologic Examination of the Lungs

The chest roentgenogram is of paramount importance in the evaluation of patients with symptoms of pulmonary disease. A plain roentgenogram of the chest not only identifies the patient who has an abnormal pulmonary condition but also frequently provides a good general indication of the type of pathology present.

Routine Examination

For patients under the age of 30 years, a single posteroanterior (PA) examination is sometimes considered adequate. Most roentgenologists prefer at least two views of the chest to provide a three-dimensional appreciation of it. A straight PA and a lateral projection are the two views most commonly employed, although some individuals routinely make stereoscopic PA roentgenograms. Ordinarily, these oblique views- are considered supplementary to standard PA and lateral projections.

Plates 1 and 2 illustrate correct positioning for the routine PA and lateral views and also for left and right anterior oblique roentgenograms. In every instance the exposure should be made at maximum inspiratory effort, and the patient should, of course, not breathe while it is made. There should be as little rotation as possible in the PA and lateral positions, and the degree of rota-

tion for oblique roentgenograms should be standard. When one is studying lung pathology, a 45 degree oblique projection is desirable, while for cardiac pathology, a 60 degree angle is preferable.

Exposures may be made utilizing 80 to 125 kv, or even in some instances 300 kv. Many roentgenologists now use higher kilovoltage techniques (125 kv) to obtain increased exposure latitude. Although the film made at these levels has less contrast and is not as pleasing to the eye, it often provides additional information and is less likely to be underexposed or need to be repeated.

While the *PA* film is easily interpreted and yields the most information about the heart, pleura, lungs and chest wall, the *lateral* roentgenogram is more revealing with regard to
(Continued)

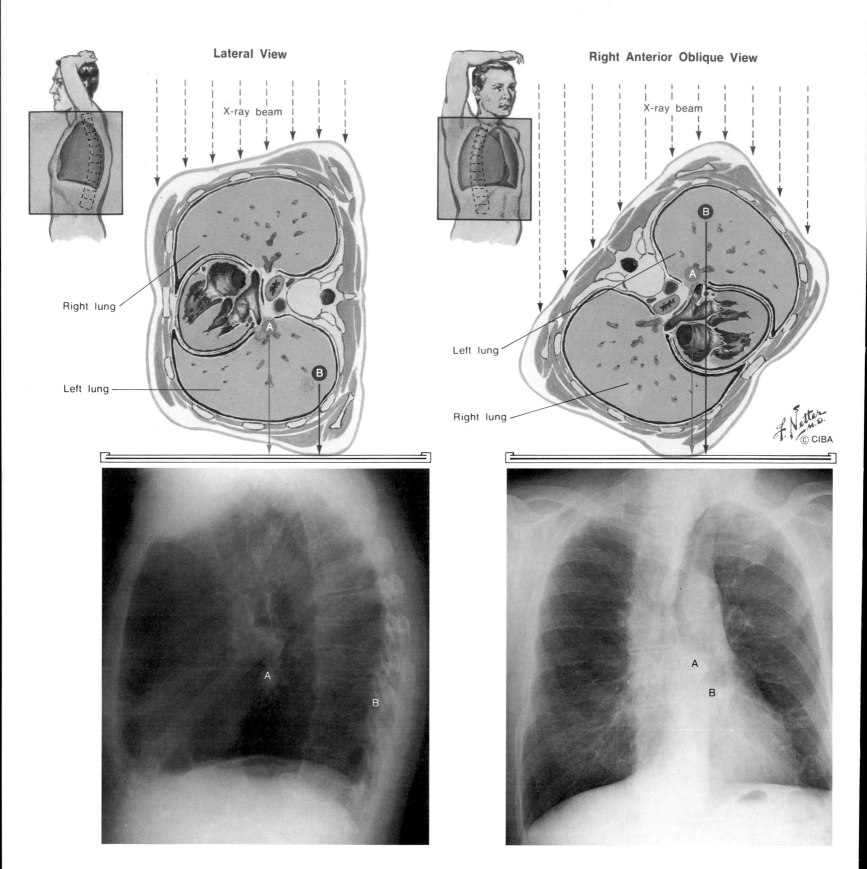

Lateral View

X-ray beam

Right lung

Left lung

A

B

Right Anterior Oblique View

X-ray beam

B

A

Left lung

Right lung

F. Netter M.D. © CIBA

A

B

A

B

Roentgenologic Examination of the Lungs
(Continued)

small lesions in the mediastinum and some masses in the anterior portions of the lung adjacent to it. Lesions of the vertebral column are generally not apparent on PA films but can readily be seen on the lateral view. Small pleural effusions often blunt the costophrenic sulci posteriorly while leaving the lateral sulci apparently clear; hence they are visible only on the lateral roentgenogram.

Oblique films are helpful in localizing a suspected lesion by projecting it free from overlying structures. They are particularly valuable in determining whether a lesion is in the lung or in the chest wall. They also aid the investigation of mediastinal lesions, especially when made with barium in the esophagus.

In the interpretation of oblique roentgenograms, it is well to remember that the heart is an anterior structure and thus moves to the left in the right anterior oblique exposure and to the right in the left corresponding exposure. The spine, a posterior structure, moves in the opposite direction. Nodules within the lung can be seen as lying anteriorly or posteriorly by their change in position relative to the heart and the vertebral col-

umn. This is a particularly useful observation in a patient in whom a nodule is identified on the PA projection but is not seen well on the lateral roentgenogram. The relative shifts in position of pulmonary densities are shown in Plates 1 and 2.

The lordotic view is useful in investigating the apical portions of the lungs, which may be partially obscured by overlying shadows of the anterior first rib and the clavicle on a routine PA roentgenogram. It is employed to confirm a suspected lesion identified in the apex. This view can be made in either an AP (anteroposterior) or a PA position. Plate 3 depicts the patient's position in the AP view, which is quite simple to obtain. An alternative method of obtaining a similar film is to

(Continued)

Roentgenologic Examination
of the Lungs
(Continued)

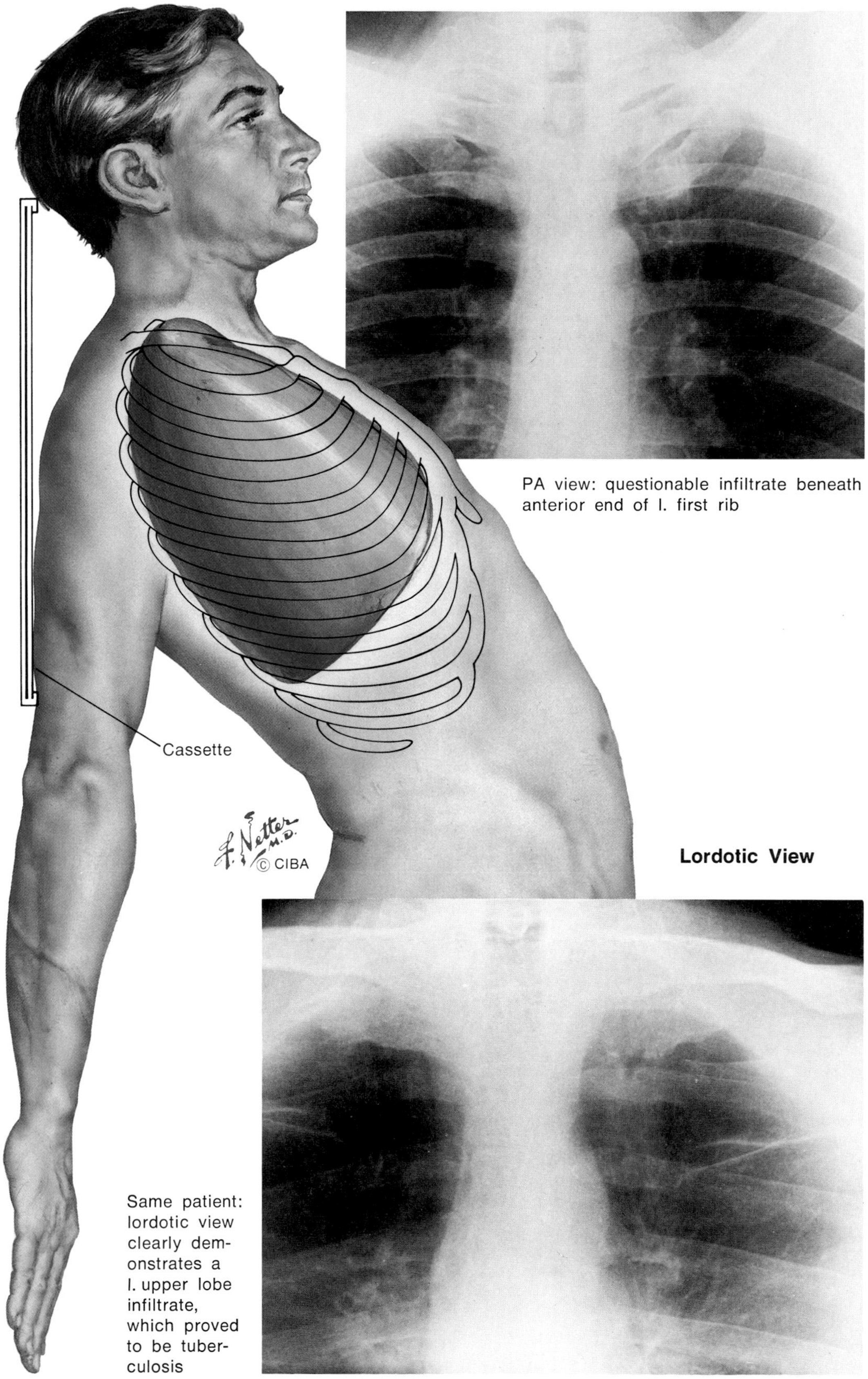

PA view: questionable infiltrate beneath anterior end of l. first rib

Cassette

Lordotic View

Same patient: lordotic view clearly demonstrates a l. upper lobe infiltrate, which proved to be tuberculosis

allow the patient to stand erect but to angle the tube 15 to 20 degrees cephalad.

The lordotic projection serves primarily to confirm a lesion suspected on a routine PA projection. It is not very useful in determining the pathologic nature of an apical lesion, nor is it generally indicated for a patient whose routine PA film is completely normal and in whom the apices are easily seen. The lordotic film may sometimes assist in evaluating middle lobe disease if there is some doubt about the presence of an abnormality in that lobe in other projections. However, a right lateral view is usually more helpful in these circumstances.

The *lateral decubitus* (lateral recumbent) view (Plate 4) is extremely important in investigating a suspected pleural effusion or in demonstrating air-fluid levels in cavities. In this projection the patient lies on one side, and the beam passes in a horizontal plane tangential to the chest wall. The side on which the patient is lying should be elevated in some fashion so that the edges of the chest wall can be adequately visualized on the film. Elevation can be accomplished by mattresses or pillows, or by using a specially constructed decubitus table. Amounts of fluid as small as 25 to 50 ml may be identified with this technique.

Stereoscopic projections of the chest may be useful in studying lesions adjacent to the mediastinum or in the lung apices, particularly for recognizing cavities. The physician experienced in stereoscopy may prefer routine PA stereoscopic roentgeno-

grams rather than PA and lateral films. He may also prefer stereoscopic views rather than lordotic or oblique projections for localization of lesions.

The *expiratory* roentgenogram helps in assessing the trapping of pulmonary air, either local or diffuse, and may confirm the presence of a pneumothorax. A finding of localized air-trapping is particularly useful in identifying an endobronchial foreign body in children, and occasionally suggests the presence of a tumor in the bronchial tree when routine inspiratory roentgenograms appear normal. An unexplained wheeze is a symptom which may suggest the need for films during both inspiration and expiration.

The *supine projection* is made when an adult is unable to sit or stand, and it is the routine projection for infants. Interpretation of the supine roentgenogram must take into consideration the magnification of mediastinal structures that occurs in the AP view and also the alteration in pulmonary perfusion that occurs with the patient on his back.

In roentgenography of large patients, a certain amount of "scatter" radiation takes place. This happens when the primary x-ray beam strikes the patient and is deflected in a different direction. If only a small number of scattered x-ray photons are
(Continued)

Lateral Decubitus View

Roentgenologic Examination of the Lungs
(Continued)

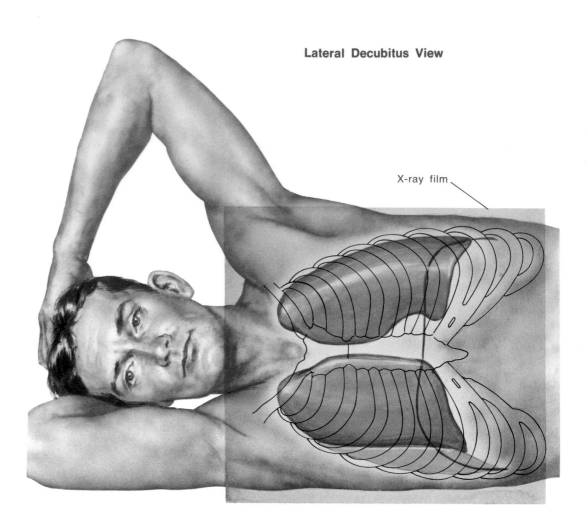

present, the roentgenogram remains relatively sharp, and no mechanism is necessary to compensate for their dispersal. However, with large patients or during longer exposures in which overpenetrated films are desired, considerable scattering of radiation occurs. In order to reduce the amount of scattered radiation reaching the film, a plate made up of a series of lead strips (grid) is interposed between it and the patient. Primary radiation will pass between the parallel strips of the grid while the scattered radiation will be absorbed. The result is a sharper image (Plate 5).

Another technique for keeping scatter from reaching the film is to interpose an air gap of 6 in. between it and the patient. To reduce magnification, a 10 ft rather than a 6 ft distance should be used between the x-ray tube and the film.

Magnification roentgenograms are made by increasing the patient-film distance and decreasing the tube-patient distance, thus magnifying pulmonary structures. A very small focal spot (0.3 mm) is necessary to preserve detail. This technique is used in investigating diffuse lung disease.

Tomography (laminography, body section radiography, planigraphy) allows roentgenographic investigation of a thin slice of the patient's anatomy, and is a useful technique in the study of chest lesions (Plate 6). In this type of examination, the film and the x-ray tube move on a fixed fulcrum to create a roentgenogram in which a plane several millimeters thick is in focus and the remaining details of the patient's anatomy are blurred.

(Continued)

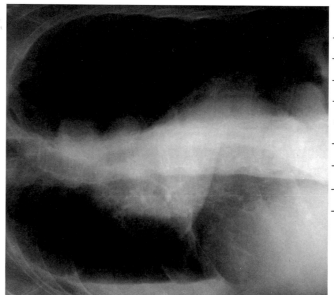

R. lateral decubitus x-ray film: fluid in r. pleural space

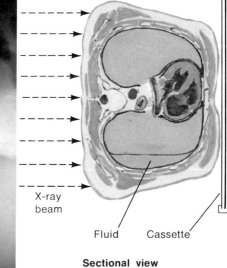

X-ray beam

Fluid   Cassette

Sectional view

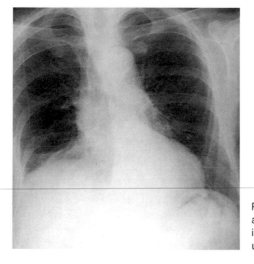

PA view of same patient. Right diaphragm appears elevated but costophrenic sulcus is sharp. Effusion not apparent in upright view

Roentgenologic Examination of the Lungs
(Continued)

Penetrated Grid Roentgenograms

Direct parallel rays (blue) pass through grid; stray scattered rays (red) cannot pass through and a sharper picture results

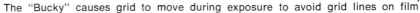

Cassette

Grid (greatly magnified)—

F. Netter
© CIBA

The "Bucky" causes grid to move during exposure to avoid grid lines on film

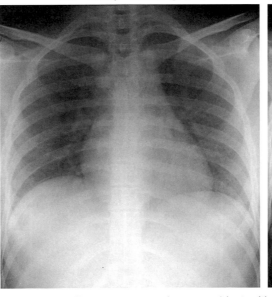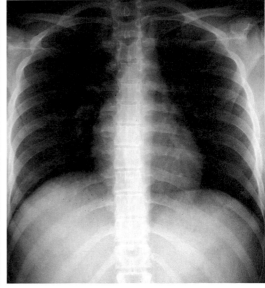

Roentgenogram of same subject without grid (left) and with grid (right)

Thus, tomography can: (1) obtain better visualization of a poorly focused density seen on the routine chest film, (2) demonstrate the presence or absence of calcification within a pulmonary nodule, and (3) demonstrate the presence or absence of cavitation within a pulmonary lesion. This last use of tomography is particularly important in the study of pulmonary tuberculosis. Favis has shown that tomography reveals cavitation in approximately 10% of patients in whom no suggestion of a cavity was seen on conventional roentgenograms. Laminography (tomography) may also demonstrate the vascular nature of an arteriovenous fistula.

Fluoroscopy of the chest aids the study of pulmonary or cardiac dynamics and is useful in localizing a pulmonary lesion which is identified in only one projection on the routine examination. Fluoroscopy may also provide information about diaphragmatic motion. A paralyzed diaphragm often indicates mediastinal involvement of the phrenic nerve. When fluoroscoping a patient for diaphragmatic paralysis, one must view the patient in both the PA and lateral projections. In the lateral projection it is often apparent that only the dome of the diaphragm is moving paradoxically, while another part, usually the posterior portion, will be seen to move normally. This discrepancy indicates localized diaphragmatic weakness (partial eventration) rather than true paralysis. True

paralysis of the diaphragm may be overlooked if fluoroscopy is done with the patient breathing quietly. Asking the patient to take a quick short "sniff" (sniff test) can demonstrate a previously unnoted paralysis.

Fluoroscopy of the heart sometimes reveals calcification in a cardiac valve or in the coronary arteries. Pericardial effusion may also be seen fluoroscopically when it is not readily apparent on a routine chest roentgenogram. A short cinefluorographic film strip can be helpful in evaluating the presence of a pericardial effusion that is difficult to identify. (Ultrasonography is much more accurate than fluoroscopy and is currently

the most useful noninvasive study for demonstrating pericardial effusion.)

The character of a mediastinal lesion may be much better understood following fluoroscopy, particularly when the patient is asked to swallow barium sulfate during the examination. The esophagus is a mobile structure and is frequently displaced by mediastinal masses. Pulsation of a mediastinal mass is another situation which can be evaluated on the fluoroscopic screen. This may be misleading and should be interpreted with great care, since a mass adjacent to a vascular structure may transmit pulsations and appear it-
(Continued)

Tomography

As x-ray tube and cassette move synchronously in opposite directions, projection of one plane (B) remains in same position on film and is therefore sharp. Projections of other planes (A and C) move on film and are therefore blurred. Position of tube is adjusted to photograph successive sharp sections through the lung

Movement of x-ray tube

A B C

C B A

Movement of cassette

Roentgenologic Examination of the Lungs
(*Continued*)

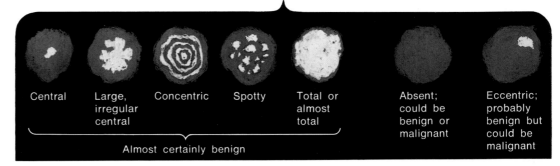

Shadow of lesion very faint in this section (5 cm cut)

Shadow distinct in this section (7 cm cut)

Shadow again hazy in this section (9 cm cut)

Types and degrees of calcification which may be demonstrated in shadows by tomography

Central | Large, irregular central | Concentric | Spotty | Total or almost total | Absent; could be benign or malignant | Eccentric; probably benign but could be malignant

Almost certainly benign

self to be pulsatile. Conversely, large aortic aneurysms often pulsate rather poorly, especially if they are filled with clot.

If the suspected mediastinal mass is a pulmonary vein or the superior vena cava, it may change its size with the Valsalva or Müller maneuver, becoming smaller with the former maneuver and larger with the latter.

In the past, fluoroscopy of the chest has been used as a screening procedure in routine examinations. This is no longer acceptable. Small pulmonary lesions can readily be missed at fluoroscopy, and there is no permanent record of the procedure for later comparative purposes. In addition, patient radiation exposure is many times greater with a short fluoroscopic examination than with standard roentgenograms. Fluoroscopy should be reserved for further evaluating a lesion previously identified on a chest roentgenogram or for studying cardiac or pulmonary dynamics.

Contrast Examinations

The routine chest roentgenogram provides major insights into pathologic processes and anatomic variations in the chest. Air in the bronchi and alveoli is a superb contrast medium. It outlines the pulmonary vasculature, the heart, the aorta and other mediastinal structures. In addition, pathologic processes in the lungs themselves characteristically disturb the usual pattern of the pulmonary vessels or the air-filled alveoli in a

fashion that is useful in making a rather accurate diagnosis of the patient's pulmonary problem, or occasionally of a generalized systemic problem.

Despite the great value of the routine chest roentgenogram, it is sometimes well to introduce contrast material into the chest to gain more information about some process which involves the lungs, the heart or a mediastinal structure. Positive contrast material can readily be introduced into the esophagus, trachea and bronchi, pulmonary vasculature, aorta and mediastinal arteries, superior vena cava and mediastinal veins, and, with some difficulty, the mediastinal lymphatics. Negative contrast material—air or other gases—

can be introduced into the pleural cavity, the peritoneal cavity, the mediastinum or the heart.

Barium Swallow. The simplest contrast examination is the barium swallow (esophageal contrast study), best carried out under fluoroscopic guidance. A suspension of barium sulfate outlining the esophageal contour demonstrates any displacement of the esophagus by adjacent mediastinal masses. Abnormalities of the esophagus itself such as achalasia or an esophageal tumor are also easily identified. The presence of unsuspected masses in the mediastinum such as metastatic lymph nodes may be shown. Analysis of cardiac
(*Continued*)

Roentgenologic Examination
of the Lungs
(*Continued*)

Bronchography: Technique

Anesthetization of pharynx and bronchial tree by spray of lidocaine or cocaine as patient inhales

Method A: Contrast medium dripped over dorsum of extended tongue

Method B: Contrast medium introduced via nasal or oral intratracheal catheter

Method C: Percutaneous tracheal catheterization through cricothyroid membrane after regional local anesthesia

Patient tipped to one side or other to achieve selective right or left bronchogram

chamber enlargement is also better accomplished by using roentgenograms in which the esophagus is outlined by barium sulfate.

Bronchography. While the trachea and major bronchi can readily be seen within the mediastinum, contrast bronchography is necessary to evaluate the smaller bronchi (Plate 7). Contrast medium for bronchography can be introduced in one of several ways: (1) following appropriate local anesthesia, contrast material can be dripped over the patient's extended tongue into the trachea; (2) it can be introduced by a catheter inserted through the patient's nose or mouth into the trachea; (3) it can be introduced by an indwelling catheter inserted into the trachea through a puncture made in the cricothyroid membrane; (4) it can be introduced into the bronchial tree by multiple punctures of the cricothyroid membrane. Careful positioning of the patient, either with or without fluoroscopy, will then distribute the contrast material into all of the bronchi (Plates 7, 8 and 9). Another, infrequently used technique is to deposit powdered tantalum on the mucosa of the trachea and bronchi by aerosol.

Since the advent of fiberoptic bronchoscopy, bronchography is seldom used to evaluate the tracheobronchial tree for tumor. Bronchoscopy yields a great deal more information by allowing the bronchoscopist to visualize the lesion directly and to take appropriate biopsies. However, the bronchoscopist cannot visualize the very small

bronchi and cannot readily make the diagnosis of bronchiectasis. The bronchogram, therefore, is used almost exclusively in evaluating bronchiectasis. The normal anatomy of the tracheobronchial tree is shown in Plates 8 and 9.

Pulmonary Angiography. Pulmonary angiography (Plate 10) is accomplished by injecting contrast material through a catheter introduced into the main pulmonary artery or its branches, the chambers of the heart or the great veins. It can also be accomplished by direct injection of contrast material into a large vein in one or both arms.

Any abnormality of the pulmonary vasculature can be studied by angiography, but its most

common use is to investigate thromboembolic disease of the lungs. Today, the much less invasive lung scan is more often employed as a screening procedure when a pulmonary embolus is suspected. When the scan is equivocal, angiography may be done to evaluate the patient better.

Congenital abnormalities of the pulmonary vascular tree, such as hypoplasia or agenesis of the pulmonary artery, arteriovenous malformation, pulmonary varix, or anomalous pulmonary venous return, are also readily identified by introducing contrast material directly into the pulmonary vascular tree.

(*Continued*)

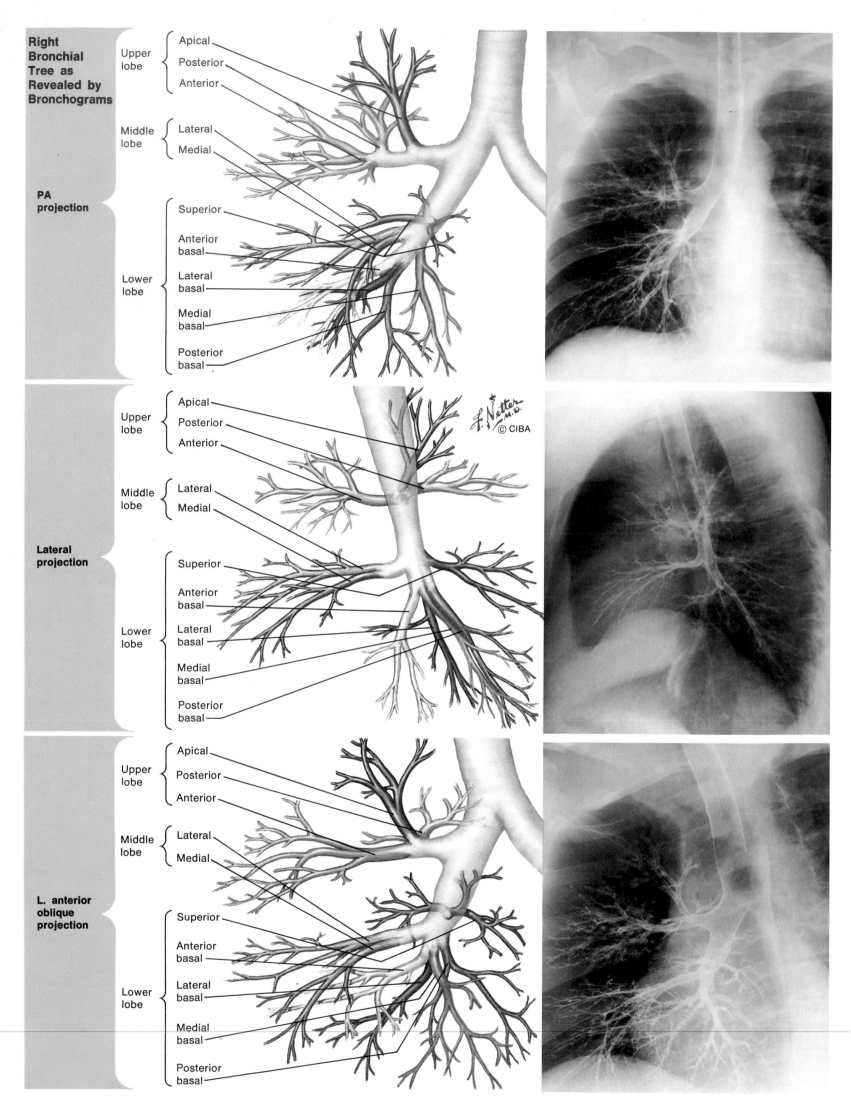

Right Bronchial Tree as Revealed by Bronchograms

PA projection

Upper lobe
- Apical
- Posterior
- Anterior

Middle lobe
- Lateral
- Medial

Lower lobe
- Superior
- Anterior basal
- Lateral basal
- Medial basal
- Posterior basal

Lateral projection

Upper lobe
- Apical
- Posterior
- Anterior

Middle lobe
- Lateral
- Medial

Lower lobe
- Superior
- Anterior basal
- Lateral basal
- Medial basal
- Posterior basal

L. anterior oblique projection

Upper lobe
- Apical
- Posterior
- Anterior

Middle lobe
- Lateral
- Medial

Lower lobe
- Superior
- Anterior basal
- Lateral basal
- Medial basal
- Posterior basal

92

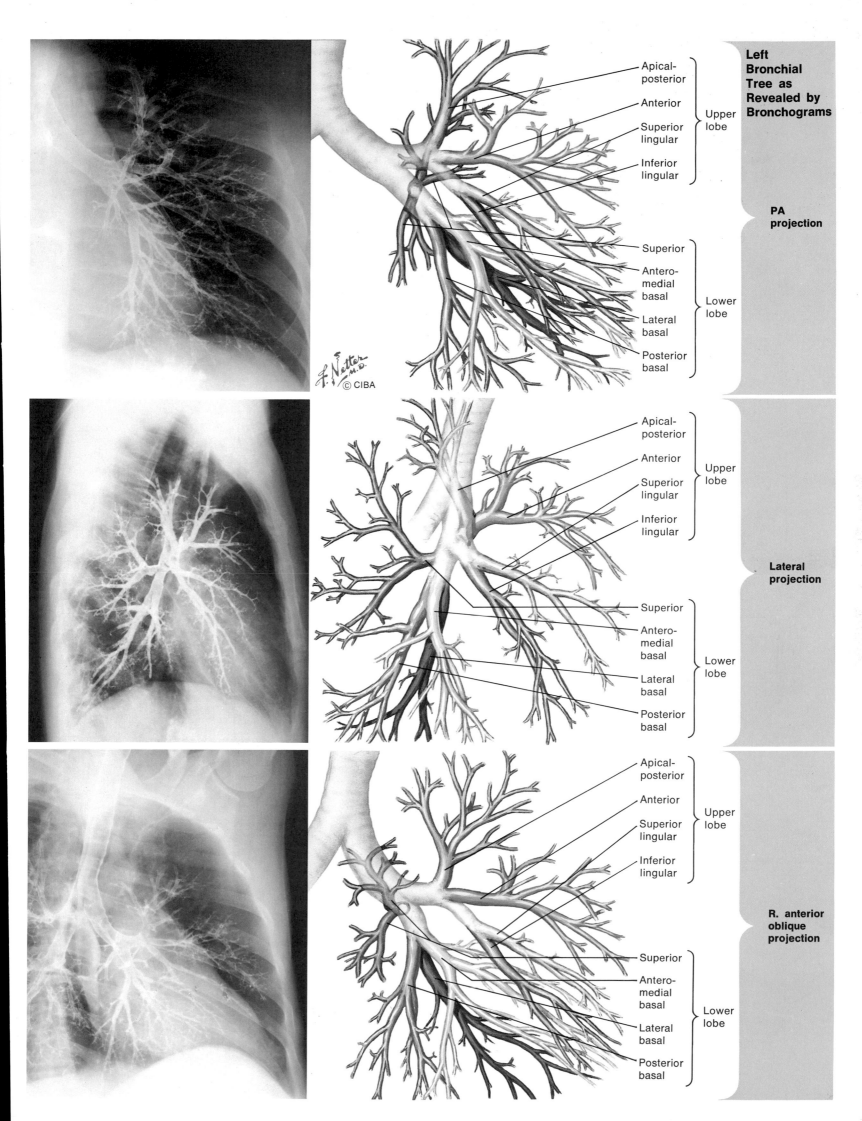

Left
Bronchial
Tree as
Revealed by
Bronchograms

Apical-
posterior
Anterior
Superior
lingular
Inferior
lingular

Upper
lobe

Superior
Antero-
medial
basal
Lateral
basal
Posterior
basal

Lower
lobe

PA
projection

Apical-
posterior
Anterior
Superior
lingular
Inferior
lingular

Upper
lobe

Superior
Antero-
medial
basal
Lateral
basal
Posterior
basal

Lower
lobe

Lateral
projection

Apical-
posterior
Anterior
Superior
lingular
Inferior
lingular

Upper
lobe

Superior
Antero-
medial
basal
Lateral
basal
Posterior
basal

Lower
lobe

R. anterior
oblique
projection

Pulmonary Angiography

Blue = Arterial Phase
Pink = Venous Phase

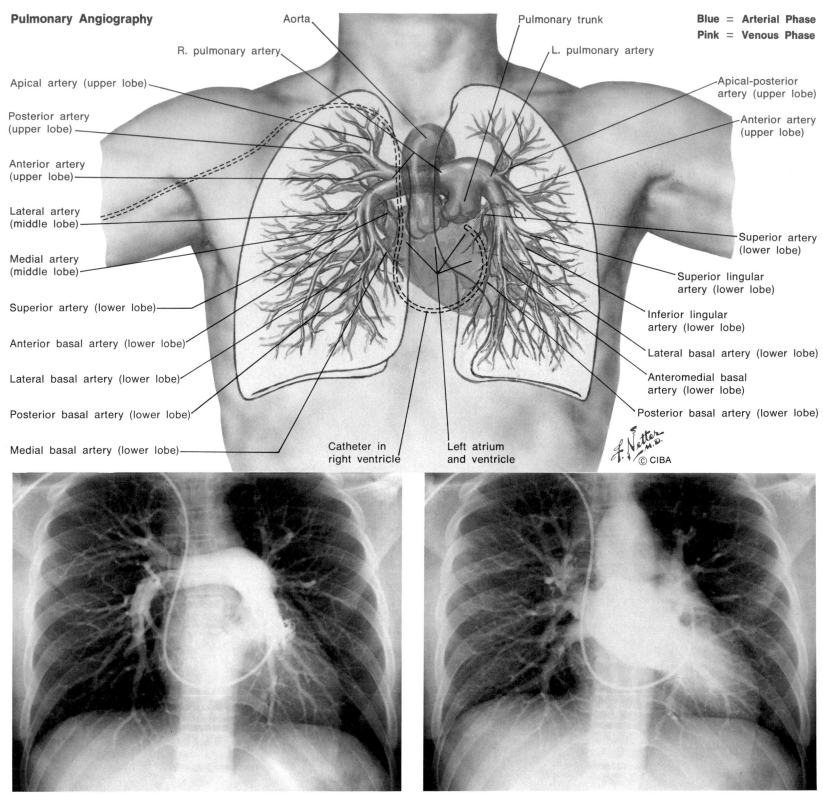

Aorta

R. pulmonary artery

Apical artery (upper lobe)

Posterior artery (upper lobe)

Anterior artery (upper lobe)

Lateral artery (middle lobe)

Medial artery (middle lobe)

Superior artery (lower lobe)

Anterior basal artery (lower lobe)

Lateral basal artery (lower lobe)

Posterior basal artery (lower lobe)

Medial basal artery (lower lobe)

Pulmonary trunk

L. pulmonary artery

Apical-posterior artery (upper lobe)

Anterior artery (upper lobe)

Superior artery (lower lobe)

Superior lingular artery (lower lobe)

Inferior lingular artery (lower lobe)

Lateral basal artery (lower lobe)

Anteromedial basal artery (lower lobe)

Posterior basal artery (lower lobe)

Catheter in right ventricle

Left atrium and ventricle

Normal angiogram (arterial phase)

Normal angiogram (venous phase)

Roentgenologic Examination of the Lungs
(Continued)

In the past, pulmonary angiography was also used to determine the resectability of primary carcinoma of the lung, but mediastinoscopy has now largely supplanted this procedure.

Aortography. It is relatively simple to make the aorta opaque by retrograde catheterization from the femoral artery using the Seldinger technique. It is also possible to inject the venous system and to visualize the aorta following passage of the contrast material through the pulmonary bed, although the latter method gives rather poor opacification and is seldom used in this age of skilled arteriographers.

Since the aorta is primarily in the middle or visceral compartment of the mediastinum, aortography is most useful in evaluating masses in this area. If the masses are vascular, this procedure will clearly demonstrate their vascular nature. Dissecting, saccular or fusiform aneurysms of the aorta, and anomalies or unusual tortuosity of the aorta or great vessels, may all be demonstrated by this technique. Any of these pathologic processes may present as a puzzling shadow on the routine chest x-ray film.

The great vessels may be selectively catheterized and studied. In addition, selective catheterization of the coronary arteries is commonly performed and yields information which may determine the advisability of coronary artery bypass surgery. Formerly, bronchial arteriography was used to study carcinoma of the lung, but it is now seldom done for this purpose.

Venography (phlebography) may also be used to study mediastinal masses. Displacement or obstruction of the superior vena cava may provide useful information in characterizing the nature of a mediastinal mass. Contrast opacification of the azygos vein may also assist in clarifying puzzling mediastinal shadows (see page 222).

(Continued)

Radioactive Scanning Methods

For perfusion scan, radioactive material is injected intravenously, and thus it is distributed to the pulmonary circulation

Roentgenologic Examination of the Lungs
(Continued)

For ventilation scan, patient inhales radioactive material injected into inspired air

F. Netter M.D. © CIBA

For both methods, distribution of radioactivity in lungs is determined by scintillation camera

Scintillation camera

Cable to console

Polaroid or other camera to photograph display

Visual display

Air Contrast Studies. Air or other gas can be injected into various compartments of the chest as a contrast medium, and may yield valuable information. Air in the pleural space (diagnostic pneumothorax) may identify a pleural lesion. However, since other techniques, such as pleural biopsy, provide more definitive and reliable data, diagnostic pneumothorax is no longer commonly done. Air in the peritoneal cavity may be helpful in evaluating a subphrenic abscess or diaphragmatic lesion. Diagnostic pneumomediastinum has been used to study mediastinal masses, particularly in searching for a thymoma, which is not identified by routine studies.

Radionuclide Scans

Scanning the lung following deposition of radioactive material in either the alveoli or the capillaries is an important clinical tool in investigating pulmonary pathophysiology (Plates 11 and 12). Two things are necessary to accomplish this purpose: (1) a radioactive material with suitable gamma emission that can be deposited in the appropriate area of interest, and (2) an instrument for recording the radioactivity.

The usual instruments for recording radioactivity in the lung are scanners and cameras. Both devices employ a sodium iodide crystal detector which detects and records radioactive emissions. The scanner uses a sodium iodide crystal with a focused collimator, moves stepwise in parallel lines across the lungs, and records the amount of radioactivity at each step. The gamma camera, a much larger crystal detector, has a series of parallel hole collimators that allow the large crystal to "see" the entire chest with a single view. Thus, a gamma camera can achieve in seconds what would take five minutes with the retrolinear scanner.

Radioisotopes may be used to depict pulmonary perfusion or pulmonary ventilation. To determine the patterns of pulmonary perfusion, small particles, which are larger than the diameter of a pulmonary capillary, are injected intravenously. The particles are trapped in the pulmonary

capillaries, and their distribution gives an accurate representation of pulmonary blood flow. The radioisotopes used initially were iodine 131 (^{131}I) or technetium 99m, tagged to macroaggregated human serum albumin. Technetium 99m is preferable because its short half-life (six hours) allows relatively large doses to be administered without undue radiation exposure. Macroaggregated serum albumin particles were not ideal because they varied in size, and some particles could pass through the pulmonary capillary bed to be picked up in the reticuloendothelial system throughout the body, particularly the liver. Currently, biodegradable albumin microspheres, with a controlled

particle size of 20 to 40 microns, are the particles of choice for perfusion scans.

To study ventilation in the lung, a gas must be used. The gas most commonly employed today is xenon 133. The patient breathes and rebreathes the gas continuously until it comes into equilibrium with the other gases in the lung (Plate 11). A series of gamma camera scans is made during this process, and areas of poor ventilation can be detected. The patient is then allowed to exhale the gas openly, and a second series of scans is made to determine whether gas is being trapped in any portion of the lung.

(Continued)

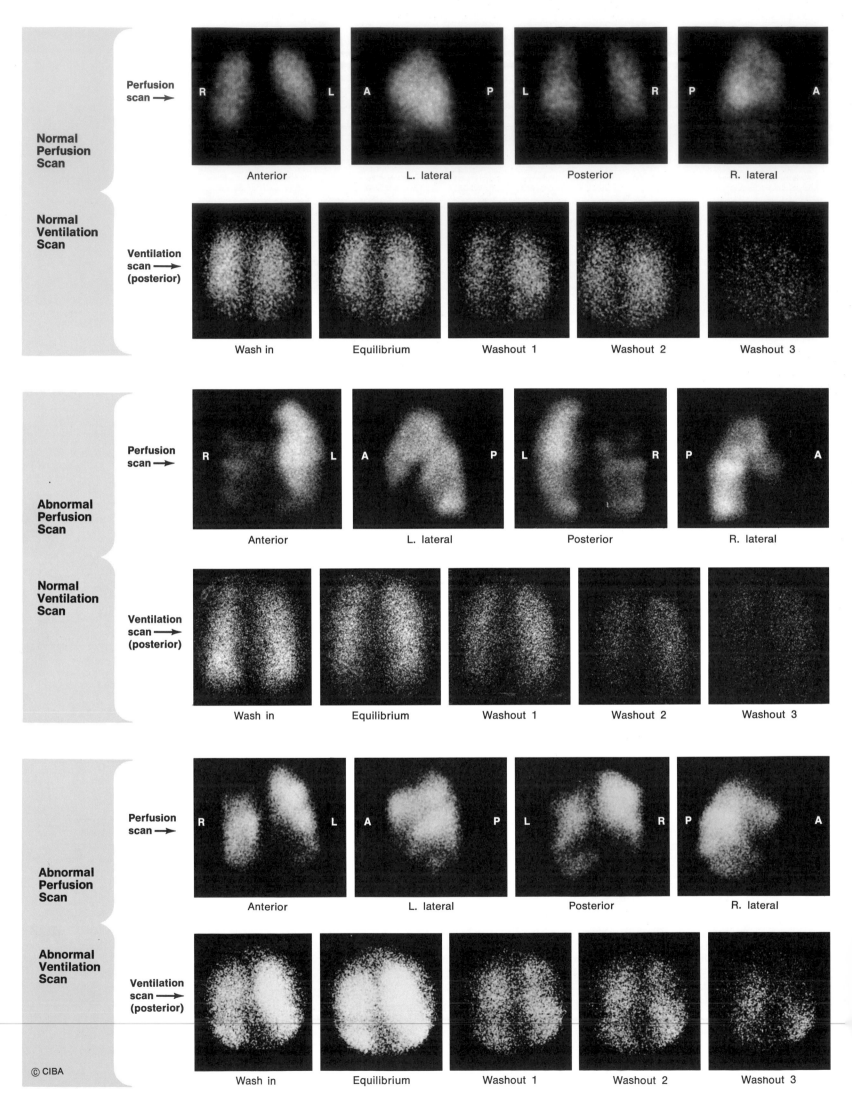

Normal Perfusion Scan

Perfusion scan →

R   L   A   P   L   R   P   A

Anterior   L. lateral   Posterior   R. lateral

Normal Ventilation Scan

Ventilation scan → (posterior)

Wash in   Equilibrium   Washout 1   Washout 2   Washout 3

Abnormal Perfusion Scan

Perfusion scan →

R   L   A   P   L   R   P   A

Anterior   L. lateral   Posterior   R. lateral

Normal Ventilation Scan

Ventilation scan → (posterior)

Wash in   Equilibrium   Washout 1   Washout 2   Washout 3

Abnormal Perfusion Scan

Perfusion scan →

R   L   A   P   L   R   P   A

Anterior   L. lateral   Posterior   R. lateral

Abnormal Ventilation Scan

Ventilation scan → (posterior)

Wash in   Equilibrium   Washout 1   Washout 2   Washout 3

Roentgenologic Examination
of the Lungs
(Continued)

The major clinical application of perfusion and ventilation scans of the lung is to detect pulmonary embolic disease. In many patients with pulmonary emboli the chest x-ray film is normal. Demonstration of one or several perfusion defects in the presence of a normal chest roentgenogram and a normal ventilation scan is diagnostic of pulmonary embolism. If the lung has an area of consolidation, both the ventilation and perfusion scans will generally be abnormal in that area. However, if the ventilation scan is normal in the remainder of the lung, but there are other areas of abnormality in a perfusion scan, this is indicative of pulmonary emboli and suggests that the area of consolidation is probably a pulmonary infarct.

If the patient has localized areas of poor perfusion coupled with similar areas of poor ventilation on radionuclide scans, it is extremely difficult to confirm the presence of a pulmonary embolus with any degree of certainty. This combination of ventilation and perfusion abnormalities occurs in patients with pulmonary emphysema. In such patients, pulmonary angiography is frequently necessary to establish the diagnosis of pulmonary embolism. Various patterns of ventilation-perfusion abnormalities are demonstrated in Plate 12.

Perfusion scans may also be helpful in evaluating the amount of perfusion to one lung, or a portion of one lung, if surgery is contemplated in a patient with poor pulmonary function. The scanning may indeed determine the advisability of surgery, for if the planned area of lung resection is very poorly perfused, resection may not greatly decrease lung function.

The perfusion scan may likewise assist in documenting abnormalities in pulmonary blood flow such as those occurring in hypoplasia of the pulmonary artery, Swyer-James anomaly or emphysema. Perfusion abnormalities are also present in patients with central carcinoma of the lung and in those with chronic inflammatory disease such as tuberculosis.

Interpretation of Roentgenographic Patterns

The scope of this section does not allow for a detailed discussion of all the pathologic processes that may be apparent on a chest roentgenogram. However, certain basic roentgenographic concepts will be discussed.

Atelectasis. Atelectasis is loss of volume of a lung, lobe or segment from any cause. Of the various mechanisms of atelectasis the most important is obstruction of a major bronchus by tumor, foreign body or bronchial plug. The other common cause of loss of lung volume is pneumonia, in which collapse occurs in the presence of patent bronchi, presumably secondary to abnormalities of surfactant.

There are several roentgenographic signs of atelectasis, or collapse, the most reliable being displacement of interlobar fissures (Plates 13 and 14). Localized increase in density of the collapsed lobe is another dependable sign of atelectasis. Indirect signs are: (1) elevation of the hemidiaphragm of the ipsilateral side, (2) deviation of the trachea and other mediastinal structures toward the side of the atelectasis, (3) compensatory hyperaeration of the remainder of the ipsilateral lung and sometimes of the contralateral lung, which may occasionally cross the mediastinum, (4) displacement of the hilar shadows toward the collapsed lobe or segment, and (5) decrease in size of the bony thorax on the involved side. These indirect signs are ordinarily seen only with atelectasis of major lung segments. They are less reliable than the direct signs, and can occasionally be simulated by normal and anatomic variations.

Certain fundamental observations can be made about lobar collapse: (1) The proximal portion of the lobe is tethered to the hilus, and consequently the roentgenographic shadows of the collapsed lung will always point toward the hilus. (2) Lobar collapse is always toward the mediastinum on the PA films. (3) On the lateral film, the upper lobe collapses anteriorly, the lower lobe collapses posteriorly, and the middle lobe symmetrically decreases in volume.

It is very important to recognize the patterns of lobar collapse since they are major indicators of primary pulmonary pathology. Recognition of a collapsed lobe may be difficult, particularly if the collapse is almost complete. Of great help in identifying its presence is the "silhouette sign," popularized by Felson. The silhouette sign may also be useful in identifying consolidation of the lung other than that caused by atelectasis. The sign is based on the premise that consolidation of a segment or lobe of lung contiguous and anterior to the border of the heart, aorta, diaphragm or mediastinum can obliterate that portion of the border on the roentgenogram. Frequently, this obliteration of a heart border or fuzziness of the diaphragm is the first clue that leads the observer to suspect the presence of atelectasis.

Alveolar vs Interstitial Disease. Pulmonary pathology can be manifested by densities occurring in the pulmonary alveoli or in the interstitial spaces of the lungs, or in both. It is often useful to distinguish alveolar from interstitial disease, although in some instances the distinction can be made only with great difficulty or not at all. In pure alveolar or interstitial disease, certain roentgenographic signs allow the investigator to tell one from the other (Plate 16).

Roentgenographic findings of alveolar disease are: (1) coalescent densities, creating large homogeneous shadows; (2) frequent presence of an air bronchogram (air is seen in the bronchial tree on account of fluid in surrounding alveoli; ordinarily the bronchial air is not visible because there is no contrast between air in the bronchi and air in the surrounding alveoli); (3) fluffy or irregular margins of localized areas of consolidation; (4) generally rapidly changing rather than static lesions.

Characteristically, alveolar disease is an acute process that occurs in localized patterns, as in a lobar or segmental distribution (pneumonia) or in a "butterfly" or "batwing" pattern (pulmonary edema).

Interstitial disease tends to be chronic rather than acute, and has several roentgenographic characteristics: (1) interstitial changes are usually discrete and sharp, not fluffy and irregular; (2) the lesions are likely to be diffuse rather than localized; (3) coalescence is not present; (4) certain typical patterns are seen—nodular, reticular and linear.

Localized Alveolar Disease. Pneumonia is the most common cause of localized alveolar infiltrates. Pneumonia may involve a single segment or several segments, a lobe, or occasionally almost all of both lungs. Various other inflammatory lesions such as tuberculosis or fungus disease may present as a localized alveolar pattern. Tumor, usually primary bronchogenic carcinoma, may also present in this way, as does alveolar cell carcinoma.

It is helpful to recognize the pulmonary segment involved by localized disease. Knowledge of the bronchographic anatomy of the lung allows one to localize the pulmonary subsegments. Plate 15 depicts the usual area seen on a PA roentgenogram by consolidation of a particular segment. This is of some importance as, for example, minimal tuberculosis almost exclusively involves the apical and posterior segments of the upper lobes and the superior segment of the lower lobe. Conversely, primary carcinoma of the lung occurs more frequently in the anterior segment of the upper lobe.

Pulmonary Nodule (Coin Lesion). While localized densities with ill-defined margins (alveolar disease) are generally inflammatory, the well-

(Continued)

Patterns of Lobar Collapse; Right Lung (after Lubert and Krause)

Horizontal (minor) fissures

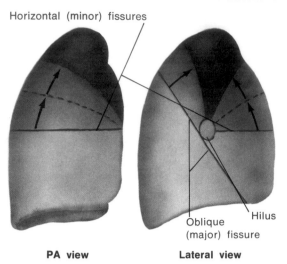

Oblique (major) fissure   Hilus

PA view   **Lateral view**

R. upper lobe collapse

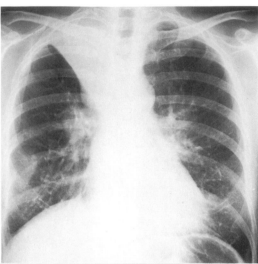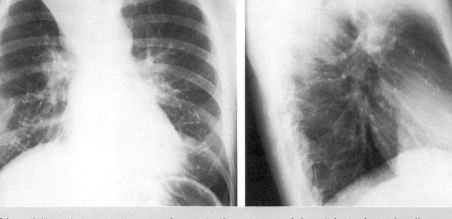

PA and lateral roentgenograms demonstrating r. upper lobe atelectasis and collapse secondary to an endobronchial carcinoma. Hilar adenopathy is also present as well as a metastasis in r. 8th posterior rib

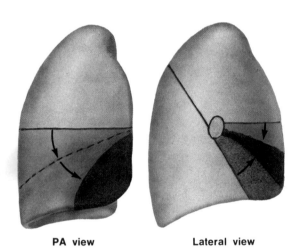

PA view   **Lateral view**

R. middle lobe collapse

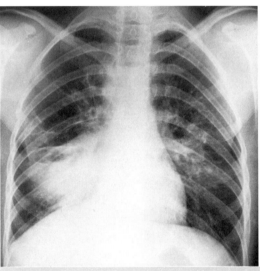

PA and lateral roentgenograms demonstrating r. middle lobe atelectasis and collapse secondary to allergic aspergillosis with bronchial obstruction by matted mycelia of aspergilli. There is an associated cavity in r. middle lobe. Some consolidation in superior segment of l. lower lobe is also present

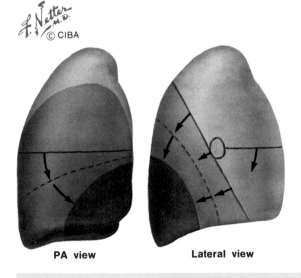

PA view   **Lateral view**

R. lower lobe collapse

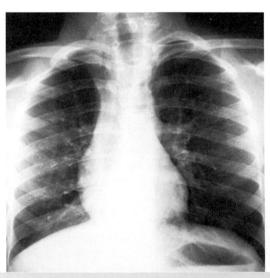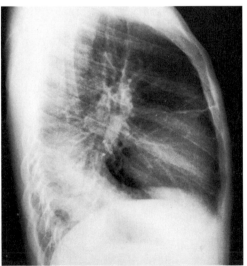

PA and lateral roentgenograms demonstrating r. lower lobe atelectasis and collapse secondary to bronchial plug in an asthmatic. On PA film, r. lower lobe collapse lies primarily behind cardiac silhouette and is seen through heart shadow. On lateral roentgenogram, posterior displacement of major fissure and blurring of sharp margin of posterior part of right hemidiaphragm are seen. Both changes indicative of consolidation and loss of volume of r. lower lobe

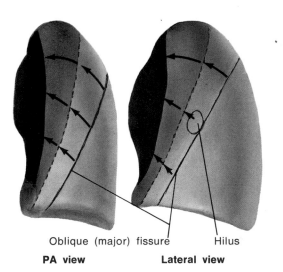

Oblique (major) fissure   Hilus

PA view   **Lateral view**

L. upper lobe collapse

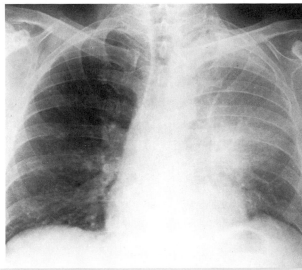

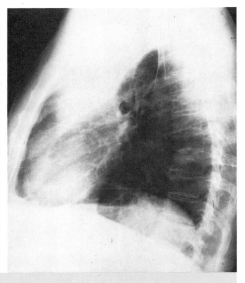

PA and lateral roentgenograms demonstrating l. upper lobe atelectasis and collapse secondary to bronchogenic carcinoma. Note loss of definition of aortic knob and left heart border (silhouette sign) caused by their relationship to atelectatic lung

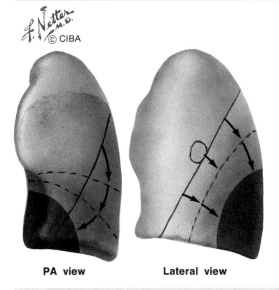

PA view   **Lateral view**

L. lower lobe collapse

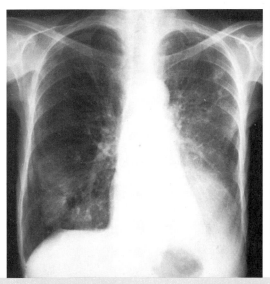

PA and lateral roentgenograms demonstrating l. lower lobe atelectasis and collapse secondary to endobronchial tumor. Other nodular lesions scattered through both lung fields represent additional metastases

Roentgenologic Examination of the Lungs
(Continued)

circumscribed pulmonary nodule (coin lesion) is more likely to be a neoplasm, especially in patients beyond the age of 35 years (see page 168). A large number of benign diseases may present as a well-circumscribed, solitary pulmonary nodule. A partial list includes tuberculous granuloma, histoplasmosis and other fungus diseases, pulmonary hamartoma, bronchogenic cyst, arteriovenous malformation (see CIBA COLLECTION, Volume 5,

pages 134 and 135), pulmonary sequestration, bronchial adenoma and necrobiotic nodule.

Laminography may be helpful in studying a solitary pulmonary nodule to identify cavitation or calcification within it. Central or concentric calcification is a strong indicator of benign disease, and usually signifies a granuloma. Multiple punctate calcification is another indicator of a benign process, and is frequently seen with a hamartoma. Eccentric calcification is of no diagnostic value since it may be seen in malignancy.

Cavitation in a pulmonary nodule seldom helps to identify the underlying disease with certainty, since either infection or tumor may cause it.

If a nodule in the lung field does not change over a long period of time, there is a strong likelihood that the lesion is benign. The physician can often obtain a previous roentgenogram and confirm that a lesion is not changing, thus saving the patient an exploratory thoracotomy. It is important to emphasize, however, that slowly growing

nodules in an older patient are very likely to be malignant. They may grow quite slowly over a period of several years.

Diffuse Alveolar Disease. Alveolar disease is characteristically an acute process and tends to be localized. However, it may be bilateral and diffuse, and is then frequently chronic. Diffuse alveolar disease often has a somewhat nodular pattern, but as a rule the nodules are ill defined or fuzzy (Plate 16). Some investigators believe these nodules represent the pulmonary acinus. When acute, a diffuse alveolar pattern is usually pulmonary edema on either a cardiac or a noncardiac basis. When chronic, a similar pattern should suggest such diagnoses as pulmonary alveolar proteinosis, alveolar cell carcinoma, "alveolar" sarcoidosis, lymphoma, metastatic carcinoma (particularly from the breast), eosinophilic lung disease, desquamating interstitial pneumonitis, and various forms of vasculitis.

(Continued)

Roentgenologic Examination
of the Lungs
(Continued)

Diffuse Interstitial Disease. Among the many causes of interstitial lung disease are:

1. Pneumoconiosis, especially silicosis and asbestosis
2. Infection
    a. Viral pneumonia
    b. Miliary tuberculosis
3. Metastatic tumor
    a. Nodular pattern
    b. "Lymphangitic spread" pattern
4. Sarcoidosis
5. Collagen disease, especially scleroderma and rheumatoid disease
6. Interstitial pulmonary edema
7. Hypersensitivity pneumonitis
8. Idiopathic pulmonary fibrosis
9. Eosinophilic granuloma

Interstitial lung disease is generally chronic and diffuse and takes three common patterns—nodular, reticular and linear (Plate 16). The nodules may be minute or appear as quite large masses, and ordinarily have sharply defined edges. Interstitial patterns typically presenting with nodules are seen in: pneumoconiosis—especially silicosis—metastatic tumor, miliary tuberculosis and sarcoidosis.

Linear densities are most commonly seen in acute rather than chronic interstitial lung disease, and are characteristic of interstitial pulmonary edema. A prominent interstitial pattern may also be seen in pneumonia secondary to infection with viral or pleuropneumonialike organisms (PPLO). Lymphangitic spread of tumor, an unusual kind of metastasis, also presents with a prominent linear pattern. Kerley lines are quite conspicuous in the linear presentation of interstitial lung disease.

A reticular or reticulonodular pattern is seen in sarcoidosis, asbestosis, and collagen disease (particularly scleroderma and rheumatoid lung), as well as being a characteristic of the "end-stage lung pattern," which is often the final result of various types of chronic interstitial disease. Notable in this group is idiopathic pulmonary fibrosis (Hamman-Rich syndrome).

Abnormalities of Air Distribution. Problems of air distribution within the lung can often be suspected from the roentgenogram, usually in patients with rather advanced disease. In the asthmatic, the chest roentgenogram is generally normal unless the patient is in status asthmaticus, in which case the lung fields are hyperinflated. Advanced pulmonary emphysema (see page 150) can be detected on the basis of pulmonary hyperinflation, bullous change and localized areas of destruction of the pulmonary vasculature. Fluoroscopy and inspiratory and expiratory films may lead to earlier detection of emphysema, but pulmonary function tests are much more reliable, so that early discovery of emphysema is not made on the basis of chest roentgenograms.

In chronic bronchitis, like asthma, the chest roentgenogram is ordinarily normal. However, the patient may have prominent vascular markings and exhibit some degree of hyperinflation.

Pulmonary Blood Flow Redistribution. The pulmonary arteries and veins are easily recognizable on the chest roentgenogram, and the careful observer can readily identify localized or generalized redistribution of pulmonary blood flow.

The pulmonary vascular bed has an extremely low resistance, allowing ready redistribution of its contents as resistance is increased locally.

Posture has a marked effect on flow distribution. In the erect position, the pulmonary vessels are seen as significantly larger in the bases than in the apices due merely to the effect of gravity. Alteration in posture obviously affects this distribution, and in a supine position, flow is relatively uniform from the apices to the bases. Thus it is of considerable importance when evaluating pulmonary vasculature to know the patient's position during roentgenography.

While alveolar pressure is generally constant throughout the lung, it may undergo regional changes due to obstruction of individual bronchi by a foreign body or perhaps mucous plugging in an asthmatic. This will result in a redistribution of blood flow away from the localized areas of increased pressure. Similar changes take place in pulmonary emphysema, although the redistribution that occurs in this disease is in greater part due to actual destruction of the pulmonary vascular bed by the pathologic process.

A pulmonary embolus may show up on the roentgenogram as a segment of oligemia distal to an obstructed pulmonary artery, although this sign is rarely seen except with occlusion of a very large vessel.

Disease processes which directly involve the pulmonary vasculature will cause recognizable patterns of blood flow redistribution. In primary pulmonary hypertension, the peripheral vessels are small and the central vessels quite large, giving the characteristic "pruned tree" appearance. In emphysema, local destruction of the capillary bed results in bizarre and unpredictable patterns of pulmonary blood flow.

Cardiac disease is the most familiar cause of pulmonary blood flow redistribution. The classic example occurs in mitral stenosis, in which it was observed early that upper lobe vessels become prominent and lower lobe vessels narrowed. However, any cardiac problem that increases left atrial pressure can cause a similar redistribution of blood flow from the bases to the apices (cephalization). This, of course, takes place in left heart failure. Interestingly, the redistribution is much more readily detectable in patients with chronic heart failure than in those with acute failure. Cephalization of pulmonary perfusion is a clue that some cardiac disease exists, and its appearance should alert the observer to look carefully at the cardiac silhouette for an explanation of this pattern of blood flow redistribution.

Pleural Disease

The chest wall is covered by a thin sheet of mesothelial cells (parietal pleura), and the lungs and fissures are similarly lined (visceral pleura). Between the parietal and visceral pleurae is a potential space which can be involved in various disease processes. Such involvement is manifested by pleural fluid, localized or diffuse pleural thickening or pleural nodules.

Intrapleural fluid appears roentgenographically as a homogeneous opacity that is usually in a dependent position in the pleural cavity. Small amounts of free fluid may be difficult to detect, but careful observation of the posterior costophrenic sulcus on the lateral roentgenogram often shows minor blunting with as little as 25 to 50 ml of fluid. A decubitus roentgenogram will confirm the presence of free fluid (Plate 4).

With larger effusions, the lateral costophrenic sulcus is also blunted on the PA roentgenogram. Sometimes the fluid becomes loculated in the pleural space and thus is difficult to differentiate from localized pleural thickening. An effusion which is rapidly loculated strongly suggests inflammatory disease of the pleura, since this occurs in effusions high in protein (exudates).

Localized or generalized fibrosis of the pleura may occur in a variety of conditions. *Localized* pleural thickening is commonly seen at the lung apices. It frequently makes one suspect tuberculosis, but apical pleural thickening is usually an unexplained phenomenon which may be related to aging. Blunting of the costophrenic sulcus may be due to a previous pleural effusion. If a costophrenic sulcus is blunted laterally on the PA film but not blunted posteriorly on the lateral film, it is extremely unlikely that free pleural fluid is present; instead, the blunting probably represents old pleural thickening.

When localized pleural change has the appearance of a nodule, this should suggest pleural tumor—either mesothelioma or metastatic malignancy.

Common causes of *unilateral* effusions are tuberculosis, pneumonia, pulmonary infarction, metastatic tumor, primary pleural tumor, lymphoma, chest trauma, and intraabdominal processes such as subphrenic abscess or pancreatitis.

(Continued)

Roentgenologic Examination of the Lungs
(Continued)

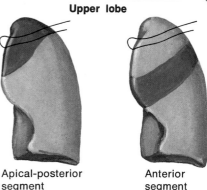

Right lung

Upper lobe

Apical segment	Posterior segment	Anterior segment

Left lung

Upper lobe

Apical-posterior segment	Anterior segment

Middle lobe

Lateral segment	Medial segment

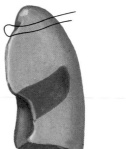

Superior lingular segment	Inferior lingular segment

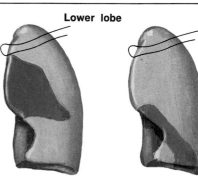

Lower lobe

Superior segment	Medial basal segment

Lower lobe

Superior segment	Lateral basal segment

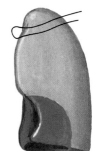

Anterior basal segment	Lateral basal segment	Posterior basal segment

Anteromedial basal segment	Posterior basal segment

The most common cause of *bilateral* pleural fluid is congestive heart failure. Other frequent causes include the collagen vascular diseases — especially lupus erythematosus and rheumatoid arthritis — metastatic tumor, and the hypoproteinemic states which are generally secondary to hepatic or renal disease. Any of the entities that cause fluid to accumulate in both pleural spaces can also result in unilateral effusion and so should be considered in its differential diagnosis.

Thoracentesis and pleural biopsy are extremely important procedures in characterizing the nature of a pleural effusion that has been identified roentgenographically.

Generalized pleural thickening in one hemithorax is usually secondary to previous tuberculosis, empyema or hemothorax. *Bilateral* pleural thickening should make one suspect asbestosis (see page 211), particularly if accompanied by pleural calcification. Asbestosis uncomplicated by mesothelioma may also sometimes present with nodular pleural thickening.

Abnormalities of Diaphragm and Chest Wall

Variations of diaphragmatic contour are frequent. While each hemidiaphragm is generally a smooth dome-shaped structure, localized bulges are common and are usually due to a deficiency of muscle in that portion (partial eventration). Fluoroscopically, paradoxical motion is often observed in such a localized segment, and in all instances this area moves less well than the normal muscle surrounding it.

The several foramina in the normal diaphragm may become enlarged and allow herniation of abdominal viscera into the chest. The paired foramina of Morgagni lie anteriorly and medially. Hernias occasionally occur through them, and are more common on the right side than on the left. Most often, herniations develop through the centrally placed esophageal hiatus. The stomach is the usual viscus to herniate through this opening, but the colon may also do so, and occasionally small bowel herniation is seen as well. Posteriorly and slightly laterally are the paired foramina of Bochdalek. Massive congenital hernias seen in newborns — though infrequently — generally bulge through a large foramen of Bochdalek, usually on the left side (see page 110). In addition to diaphragmatic hernias, a tumor of the diaphragm sometimes presents as a mass on the chest roentgenogram.

Abnormalities of the thoracic cage are identified as a rule by destruction of ribs and protrusion of a mass into the lung, creating a characteristic pattern. Most abnormalities in this location are metastatic tumors, but primary tumors of the
(Continued)

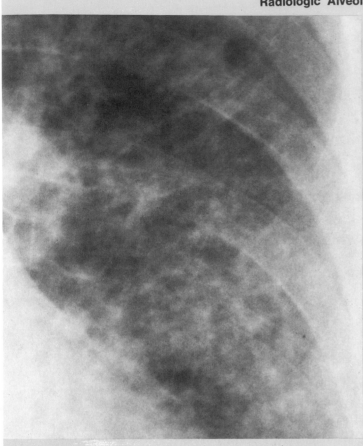

A. Somewhat nodular diffuse pattern (diffuse alveolar cell carcinoma)

B. Acinar shadows with tendency to perihilar, "butterfly," pattern (pulmonary edema)

© CIBA

Roentgenologic Examination of the Lungs
(Continued)

ribs or soft-tissue sarcomas may also be recognized. Almost invariably, these lesions indicate their presence by destroying or eroding the ribs. Their protrusion into the lung causes a shadow with very smooth margins and tapering edges; it is likely to be seen well in only one of the two routine roentgenograms of the chest. This characteristic configuration has been designated the "extrapleural sign" by Felson. Since it may be mimicked by many pleural lesions, bone destruction is the key to accurate identification of an extrapleural mass.

Occasionally, densities appear on roentgenograms of the chest wall that are due to lipomas. Fat pads may also cause densities without any rib involvement.

Abnormalities of Mediastinum

Mediastinal structures are visualized indirectly on the chest roentgenogram, since all of them, except the trachea, are of water density and cannot readily be differentiated one from another. Indirect visualization is provided by the air in the surrounding lung. Various inferences can be drawn about the anatomy and pathology of these structures based on their impression on the surrounding lungs (see page 172).

Introduction of barium into the esophagus gives additional information about the esophagus itself and its adjacent mediastinal contents. More invasive techniques such as arteriography or venography may yield further data.

In anatomical texts, the mediastinum has been divided into a superior and an inferior compartment and the latter into anterior, middle and posterior subdivisions. A slight departure from the usual anatomic division allows unification of thought when one is attempting to classify mediastinal lesions seen on roentgenography.

The anterior compartment is bounded anteriorly by the sternum and posteriorly by the heart, aorta and innominate vessels. The middle compartment contains the heart, great vessels, trachea and its branches, esophagus and descending aorta. This is a slight variation from the anatomic classification, in which portions of esophagus and descending aorta lie in the posterior mediastinum.

In the radiologic division of the mediastinum, the posterior boundary of the middle mediastinal compartment is the anterior spinal ligament; thus everything anterior to this lies in one large compartment, which can be designated the middle or visceral compartment. The posterior compartment therefore contains only the vertebrae and the paravertebral sulci. Using this basis for division,

radiologically detected lesions within the mediastinum can be readily categorized. The usual masses found in the *anterior compartment* are lymph node enlargement from any cause, substernal goiter, the thymus and thymic tumors, and teratoid tumors. Thyroid masses almost invariably appear high in the anterior mediastinum and displace the trachea in some way. Thymomas and teratoid tumors lie below the aortic arch in most instances and each presents as a single, well-demarcated mass. Lymph node enlargement is usually diffuse, with a rather nodular or lumpy character. It can have a number of causes, mainly metastatic tumor, lymphoma, sarcoidosis, primary tuberculosis and occasionally other inflammatory lesions.

The *middle compartment* of the mediastinum contains all the viscera; thus the common abnormalities arising from them are located in this region. Again, lymph node enlargement is a frequent finding which usually presents as a diffuse expansion of the zone, often associated with enlargement of one or both hilar shadows. Anomalies or aneurysms of the aorta or the great vessels, and duplication cysts of the esophagus and tracheobronchial tree may present as localized densities in this location. The esophagus itself may appear as a long tubular shadow, and tumors or diverticula of the esophagus may be seen as localized mediastinal masses. Pericardial cysts or tumors also occur in the middle mediastinum.

The only common masses of the *posterior compartment* are neurogenic tumors, but tumors or infections of the vertebral column may also occasionally present in a similar location.

(Continued)

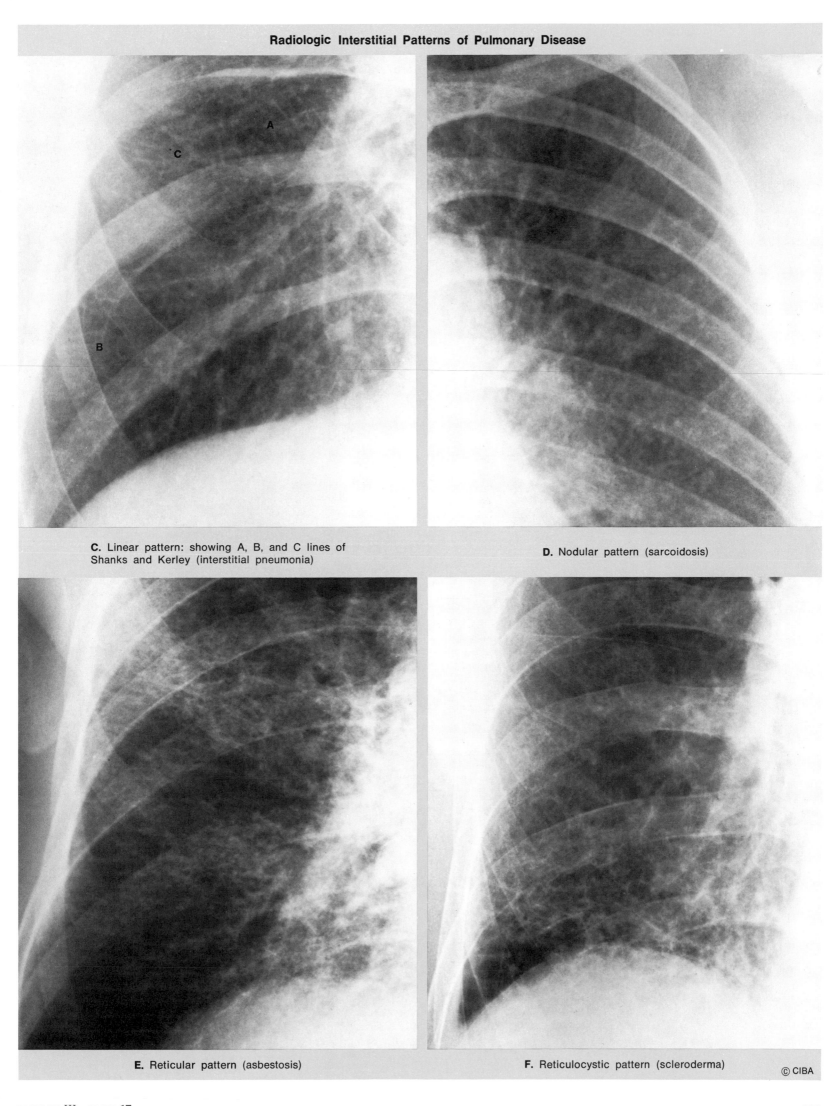

C. Linear pattern: showing A, B, and C lines of Shanks and Kerley (interstitial pneumonia)

D. Nodular pattern (sarcoidosis)

E. Reticular pattern (asbestosis)

F. Reticulocystic pattern (scleroderma)

© CIBA

Roentgenologic Examination of the Lungs
(Continued)

Computerized Tomography

Computerized tomography is a new and important roentgenographic tool. In this technique, a series of pencil-thin or fan-shaped x-ray beams traverses the patient, and the transmitted radiation from each beam is measured by a crystalline detector instead of impinging on a film. As the machine rotates circumferentially around the patient the process is repeated, and a computer reconstructs the amount of transmitted radiation for each small area of the body examined by the x-ray beam. Several hundred thousand individual measurements are made. The resultant information can be displayed as a series of numbers, or as a reconstructed image of the patient (CT scan) quite similar to a roentgenogram (Plate 18).

The major advantage of computerized tomography is its ability to detect differences in x-ray density of as low as 1 to 2%; standard techniques detect density differences of 5%. Thus, minor variations in soft tissue which cannot be appreciated by ordinary roentgenographic techniques can be readily demonstrated by computerized tomography. Density differences may also be enhanced by administering intravenous contrast material to the patient.

The initial and most valuable thrust in computerized tomography was in neuroradiology. This technique allowed visualization of the brain, ventricles and subarachnoid spaces by an entirely noninvasive technique. Subsequent development of computerized tomography has shown it to be most useful in other parts of the body, especially in the abdomen.

In the thorax, the impact of computerized tomography has been less great. This is primarily due to the fact that a routine chest roentgenogram allows good visualization of intrathoracic structures, due to the air contrast present. Pathologic processes within the lung itself are readily visible and abnormalities of the heart, mediastinum, pleura and chest walls are generally recognizable due to impressions on the air-containing lung. Nonetheless, CT scanning is a more sensitive means of studying chest pathology and has proven useful in various situations.

Pulmonary Nodules. Computerized tomography is much more effective than standard chest roentgenography or tomography in identifying pulmonary nodules. It has thus proven useful in evaluating the presence of metastases or the extent of metastatic disease in a patient with known malignancy. Unfortunately, the mere detection of a nodule does not indicate its pathologic nature, and computerized tomography detects many small and possibly innocent granulomas which would not have shown up using conventional techniques, and which cannot be differentiated from metastatic tumors.

Computerized Tomography (CT Scans) in Thoracic Diagnosis

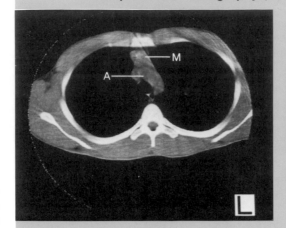

A. Thymoma. Mediastinal mass (M) containing small amount of calcification seen lying anterior to ascending aorta (A) in right side of superior mediastinum. Trachea with contained air lies behind and to left of ascending aorta

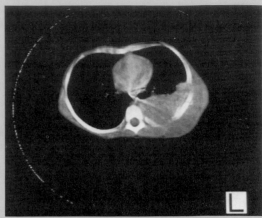

B. Chest wall sarcoma invading lung and bone. Large mass in left posterior hemithorax destroying ribs and extending beyond rib cage into soft tissues of chest wall, which are consequently much larger than those in corresponding position on right side

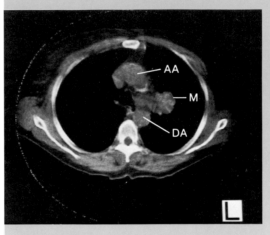

C. Carcinoma of lung invading mediastinum. Large mass (M) apparent in left lung invading mediastinum in area of aortic arch (AA). Aortic arch visualized in its entirety with beginning of descending aorta (DA) lying posteriorly

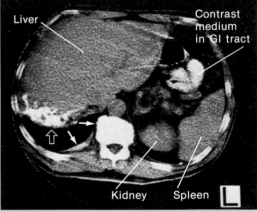

D. Asbestosis with pleural plaques. In right hemithorax calcification seen in right hemidiaphragm (open arrow) and calcified pleural plaques in parietal pleura of posterior costophrenic sulcus (solid arrows). Scan also shows portions of abdominal viscera

© CIBA

Mediastinal Masses. Computerized tomography has proven useful in establishing the extent of a mediastinal mass and, in some instances, in determining its identity. It is particularly useful in distinguishing fat from lymphadenopathy in a widened mediastinum. The CT scan may identify a mediastinal mass even in the absence of positive findings on the chest roentgenogram. This is a useful technique in searching for mediastinal adenopathy in a patient with primary lung carcinoma or in searching for a thymoma in a patient with myasthenia gravis.

Carcinoma of the Lung. Computerized tomography is useful in evaluating the size of lung carcinomas and their extension into the mediastinum or chest wall. As previously mentioned, it is also valuable in identifying mediastinal adenopathy not seen on the standard chest roentgenogram. Unfortunately, the value of a CT scan is limited, because a negative result does not exclude enlargement of hilar nodes and thus does not obviate the need for mediastinoscopy in staging lung carcinoma.

Pleural Lesions. The CT scan is very sensitive in detecting small pleural effusions and small pleural nodules. It is useful for identifying pleural metastatic disease or pleural plaques in patients with asbestos exposure.

Chest Wall Lesions. Computerized tomography is quite valuable in demonstrating the extent of lesions which have arisen primarily in the chest wall (*e.g.*, soft-tissue sarcoma) and in identifying invasion of the chest wall by other malignancies. Bone destruction which is not appreciated on the ordinary roentgenogram can often be demonstrated by CT scanning.

Vascular Lesions. The new fast scanners with a scan time of five seconds or less can permit imaging of vascular lesions involving the aorta and its branches or pulmonary vessels. This is particularly useful in identifying aortic aneurysms and abnormalities of central vascular structures.

Diffuse Lung Disease. CT numbers rather than scans are useful for the measurement of the density of the structure being studied and have the potential advantage of indicating the presence of subradiographic diffuse lung disease. However, differences in density caused by inspiration and expiration, pulmonary blood flow alterations that occur in positioning the patient, and other problems of variability within the lung itself have made this technique unreliable at present.

Section IV

Diseases and Pathology

Frank H. Netter, M.D.

in collaboration with

Mary Ellen Avery, M.D. and Lynne M. Reid, M.D.   *Plates 48-49, 137-139*

Howard A. Buechner, M.D.   *Plates 81-87, 105-106*

Howard A. Buechner, M.D. and Charles V. Sanders, Jr., M.D.   *Plates 79-80*

Robert W. Colman, M.D.   *Plates 107, 109, 121*

Paul E. Epstein, M.D.   *Plates 50-59, 61-65*

Alfred P. Fishman, M.D.   *Plates 2-3, 114-120, 124-125*

Roland H. Ingram, Jr., M.D.   *Plates 28-45*

Victor J. Marder, M.D.   *Plate 111*

Wallace T. Miller, M.D.   *Plates 60, 110*

Roger S. Mitchell, M.D.   *Plates 88-96*

W. Spencer Payne, M.D.   *Plate 122*

Giuseppe G. Pietra, M.D.   *Plate 123*

Max L. Som, M.D.   *Plates 10-12*

D. Eugene Strandness, Jr., M.D.   *Plates 112-113*

Morton N. Swartz, M.D.   *Plates 66-76*

Alvin S. Teirstein, M.D. and Jacob Churg, M.D.   *Plates 140-149*

Joseph J. Timmes, M.D.   *Plates 1, 4-9, 126-136*

Earle B. Weiss, M.D.   *Plates 13-27*

William Weiss, M.D.   *Plates 46-47, 77-78*

J. Edwin Wood, III, M.D.   *Plate 108*

Morton M. Ziskind, M.D.   *Plates 97-104*

Congenital Deformities of Thoracic Cage

Pectus Excavatum. Pectus excavatum is also called funnel chest, chonechondrosternon or trichterbrust. It is a deformity of the anterior chest wall characterized by depression of the lower sternum and adjacent cartilages. The lowest point of the depression is at the junction of the xiphoid process and the body of the sternum. The trait is inherited and may coexist with other musculoskeletal malformations such as clubfoot, syndactyly and Klippel-Feil syndrome. The etiology of funnel chest remains obscure. A short central tendon and muscular imbalance of the diaphragm have been blamed. Most current writers attribute the deformity to unbalanced growth in the costochondral regions.

Symptoms are very uncommon. However, a child, particularly a male, with a deformity that is all too obvious suffers unfortunate psychological effects and often becomes shy, withdrawn and depressed. Funnel chest is usually associated with postural disorders such as forward displacement of the neck and shoulders, upper thoracic kyphosis and protuberant abdomen. Functional heart murmurs and benign cardiac arrhythmias are not infrequently seen, and the electrocardiogram may show right axis deviation because of the displacement of the heart. In older patients there may be an appreciable incidence of chronic bronchitis and bronchiectasis.

Depression of the sternum begins typically at the junction of the manubrium and the gladiolus. The xiphoid process may be bifid, twisted or displaced to one side. Costal cartilages are angulated internally, beginning with the second or third and extending caudally to involve the remainder. In general, the defect tends to be symmetric, but one side may be more depressed than the other, so that the sternum deviates from the middle line. An estimate of the cavitary volume may be obtained by filling the depression with water while the patient lies supine. Standard x-ray films reveal that the heart is displaced toward the left side, and lateral films show the displacement of the body of the sternum posteriorly.

In patients who are symptomatic or who show a significant progression of pectus excavatum, the deformity should be corrected surgically. As most of the operations are carried out with a cosmetic end in mind, the results are best when surgery is performed between the third and seventh year of age. Surgical correction consists of excision of the hypertrophied costal cartilages on both sides, osteotomy of the sternum at the junction of the manubrium and body, and then internal fixation by pins or rods, which are removed later. Fixation by a metal strut or wire is required in older patients to prevent recurrence of the deformity which, in some degree, may occur despite initial overcorrection.

Pectus Carinatum. Also known as pigeon breast, chicken breast or keel breast, this is a protrusion deformity of the anterior chest wall, unrelated to pectus excavatum and occurring about one-tenth as often. Two principal types are recognized: (1) chondromanubrial, in which the protuberance is maximal at the xiphoid, and the gladiolus is directed posteriorly so that a secondary saucerization is evident, and (2) chondrogladiolar,

Pectus excavatum

Pectus carinatum

Bifid sternum

in which the greatest prominence is at, or near, the gladiolus. The pathogenesis is no better understood than that of pectus excavatum, but the theory of unbalanced or excessive growth of the cartilages is attractive. While functional cardiac and respiratory difficulties have been observed, the chief reason for surgical correction is cosmetic. If the deformity is minor, no treatment is required. When operation is necessary, the procedure should be tailored to the particular deformity, taking into account the full life-circumstances of the patient. When the deformity causes embarrassment, the surgical procedure is aimed at achieving psychological as well as physiologic improvement.

Bifid Sternum. Failure of fusion of the sternal bands may occur, creating a defect of the anterior chest wall. Separation of the sternum may be complete or incomplete and may be associated with an ectopia cordis. When the defect is incomplete, surgical correction of the abnormality may be accomplished. If the repair cannot be effected by primary approximation of the sternal segments, a prosthesis or a cartilage autograft may be used.

Other deformities of the chest wall occasionally seen include cervical ribs (with or without compression of the brachial plexus and artery), partial absence of ribs, supernumerary ribs, and thoracic-pelvic-phalangeal dystrophy.

Kyphoscoliosis

Kyphoscoliosis has long been recognized as a cause of cardiorespiratory failure. Only in recent years, however, has the combination of clinical picture, physiologic measurements and anatomic observations at autopsy clarified the natural history of the cardiorespiratory disorder.

Unless there is independent lung disease, such as bronchitis and emphysema, only patients with severe spinal deformities are candidates for cardiorespiratory failure. Subjects with mild deformities are consistently asymptomatic. In contrast, those with severe degrees of deformity, particularly if considerable dwarfing has occurred, are often restricted in their activities by dyspnea on exertion. They are the ones most prone to cardiorespiratory failure if an upper respiratory infection should supervene. From the point of view of disability and the likelihood of cardiorespiratory failure, the nature of the deformity—*i.e.,* kyphosis or scoliosis or both—is unimportant when compared to the severity of deformity and dwarfing.

One approach to classifying kyphoscoliotic subjects is on the basis of lung volumes. The more normal the total lung capacity, vital capacity and tidal volume, the more the subject tends to remain asymptomatic. In persons with severe reduction in lung volumes, the stage is set for cor pulmonale.

Estimates of the work of breathing, using pressure-volume loops, show an inordinate work load (and energy expenditure) attributable to the severe limitation of distensibility of the chest wall, which produces markedly reduced compliance. As a consequence of the high cost of breathing, the individual adopts a pattern of rapid, shallow breathing. Although this pattern is economical in terms of the work and energy required, it sacrifices alveolar ventilation for the sake of deadspace ventilation. The resultant alveolar hypoventilation brings about arterial hypoxemia, hypercapnia and respiratory acidosis by hyperventilating the conducting airways and hypoventilating the alveoli. Thus, the asymptomatic kyphoscoliotic person consistently manifests normal arterial blood gases, whereas the severely deformed kyphoscoliotic person is often cyanotic and shows not only arterial hypoxemia but also hypercapnia. Between these two extremes are the patients who remain breathless on exertion and whose arterial blood gases hover at the brink of important hypoxemia and hypercapnia. They are easily toppled into a state of cardiorespiratory failure by a bout of bronchitis or pneumonia.

In asymptomatic persons the pulmonary arterial pressure is normal at rest and increases to clinically insignificant levels during exercise. In contrast, the pulmonary arterial pressure in the

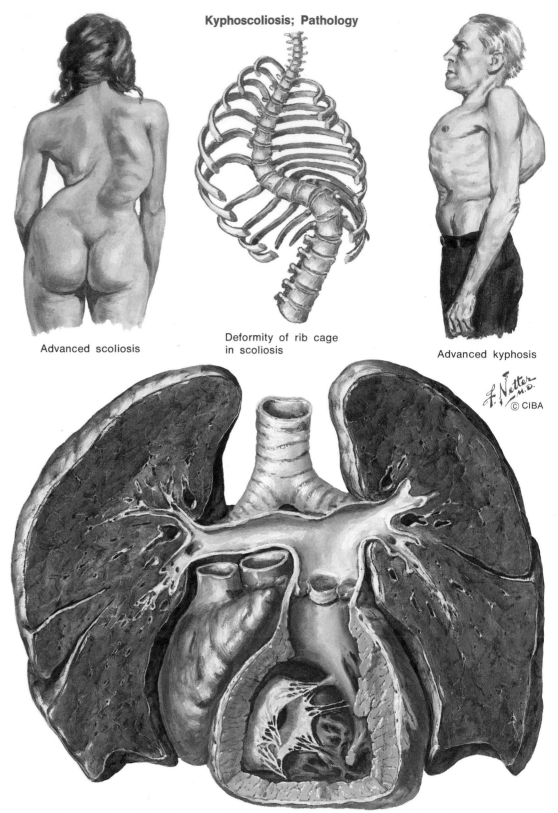

Kyphoscoliosis; Pathology

Advanced scoliosis

Deformity of rib cage in scoliosis

Advanced kyphosis

Characteristic cardiopulmonary pathology in kyphoscoliosis: hypertrophy and dilatation of right ventricle (and atrium); lungs atelectatic and reduced in volume with little or no emphysematous changes

severely deformed not only may be high at rest but also increases precipitously during modest exercise. The basis for this pulmonary hypertension is generally twofold: (1) a restricted pulmonary vascular bed due to the compressing and distorting effects of the deformity on the lungs and on the pulmonary vasculature, and (2) the pulmonary pressor effects of hypoxia. These two effects are most marked during exercise because of the increase in pulmonary blood flow into the restricted vascular bed and the pulmonary vasoconstriction elicited by the exercise-induced hypoxemia. The patients show enlargement of the right ventricle at autopsy. During an upper respiratory infection

the pulmonary pressor effects of the arterial hypoxemia may be sufficiently severe to raise pulmonary arterial pressure to very high levels and to precipitate right ventricular failure.

In patients in whom chronic alveolar hypoventilation has caused sustained pulmonary hypertension, hypercapnia consistently accompanies the arterial hypoxemia. Hypercapnia contributes to pulmonary hypertension by way of the respiratory acidosis that it causes, since acidosis acts synergistically with hypoxia in causing pulmonary vasoconstriction. However, hypercapnia exerts its predominant effects on the central nervous system

(Continued)

Pulmonary Function in Kyphoscoliosis

Kyphoscoliosis
(Continued)

rather than on the heart or circulation. In kyphoscoliotic subjects who are chronically hypercapnic there is generally no clinical manifestation of the hypercapnia *per se*. Ventilatory response to inhaled carbon dioxide is depressed when compared to that of asymptomatic or nonhypercapnic kyphoscoliotic persons, reflecting impaired responsiveness to the major chemical stimulus to breathing. As a corollary, greater reliance is placed on the hypoxic drive via the peripheral chemoreceptors. But, if a kyphoscoliotic subject develops acute hypercapnia during an upper respiratory infection, or exaggerates the preexisting degree of hypercapnia, he may manifest personality changes, become unresponsive to conventional stimuli, and lapse into coma. Accompanying these clinical disorders are cerebral vasodilation, cerebral edema and an increase in cerebrospinal fluid pressure. The increase in intracranial pressure may be so large as to cause choking of the optic discs, simulating a brain tumor.

All of the disturbances in uncomplicated kyphoscoliosis are greatly exaggerated by intrinsic lung disease. Therefore, smoking and its attendant bronchitis increase the risk of respiratory insufficiency in the kyphoscoliotic person. Pneumonia may be disastrous.

From these observations it is possible to reconstruct the pathogenesis of alveolar hypoventilation and cor pulmonale in kyphoscoliosis. The sequence begins with severe thoracic deformity, reducing the compliance of the thoracic cage and lung expansion. The work and energy cost of breathing is thus greatly increased. In order to minimize this work, the patient unconsciously adopts a pattern of rapid, shallow breathing, which results in chronic alveolar hypoventilation. Not only do the small, encased lungs contribute to the increased work of breathing, but they also limit the capacity and distensibility of the pulmonary vascular bed. Pulmonary arterial hypertension is caused by a disproportion between the level of pulmonary blood flow—which is normal for the subject's metabolism—and the restricted vascular bed. Once arterial hypoxemia is corrected, polycythemia, hypervolemia and a rise in cardiac output help to sustain the pulmonary hypertension. The end result of the chronic pulmonary hypertension is enlargement of the right ventricle (cor pulmonale). In this situation any additional mechanism for pulmonary hypertension, particularly an upper respiratory infection, may precipitate heart failure.

Hypercapnia goes hand in hand with the arterial hypoxemia. This is generally well tolerated unless alveolar hypoventilation is acutely intensified, so that carbon dioxide elimination is further impaired. The acute increase in arterial P_{CO_2} may evoke serious derangements in the central nervous system as well as contribute to the pulmonary hypertension and right ventricular failure.

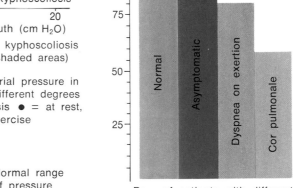

Total lung capacity, vital capacity, and tidal volume progressively reduced, and residual volume increased in relation to severity

Lung volumes and capacities in normal and progressive degrees of kyphoscoliosis

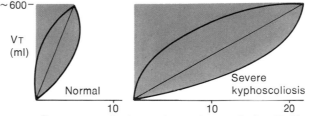

Pressure-volume loops in normal and severe kyphoscoliosis showing increased work of breathing (pink shaded areas)

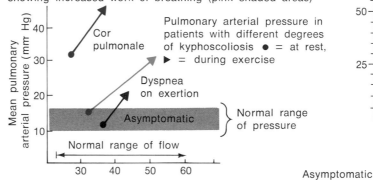

Pulmonary arterial pressure in patients with different degrees of kyphoscoliosis ● = at rest, ▸ = during exercise

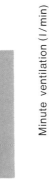

Pa_{O_2} of patients with different degrees of kyphoscoliosis compared to normal

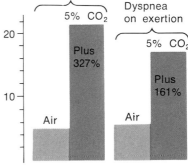

Pa_{CO_2} of patients with different degrees of kyphoscoliosis compared to normal

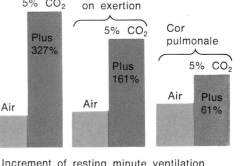

Increment of resting minute ventilation in patients with different degrees of kyphoscoliosis when breathing 5% CO_2 compared to breathing air. Normal increment = 200 to 400%

Treatment of cardiorespiratory failure is directed toward reversing the pathogenetic sequence. In this emergency, generally precipitated by an upper respiratory infection, assisted ventilation may be required in conjunction with slightly enriched oxygen mixtures (up to 25 to 40%) to achieve tolerable levels of blood gases. The ventilatory insensitivity of the chronically hypercapnic patient to an increase in arterial P_{CO_2}, as well as his reliance on hypoxic stimulation of the peripheral chemoreceptors for an important part of the ventilatory drive, imposes a need for caution against using excessively high oxygen mixtures. Respiratory depressants are also hazardous, since they may cause

breathing to stop completely. Antibiotics and supportive measures usually suffice to tide the patient over the crisis brought on by acute respiratory infection. The goal of treatment is to restore the patient to the clinical state that existed prior to the acute episode. The kyphoscoliotic individual who was dyspneic on exertion before an acute episode of cardiorespiratory failure can be expected to return to that condition after the crisis has passed. For many patients who are severely kyphoscoliotic, modest arterial hypoxemia and slight hypercapnia may remain. However, it is remarkable how successful adequate therapy can be in restoring the kyphoscoliotic to the precrisis state of health.

Congenital Diaphragmatic Hernia

The diaphragm is a septum that separates the thoracic from the abdominal cavity. A domelike structure, it consists of muscular and tendinous elements having their origin in costal, sternal and lumbar sources. The sternal portions are two flat bands, which arise from the posterior aspect of the body of the sternum. Costal elements arise from the lowest six ribs and interdigitate with the transversus abdominalis muscles. The lumbar portions arise from the lateral and medial lumbar costal arches. The complex embryogenesis of the diaphragm is presented in CIBA COLLECTION, Volume 3/II, page 3.

True congenital diaphragmatic hernias resulting from defects in embryogenesis are through: (1) the hiatus pleuroperitonealis (foramen of Bochdalek) without an enclosing sac, (2) the dome of the diaphragm, (3) the foramen of Morgagni and (4) a defect caused by the absence of the left half of the diaphragm. The two more common types of congenital diaphragmatic hernias are those through the foramen of Bochdalek and the foramen of Morgagni. Foramen of Bochdalek hernias constitute approximately 90% of diaphragmatic hernias in infants and young children, and the left side is involved in four-fifths of the cases, probably because the liver forms an effective barrier on the right. The stomach, portions of the small and large intestines, the spleen and the upper pole of the kidney may herniate through the defect into the pleural cavity and ascend freely to the apex of the chest. On the involved side the lung remains in its fetal atelectatic state, and the shifting of the mediastinum toward the uninvolved side causes some compression of that lung as well. The result is a cyanotic, dyspneic and tachycardiac newborn who cannot nurse effectively. A diaphragmatic hernia is one of the causes of neonatal respiratory distress. Few infants with this malformation survive without early surgical intervention.

The presumptive diagnosis can be made from the occurrence of cyanosis and dyspnea soon after birth, with unusual physical findings in the chest. Peristaltic sounds may be heard in the thorax, and at the same time the abdomen is found to be soft and scaphoid in contour.

Standard x-ray films are usually sufficient to establish a firm diagnosis. They will show a shift of the mediastinum to the right and bowel loops occupying the entire left hemithorax. The differential diagnosis includes such common causes of neonatal respiratory distress as eventration of the diaphragm, cystic disease of the lungs, and loculated hydropneumothorax. Hernias that occur on the right side may simulate pleural and mediastinal tumors. However, the posterior location of the mass in the lateral projection and the shift of the heart are helpful findings.

A foramen of Bochdalek hernia is a true emergency, and the infant should be operated upon before massive distention of the intrathoracic gastrointestinal tract causes lethal consequences. (See CIBA COLLECTION, Volume 3/II, page 124, for

Congenital Diaphragmatic Hernia

Sites of herniation

Foramen of Morgagni

Esophageal hiatus

A large part or all of diaphragm may be congenitally absent

Foramen of Bochdalek (most common site)

Trachea (deviated)

Right lung (compressed)

Left lung (atrophic)

Heart

Diaphragm

Liver

Small bowel

Colon

Omentum

Stomach

Spleen

Foramen of Bochdalek

Cecum (malrotation of bowel often associated)

surgical repair of diaphragmatic hernia.) A nasogastric tube attached to low suction should be inserted, as well as a rectal tube. The child should be given appropriate concentrations of oxygen, and surgical correction should be carried out either through the thorax or through the abdomen. Most surgeons prefer a subcostal incision; it is easier to pull the intestinal contents down out of the chest than to stuff them into the peritoneal cavity from above. During surgery it is helpful to insert an open catheter through the foramen in order to abolish the negative intrapleural pressure. Postoperatively, a catheter should be left in the chest for drainage and mild underwater

suction. The fetal atelectatic lung should not be forcefully inflated; within 7 to 10 days it will be fully aerated and resemble a normal lung.

Congenital defects in the anterior parasternal region (Laney's space) may result in the formation of a foramen of Morgagni hernia. A sac is present which usually contains omentum, and the colon is also present in over 50% of the cases. The hernia must be differentiated from a pericardial cyst. The distinction is readily made by barium enema, if colon is present in the sac. As with foramen of Bochdalek hernias, effective surgical closure can easily be done from the thoracic or abdominal approach.

Tracheoesophageal Fistulas and Tracheal Anomalies

Tracheoesophageal fistula and esophageal atresia rarely occur as separate entities, but they are often seen in various combinations: esophageal atresia with (a) upper fistula, (b) lower fistula and (c) double fistulas. Type b accounts for 90% of all tracheoesophageal fistulas. The etiology of these congenital anomalies is not well understood, but it is assumed that systemic infection of the mother during pregnancy plays a role.

In the common form, the diagnosis can be suspected immediately when it is noted that the newborn infant has excessive mucus and cannot handle his secretions adequately. Suction provides temporary relief, but the secretions continue to accumulate and overflow, resulting in aspiration and respiratory distress. Feedings are also regurgitated and aspirated. Formerly the diagnosis was made by using a contrast study with barium or Gastrografin (meglucamine diatrizoate). However, with these substances there is danger of aspirating foreign material into the lungs. The diagnosis can readily be made by passing a fairly large radiopaque plastic catheter through the nose and down into the pouch. When the catheter cannot be advanced into the stomach, the diagnosis is immediately evident. The catheter should then be taped in place and put on constant gentle suction. This keeps the pouch free of saliva and minimizes the chances of aspiration pneumonitis. On the chest x-ray film it will be noted that the tip of the catheter is usually opposite T2-3. If the surgeon prefers a contrast study, no more than 0.5 ml of contrast material should be introduced through the catheter, with the child in the upright position. X-ray study will show the typical esophageal obstruction, and the contrast material should then be immediately aspirated.

In infants who have esophageal atresia without a distal tracheoesophageal fistula the abdomen remains flat. If there is a fistula in the lower esophageal segment, the abdomen usually becomes distended with air.

In the case of a fistula without esophageal atresia, the diagnosis may be difficult even with repeated x-ray examination. Cinefluorography to show simultaneous filling of the trachea and esophagus during a contrast study may be necessary to establish a diagnosis.

Treatment is by surgical correction. Ideally, if a diagnosis is made promptly and a large tube placed in the esophageal pouch to avoid aspiration, operation may be performed safely, even on a premature infant. Once pneumonitis has occurred, the infant should be treated by constant esophageal suction, antibiotics and fluid replacement until the pneumonic process has cleared, after which an elective operation can be carried out. In the latter case, gastrostomy, under local anesthesia, should be performed for feeding purposes. The ideal surgical procedure consists in disruption of the fistula and an end-to-end anastomosis of the esophagus. It is advantageous to perform the surgery by an extrapleural route, so that if leakage occurs at the anastomotic site it will be easier to handle.

A. Most common form (90 to 95%) of tracheoesophageal fistula. Upper segment of esophagus ending in blind pouch; lower segment originating from trachea just above bifurcation. The two segments may be connected by a solid cord

B. Upper segment of esophagus ending in trachea; lower segment of variable length

C. Double fistula

D. Fistula without esophageal atresia

E. Esophageal atresia without fistula

F. Aplasia of trachea (lethal)

G. Stricture of trachea — Web, Hourglass

H. Absence of cartilage — Inspiration, Expiration

I. Deformity of cartilage

J. Abnormalities of bifurcation — To upper lobes, To lower lobes, Left bronchus, Right bronchus

Anomalies and Strictures of the Trachea. Tracheal anomalies are very rare. With stricture of the trachea there is local obstruction to the passage of air. In the absence of cartilage the trachea can collapse and therefore obstruct on expiration. With deformity of cartilage there is obstruction on inspiration and expiration. When abnormal bifurcations are present, the right upper and/or left upper lobe bronchi arise independently from the trachea. (See also CIBA COLLECTION, Volume 3/I, page 138.)

Clinically, stenosis may be localized or diffuse. The localized form is caused by a web of the respiratory mucosa or by excessive growth of tracheal cartilage. The diffuse form is due to a congenital absence of elastic fibrous tissue between the cartilage and its rings in the trachea, or to an absence of cartilage. Clinically, obstruction of the trachea causes chronic dyspnea; cyanosis, especially on exercise; and repeated attacks of respiratory tract infection. The diagnosis is established by bronchoscopy and by roentgenography.

For localized obstruction, surgery is advisable, either dilatation or excision with end-to-end anastomosis. Resection and anastomosis of the trachea can be carried out including up to six tracheal rings. For generalized stenosis, only supportive therapy is available.

Pulmonary Agenesis, Aplasia and Hypoplasia

Three different degrees of arrested development of the lungs may occur: (1) *agenesis,* in which there is a complete absence of one lung or both lungs and no trace of bronchial or vascular supply or parenchymal tissue; (2) *aplasia,* in which there is a suppression of all but a rudimentary bronchus ending in a blind pouch—there are no pulmonary vessels and no parenchyma; and (3) *hypoplasia,* in which the bronchus is fully formed but reduced in size and, because of failure of alveolar development, ends in a fleshy mesenchymal structure usually lying within the mediastinum. Alternatively, a segmental bronchus, commonly the apical or posterior segmental bronchus of the right upper lobe, may fail to grow, but the defect is so fully compensated for by the development of the associated segmental bronchi that the condition is not clinically apparent.

The incidence of this anomaly is low. There is no clear-cut sex predominance; neither does it occur more frequently on one side or·the other. Experimental work in the rat fetus has shown that mothers deprived of vitamin A have a greater incidence of pulmonary agenesis, suggesting such deprivation as a contributing etiologic factor. However, a similar degree of malnutrition of this type is unlikely to occur in humans. Although absence of the lung is often associated with other congenital defects which terminate life in infancy, many patients with a single lung have lived well into adult life. Sixty percent of patients with agenesis of the lung are found to have other congenital anomalies. The most frequently associated anomalies are: patent ductus arteriosus, tetralogy of Fallot, anomalies of great vessels, and bronchogenic cysts. Since one normal lung is more than adequate to sustain life, and since a single lung probably hypertrophies as the infant lung may do, the condition alone is not symptomatic. Obviously, however, pulmonary function can more easily be compromised by pneumonia, foreign body or other insults if there is only one functional lung present.

The finding in cases of agenesis, aplasia or whole-lung hypoplasia is, as might be expected, total or almost total absence of aerated lung. The marked loss of volume is indicated by approximation of the ribs, elevation of the ipsilateral hemidiaphragm, and shift of the heart and mediastinum into the unoccupied hemithorax. However, because of distention and herniation of the remaining functioning lung tissue across the mediastinum, breath sounds may be audible bilaterally, and auscultation alone may not be diagnostic. The diagnosis depends on bronchoscopic and bronchographic determination, along with tomography and angiography to demonstrate the absence of the main bronchus on the affected side, together with the absence of the pulmonary artery. On histologic study of hypoplastic lung, a pleural surface can be seen under

A. Complete unilateral agenesis. Left lung and bronchial tree are absent. Right lung is greatly enlarged with resultant shift of mediastinum to left, elevation of left diaphragm, and approximation of ribs on that side

B. Aplasia of left lung. Only rudimentary bronchi on left side, which end blindly

C. Hypoplasia of left lung

Hypoplastic lung contains some poorly developed bronchi but no alveolar tissue

which there is a small, poorly developed bronchus but no bronchial or alveolar tissue.

Congenital absence of a pulmonary lobe presents similar but less dramatic findings. Physical and x-ray examinations show diminished volume of the affected hemithorax, shift of the heart and mediastinum into the affected side, and ipsilateral elevation of the hemidiaphragm. Bronchography establishes the diagnosis by proving the absence of the bronchus to the missing lobe, and angiography is confirmatory.

Newborn infants with diaphragmatic hernia of the Bochdalek type have hypoplasia of the lung on that side, but this lung usually expands to normal size within two weeks of repair of the hernia. However, it is possible to have a diaphragmatic hernia with agenesis of the lung.

In "horseshoe lung," a rare congenital anomaly, there is a partial fusion of both lungs behind the pericardial sac. In this condition one lung is smaller than the other, but both are supplied by separate bronchi.

Treatment consists in managing intercurrent diseases as they arise. Patients must take extreme precautions to avoid infection, and their prognosis is always guarded, since those who survive into adult life have progressively decreased pulmonary function.

Congenital Bronchogenic and Pulmonary Cysts

Congenital cysts of the lung may be differentiated into three groups.

The *bronchogenic cell type* of cyst is a rare congenital anomaly resulting from abnormal budding and branching of the tracheobronchial tree during its development. Bronchogenic cysts are characterized by respiratory cell mucosa composed of either columnar or cuboidal ciliated cells which line the cavity. These cysts do not communicate with the tracheobronchial tree unless they become infected. Bronchogenic cysts must be distinguished from acquired bronchiectasis, which is more common in the dependent portions of the lung; in multiple congenital cysts, the upper lobes are often the site of the disease.

Bronchogenic cysts may be pulmonary or mediastinal. The pulmonary variety appears as sharply circumscribed, solitary, round or oval shadows on x-ray examination, usually in the middle third of the lungs. The majority of uninfected bronchogenic cysts cause no symptoms and are discovered by accident on a screening chest roentgenogram. When symptoms do occur—usually hemoptysis and expectoration of purulent secretions—they indicate the presence of infection. In neonates, communication between a cyst and the tracheobronchial tree may incorporate a check valve mechanism, which may result in rapid expansion of the cyst. Such an airspace sometimes becomes so large as to compress the mediastinum, with resulting cardiac embarrassment and death.

Mediastinal bronchial cysts may occur in the paratracheal, carinal, hilar or paraesophageal areas. The most common location for a bronchogenic cyst is in relation to the carina. It usually presents as a clearly defined mass of homogeneous density just inferior to the carina, often protruding slightly to the right, and overlapping the right hilar shadow. Unlike pulmonary bronchogenic cysts, mediastinal cysts rarely communicate with the tracheobronchial tree. They are always solitary, but many are multiloculated. These cysts also may become very large without causing symptoms. However, in the subcarinal area they can cause pressure symptoms even when they are quite small. When they become infected, they may break through into a bronchus.

Pulmonary sequestration, the second type of cyst, is illustrated in Plate 8.

The *alveolar cell type* is the third category of cyst. The cysts are lined with flat squamous cells and may be solitary or multiple. They occur more frequently in infants and children and usually have a single bronchial communication. The clinical manifestations depend largely on whether or not there is a communication with a bronchus. If the bronchus is patent, infections cause cough, purulent sputum and, rarely, hemoptysis. Pulmonary cysts may become infected by extension from adjacent diseased lung tissue without a bronchial communication, although solitary lesions can remain asymptomatic for long periods.

Histologic examination shows that a congenital cyst may be lined with ciliated epithelium and contain mucous glands and cartilage as in the

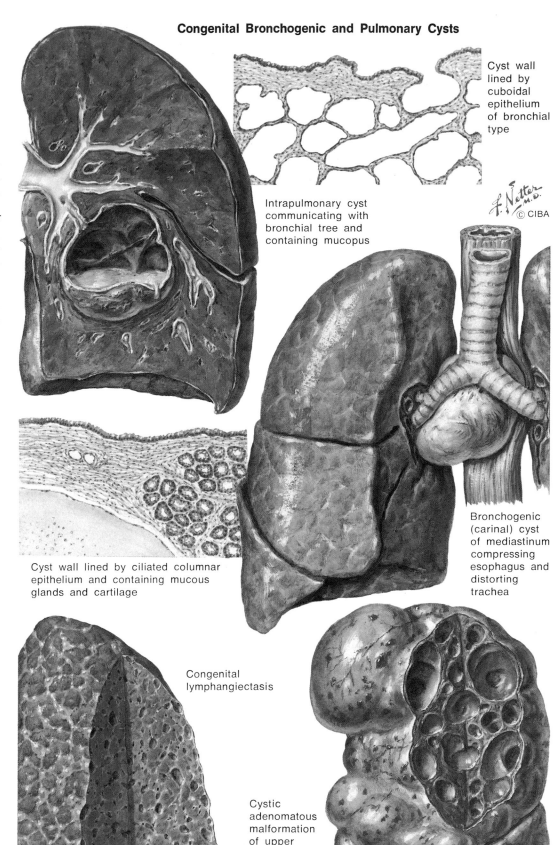

Cyst wall lined by cuboidal epithelium of bronchial type

Intrapulmonary cyst communicating with bronchial tree and containing mucopus

Cyst wall lined by ciliated columnar epithelium and containing mucous glands and cartilage

Bronchogenic (carinal) cyst of mediastinum compressing esophagus and distorting trachea

Congenital lymphangiectasis

Cystic adenomatous malformation of upper lobe of a lung

normal bronchial wall. Or, the bronchogenic cyst may be lined by cuboidal epithelium of the bronchial type. The epithelial lining also may be nonciliated, and the cyst may connect directly with the alveolar spaces.

Cystic Adenomatous Malformation. This lesion is somewhat similar to sequestration (Plate 8), and it too causes air-trapping and displacement of the mediastinum. A chest x-ray study will show prominent air-trapping or multiple cysts filled with air-fluid levels. Mechanical problems lead to respiratory distress and deviation of the trachea. At surgery a lobe is found that is diffusely cystic and will not collapse, even with firm pressure.

Pathologic examination reveals that the abnormal lung tissue contains no cartilage.

Congenital Pulmonary Lymphangiectasis. In this condition there is dilatation of the lymphatic vessels of the lungs, which may be associated with lymphedema in other portions of the body. Infants with this problem have respiratory distress with cyanosis, and the majority succumb very early. Radiologic findings include a ground-glass appearance with fine, diffuse, granular densities representing dilated lymphatics. On examination, the lungs are bulky, with pronounced lobulation, and they contain many thin-walled cystic spaces—dilated lymphatic vessels.

Bronchopulmonary Sequestration

Bronchopulmonary sequestration is a congenital malformation in which a mass of pulmonary tissue is detached from the normal lung, has no communication with an airway, and receives its blood supply from a systemic artery. The systemic artery usually arises from the aorta either above or below the diaphragm, or occasionally from an intercostal artery or, rarely, from the brachiocephalic (innominate) artery. The sequestered tissue presents itself in two forms: (1) *intralobar* and (2) *extralobar.* The sequestered lung often contains air that has apparently reached it through minute alveolar connections rather than through a major normal airway.

Intralobar Sequestration. This type comprises a nonfunctioning portion of lung within the visceral pleura of a pulmonary lobe. In the majority of cases it derives its systemic arterial supply from the descending thoracic aorta or the abdominal aorta. The venous drainage is invariably by way of the pulmonary veins, producing an arterioarterial communication. Embryologically, it appears to be a failure of the normal pulmonary artery to supply a peripheral portion of the lung; hence the arterial supply is derived from a persistent ventral branch of the primitive dorsal aorta. As a rule the sequestered portion is situated in the left paravertebral gutter. Intralobar sequestration is never seen in neonates at autopsy. Classically, the sequestered segment is a closed system and not connected to the normal bronchus.

On pathologic examination, the affected mass is cystic, and the spaces are filled either with mucus or, if infected, with purulent material. The cystic spaces are lined by either columnar or flat cuboidal epithelium. The anomalous vessel usually enters the lung through the lower part of the pulmonary ligament and is characteristically much larger than would be expected to supply such a limited amount of lung. On histologic examination, the vessel demonstrates arteriosclerotic changes.

On roentgenologic examination, the appearance depends upon the presence or absence of infection, which usually results in communication with the airways of the contiguous lung tissue. When no communication exists, the anomalous tissue appears as a homogeneous mass in the posterior portion of the lower lobe, usually to the left and almost always adjacent to the diaphragm. As a result of infection, the cystic mass communicates with the bronchial tree and presents an air-containing cyst, with or without fluid levels. Diagnosis can be suspected from the x-ray film appearance, but a definite diagnosis can be made only by visualization of the aberrant artery by cineradiography.

Extralobar Sequestration. This malformation differs from the intralobar varieties in the following respects: (1) It develops as a complete segment of pulmonary tissue in the form of an accessory lobe or segment which is enclosed in its own visceral pleura. Basically, it is a primitive accessory lung. (2) Anatomically, it is related to the left hemidiaphragm in over 90% of cases. It may be situated between the diaphragmatic surface of the

lower lobe and the diaphragm, or within the substance of the diaphragm. (3) Venous drainage is into the systemic venous system, creating a left-to-right shunt. (4) The systemic arterial supply is commonly from the abdominal aorta or one of its branches. (5) In contrast to intralobar sequestration, the extralobar form is often seen at autopsy in neonates and is frequently associated with other congenital anomalies.

Clinically, the extralobar variety is often asymptomatic and is usually discovered during other diagnostic procedures or surgical exploration. Occasionally, it is discovered together with a congenital diaphragmatic hernia. When it is not

Extralobar sequestered lobe of left lung. Arterial supply from thoracic or abdominal aorta, venous return to hemiazygos vein

Intralobar sequestration with cavitation. Arterial supply from thoracic or abdominal aorta; venous return to pulmonary veins

Extralobar sequestered lobe supplied by accessory bronchus

Extralobar sequestered lobe with communication from esophagus (communication with cardia of stomach has also been observed)

infected, the ectopic lung tissue rarely causes symptoms unless the sequestration exists in the wall of the esophagus, where it may cause dysphagia and hematemesis.

When the sequestered lung becomes infected, it often appears to be a chronic pulmonary abscess, accompanied by episodes of fever, chest pain, cough and bloody mucopurulent sputum.

Treatment for either type consists of surgical resection. Because of the constant threat of secondary infection and hemorrhage, surgery should be recommended even though the patient is asymptomatic at the time. Once infection occurs, complete removal is mandatory.

Congenital Lobar Emphysema

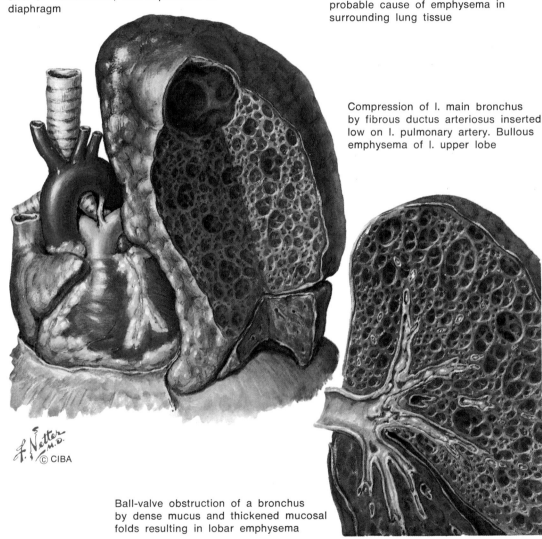

Congenital emphysema of middle lobe of right lung evidenced by hyperlucency with compression of r. upper and middle lobes, shift of mediastinum, and depression of diaphragm

Section showing a fairly large bronchus with almost no cartilage in its wall: a probable cause of emphysema in surrounding lung tissue

Compression of l. main bronchus by fibrous ductus arteriosus inserted low on l. pulmonary artery. Bullous emphysema of l. upper lobe

Ball-valve obstruction of a bronchus by dense mucus and thickened mucosal folds resulting in lobar emphysema

Sometimes immediately after birth, but usually during the first few weeks of life, congenital lobar emphysema can cause severe pulmonary problems with all the features of obstructive emphysema. The overdistended lobe or lobes cause compression of the remaining normal ipsilateral lung and a marked shift of the mediastinum to the opposite side, so that a ventilatory crisis results with dyspnea, cyanosis and sometimes circulatory failure. In some infants, clinical manifestations do not appear until the sixth month, but rarely thereafter.

Physical examination usually reveals hyperresonance and bulging of the affected hemithorax with a contralateral displacement of the trachea and mediastinum. Hyperlucency of the diseased side is seen on roentgenogram, the ribs are spread farther apart, the diaphragm is lower than normal and flattened, and the uninvolved lobe or lobes may be atelectatic. There is displacement of the mediastinum to the opposite side where the lung appears relatively radiopaque, but the diaphragm is not elevated as would be seen with atelectasis. In the involved lung, vascular markings may distinguish the abnormality from a pneumothorax.

The pathogenesis of congenital lobar emphysema falls into three categories. In the first group, there are defects in the bronchial cartilage with absent or incomplete rings; the abnormality has also been described in chondroectodermal dysplasia, or Ellis-Van Creveld syndrome. In the second group, there is an obvious mechanical cause of bronchial obstruction — for example, a fold of mucous membrane acting as a ball valve, an aberrant artery or fibrous band, tumors or a tenacious mucous plug. In the third and largest group, no local pathologic lesions other than overdistention of the lobe can be seen, but unrecognized bronchiolitis has been thought to be a possible cause. In each instance the lobe inflates

Congenital abnormalities of the pulmonary circulation are not discussed here; they are covered in CIBA COLLECTION, Volume 5, pages 127-130, 134, 135, 148-152, 155, 158-163.

normally as the bronchus widens during inspiration, but the obstruction to it during expiration results in air trapping and overdistention. Even with the chest open, the lung cannot be collapsed.

The upper lobes are most commonly involved, particularly on the left side, and the middle lobe is second in order of frequency. Multilobar bilateral involvement rarely occurs. Differential diagnosis from endobronchial pneumothorax, diaphragmatic hernias, tension cysts and endobronchial foreign bodies must be made.

Lobectomy is urgently indicated for this usually acute respiratory emergency. It is important that the child be anesthetized by a technique that

does not require assisted ventilation and muscle relaxants, as the resulting hyperventilation will increase the amount of emphysema because of the check valve mechanism present. The chest should be opened rapidly and the overdistended lobe displaced outside the chest. Anesthesia may then proceed normally; once the chest is open, the trapped air no longer causes any further trouble. The prognosis with surgery is excellent. Occasionally a congenital cardiac anomaly is found to coexist. Postoperatively some patients have manifested chronic bronchitis and asthma; however, the majority of infants develop normally without further respiratory tract difficulties.

Laryngeal Granuloma and Tracheal Stenosis

The use of cuffed endotracheal and tracheostomy tubes for mechanical ventilation is an important therapeutic measure which is often lifesaving. Unfortunately, in some instances the use of these devices has serious sequelae—namely, tracheal erosion, tracheomalacia and tracheal stenosis. Various modifications of the apparatus and of the procedure have been proposed, therefore, including low-pressure cuffs and methods of inflating the cuff only on the inspiratory cycle of assisted ventilation. It has also been recommended that the cuff be deflated at intervals to avoid an excessively prolonged compression of the tracheal mucosa. The problem with the latter method is that the cuff may not empty completely, and if it is reinflated with the minimal fixed volume of air recommended for filling, overinflation occurs. Best results are obtained by inflating under auscultatory control until the leak stops.

Even brief endotracheal intubation, as for anesthesia, may result in some morbidity. In adults, the tube impinges on the vocal processes of the arytenoid cartilages, and this pressure plus the movement and pulsation of the tube with each ventilatory cycle may cause erosion, leading to formation of laryngeal granulomas. In children, because of the smaller size of the larynx, the tube rests in the interarytenoid space, and the resultant laryngeal granuloma may be subglottic.

The consequences of tracheal stenosis and tracheomalacia are more serious. In the anterior and lateral tracheal walls, the vertical blood vessels course between the mucosa and the cartilage rings, and they may be readily compressed by a distending balloon. The posterior tracheal wall is devoid of cartilage and yields easily, so that the vessels are less likely to be compressed in that site. With excessive and prolonged pressure, however, they also can be compromised.

Thus, in about 50% of cases of postendotracheal or tracheostomy balloon stenosis, the posterior tracheal wall is spared, and only the anterior and lateral walls are affected by avascular ulceration, perichondritis and fragmentation of the cartilage. The resultant stricture often has a triangular configuration on transverse section, due to anterior weakening of the cartilaginous arch with lateral collapse. In the remaining cases the entire circumference of the trachea is compromised.

The stricture caused by ischemic necrosis may be narrow and weblike, involving only the area of one tracheal ring. In other instances the stenotic segment is longer, involving two to five tracheal rings, and has tapering margins. The characteristics and extent of the stenosis may be demonstrated by tomography in the frontal and lateral projections. Contrast tracheography using propyliodone further delineates the length and shape of the stricture. Sometimes the affected segment is yielding so that it will collapse only on inspiration. Consequently, there is greater functional impairment than is apparent radiographically. A flow-volume loop may show reduction in the inspiratory flow rate.

X-ray studies serve to localize the exact location and extent of the stenosis. In some cases, multiple stenoses may occur, especially after the use of tubes of different lengths or tubes with double cuffs. For this reason the latter are no longer popular.

Postintubation Laryngeal Granuloma

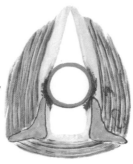
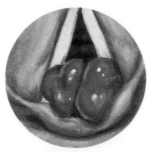
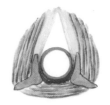

Laryngeal granulomas following endotracheal intubation. These often regress spontaneously

Etiology. In adults, tube impinges on vocal processes of arytenoid cartilages, causing erosion by pressure and by movement and pulsation of tube with intermittent positive pressure ventilation

In children, because of smaller larynx, tube lies in interarytenoid space and subglottic granuloma may result

Postintubation and Posttracheostomy Balloon Stenosis

Blood supply of upper trachea

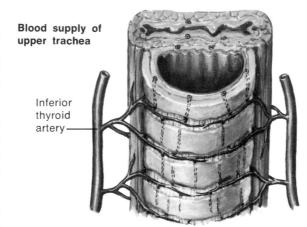

Inferior thyroid artery

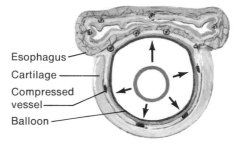

Esophagus
Cartilage
Compressed vessel
Balloon

Tracheoesophageal branches from inferior thyroid arteries send circumferential vessels to intercartilaginous spaces, with vertical ascending and descending branches beneath mucosa

Vertical submucosal vessels may be readily compressed against cartilage rings of anterior and lateral tracheal walls by a distended endotracheal balloon, with resultant erosion followed by avascular ulceration and perichondritis, collapse, and stenosis. Posterior fibromuscular wall, however, is yielding, and vascular compression is therefore less likely here, so that this wall is often spared

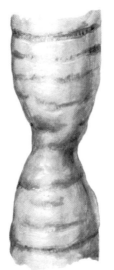

Hourglass constriction of trachea; cartilage rings obscured by perichondritis, so that serial transverse cuts may be required to determine limits of normal tissue

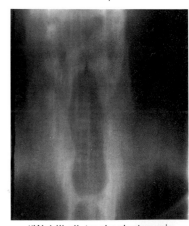

Section through excised specimen viewed from above, showing fragmentation of cartilage and complete concentric stenosis with ulcerations

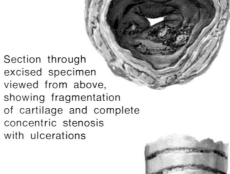

Stenosis involving only anterior and lateral cartilaginous walls; posterior fibromuscular wall intact

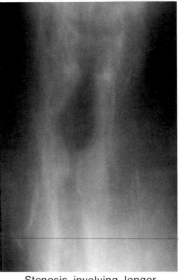

"Weblike" tracheal stenosis

Stenosis involving longer segment of trachea

Tracheal Resection and Anastomosis

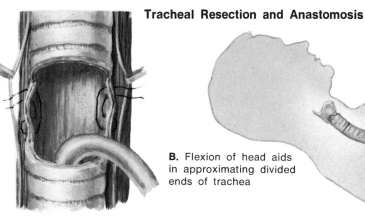

A. If only anterior and lateral walls of trachea are involved in stenosis, those portions are excised. A Stewart or Connell stitch is taken in each margin of intact posterior wall, with care not to injure recurrent laryngeal nerves

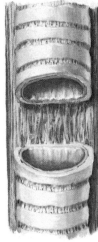

B. Flexion of head aids in approximating divided ends of trachea

C. End-to-end anastomosis accomplished with fine wire

D. If entire circumference of trachea is involved, complete transection with excision of stenosed segment is necessary

E. If only 2 or 3 rings require excision, approximation and suture may be accomplished with aid of head flexion

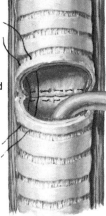

F. If more extensive excision is required, approximation may not be readily accomplished without undue tension on suture line, and measures to bring ends of trachea together become necessary

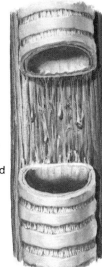

G. Release of tension may be achieved by lengthening remaining trachea by hemicircumferential incisions of alternate intercartilaginous ligaments, with care not to injure underlying mucosa

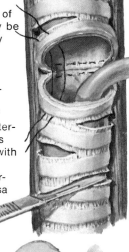

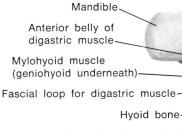

Mandible

Anterior belly of digastric muscle

Mylohyoid muscle (geniohyoid underneath)

Fascial loop for digastric muscle

Hyoid bone

Cut ends of sternohyoid and omohyoid muscles

Thyrohyoid membrane divided

Thyrohyoid muscle divided

Thyroid cartilage

Cut end of sternothyroid muscle

Trachea

Hyoglossus muscle

Stylohyoid muscle

Posterior belly of digastric muscle

Middle constrictor

Superior laryngeal nerve and artery

Inferior constrictor

Esophagus

If additional tracheal relaxation is necessary, larynx may be dropped by cutting thyrohyoid muscle and thyrohyoid membrane plus upper fibers of inferior constrictor below hyoid bone, avoiding superior laryngeal nerve and artery. Alternatively, muscles above hyoid bone may be divided (broken line)

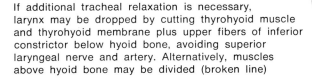

Low intrathoracic tracheal lesions may be approached via posterolateral thoracotomy as described by Grillo. This approach also permits additional tracheal relaxation by cutting pulmonary ligaments

Tracheal Resection and Anastomosis

In most cases of symptom-producing, so-called balloon stenosis of the trachea, conservative therapy, consisting of repeated dilatations, has proved to be ineffective. Consequently, surgical correction is necessary. The procedure of choice is excision of the stenotic tracheal segment with end-to-end anastomosis (see illustration).

Resection with reanastomosis is more readily accomplished if the lesion is in the cervical portion of the trachea than if it is within the mediastinum. In the former instance, the approach is via a transverse cervical incision; in the latter case, a median sternotomy may be required. In anticipation of such problems, when a tracheostomy is indicated for prolonged intubation, it should be performed at a high level. Then, if stenosis occurs later at the site of the cuff 1.5 to 2.0 cm below the tracheostomy, a similar corrective procedure may be used.

Although preoperative study of the location and extent of the lesion is essential, the situation must be further evaluated at the time of surgery. Usually, the stenotic segment may be identified by the "hourglass" constriction of the outer tracheal wall. Nevertheless, the lumen must be examined via a transverse incision at the lower end of the constriction to determine whether the stenosis is circumferential or confined to the anterior and lateral cartilaginous walls of the trachea. It may also be necessary to make serial transverse incisions through successive cartilages to determine the full extent of the lesion.

Low intrathoracic tracheal lesions must be approached through a posterolateral thoracotomy. Such lesions usually result from direct external or penetrating trauma rather than from intubation.

Plastic Tracheal Reconstruction

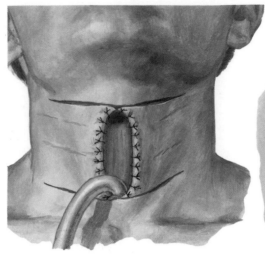

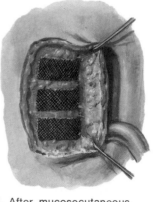

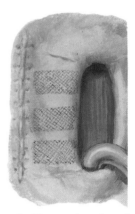

Plastic Reconstruction of Anterior Two-thirds of Trachea with Intact Posterior Wall

A. After excision of long segment of anterior and lateral tracheal walls (4 to 6 tracheal rings) skin flaps created on each side of defect, undermined, and sutured to margins of intact posterior tracheal wall

B. After mucosocutaneous healing, incision made lateral to tracheostoma, and tantalum or Marlex mesh strips inserted subcutaneously

C. Flap replaced and allowed to heal over buried tantalum or Marlex strips

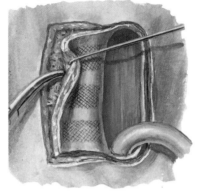

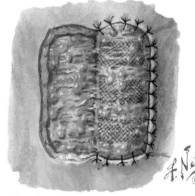

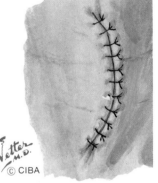

D. Hinged flap later undermined deep to mesh strips, almost to margin of tracheostoma, with incision encircling tracheostoma

E. Mesh shaped convexly outward, flap rotated and sewed over tracheal opening

F. Skin defect closed by undermining and rotating skin flap

Reconstruction After Circumferential Excision of Long Tracheal Segment

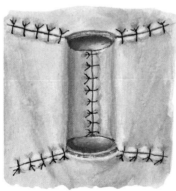

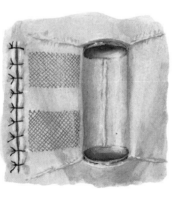

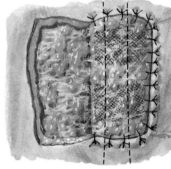

A. Skin flaps sutured in midline to create new posterior wall of skin-lined trachea

B. Marlex strips subsequently buried subcutaneously lateral to tracheal defect

C. Mesh shaped convexly and flap turned over to form anterior tracheal wall; skin defect closed as above. Intratracheal tube in place until seal is airtight

---

Tracheal stenosis is occasionally extensive, involving four to five rings and making necessary the resection of this relatively long segment. In such cases it may be impossible to perform end-to-end anastomosis without undue tension, even if measures are taken to lengthen the remaining tracheal segments. Plastic reconstruction of the trachea must then be accomplished in order to achieve a continuous airway.

If only the anterior and lateral tracheal walls, which constitute the cartilaginous portion, have been resected and the posterior wall remains intact, the following procedure is employed: A T-shaped incision is made above the original collar exploratory incision, with its vertical limb joining the latter in the midline. Skin flaps are then elevated on each side of the midline vertical incision and sutured to the lateral margins of the intact posterior tracheal wall for the full extent of the defect, with openings into the trachea above and below. After healing of the mucocutaneous suture lines, a vertical incision is made laterally to one side of the extensive tracheostoma and the skin undermined medially almost up to the margin of the mucocutaneous junction. Several strips of tantalum or Marlex mesh are buried there subcutaneously, and the skin flaps are replaced. After allowing about three weeks for healing, the vertical scar is excised and the incision carried horizontally to the upper and lower limits of the tracheostoma. The resulting skin flap with its contained Marlex or tantalum mesh strips is then elevated deep to the fascia. The contralateral mucocutaneous junction is

incised, and the hinged, doorlike flap, with its mesh shaped convexly outward, is turned over to cover the tracheostoma and sutured to the opposite margin of the posterior tracheal mucosa. The skin lateral to the flap site is undermined, the platysma and subcutaneous tissue are employed as a secondary closure line, and finally the skin is drawn over to cover the raw area.

When it is necessary to perform a complete circumferential excision of an extensive portion of the cervical trachea and preservation of the posterior wall is not possible, the skin flaps created as described above are brought together in the midline to form the posterior wall for a new skin-lined tracheal segment. Marlex or tantalum strips are buried subcutaneously, and the flap containing them is turned over to complete the anterior and lateral tracheal walls. The exposed area is covered by platysma, subcutaneous tissue and skin as previously described. A lower tracheostomy is not feasible in such cases, and a noncuffed endotracheal tube is left in place for 24 or 48 hours—*i.e.*, until an airtight seal is obtained.

By means of these methods, a well-functioning airway has been reestablished and the adequacy of the lumen demonstrated roentgenographically in a number of cases when direct end-to-end anastomosis was not possible.

Bronchial Asthma

Bronchial asthma, which affects an estimated 6 to 8 million Americans, is a clinical state of heightened reactivity of the tracheobronchial tree to numerous stimuli. Episodes of dyspnea and wheezing—symptoms of airway obstruction—are characteristic features of the disorder. In some patients, cough, with or without tenacious sputum, may occur. Asthmatic symptoms are results of obstructive bronchospasm, bronchial wall edema and inflammation, and hypersecretion by mucous glands, leading to hyperinflation, gas exchange defects and increased respiratory work. Asthmatic episodes may be continuous or paroxysmal with impaired respiratory function ranging from modest disability to life-threatening asphyxiation—status asthmaticus. A major feature of asthma is that it is *reversible* to some extent either spontaneously or through treatment.

Clinical Forms of Bronchial Asthma

Clinically, patients can exhibit several forms of asthma. The most common classification is based on etiologic factors but also takes account of both clinical variations and therapeutic implications.

Extrinsic Asthma. Also called *allergic asthma,* extrinsic asthma usually affects children and young adults (Plate 13). It is characterized by reversible paroxysms of bronchospasm with wheezing, dyspnea and other symptoms of respiratory distress following exposure to causative allergens. These episodes are usually of sudden onset and brief duration, and between them the patient may be relatively symptom free. A personal history of other allergic manifestations such as hay fever or eczema *(atopy)* is common, as is a family history of atopy. Dermal reactivity to offending allergens is significant, with immunoglobulin E (IgE) playing a role. Response to medical therapy is generally favorable and long-term prognosis is good. However, in adult life a number of patients experience recurrences.

Intrinsic Asthma. Intrinsic asthma usually develops in middle age (Plate 14). Immunologic factors have no apparent role in etiology, and respiratory tract infection is a frequent causative factor; this form is also called *idiopathic* or *infective* asthma. Occasionally there is a history of atopy.

Often in the initial presentation intrinsic asthma is clinically indistinguishable from allergic asthma, although sputum production (purulent) and cough may be more severe in patients with infective asthma. Obviously, factors such as age or infection in the sinuses or bronchial tree will favor intrinsic asthma, but once the acute

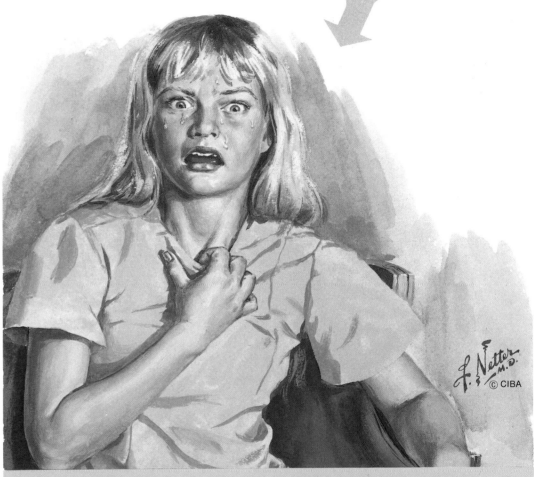

Extrinsic Allergic Asthma: Clinical Features

Young patient: child or teenager

Family history usually positive

Attacks related to specific antigens — Pollens, Foods, Drugs, Dusts, Danders

Skin tests usually positive

History of eczema in childhood

"Allergic shiner" may be present

Favorable response to hyposensitization

IgE–associated

Attacks acute but usually self-limiting; prognosis favorable; condition often outgrown but may become chronic; death rare

Features common to both extrinsic allergic and intrinsic asthma:
Respiratory distress, dyspnea, wheezing, flushing, cyanosis, cough, flaring of alae, use of accessory respiratory muscles, apprehension, tachycardia, perspiration, hyperresonance, distant breath sounds and rhonchi, eosinophilia

espisode has subsided, the more precise form can then be determined by a complete and accurate history and laboratory data.

Therapy for intrinsic asthma is not always fully effective, and the prognosis is generally poorer than for the allergic variety. Moreover, intrinsic asthma has a greater tendency to become chronic, with continuous cough and sputum production.

Other Forms of Asthma. The clinical course of asthma is variable, so patients often cannot be unequivocally classified as having the extrinsic or intrinsic type.

Mixed asthma refers to a combination of variable allergic and infective factors, which can affect even one patient. In addition, a number of clinical subtypes of asthma exist:

Chronic Asthmatic Bronchitis. Asthma coexists with chronic bronchitis; allergic factors are not necessarily identifiable. Therapy for bronchitis is supplemented with bronchodilators.

Asthma, Aspirin Sensitivity and Nasal Polyposis. Symptoms of asthma develop within 20 minutes of ingestion of aspirin, with or without nasal polyposis. Most patients have intrinsic asthma with perennial symptoms. Coexisting eosinophilia can be severe. An estimated 10% of adult asthmatics have an intolerance to salicylates *(Continued)*

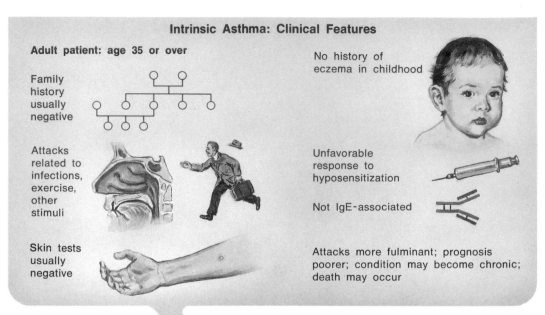

Intrinsic Asthma: Clinical Features

Adult patient: age 35 or over

Family history usually negative

Attacks related to infections, exercise, other stimuli

Skin tests usually negative

No history of eczema in childhood

Unfavorable response to hyposensitization

Not IgE-associated

Attacks more fulminant; prognosis poorer; condition may become chronic; death may occur

Bronchial Asthma
(Continued)

which does not appear to be immunologically induced. Bronchial sensitivity to indomethacin, yellow dye No. 5 (tartrazine) and other drugs may also be present.

Exercise-induced Asthma. This variant of asthma is precipitated following moderate to severe exercise, particularly in young atopic individuals, becoming maximal 10 minutes after the start of exertion such as running. Bronchodilators or cromolyn sodium may be used prophylactically or precipitating levels of physical exertion avoided. Tracheal loss of heat and moisture may be important in its etiology.

Dual Type I and Type III Reactions. More than one immune mechanism can lead to asthma. For example, sensitivity to the saprophytic mold *Aspergillus fumigatus* can induce a typical Type I "immediate hypersensitivity" asthma reaction (within 10 to 30 minutes of exposure), or Type III "Arthus type" reaction (two to six hours after exposure), or both Type I and Type III reactions combined. Patients with a dual reaction will develop an acute episode of wheezing and dyspnea with a fall in FEV_1 within 10 to 15 minutes of exposure to the allergen. These findings may subside, to be followed by a relapse two to six hours later. The second reaction develops more slowly and is characterized by progressively severe airway obstruction, dyspnea and, in some patients, pulmonary inflammatory infiltrates. Late (Type III) bronchial reactions can also occur alone and even in nonatopic patients. Both immediate and late skin sensitivity may be found in association with reaginic IgE and precipitating IgG antibodies in the serum, suggesting that the pathogenesis is a consequence of immune processes involving these two immunoglobulins in addition to serum complement and polymorphonuclear cells. Dual reactions can also occur in response to other substances, including avian allergens, mites and wood dusts. Cromolyn sodium may inhibit the sequence. Therapy consists in avoidance of the cause. If this is not possible, corticosteroids may be used.

Status Asthmaticus. This is a severe clinical stage of asthma, refractory to the usual drug therapy for acute episodes, and distinguishable both pathologically and pharmacologically from milder episodes of acute asthma. It is a medical emergency, even in the early phases, since if not treated adequately and promptly, death may result from hypoxia and/or respiratory acidosis (see page 131).

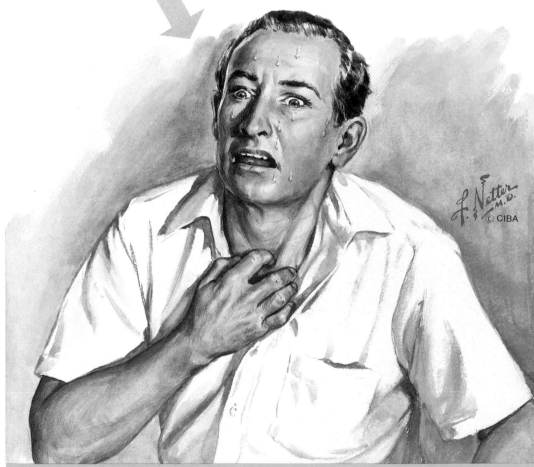

Features common to both extrinsic allergic and intrinsic asthma:
Respiratory distress, dyspnea, wheezing, flushing, cyanosis, cough, flaring of alae, use of accessory respiratory muscles, apprehension, tachycardia, perspiration, hyperresonance, distant breath sounds and rhonchi, eosinophilia

Pathogenesis of Asthma

Theories about asthma generally explain the hyperreactivity of the airways as an exaggeration of the normal defense response of the respiratory tract. This can result from abnormal tissue reactions in the airways, which may be immunologically induced, or from a biochemical or neurohumoral imbalance of other normally functioning responses. Because of the diverse stimuli known to produce asthma, no single current theory satisfactorily explains all types and cases (Plate 15).

Immediate Hypersensitivity (Type I) Reaction. Allergic bronchial asthma (extrinsic asthma) and other allergic diseases like hay fever and anaphylaxis are examples of immediate hypersensitivity (Type I) reactions (Plate 16). Such allergic reactions take place in specific target organs—the lungs, gastrointestinal tract or skin. These immune processes leading to a hypersensitivity reaction represent the disease state referred to clinically as "allergy."

Immediate hypersensitivity reactions can lead to a simple acute inflammatory response (*urticaria*), or can cause complex reactions that may be systemic (*anaphylaxis*) or chiefly limited to bronchial smooth muscle (*asthma*). The immune
(Continued)

Postulated Mechanisms of Airway Hyperreactivity Causing Asthma

A. Immunologic response

Antigen

B. β-adrenergic blockade caused by

Infection

Metabolites

Adenylcyclase deficiency

Drugs

C. Cholinergic dominance

Central influences ?

D. β-adrenergic amine deficiency

E. Intrinsic smooth muscle defect

Antigen-antibody reaction

Block

Sympathetic nerves

Vagus nerves

Reflex bronchospasm

Sensitized mast cell

Vagus efferent — Vagus afferent

Nonantigenic stimuli or antigenically modulated stimuli

Release of pharmacologic mediators (histamine, SRS-A, etc.)

Block

β β β

Direct action on end-organs (glands, smooth muscle, blood vessels)

F. Multiple factors

Bronchial Asthma
(Continued)

sequence consists of the sensitization phase, followed by a challenge reaction which produces the clinical syndrome concerned.

In the *sensitization phase,* a genetically atopic patient is exposed to antigen—*e.g.,* ragweed pollen. Lysozymes from the respiratory mucosa digest the outer lipid-polysaccharide coating of the pollen, releasing water-soluble proteins. As these proteins are absorbed, plasma cells within the lymphoid tissues of the upper or lower respiratory mucosa respond by forming a specific cytotropic antibody of the IgE class *(reagin).* The IgE molecules attach to the surfaces of the mast cells, or other cells such as basophils. (This affinity of the IgE molecules for certain cells is known as *homocytotropism* [cytotropism], and is species specific.) The mast cells containing IgE are distributed in the mucosa of the upper and lower respiratory tract and perivascular connective tissues of the lung.

After a variable latent interval (days to months), a reexposure of the patient to the specific antigen may result in a *challenge (allergic) reaction.* IgE-sensitized mast cells in contact with the specific antigen secrete preformed pharmacologically active substances including histamine, slow-reacting substance of anaphylaxis (SRS-A), various kinins, eosinophil chemotactic factor (ECF), serotonin and probably prostaglandins. Calcium and magnesium ions are required for the reaction to occur, and each antigen molecule has to bridge at least two of the IgE molecules bound to the surface of the cell. Muscle contraction, vasoconstriction and hypersecretion of mucus, together with an inflammatory response of increased capillary permeability and cellular infiltration with eosinophils then follow, producing the clinical symptoms of bronchial asthma. Also, because of the inflammatory response, the cilia of the mucosal cells fail to function normally *(ciliostasis).* Particle retention results and may reflexly cause additional bronchoconstriction. Cell necrosis aggravates the picture and may facilitate increased permeability of the tissues to the inciting antigen. Continued sensitization and reaction may then occur.

Immunoglobulin E, the antibody mediator of the immediate hypersensitivity reaction, is a heat-labile gamma-l-glycoprotein with a molecular weight of 200,000. Synthesized by plasma cells in the mucosa of the nose, respiratory and gastrointestinal tracts, and lymphoid tissues, it is found in various tissues, in body fluids and in nasal and

bronchial secretions of allergic individuals. Serum concentrations of IgE average 300 ng/ml; the half-life is about two days, indicating active formation. IgE levels are increased in patients with parasitic infestations, allergic aspergillosis, seasonal rhinitis, eczema, food sensitivities and particularly in extrinsic bronchial asthma (60% of cases with allergen-induced asthma have elevated serum IgE levels). However, such increased serum concentration is not necessarily a specific indicator of the extent or severity of allergy in the individual concerned.

A unique property of human IgE is its antigenic determinants, which lead to *specific tissue binding.* This property is absent from other human

immunoglobulins. Historically, demonstration of the affinity of IgE for skin by direct skin tests leads to the term *skin-sensitizing antibody.* However, lung tissue can also be actively sensitized. While IgE levels can be measured in body fluids, methods for estimating levels of tissue-bound IgE are currently limited. Radioimmunoassay is the method of choice for measuring antibody activity: the RIST (radioimmunosorbent test) measures total IgE; the RAST (radioallergoabsorbent test) is the best test suited for large-scale clinical use. Radiolabeled, purified anti-IgE antiserum is used to detect specific IgE antibody that reacts with allergen in the serum of allergic patients. The
(Continued)

Bronchial Asthma
(Continued)

RAST seems to correlate with skin test reactivity and leukocyte histamine release.

While immunologic mechanisms may have a significant role in the causation of asthma, the regulation of the release and generation of mediators, as well as the expression of their effects, is under significant neurogenic controls. An understanding of the beta adrenergic system and cholinergic factors is necessary for a fuller appreciation of the etiology and pathogenesis of asthma. It also provides a foundation for a rational approach to therapy.

Adrenergic Receptors. The sympathetic nerves are poorly represented in the lung by direct innervation, except to the vasculature. However, *circulating catecholamines* probably have a marked influence in the lung. Pharmacologic studies indicate that there are two basic types of adrenergic receptors, alpha and beta. The alpha receptors are located primarily in smooth muscle and exocrine glands. Beta receptors have been differentiated pharmacologically into beta$_1$, located in the heart, and beta$_2$, located in smooth muscle throughout the body, including the bronchial and vascular smooth muscle (Plate 17; see also page 22).

Generally, alpha stimulation is excitatory. Beta stimulation may be either inhibitory (relaxation of bronchial smooth muscles) or excitatory (increase in both heart rate and force of contraction). Certain tissues contain both alpha and beta receptors. The results of stimulation depend on the nature of the stimulating catecholamine, and the relative proportion of the two types of receptors present. For instance, in the lungs, beta stimulation causes bronchodilatation and possibly decreased secretion of mucus; alpha stimulation causes bronchoconstriction.

In humans, three principal catecholamines are formed: dopamine, norepinephrine and epinephrine. *Dopamine* is chiefly a neurotransmitter in the extrapyramidal nervous system. *Norepinephrine,* a metabolic precursor of epinephrine, is the main neurotransmitter of the postganglionic sympathetic fibers. *Epinephrine* is the major hormone of the adrenal medulla. A number of synthetic catecholamines have been developed. Of these, *isoproterenol* (or its derivatives) is most often used in the treatment of asthma. The role of circulatory neurohormones in bronchial asthma is concerned with (1) inhibition of mast cell mediator release and (2) bronchial smooth muscle relaxation.

Beta Adrenergic Blockade. In the normal individual, airway tone and patency represent a bal-

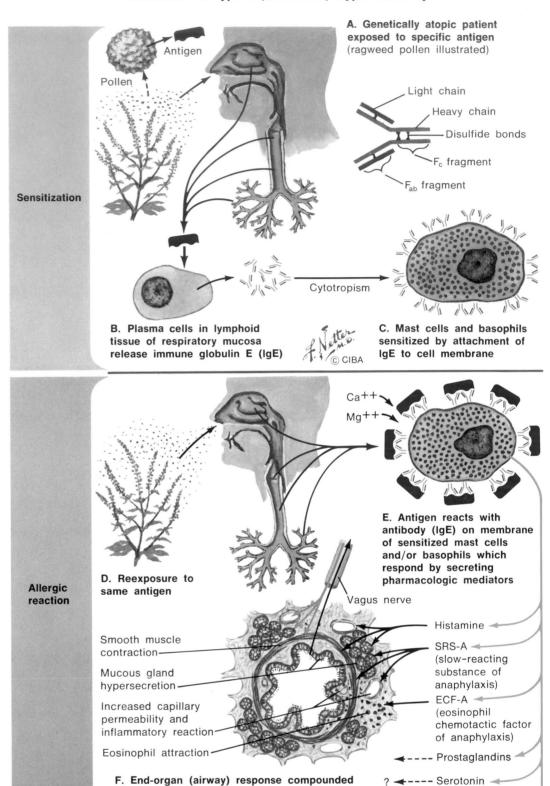

A. Genetically atopic patient exposed to specific antigen (ragweed pollen illustrated)

Light chain
Heavy chain
Disulfide bonds
F$_c$ fragment
F$_{ab}$ fragment

Sensitization

Pollen
Antigen

Cytotropism

B. Plasma cells in lymphoid tissue of respiratory mucosa release immune globulin E (IgE)

C. Mast cells and basophils sensitized by attachment of IgE to cell membrane

Allergic reaction

D. Reexposure to same antigen

Ca++
Mg++

E. Antigen reacts with antibody (IgE) on membrane of sensitized mast cells and/or basophils which respond by secreting pharmacologic mediators

Vagus nerve

Smooth muscle contraction
Mucous gland hypersecretion
Increased capillary permeability and inflammatory reaction
Eosinophil attraction

Histamine
SRS-A (slow-reacting substance of anaphylaxis)
ECF-A (eosinophil chemotactic factor of anaphylaxis)
Prostaglandins
? Serotonin
? Kinins

F. End-organ (airway) response compounded by nonspecific reactions (ciliostasis, particle retention, and cell injury)

ance between bronchorelaxation forces induced by beta adrenergic stimuli and bronchoconstrictive tendencies caused by vagal impulses (and possibly by alpha adrenergic stimuli), although other factors already cited can also have some influence (Plate 18).

Beta adrenergic stimulation activates *adenylcyclase,* an enzyme thought to be closely associated with but not necessarily identical to the beta receptor which is located in the cell membrane of the muscle or mast cell. This is produced by a circulating hormone or drug—the first messenger—linking with these selective receptors which are responsible for hormonal specificity in tissues. Adenylcyclase catalyzes the

synthesis of cyclic adenosine monophosphate (cyclic 3′, 5′-AMP, or cAMP) from adenosine triphosphate (ATP). Cyclic AMP then diffuses into the cell where it has a number of functions. Its most important function for the bronchial smooth muscle cell is activation of mechanisms that prevent contraction or induce relaxation of the muscle. In the mast cell, cAMP serves to inhibit mediator release.

These receptors modulate the activity of adenylcyclase, which controls the level of cAMP activity and hence of the metabolic functions according to the enzyme profile of the cell. Functionally opposing biologic transmitters also

(Continued)

Catecholamine Action on α and β Receptors of Heart and Bronchial Tree

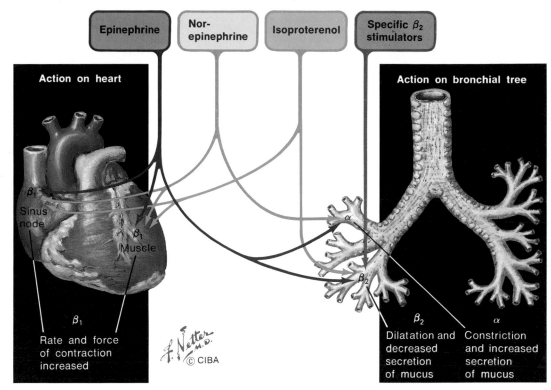

Bronchial Asthma
(*Continued*)

stimulate specific cell membrane receptors and activate the nucleotide cyclic 3', 5', guanosine monophosphate (cGMP). Acetylcholine is a major cause of increased tissue cGMP.

Beta adrenergic blockade may occur because of a malfunction or deficiency of the adenylcyclase system within the smooth muscle cells of the airway, glands, blood vessels of the lungs and tissue mast cells.

Such deficiency may be acquired from infection or arise from certain metabolites, or it may be inherited. It causes normal beta adrenergic responses to various stimuli to become inadequate, and bronchoconstriction occurs by autonomic imbalance (or other similar influences). Alternatively, the same result could develop when beta adrenergic responses are initially adequate, but the ability of adenylcyclase to catalyze production of cAMP is limited. Hence, in the airway, excessive or prolonged tonic constrictive stimulation would eventually overcome the counterbalancing bronchorelaxing effects of beta adrenergic stimulation; in the mast cell these events would lead to mediator release. Beta adrenergic blockade may also be caused by adrenergic blocking agents, such as *propranolol*.

Role of the Vagus. As discussed above, bronchial constriction is partly an autonomic reflex. The afferent fibers of the arc arise from receptors in the tracheobronchial tree or, at times, in the nose and sinuses. The efferent motor fibers of the reflex arc return to the lung, also via the vagus nerve, to terminate on the bronchial smooth muscle. Initiation of the reflex originates with stimulation of epithelial "irritant receptors." Concurrently, airway caliber can also be altered by regional changes in oxygen or carbon dioxide tension, which may occur with pulmonary embolus or asthma, or by a direct action on smooth muscle from chemical mediators of the allergic reaction released by mast cells. In addition, it is possible that central nervous system activity, including stimuli arising in higher centers, can contribute to bronchomotor tone and induce bronchial constriction.

Recently, the role of these vagally mediated cholinergic influences in causing asthma has received renewed emphasis. It is suggested that vagally mediated responses to various stimuli are exaggerated in the asthmatic patient compared with a normal person. In other words, the bronchi of the asthmatic patient react more severely to mild degrees of both antigenic and nonantigenic stimuli than do normal bronchi. An increased sensitivity of the irritant receptors is proposed as

Neurohumoral Control of Bronchial Musculature, Glands, and Vessels

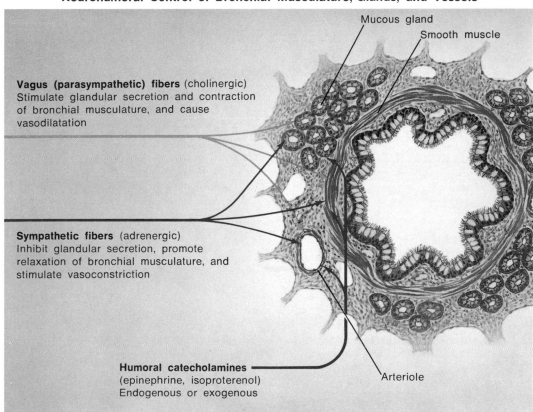

the mechanism of asthma in these cases. This effect might be partially due to increases in the amounts of cGMP released from mast cells following cholinergic discharge. Or it might have a neurogenic basis, provoking hyperresponse of the receptors or of the airway smooth muscle. Pharmacologically, bronchial constriction produced by this autonomic reflex pathway can be blocked by atropine or vagotomy whether induced by specific antigenic stimuli or nonspecific irritants.

Mediator Release and Activity. As described above, the challenge reaction of the immune sequence is characterized by the release of pharmacologic mediators from either mast cells lo-

cated in the respiratory mucosa or circulating basophils. Complement is probably not generally involved in the challenge reaction, and cytolysis does not result. The secretory release of mediators from the mast cell is influenced by the intracellular cyclic nucleotides, cAMP and probably cGMP.

Increased cAMP levels *inhibit* mediator release from mast cells and also prevent the contraction or facilitate the relaxation of the smooth muscle of the airway (Plate 18). Increased cGMP occurs when the cholinergic receptor is stimulated by acetylcholine. Increased cGMP *augments* the release of mediator from mast cells. Thus, cyclic
(*Continued*)

Theory of Catecholamine Effects and β-Adrenergic Blockade

Bronchial Asthma
(Continued)

nucleotides modulate both the release of mediators from sensitized mast cells and the patency of the airway by an action on the airway musculature. Therapeutic agents that stabilize the plasma membrane or modify the cAMP-cGMP balance can act to inhibit mediator release and hence can interrupt the immunologic asthmatic sequence.

Histamine is a vasoactive amine widely distributed in body tissues, particularly the lung, where it is concentrated as granules within tissue mast cells, especially those in proximity to capillary endothelium in the bronchial submucosa. It is also present in circulating basophils and neutrophils. However, the respiratory mucosa and perivascular sites are particularly rich in mast cells and are thus responsible for the propensity for allergic lung reactions following challenge by airborne allergens.

The release of histamine causes increased capillary permeability and vasodilatation, with resulting edema and infiltration by inflammatory cells (Plate 16). Contraction of airway smooth muscle and increased secretion from mucous glands also take place. Parenthetically, aerosol administration of histamine to asthmatic patients usually produces typical bronchospasm, whereas in normal subjects only minor effects occur at equivalent concentrations. *In vitro,* histamine release can be demonstrated in leukocytes or lung tissue of allergic individuals on exposure to appropriate antigens; blood histamine levels also rise in sensitive subjects after antigen inhalation. *In vivo* observations, however, including the minor clinical response to antihistamine drugs, suggest that histamine is not the sole mediator in human asthma. Histamine may have a dose-dependent action: low doses acting through vagal reflexes and higher concentrations directly stimulating both peripheral and central airway smooth muscle.

The *slow-reacting substance of anaphylaxis (SRS-A)* is an acidic, thermostable (at alkaline pH) substance which appears to be a major mediator. Its pharmacologically significant features are a delay in maximal effect on bronchial contraction, and a more prolonged action than histamine has. Moreover, its actions are uninfluenced by antihistamine drugs. Its role in man is unclear.

In addition, the "kinin system" may be operative in producing inflammatory responses and smooth muscle contraction, although its exact role is also unclear. *Bradykinin,* considered the most important mediator, is a potent nonapeptide yielding bronchoconstriction in animals and man.

The roles of several other substances may be noted. *Acetylcholine* is not a direct mediator, but as a neurotransmitter it is involved in the vagally

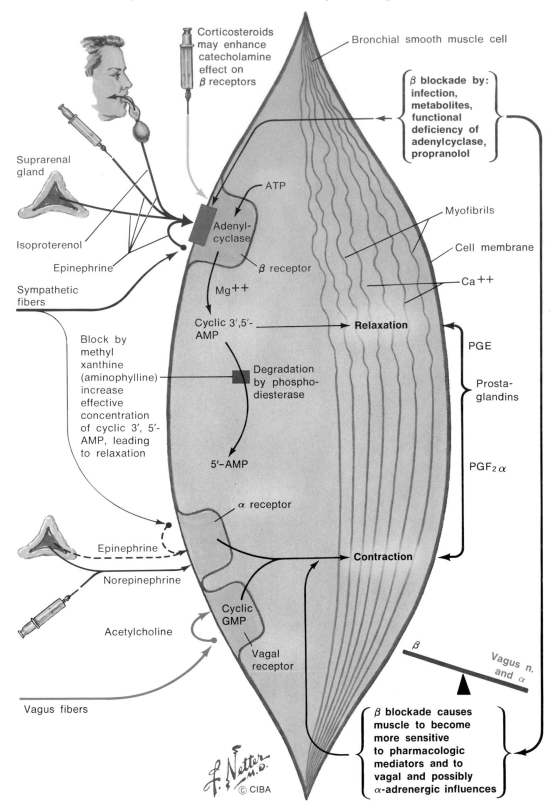

mediated reflexes. *Anaphylatoxins,* C3a and C5a, derivatives of the complement system, have been described in a limited number of patients after antigen challenge. The *eosinophil chemotactic factor of anaphylaxis (ECF-A)* produced in lungs after challenge with antigen is implicated in attracting eosinophils to the allergic site. A *neutrophil chemotactic factor* has also been identified. *Serotonin* increases capillary permeability and constricts smooth muscle; however, its local lung concentrations are negligible, and aerosol challenges are ineffective. *Prostaglandins (PG),* metabolites of arachidonic acid, are released in the lung under a variety of stimuli, including antigen exposure. They exert contractile or relaxant effects on the

smooth muscles of the airways and vasculature. PGE has a bronchodilator action, while PGF_{2a} and thromboxanes act as bronchoconstrictors. Their relatively high potency suggests that the ratio of tissue PGE/PGF_{2a} may be important in influencing tension responses in airway smooth muscle. Aerosol PGE has been shown to be an effective bronchodilator in some patients with asthma. Increased serum levels of PGF_{2a} have been found following allergen inhalation in other asthmatic patients. The full biologic and potential therapeutic roles for prostaglandins or other metabolites such as thromboxanes are yet to be established.

(Continued)

Corticosteroid Actions in Bronchial Asthma

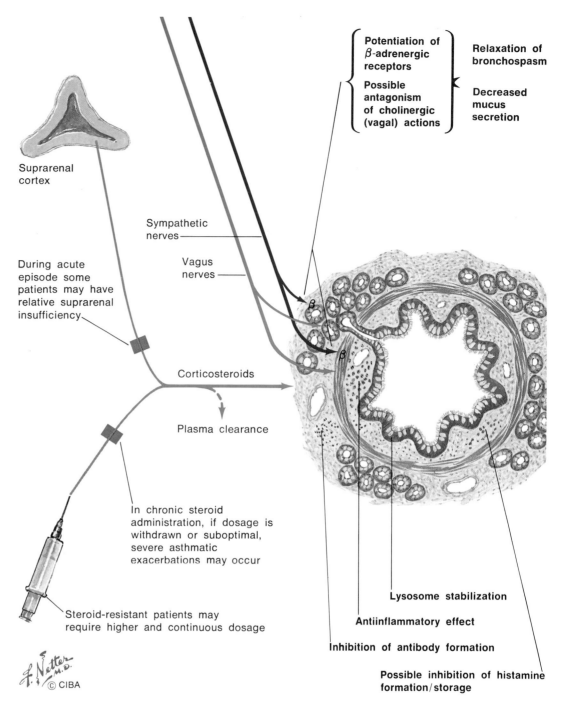

Suprarenal cortex

Sympathetic nerves

Vagus nerves

During acute episode some patients may have relative suprarenal insufficiency

Corticosteroids

Plasma clearance

In chronic steroid administration, if dosage is withdrawn or suboptimal, severe asthmatic exacerbations may occur

Steroid-resistant patients may require higher and continuous dosage

Potentiation of β-adrenergic receptors

Possible antagonism of cholinergic (vagal) actions

Relaxation of bronchospasm

Decreased mucus secretion

Lysosome stabilization

Antiinflammatory effect

Inhibition of antibody formation

Possible inhibition of histamine formation/storage

Bronchial Asthma
(Continued)

Complex biologic interactions between these mediators appear to exist. For example, histamine-stimulated contractions can be potentiated by SRS-A or prostaglandin intermediates; inhibition of mediator generation or release may be influenced by histamine or PGE by its action on cellular cyclic nucleotides.

Adrenal Corticosteroids. The role of the adrenal-pituitary axis in bronchial asthma is difficult to assess during acute attacks. Nevertheless, adrenocortical function must be considered, primarily because of the important actions of the adrenal corticosteroids. These include an antiinflammatory effect, decreased mucus secretion, lysosome stabilization, inhibition of antibody formation, possible depletion of tissue histamine, and potentiation of bronchodilator agents (Plate 19). Most asthmatic patients including those who have taken corticosteroid medication on a *short-term* basis have normal adrenal function. As would be expected, continuous *long-term* therapy with corticosteroids may suppress the function of the adrenal cortex. Asthmatic patients on chronic corticosteroid therapy are likely to have more severe asthmatic episodes, including status asthmaticus, apparently because of suppressed adrenocortical function. In some patients with severe asthma not on such medication, there is also a limited response to ACTH. Similarly, the anticipated increase in urinary excretion of 11-hydroxycorticosteroids in response to stress does not occur. Therefore, these patients may be more vulnerable to stress and more susceptible to allergic challenge.

Therapeutic Implications. Briefly, the activation of adenylcyclase by catecholamines (or sympathomimetic amines) provides a biochemical rationale for their clinical use. cAMP is degraded to 5'-AMP by the cytoplasmic enzyme phosphodiesterase. Hence, the increase in cAMP that results from methyl xanthine competitive inhibition of phosphodiesterase yields a synergistic action with the beta stimulant drugs. Corticosteroids have many effects and among them they are able to potentiate the action of adrenergic bronchodilators. Beta blocking agents—propranolol, for example—cause an expected worsening of asthma. Concurrently, cellular cGMP is influenced by vagal activity. Thus, for an asthmatic patient, drug action influences the biochemical and physiologic events in the mast cells and/or smooth muscle leading to inhibition of chemical mediator release and hence to muscle relaxation.

Finally, physical changes may be important factors in hyperresponsiveness. Patients with

chronic asthma have increased airway smooth muscle, which might be a contributing factor. Also, a precontracted airway (by Poiseuille's law) might contract more easily, offering a lower threshold for further airway obstruction. Clearly, one or many factors could contribute to the hyperirritant process.

General Causes of Asthma

Common precipitating factors in asthma are illustrated in Plate 20.

Allergic Stimuli. In allergic asthma, acute episodes may be precipitated by inhaled or ingested *allergens.* Airborne allergens such as house dusts, feathers, animal danders, insect fragments, furniture stuffing, fungal spores and various plant pollens are substances that may be inhaled. Allergenic foods like cow's milk, fish, eggs, various nuts, chocolate, shellfish and tomatoes are less culpable as a cause of asthma. In some patients, various allergens may have an additive or even synergistic effect. Allergens causing sensitivity in a patient are unpredictable and variable; the re-

sponse can change, and often decreases in severity from childhood to adult life.

Toxic and Irritative Stimuli. Many irritative factors in the inhaled air may evoke or aggravate an asthmatic attack. Obvious examples are tobacco smoke, air pollutants including automobile exhaust and industrial fumes, and volatile substances such as paint or gasoline. Chemicals such as TDI (toluene diisocyanate) and metals such as platinum or nickel can also provoke an attack.

Infection. Although infection (viral, bacterial or fungal) is often the precipitating stimulus in infective asthma, it can also be a significant factor in allergic asthma. Thus, bacterial sinusitis or a common cold may trigger an asthmatic episode, or infection may complicate an attack that began on a purely allergic basis. In man, experimental or naturally induced respiratory viral infections increase bronchoconstrictive responses to inhaled irritants or cholinomimetic drugs.

Medications. Drugs may initiate acute asthma either by pharmacologic action (beta adrenergic *(Continued)*

Common Precipitating Factors in Etiology of Bronchial Asthma

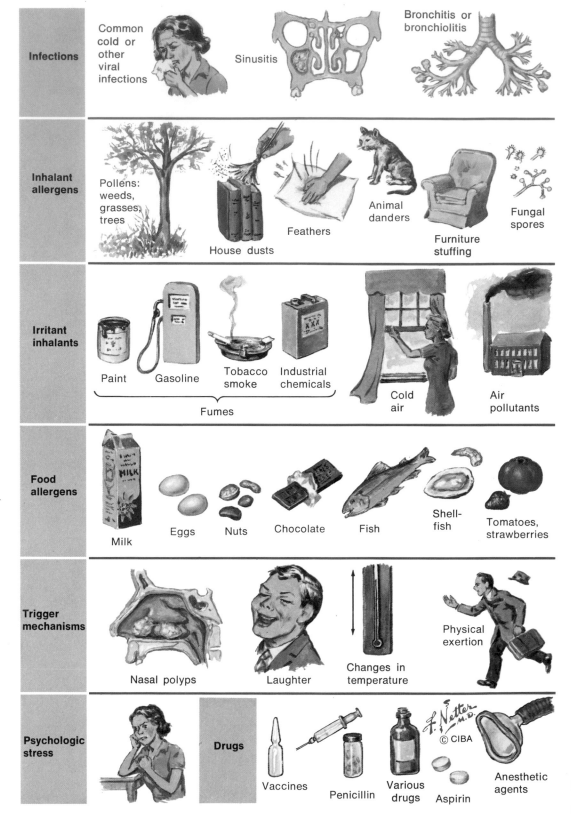

Bronchial Asthma
(*Continued*)

blockade) or by an allergic response, as with penicillin and vaccines. In patients with aspirin sensitivity, symptoms may occur within 20 minutes after ingestion.

Other Causes and Contributing Factors. Psychological and physical stress may contribute to an asthmatic episode in susceptible individuals. Similarly, trigger mechanisms such as breathing cold air, rapid changes in temperature or humidity, physical exertion or even laughing may cause an acute episode of bronchospasm and respiratory distress.

Pathologic Changes in Asthma

Gross and Microscopic Changes. The major pathologic features of bronchial asthma are generally limited to those observed in association with severe episodes (status asthmaticus). However, it may be inferred that lesser degrees of characteristic findings occur during attacks of a milder nature.

In status asthmaticus (Plate 21), the bronchi and bronchioles exhibit mucosal and submucosal edema, thickening of the basement membrane, a profuse leukocyte infiltration (particularly with eosinophils), intraluminal mucous plugs and smooth muscle hyperplasia and contraction. Grossly, the pale lungs are overdistended, often with regional parenchymal zones of hyperinflation alternating with areas of atelectasis caused by creamy, thick, tenacious, intraluminal mucous plugs. Especially if dehydration is clinically evident, the mucous plugs are viscous and adhere to the bronchial wall, narrowing the airway lumen. The process is compounded by enfolding of the epithelial surface from contraction of hyperplastic and possibly hypertrophied smooth muscle. Collectively, these actions cause the major increases in airflow resistance.

The mucous plugs (often contiguous with intracellular mucus) contain a PAS-positive matrix, polymorphonuclear cells, eosinophils and Charcot-Leyden crystals, which are degenerative crystalloids of eosinophils. Also characteristic are tiny whorls arising as casts within the smaller airways, so-called Curschmann's spirals. Extensive denuded and sloughed areas of the epithelial surface are common. Detached epithelial fragments may be seen in the lumen or sputum as clusters of ciliated cells (Creola bodies).

Submucosal gland hypertrophy is not as severe as in chronic bronchitis, yet a typical finding is goblet cell metaplasia, especially in the peripheral airways. The basement membrane is frequently thick and hyalinized. Partial atrophy of cartilage

can occur. Tissue mast cells are sparse, but their histologic detection may be hindered by degranulation. Limited immunoglobulin deposition is described.

It should be emphasized that the alveolar destructive changes which are found in patients with pulmonary emphysema are absent, as are severe permanent pathologic sequelae.

Pathophysiologic Effects of Asthma

The pathophysiologic effects of airway obstruction on respiratory function and hence on blood gases and pH values occur regardless of the specific mechanisms producing asthma. In status asthmaticus, severe gas exchange defects represent

the greatest immediate danger, and their improvement demands therapeutic priority.

Spirometry and Ventilatory Function in Asthma. In asthma, the prime physiologic disturbance is obstruction to airflow, which is more marked in expiration. This obstruction is variable in severity and in its site of involvement and is, by definition, reversible to some degree. Various combinations of smooth muscle spasm, inflammation, edema and mucus hypersecretion produce this airflow impediment. In addition, low lung volumes with terminal airspace collapse may compound the airway obstruction. In the larger airways there are the rigid cartilaginous rings

(*Continued*)

Pathology of Status Asthmaticus

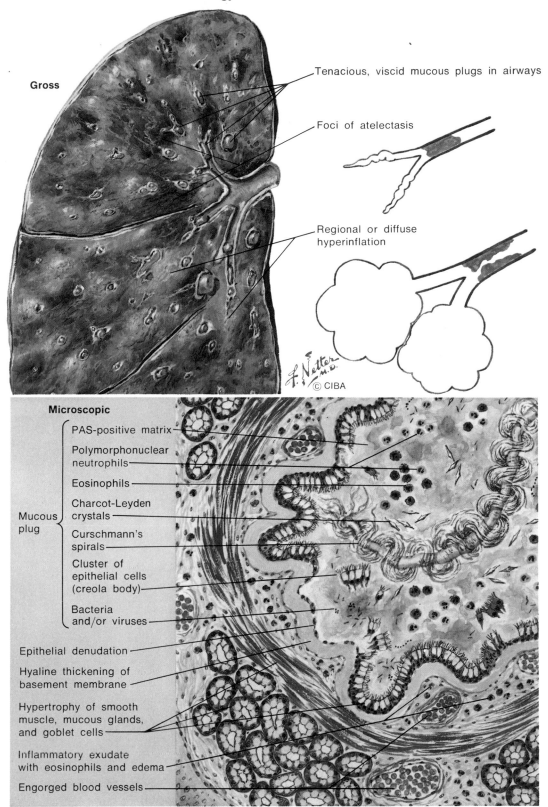

Gross

Tenacious, viscid mucous plugs in airways

Foci of atelectasis

Regional or diffuse hyperinflation

F. Netter M.D.
© CIBA

Microscopic

Mucous plug
- PAS-positive matrix
- Polymorphonuclear neutrophils
- Eosinophils
- Charcot-Leyden crystals
- Curschmann's spirals
- Cluster of epithelial cells (creola body)
- Bacteria and/or viruses

Epithelial denudation

Hyaline thickening of basement membrane

Hypertrophy of smooth muscle, mucous glands, and goblet cells

Inflammatory exudate with eosinophils and edema

Engorged blood vessels

Bronchial Asthma

(Continued)

which help maintain patency. In the peripheral airways, however, there is little opposition to the smooth muscle action because of the paucity of cartilage. Instead, the patency of these airways is influenced by lung volume because they are imbedded in and partially supported by the lung parenchyma.

At the onset of an asthmatic attack, or in mild cases, obstruction is not extensive. Only minor abnormalities in FVC or expiratory flow derivatives may occur, with spirometric change being limited to a fall in $FEF_{25-75\%}$. As asthma progresses and involves more of the bronchial tree, airways resistance significantly increases. Although inspiratory resistance also rises, the abnormality is more pronounced during expiration, because of closure of the airways as the lung empties. At this point, further expiratory effort does not produce any increase in expiratory flow rate and may even intensify airway collapse.

Because of these mechanical resistances, the respiratory muscles must produce a greater degree of chest expansion. More important, the elastic recoil of the lungs is insufficient for "passive" expiration. The respiratory muscles, therefore, must now play an active role in expiration. If obstruction is severe, air trapping will occur, with a rise in RV and FRC.

Airway obstruction is uneven and results in unequal distribution of gases to alveoli. This and other stimuli result in tachypnea and a consequently shortened respiratory cycle, even though the bronchial obstruction requires a lengthened respiratory time for adequate ventilation. These conflicting demands cannot be reconciled while the asthmatic attack continues.

The severity of the obstruction is reflected in the spirometric measurements of expiratory volume and airflow. The vital capacity (VC), forced expiratory vital capacity (FVC), inspiratory reserve volume (IRV) and inspiratory capacity (IC) are reduced during an acute attack.

The peripheral airways have a proportionately large total cross-sectional area. For this reason, the resistance of the peripheral airways normally accounts for only 20% of the total airway resistance. Thus extensive obstruction in these smaller airways may go undetected if the physician relies only on clinical findings. The reduction in FVC and FEV_1 shows a good correlation with the fall in Pa_{O_2}, while carbon dioxide retention does not occur until the FEV_1 is about 1 liter or 25% of the level predicted.

The extent of reversibility is measured from spirometric tracings at maximal expiratory flow-volume curves after the administration of an

aerosolized bronchodilator. A 15 to 20% increase in FEV_1, $FEF_{25-75\%}$ or even FVC is considered evidence of reversibility of bronchospasm. A limited response to bronchodilators indicates either that factors other than bronchospasm (*e.g.*, loss of lung parenchyma) are responsible or that the obstruction is temporarily refractory to bronchodilators because of secretions or receptor blockade. Similarly, serial determinations of FVC, FEV_1 or $FEV_{25-75\%}$ help assess both the course of the asthmatic attack and the response to therapy.

With progressive obstruction, expiration becomes increasingly prolonged. Increases in RV and FRC occur. These volume changes may represent an inherent physiologic response by the patient, since breathing at higher lung volumes prevents the closure of terminal airways. The overall effect of these events is alveolar hyperinflation, which tends to further increase the diameter of the airways by exerting a greater lateral force on their walls. This hyperinflation may partially preserve gas exchange. It is disadvantageous because much more work is required. Moreover, such a state compromises IC and VC. Additional consequences are an increase in O_2 consumption and the development of pulsus paradoxus. The symptoms of dyspnea and fatigue may also arise in part from this process. Finally, the effectiveness of

(Continued)

Representative Differential Diagnosis of Bronchial Asthma

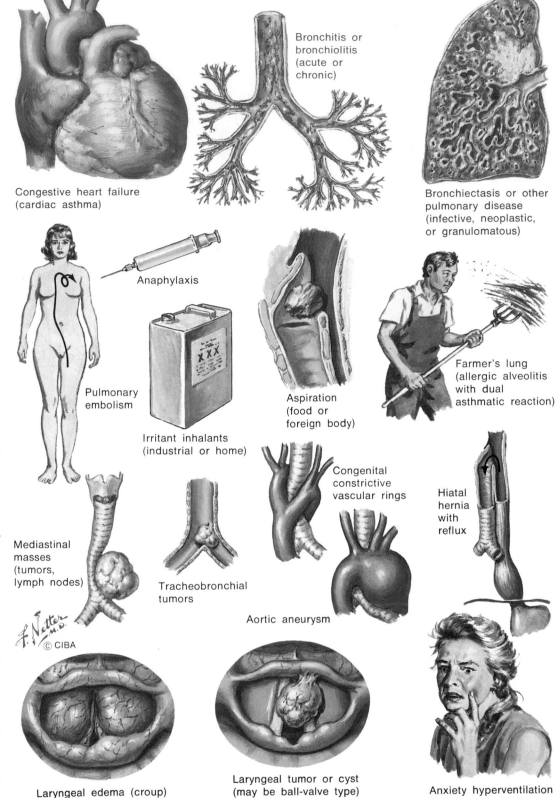

Congestive heart failure (cardiac asthma)

Bronchitis or bronchiolitis (acute or chronic)

Bronchiectasis or other pulmonary disease (infective, neoplastic, or granulomatous)

Anaphylaxis

Pulmonary embolism

Irritant inhalants (industrial or home)

Aspiration (food or foreign body)

Farmer's lung (allergic alveolitis with dual asthmatic reaction)

Mediastinal masses (tumors, lymph nodes)

Tracheobronchial tumors

Congenital constrictive vascular rings

Aortic aneurysm

Hiatal hernia with reflux

Laryngeal edema (croup)

Laryngeal tumor or cyst (may be ball-valve type)

Anxiety hyperventilation

Bronchial Asthma
(Continued)

cough is impaired since the velocity of respiratory airflow is seriously reduced.

Clinically, hyperinflation is estimated by physical examination of the chest, by chest x-ray studies or, if possible, by standard gas dilution techniques. Serial measurements of RV objectively assess the degree of pulmonary hyperinflation. Pulsus paradoxus, a useful clinical index of pulmonary overdistention (as is sternocleidomastoid muscle retraction), is usually present if the FEV_1 is less than 1.25 liters.

As a result of the nonhomogeneous airways obstruction in asthma, the distribution of inspired air to the terminal respiratory units is not uniform throughout the lungs. Alveoli which are hypoventilated because they are supplied by obstructed airways are interspersed with normal or hyperventilated alveoli; hence, the severity of asthma is directly related to the ratio of poorly ventilated to well-ventilated alveolar groups. Arterial hypoxemia, which is the primary defect in gas exchange in asthma, is due to this $\dot{V}_A/\dot{Q}_C$ nonhomogeneity. As the population of alveolar units with a low $\dot{V}_A/\dot{Q}_C$ ratio increases (because of advancing obstruction), the degree of arterial hypoxemia also intensifies. The $\dot{V}_A/\dot{Q}_C$ disturbance is compounded if some airways are completely obstructed. The right-to-left intrapulmonary shunt effect results in arterial hypoxemia.

Carbon dioxide elimination is not impaired when the number of alveolar-capillary units with normal $\dot{V}_A/\dot{Q}_C$ ratios remains large relative to the number of those with low $\dot{V}_A/\dot{Q}_C$ ratios. As airway obstruction progresses, there will be more and more hypoventilated alveoli. Simultaneously, appropriate increases in respiratory work, rate and depth occur. Such a response initially minimizes the increase in physiologic dead space but eventually becomes limited, and alveolar ventilation finally fails to support the metabolic needs of the body. Carbon dioxide retention now occurs together with increasing hypoxemia. This is a state of ventilatory failure, and commonly arises when the FEV_1 is less than 25% of that predicted.

Perfusion lung scan studies in asthma reveal transient areas of regional hypoperfusion which morphologically parallel the zones of hypoventilation. The hypoperfusion occurs because of regional hyperinflation or pulmonary vascular reactivity; it is migratory and fully resolves with remission of the asthmatic episode. (It may be confused with pulmonary embolism.) The pulmonary hypertension in asthma is not very severe or sustained, and chronic cor pulmonale, as seen with chronic bronchitis and emphysema, is generally absent. Diffusion limitations do not play a major role in asthma.

Clinical and Laboratory Considerations

Symptoms and Clinical Findings. Symptoms and signs of bronchial asthma range from acute, discrete episodes of shortness of breath, wheezing and cough, followed by significant remission, to more or less continuous, chronic symptoms which wax and wane in severity. For any patient, symptoms may be mild, moderate or severe at any given time. An asthmatic attack can be a terrifying experience, especially for patients who are aware of its potentially progressive nature.

Symptoms of an asthmatic episode may develop gradually or suddenly, and are at times preceded by an episode of allergic rhinitis or upper respiratory tract infection. Many patients complain of a sensation of retrosternal chest tightness and mention greater difficulty in breathing in than out. Expiratory and often inspiratory wheezing is audible and is associated with variable degrees of dyspnea. Cough is likely to be present and may be productive of sputum. The inability to raise secretions is ominous, and indicates severe and widespread bronchiolar plugging with tenacious mucus, often exacerbated by dehydration.

The patient prefers to sit upright; visible nasal alar flaring and use of the accessory respiratory muscles reflect the augmented work of breathing. Anxiety and apprehension generally relate to the

(Continued)

Sputum in Bronchial Asthma

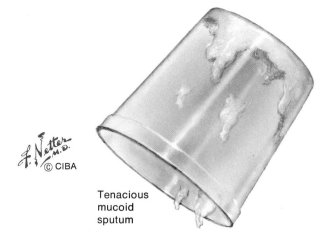

Tenacious mucoid sputum

Purulent sputum

Bronchial Asthma
(Continued)

intensity of the attack. Tachypnea may be the result of fear, airway obstruction or changes in blood and tissue gas tensions or pH. Hypertension and tachycardia both reflect increased catecholamine output, although a pulse rate greater than 110 to 130 beats/minute may indicate significant hypoxemia (Pa_{O_2} <60 mm Hg) and the seriousness of the episode. Pulsus paradoxus (10 mm Hg or higher) accompanies pulmonary hyperinflation, occurring when the FEV_1 is 1.25 liters or less. Flushing or perspiration and monosyllabic speech also signal the gravity of the attack. If severe hypoxemia and hypercapnia with respiratory acidosis supervene, the patient is usually cyanotic, fatigued, confused and agitated, or may show neuromuscular abnormalities such as asterixis and papilledema.

Chest examination reveals a hyperresonant percussion note, a low lying diaphragm, and other evidence of hyperinflation. Breath sounds can be coarse and loud, with vesicular features, but are often quite distant. Expiration is prolonged. Because of secretions, musical coarse rhonchi may be heard superimposed on this background of generalized inspiratory and expiratory wheezing. Focal areas of rales and evidence of consolidation should suggest atelectasis or pneumonia. With low-grade obstruction, wheezing may be slight or even absent but can be accentuated by rapid, deep breathing. Its pitch tends to rise with progressive obstruction, but when this is extensive, airflow is severely reduced and the chest may become paradoxically silent. This ominous finding may be inadvertently induced or worsened by administration of hypnotics, tranquilizers or sedatives which depress respiration. At the point where airflow is so decreased that the chest becomes silent, cough becomes ineffective and ventilatory failure supervenes. This requires immediate intensive therapy.

Complicating diseases such as pneumonitis, pleurisy, atelectasis, heart failure, pulmonary emboli or pneumothorax can contribute additional characteristic physical findings. Cardiac auscultation is frequently limited by the adventitious noises within the chest and by the increase in residual air. However, tachycardia and accentuated pulmonic second sound are often discernible. Laryngeal stridor or central airway obstruction from tracheal masses (*e.g.,* tumors) should not be confused with diffuse asthmatic obstruction. The primary clue here is a monophonic wheeze of similar sound quality throughout the thorax, loudest at its point of upper airway origin. In elderly patients, heart failure is readily diagnosed when the typical findings are present. These include prominent neck

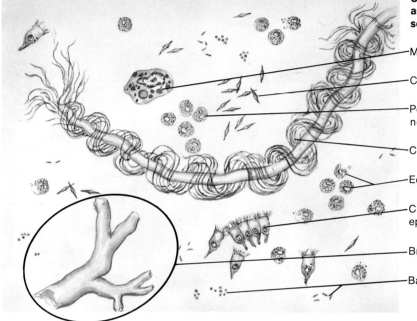

Unstained smear of asthmatic sputum; schematic (low power)

— Macrophage

— Charcot-Leyden crystals

— Polymorphonuclear neutrophil

— Curschmann's spirals

— Eosinophils

— Cluster of bronchial epithelial cells

— Bronchial cast (gross)

— Bacteria

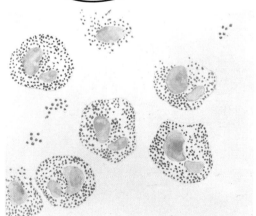

Eosinophils and staphylococci in stained smear

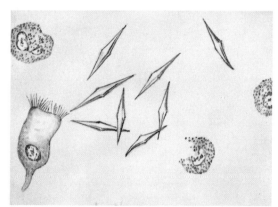

Charcot-Leyden crystals, eosinophils, and epithelial cell under high power

veins, basilar rales, cyanosis, cardiomegaly, gallop rhythm and peripheral edema. Finger clubbing is unusual in asthma, and its presence should alert the physician to possible suppurative, neoplastic or other hypoxemic disease processes. The careful evaluation of the ears, nose, sinuses, skin, abdomen and extremities is essential, and may disclose such complicating or precipitating processes as sinusitis, nasal polyps, hiatal hernia with aspiration or sources for pulmonary emboli.

Differential Diagnosis

The erroneous concept that wheezing is synonymous with asthma is still regrettably prevalent. Accordingly, the cliché "all that wheezes is

not asthma" serves as a reminder that wheezing is not pathognomonic of asthma. For the patient who is wheezing, a combination of history, physical examination and laboratory findings should establish a diagnosis. Diseases to be considered in the differential evaluation are depicted in Plate 22. Pulmonary disorders other than those illustrated include cystic fibrosis, pneumoconiosis and systemic vasculitis involving the lungs. In addition, wheezing episodes have been described following exposure to cotton fibers or inhalation of toluene diisocyanate in plastics manufacturing (polyvinyl chloride in meat wrappers), or baker's asthma from wheat flour sensitivity. In these cases

(Continued)

Bronchial Asthma
(*Continued*)

a history of specific occupational exposure and laboratory appraisal will aid in diagnosis.

Specific therapy of acute asthma is aided by various laboratory diagnostic tests which evaluate pulmonary function, assess the relative roles of infection and allergy, and determine whether complicating conditions coexist.

Radiography. The primary value of radiography is to exclude other diseases and to determine whether pneumonia, atelectasis, pneumothorax, pneumomediastinum or bronchiectasis exists. In mild asthma, the chest x-ray film will show no abnormalities. With severe obstruction, however, a characteristic reversible hyperlucency of the lung is evident, with widening of costal interspaces, depressed diaphragms and increased retrosternal air. In contrast to pulmonary emphysema in which vascular branching is attenuated and distorted, vascular caliber and distribution in asthma are generally undisturbed. Heart size remains normal or small unless cardiac disease coexists.

Focal atelectasis, a complication of asthma, is caused by impaction or inspissation of mucus. In children, even complete collapse of a lobe may be observed. Atelectatic shadows may be transient as mucus impaction shifts from one lung zone to another. When sputum is appropriately liquefied and mobilized, these patterns resolve.

Radiography is also useful in evaluating coexisting paranasal sinusitis. An upper gastrointestinal series is indicated if hiatal hernia with recurrent aspiration is suspected. Lung scans or angiography may be required if pulmonary emboli are believed to mimic asthma.

Sputum. Tracheal mucus velocity is impaired because of changes in viscosity, volume or chemical alterations. Gross and microscopic examination of any expectorated sputum is valuable for assessing airway pathology (Plate 23).

Sputum may be mucoid, frankly purulent or a mixture of both. *Mucoid sputum* is an opalescent or white gelatinous substance, generated in purely allergic insults and often very difficult to expectorate. It is quite adhesive to contiguous structures, and is internally viscous because of the presence of mucopolysaccharide and glycoprotein fibers, as well as transudated serum albumin. The more water mucoid sputum contains, the less viscous and adhesive it is. Recognition of mucoid sputum is based on its color, tenacity and adherence (*i.e.,* to the patient's tongue or sputum jar). Clinically, these qualities promote stasis and impaction of secretions leading to critical airway plugging and obstruction and often to secondary infection.

Purulent sputum is yellow, gray or green and may be produced in large volumes. Like mucoid

sputum, it can be thick or viscous, a property resulting from deoxyribonucleic acid fibers arising in necrotic debris of inflammatory cells, bacteria or parenchymal cells.

Sputum should be examined microscopically, stained with aqueous crystal violet, or viewed simply as a wet preparation under a coverslip. Thin spiral bronchiolar casts (Curschmann's spirals), measuring up to several centimeters in length, are often detected grossly and are strongly indicative of asthma. Ciliated columnar bronchial epithelial cells are frequently found. They may be recognized by their cilia and by the ovoid, basally displaced nucleus, granular cytoplasm and tapered base or tail which represents the attachment of the cell to the basement membrane. Creola bodies are clumps of such bronchial epithelial cells with moving cilia; they are very characteristic of severe asthma. Another cell easily recognized by its granular cytoplasm and, in wet preparations, by its brownian movement, is the polymorphonuclear neutrophil leukocyte (PMN), 10 to 15 microns in diameter. In purely infectious exacerbations of asthma, the PMN is the predominant cell.

In allergic asthma, eosinophils are stimulated and may constitute 10 to 90% of the sputum cell population. Eosinophils are structurally similar to PMN's except that the nucleus is often bilobed and the cytoplasmic granules are larger, more uniform and highly refractile. The latter property can be detected by focusing the microscope up and down. Large numbers of crystalloid derivatives of eosinophils can also be identified. These colorless fragments (20 to 40 microns in length), called Charcot-Leyden crystals, are elongated and octahedral. Macrophages are large cells (10 to 40 microns in diameter) and have numerous inclusion bodies. Adequate numbers (greater than 10 to 15% of the cell population) reflect appropriate cellular defenses.

Brown plugs or casts in sputum may be caused by allergic aspergillosis and should prompt a search for such fungi. Finally, examination of a gram stain preparation is important because it can guide initial antimicrobial therapy pending results of specific bacterial cultures and sensitivities.

The amount of sputum raised often indicates the effectiveness of secretion mobilization. Early in status asthmaticus sputum is likely to be sparse, emphasizing the need for therapeutic mobilization of secretions. This feature is also responsible, in part, for the slow lysis of an asthmatic paroxsym compared to the rapid reversibility achieved with bronchodilator drugs when smooth muscle spasm is the dominant abnormality. A significant finding indicating lysis of an asthmatic attack is the appearance of increased quantities of sputum. Supportive measures are mandatory to assist an ineffective cough, promote sputum clearance and prevent exhaustion.

Blood Tests. Because of stress, dehydration or infection, leukocytosis may occur. An increase (15,000/mm³) in PMN's indicates superimposed infection. A low blood eosinophil count may be seen in the early stages of the asthmatic episode or when infection is present; a count of greater than 5% may imply an allergic cause. Total eosinophil counts (TEC) are more quantitative and of greater clinical significance. They can be used serially to judge the efficacy of treatment, particularly with

corticosteroid drugs. TEC values higher than the normal 250/mm³ (often 800 to 1000/mm³) suggest a severe allergic reaction. TEC's of 4000/mm³ are often due to parasitic infection. Conversely, the absence of eosinophils does not exclude asthma. If during therapy with corticosteroids the eosinophil count does not fall, steroid-resistant bronchial asthma may exist, necessitating still higher doses of these drugs for resolution.

Usually, blood chemistry findings are normal unless secondary complications develop — vomiting, diarrhea or severe dehydration. In patients receiving diuretics or corticosteroids, complicating hypochloremic hypokalemic alkalosis may contribute to ventilatory depression. If pulmonary emboli, heart failure or connective tissue disorders are masquerading as bronchial asthma, appropriate blood tests may be of diagnostic value. When recurrent infections appear to be causative, immunoglobulins should be assayed. A sweat test for cystic fibrosis or stool examination for ova and parasites are indicated, if these are suspected.

Electrocardiogram. A tachycardia of greater than 120 beats/minute may indicate serious hypoxemia (Pa_{O_2} <40 to 60 mm Hg). The sinus tachycardia of an asthmatic attack will revert to normal with remission. During a severe episode, pulmonary hypertension may cause reversible right ventricular strain with right axis shift, right bundle-branch block and prominent right atrial P waves. Differentiation from pulmonary hypertension caused by embolization can be difficult. In elderly patients dysrhythmias or myocardial ischemia may be precipitated. Dysrhythmias can also be produced by heart-stimulating drugs such as epinephrine or isoproterenol, particularly in the hypoxemic individual with coronary artery disease, valvular disorders or a cardiomyopathy.

Principles of Management

Prompt treatment of an acute asthmatic episode is imperative, but *prevention* of asthma is basic to any therapeutic program. Each patient must be thoroughly evaluated to determine all possible causative and contributing factors, as long-term management depends on their elimination or control. The acute attack requires prompt specific drug therapy since any episode may progress to life-threatening status asthmaticus.

Treatment of Acute Episode

Aqueous epinephrine is preferred for its rapid and predominant beta stimulatory action (Plate 24). Formulations of epinephrine that provide more prolonged relief also have slower absorption; aerosol preparations are available but have generally been replaced by selective beta₂ adrenergic drugs.

Aerosolized isoproterenol, the most potent sympathomimetic amine, can also be used in an acute attack. An unexpected bronchoconstrictive effect has been reported with isoproterenol which may be related to the formation of a metabolite with a beta blocking action, and a paradoxical fall in arterial oxygen tension may be observed in some patients.

Beta₂ selective adrenergic bronchodilators have a preferential airway effect with a longer duration of action than isoproterenol, and are reputed to
(Continued)

Bronchial Asthma
(*Continued*)

cause fewer cardiovascular side effects and less hypoxemic induction. These include such agents as isoetharine or metaproterenol sulfate, available in aerosol form, and terbutaline sulfate, which is given by subcutaneous injection or orally. Ephedrine's usefulness is limited in an acute attack because of a slower and less potent action; it may be of value orally for maintenance therapy. In the hypertensive, hyperthyroid or cardiac patient, epinephrine must be used with caution or preferably not at all. Intravenous epinephrine is never recommended because ventricular dysrhythmias or cerebral hemorrhage may occur.

The initial response to epinephrine may be inadequate, or the patient may exhibit refractoriness with repeated use. Initial therapeutic resistance has been ascribed in part to coexisting respiratory acidosis, which is partially reversible by intravenous administration of bicarbonate. When this is persistent, repeated injections are of no value and may be detrimental because of side effects. In this event, aminophylline, which is longer acting and may have an additive effect with sympathomimetic drugs, can be administered intravenously, *very slowly* over 15 minutes. Too rapid administration can cause hypotension and even death, but other routes are seldom effective in an acute attack. The bronchodilating activity of aminophylline is generally related to its plasma concentration; effective levels range from 10 to 20 μg/ml. Although aminophylline is preferred for older patients, those with liver disease or heart failure should be monitored carefully since toxic reactions become more likely. Overdosing can be associated with convulsions, coma, cardiac irregularities or fatality.

When an asthmatic attack does not respond to the therapy described above, a short course of corticosteroids may be added, although their peak action usually does not occur until 6 to 12 hours after intravenous or intramuscular administration.

Important supportive measures in an acute episode include appropriate antimicrobial therapy if infection is present, adequate hydration and oxygen. Expectorants and oral ephedrine may be added.

Status Asthmaticus

Status asthmaticus is a medical emergency in which respiratory distress reflects refractoriness to conventional pharmacologic therapy for an acute asthmatic attack. Because of the nursing care and continuous monitoring required, hospitalization in an intensive care unit is mandatory. It is the stage of asthma with the most severe gas exchange

Management of Acute Asthmatic Attack

1. Give aqueous epinephrine 1:1000 subcutaneously, 0.1 ml for children, 0.3 ml for adults; if initial response is adequate, repeat at 30 to 60 minute intervals as needed; oxygen as indicated; in hypertensive, hyperthyroid, and cardiac patients use epinephrine with extreme caution (aminophylline and oxygen preferable)

2. If response to epinephrine is inadequate or if patient becomes refractory, give aminophylline intravenously very slowly; administer oxygen

3. If necessary, corticosteroids, which act more slowly, also can be given

4. Hospitalization is indicated if patient fails to respond to drugs

defects and accounts for its greatest morbidity and mortality. It may be defined as an attack resistant to several standard doses of epinephrine and/or aminophylline within a reasonable period of time. Multiple factors are often responsible for the extreme degree of airway obstruction seen, and every effort must be made to identify and correct them.

Changes in Blood Gases and pH. As a consequence of advanced airway obstruction, serious ventilation-perfusion disturbances arise, causing major changes in arterial oxygen and carbon dioxide tensions and pH (Plate 25). In fact, dangerous levels of hypoxemia sometimes develop with alarming rapidity and, at least initially,

without retention of carbon dioxide. This phenomenon may lead to sudden death.

These changes in blood gases and pH cannot be quantitated by simple clinical observation, but certain findings may be correlative. The degree of arterial hypoxemia will roughly correlate with the severity of airways obstruction. Hypercapnia is generally not seen until the FEV_1 is less than 1 liter (or 25 to 30% of that predicted). Precise documentation of blood gas and pH measurements must be obtained and followed repeatedly to evaluate serial changes in gas exchange and the response to therapy. There may be rapid

(Continued)

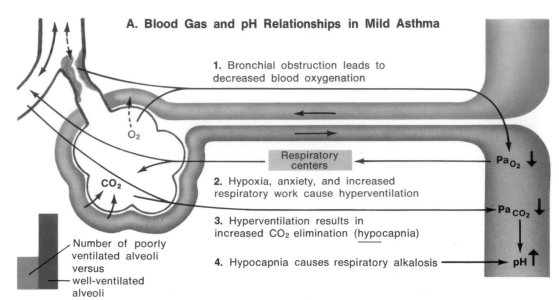

A. Blood Gas and pH Relationships in Mild Asthma

1. Bronchial obstruction leads to decreased blood oxygenation

Respiratory centers

2. Hypoxia, anxiety, and increased respiratory work cause hyperventilation

3. Hyperventilation results in increased CO_2 elimination (hypocapnia)

4. Hypocapnia causes respiratory alkalosis

Pa_{O_2} ↓

Pa_{CO_2} ↓

pH ↑

Number of poorly ventilated alveoli versus well-ventilated alveoli

O_2

CO_2

B. Crossover Phase

pH 7.5   50 Pa_{CO_2} (mm Hg)

Crossover

40   7.4

Caution

30   7.2

Time

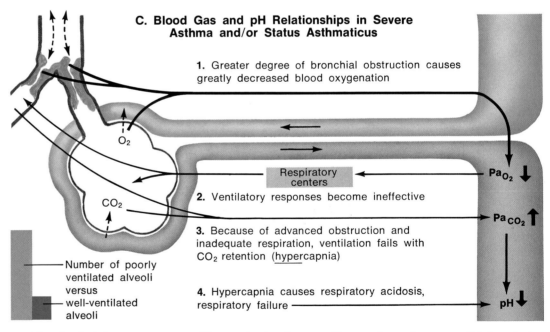

C. Blood Gas and pH Relationships in Severe Asthma and/or Status Asthmaticus

1. Greater degree of bronchial obstruction causes greatly decreased blood oxygenation

Respiratory centers

2. Ventilatory responses become ineffective

3. Because of advanced obstruction and inadequate respiration, ventilation fails with CO_2 retention (hypercapnia)

4. Hypercapnia causes respiratory acidosis, respiratory failure

Pa_{O_2} ↓

Pa_{CO_2} ↑

pH ↓

O_2

CO_2

Number of poorly ventilated alveoli versus well-ventilated alveoli

Bronchial Asthma
(*Continued*)

progression from normal values to severe hypoxemia, hypercapnia and respiratory acidosis.

In an early stage, hypoxemia (Pa_{O_2} 55 to 75 mm Hg) and hypocapnia (Pa_{CO_2} <35 mm Hg) may be noted, leading to respiratory alkalosis with a variable degree of compensation.

Spirometry may show only moderately impaired breathing capacity, and this phase will often respond favorably to bronchodilators or other drugs.

With more severe obstruction, Pa_{O_2} decreases to the range of 50 to 55 mm Hg and Pa_{CO_2} is less than 30 mm Hg; respiratory alkalosis (pH >7.50) is apparent. This profile is associated with an acute, moderately severe episode of status asthmaticus. Flow and volume indexes are significantly impaired, and response to bronchodilators is variable. At this point, all therapeutic efforts must be intensified.

Frank ventilatory failure is associated with severe hypoxemia (Pa_{O_2} <55 mm Hg); hypercapnia (Pa_{CO_2} >45 mm Hg) and respiratory acidosis (pH <7.35). This profile is typical of advanced status asthmaticus with its limited or absent response to bronchodilators. Tracheal intubation and ventilatory support will be required.

Management of Status Asthmaticus

Because the primary basis for the arterial blood gas and pH changes in status asthmaticus is airway obstruction, establishing and maintaining airway patency is fundamental to the clearing of secretions.

Mobilizing Secretions and Clearing the Airway. In conjunction with control of allergy and infection (including possible ear and paranasal sinus infection), rapid mobilization of secretions and cellular debris will help terminate the asthmatic episode. Multiple approaches are established in therapy:

1. Adequate hydration: dehydration resulting from limited fluid intake, insensible water loss and fever contributes to secretion retention, and hypovolemia increases the mortality. Replacement and maintenance fluids are essential.

2. Expectorant agents: hydration and airway humidification are most effective for mobilizing secretions. Oral SSKI, sodium iodide by infusion or oral glyceryl guaiacolate may be tried. Aerosolized N-acetylcysteine lyses mucoproteins but should be used with caution in asthma, which it may aggravate, and always with a bronchodilator agent.

3. Mechanical measures: once the patient is hydrated, the raising of secretions may be encour-

aged by physical therapy measures. Nasotracheal suctioning and occasionally bronchoscopy may be necessary.

4. Oxygen: well-humidified oxygen should be provided throughout to maintain a Pa_{O_2} of 70 to 80 mm Hg. Oxygen-induced hypoventilation can be controlled by mechanical ventilation.

5. Bronchodilators: the effectiveness of epinephrine may be limited by pharmacologic refractoriness. Isoproterenol aerosol can be provided by a hand bulb or compressor-driven nebulizer or with IPPB. Isoproterenol may reduce airway resistance and alleviate respiratory overwork, but by inducing a $\dot{V}_A/\dot{Q}_C$ mismatch it may occasionally aggravate hypoxemia; hence increased supplemental oxygen may be required. Aminophylline

is generally a major and most useful foundation for bronchodilator therapy. Isoetharine, terbutaline or other bronchodilators may also prove valuable. In children (and in a limited number of adults), intravenous isoproterenol has been advocated as an added form of therapy with the rationale that it saves time in allowing corticosteroids to become maximally effective. Thus the need for tracheal intubation and ventilation and their attendant complications are minimized. This approach must be conducted with continuous, adequate cardiac and blood gas monitoring.

6. Sedatives: sedatives are absolutely contraindicated unless supportive mechanical ventilation is to be used.

(*Continued*)

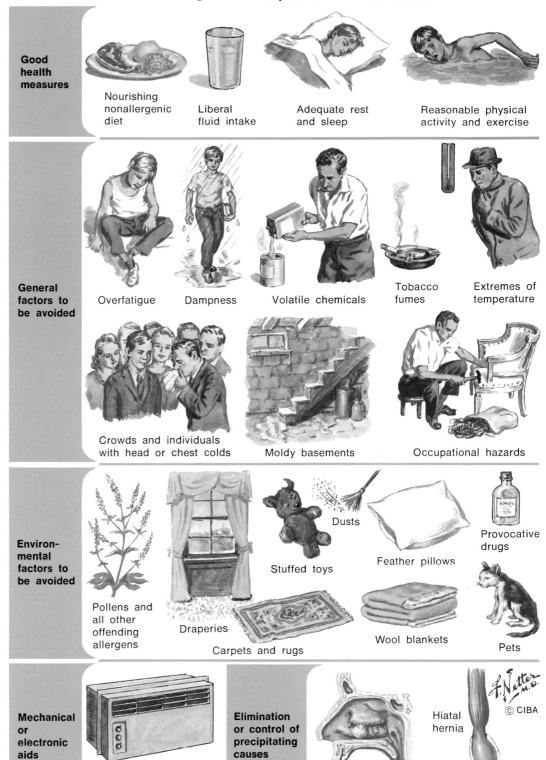

Bronchial Asthma
(Continued)

7. Mechanical ventilation: details are described elsewhere (see page 294). Ventilatory failure is a dangerous and often lethal phase of status asthmaticus. Indications for tracheal intubation and mechanical ventilation include (a) apnea, (b) rising Pa_{CO_2} of 5 to 10 mm Hg/hour despite full therapy, (c) patient exhaustion, (d) absolute Pa_{CO_2} of 50 mm Hg or greater with respiratory acidosis, (e) refractory hypoxemia. Volume-limited ventilators are preferred. Serial blood gas samples and pH measurements are necessary for optimal management.

8. Antibiotics: if evidence of infection exists, administer antibiotics preferably based on sputum culture results if available.

9. Adrenal corticosteroids: by several actions (Plate 19), corticosteroids significantly relieve otherwise uncontrollable asthmatic symptoms and may be lifesaving. Pharmacologically, they restore and potentiate the effectiveness of catecholamines on beta adrenergic receptors and also inhibit the enzyme phosphodiesterase. Early administration in high doses is advisable, particularly for critically ill patients, or those who have been on prior corticosteroid therapy.

The exact dosage or type of corticosteroids in status asthmaticus is unresolved, but generally moderate doses by the parenteral route are preferred. Treatment should be sustained until clinical improvement warrants a gradual reduction and eventual elimination of corticosteroid therapy. This precaution is particularly important for children because adrenal suppression may occur more rapidly than in adults. ACTH is not recommended in status asthmaticus because, presumably, the adrenal cortex is already maximally stimulated.

Undesirable side effects of corticosteroid medication are not usually encountered in short-term therapy.

Long-term Management of Asthma

Long-term management is required to prevent the occurrence of asthma or control its symptoms. As many diverse stimuli can interact to produce asthma, multiple therapeutic approaches are essential.

General Principles. The patient must practice moderation in daily activities and avoid exposure to precipitating agents. The home environment, particularly the bedroom, should have the factors which are shown in Plate 26 eliminated. Humidifiers are particularly important during the winter when decreased humidity may cause irritation to mucous membranes or drying of se-

cretions. A relative humidity of 50% or greater is desirable. Nose, sinus or throat infection or polyps must be appropriately treated.

Avoidance of all precipitants is not always possible (Plate 20). Incriminated drugs or foods are easier to avoid than airborne inhalants. If only one allergen such as dust or dog dander is causative, avoidance may be beneficial. Exposure and activity should be limited during periods of high air pollution.

Psychologic Management. The physician should understand the patient's mechanisms for coping with his stressful disease and encourage rapport and open communication as well as provide adequate instruction about its general nature. A

pleasant home environment and an understanding family are essential, particularly with children. Because extrinsic asthma often abates with growth, an optimistic attitude should be fostered. Parental resentment or excessive protectiveness should be minimized. Counseling with the child's teachers may also help. If serious emotional disturbances or socioeconomic or occupational problems exist, proper evaluation and counseling are indicated.

Apprehension and fear are seen in almost every patient during an acute episode and at times may be perpetuating or even precipitating factors. However, in severe asthma or status asthmaticus,
(Continued)

Bronchial Asthma
(*Continued*)

psychogenic factors must be considered secondary rather than primary causes.

Ambulatory Medication. Medications include bronchodilators (orally or by aerosol), antihistamines, corticosteroids, decongestants and expectorants. Daily use of drugs will prevent attacks and lessen chronic symptoms, although if corticosteroids have to be used, an alternate-day regimen is preferred.

Patients with moderate asthma respond well to maintenance therapy with aminophylline preparations administered orally. Aminophylline is the foundation of long-term ambulatory management and should be individualized. Some patients may benefit from a trial of antihistamines.

Aerosol preparations containing either epinephrine, isoproterenol or isoetharine are generally not primary forms of drug therapy and should never be dispensed without appropriate instruction about correct usage, proper dose and danger of overdosing. A patient may become dependent and overuse aerosol nebulizers, prompted by habit rather than by therapeutic need. The dangers of overdosage are increased, and drug propellant—induced cardiotoxic effects are more likely. Sudden death can occur in severe asthma, and, in one survey done in Great Britain, this was noted especially in children between 10 and 14 years of age who had overused gas-propelled isoproterenol nebulizers. A direct cardiotoxic effect of the propellant may have been responsible, or the deaths may have resulted from drug overdose leading to cardiac arrhythmias or a significant, paradoxical fall in Pa_{O_2}. Most of these children had severe, diffuse, secretional obstruction of their airways, and the relationship of death to treatment is uncertain. Thus, proper instruction about avoidance of the excessive use of nebulizers is imperative. Patients should notify their physicians whenever increased use of nebulizers is associated with decreased response.

Selective beta$_2$ stimulating drugs theoretically are expected to have fewer adverse cardiovascular effects, because beta$_2$ receptors are absent from the heart. Two such agents, terbutaline and salbutamol, have more prolonged action than isoproterenol.

At the first sign of an acute bacterial infection, culture specimens should be obtained and antimicrobial therapy started. Tetracycline or erythromycin may be used initially, but other antimicrobials can be substituted later, as indicated by the results of cultures and sensitivity studies. The various penicillins must be used cautiously because of the danger of drug allergy. In some patients, chronic or recurrent infection is a causative factor, and for them viral vaccines have been used prophylactically. However, their effectiveness and that of stock or autogenous bacterial vaccines remains disputed.

For ambulatory patients with severe asthma, corticosteroids are prescribed under close medical supervision (see page 133). They should be used on a long-term basis only if the response to comprehensive conventional therapy fails.

Chronic therapy may cause adrenal suppression, edema, hypertension, aggravation of diabetes mellitus, exacerbation or spread of infection, osteoporosis, myopathy, aseptic necrosis of the femoral or humeral heads, subcapsular cataracts, peptic ulceration with bleeding, psychosis, pseudotumor cerebri and hypokalemic alkalosis. To prevent these adverse effects, potassium supplements should be given; sodium restricted to less than 1 g/day; serum electrolytes and blood sugar monitored; and antacids prescribed. More important, for long-term use the drug should be administered on an alternate day schedule or by aerosol. Only careful and continuous follow-up of the patient will minimize these adverse sequelae.

In recent years new drugs have been introduced which may be of benefit in long-term management and in the prevention of acute attacks. Cromolyn sodium, a derivative of the smooth muscle relaxant khellin, acts by stabilizing the mast cell membrane and thus inhibiting the release of bronchoconstricting mediators. It is thus not a bronchodilator and is of no use in reversing established bronchospasm. It needs to be used in strictly prophylactic fashion, by inhalation using a special hand-held inhaler. Particularly in younger patients, both allergen- and exercise-induced asthma can be prevented when cromolyn sodium is given prior to such challenges. A major advantage is its ability to permit reduction or complete elimination of corticosteroids.

Aerosol preparations of corticosteroids are deposited directly in the airways and produce an adequate therapeutic response. Since they are not significantly absorbed, this topical route may reduce the need for oral administration and the complications of this type of treatment, including adrenal suppression. However, it must be clear that maintenance doses of aerosol corticosteroids do not have the same pharmacologic actions as sympathomimetic bronchodilators and therefore should not be used for the same purpose. In children, a major benefit has been a reduction in the incidence of steroid-caused growth retardation.

Hyposensitization. For patients in whom allergy plays a significant role, specific hyposensitization is an important element in long-term management. Such a program causes some discomfort, is time-consuming, and can be costly. Hence, it should be undertaken only if the asthma is sufficiently problematic, and if general avoidance measures and drug therapy are ineffective.

A hyposensitization program depends on results of skin testing and the exposure history.

Since many antigens are available for skin testing, the physician must use clinical judgment in selecting those most likely to be allergenic for a particular patient.

Preferably, skin tests are performed by a scratch (prick) technique (Plate 27) using commercial aqueous extracts of common antigens—molds, pollens, fungi, house dusts, feathers, foods or animal danders. Mixtures of unrelated antigens should not be used. If skin-sensitizing antibodies to the antigen are present, a wheal-and-flare reaction develops within 15 to 30 minutes; a control test with saline diluent should show little or no reaction.

Optimally, both the history and dermal reactivity will give corresponding results. However, some patients have positive histories but negative or questionable skin tests. In other patients negative histories and positive skin tests indicate immunologic reactivity which is clinically insignificant. Equivocal results require careful evaluation. If further testing is called for because scratch test results were inconclusive, intradermal tests may be indicated. This approach is more sensitive than scratch tests, but it is time-consuming and more likely to produce systemic or acute asthmatic reactions.

Bronchial provocation tests (BPT) are a more direct method of determining the causative role of a specific airborne allergen when a patient with a negative skin reaction has a strongly positive clinical history. Serial measurements of pulmonary function (spirometry or body plethysmography) are made after inhalation of a suspected aqueous antigenic aerosol. There appears to be good correlation among skin tests, specific serum IgE antibodies and bronchial provocation test reactions. BPT are also useful in documenting late asthmatic reactions. Here, an early fall in FEV$_1$ is followed several hours later by a further drop which is often more severe and of longer duration. Another diagnostic maneuver is the inhalation of aerosolized methacholine. Patients with asthma will exhibit a noticeable increase in airway resistance at dilutions which do not affect normal subjects.

During any type of testing, a syringe of epinephrine and a tourniquet which can be applied proximal to the test site should be available in case of a systemic (anaphylactic) or asthmatic reaction. Also, intravenous fluids, oxygen, emergency drugs (corticosteroids, aminophylline, vasopressors) and equipment to establish an airway should be readily accessible.

Results of skin or inhalation tests must be correlated with the clinical history. Best responses can be anticipated when pollens are the offending agents. Weekly injections of dilute extracts of antigen are administered under the supervision of a physician in gradually increasing doses until maximum protection is achieved. Hyposensitization schedules may be perennial, coseasonal or preseasonal. The patient's responses must be reevaluated periodically; if they are less than expected, new sensitivity to other antigens should be considered.

Formation of a blocking antibody (IgG) is postulated to occur in response to the injections of antigen. The affinity of IgG for the antigen is greater than that of IgE, and therefore, it combines with the antigen more readily. A correlation between IgG titer and clinical improvement in

(*Continued*)

Bronchial Asthma
(Continued)

hay fever victims seems to exist. Serum IgE levels in treated patients are apparently decreased, possibly by IgG feedback. Or inhibition of IgE may be related to T cell function, which appears necessary for IgE antibody synthesis. A reduction in the cellular release of histamine may be another mechanism of immunotherapy.

In controlled trials, up to 70% of patients with allergy to selected pollens have been shown to improve substantially with hyposensitization. The best responses may be expected in young asthmatics, but even adults should have a therapeutic trial if that is clinically indicated.

Other Considerations. Some patients with refractory asthmatic symptoms may benefit by relocation to another climate. Because no geographic area is devoid of airborne allergens or irritants, the response to such a move is highly variable. However, living in a less humid or less industrialized area often proves beneficial. Optimally, a trial vacation or a period of residence in the prospective region will facilitate this decision.

Physical therapy benefits certain patients. This includes breathing exercises to improve effort tolerance and relaxation techniques to temper the distress of an acute attack. Postural drainage can also be used by patients with copious secretions.

Surgical procedures are rarely indicated for asthma.

Conclusions

Of the 6 to 8 million asthmatics in the United States, between 4000 and 7000 die each year. Of this total, 1.5 million are children, yet less than 200 children die annually of causes related to asthma. The greatest danger of death occurs during severe attacks or in status asthmaticus. Prevention of such deaths requires intensive, individualized treatment based on the principles presented. Young asthmatic patients can anticipate significant relief of symptoms by the time they reach puberty. Even in adults, symptoms can be substantially alleviated by treatment.

Long-term management is based on *prevention* and requires an individualized therapy program for each patient. This program depends on the identification of the particular causes of asthma and mandates open communication and trust between patient, physician and other family members. Bronchial asthma is reversible with proper management, and its progression to permanent respiratory disability can be prevented.

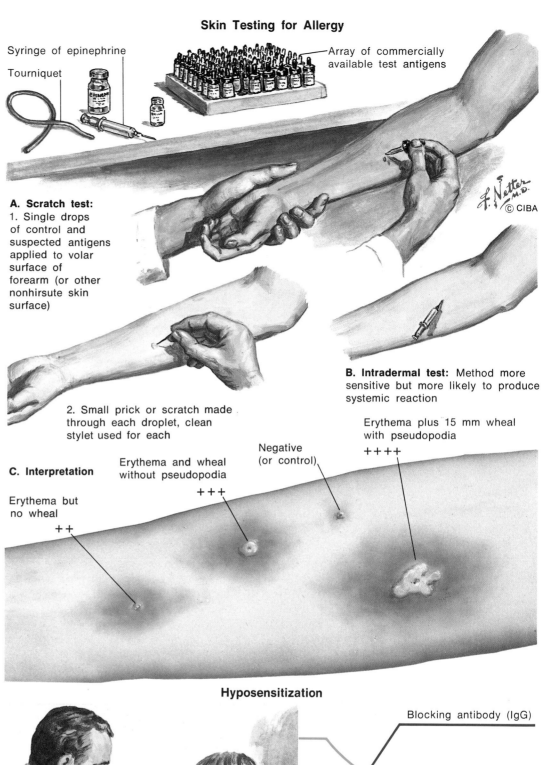

Skin Testing for Allergy

Syringe of epinephrine

Tourniquet

Array of commercially available test antigens

A. Scratch test:
1. Single drops of control and suspected antigens applied to volar surface of forearm (or other nonhirsute skin surface)

2. Small prick or scratch made through each droplet, clean stylet used for each

B. Intradermal test: Method more sensitive but more likely to produce systemic reaction

C. Interpretation

Erythema but no wheal
++

Erythema and wheal without pseudopodia
+++

Negative (or control)

Erythema plus 15 mm wheal with pseudopodia
++++

Hyposensitization

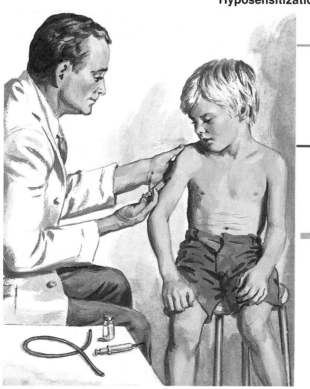

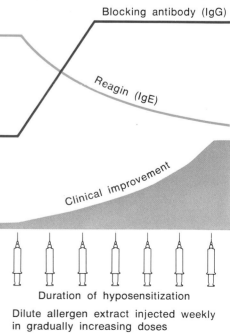

Blocking antibody (IgG)

Reagin (IgE)

Clinical improvement

Duration of hyposensitization

Dilute allergen extract injected weekly in gradually increasing doses

Tourniquet and syringe of epinephrine readily available

Chronic Obstructive Pulmonary Disease

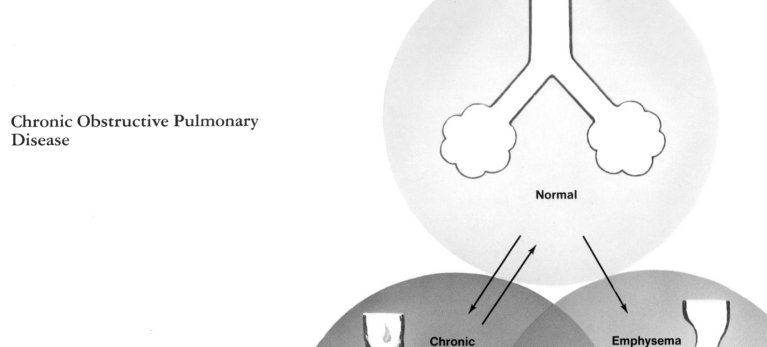

Chronic obstructive pulmonary disease (COPD), consisting of some combination of chronic bronchitis and emphysema, is the most common chronic disease of the lungs (Plate 28). It occurs far more often than carcinoma of the lung, and in contrast to the patient with carcinoma, the patient afflicted with COPD usually lives a number of years with progressive disability and multiple acute exacerbations. Thus the physician is likely to become involved for many years in the assessment, treatment and education of a patient with COPD.

Although generally present in combination, chronic bronchitis and emphysema are two distinct processes. Chronic bronchitis can be diagnosed only by taking a history; emphysema can be diagnosed with certainty only by examination of sections of whole lung fixed at inflation. Chronic bronchitis is characterized by cough and sputum production for at least three months of the year for more than two consecutive years in the absence of other kinds of endobronchial disease such as bronchiectasis. Emphysema is defined as overinflation of the distal airspaces with destruction of alveolar

septa. With each process defined from opposite extremes of the clinical spectrum—*i.e.*, chronic bronchitis from the history and emphysema from the postmortem examination—it is not surprising that radiographic, pathologic, pathophysiologic and clinical correlations have been sought to evaluate the relative contribution of each process to the disability of a given patient. In the pages that follow, an attempt will be made to clarify the structure-function relationships in both diseases, the clinical methods of assessing the mechanisms of airway obstruction, and the therapeutic and prognostic value of making such assessments.

Pathology

Chronic Bronchitis. Chronic bronchitis (Plate 29) is associated with hyperplasia and hypertrophy of the mucus-secreting glands found in the submucosa of the large cartilaginous airways. Because the mass of the submucous glands is approximately 40 times greater than that of the intraepithelial goblet cells, it is thought that these glands produce most airway secretions. The degree of hyperplasia is

quantitatively assessed as the ratio of the submucosal gland thickness to the overall thickness of the bronchial wall from the cartilage to the airway lumen. Such a ratio is known as the *Reid index*. Although the Reid index is often low in the bronchi of patients who do not have symptoms of chronic bronchitis during life and is frequently high in chronic bronchitics, there is sufficient overlap of Reid index values to suggest that a gradual change in the submucous glands may take place. Thus the sharp distinction of the clinical definition of chronic bronchitis cannot correlate completely with the pathologic changes in large airways.

In addition to changes in submucous glands, hyperplasia of the intraepithelial goblet cells, denudation of the mucosa and regions of epithelium that have undergone squamous metaplasia are frequently found in chronic bronchitis. Hyperplasia of the goblet cells is most apparent in the smaller noncartilaginous airways (bronchioles) that do not contain submucous glands. These smaller airways may be narrowed by intraluminal mucous plugs,

(Continued)

Chronic Obstructive Pulmonary Disease
(*Continued*)

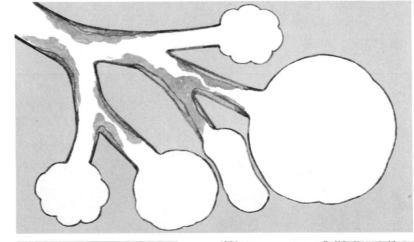

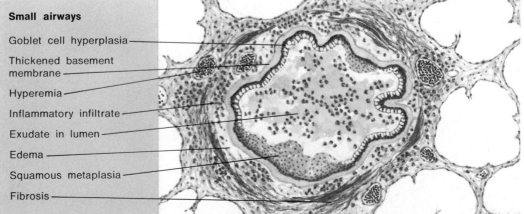

Chronic Bronchitis

Large cartilaginous airways

Mucous gland hyperplasia (elevated Reid index)

Dilated duct of gland

Thickened basement membrane

Squamous metaplasia

Inflammatory infiltrate

Hyperemia

Edema

Fibrosis

Profuse exudate in lumen

Epithelial desquamation

Cartilage intact

Airways partially or completely blocked or "one-way" valve effect by mucoid or mucopurulent secretions, with impaired or non-uniform distribution of ventilation

Small airways

Goblet cell hyperplasia

Thickened basement membrane

Hyperemia

Inflammatory infiltrate

Exudate in lumen

Edema

Squamous metaplasia

Fibrosis

mucosal edema, smooth muscle hypertrophy, inflammatory changes in the walls and peribronchiolar fibrosis. It is quite likely that the diffuse changes in small airways contribute more to the obstruction and maldistribution of inspired gas than do the more obvious abnormalities in large airways.

Emphysema. The several types of emphysema are classified according to patterns of septal destruction and dilatation within terminal respiratory units, or acini (Plate 30). The normal acinus is supplied by a *terminal bronchiole*. The terminal bronchiole undergoes three orders of branching, first into *respiratory bronchioles* with alveolate walls, then into *alveolar ducts* and finally into *alveolar sacs*.

If the septal destruction and dilatation are limited to the central portion of the acinus in the region of the terminal bronchiole and respiratory bronchioles, the disorder is called *centriacinar* or *centrilobular emphysema* (Plate 31). Because of septal destruction, there is free communication between all orders of respiratory bronchioles. Alveolar sacs at the periphery of the acinus lose volume as the
(*Continued*)

Chronic Obstructive Pulmonary Disease
(Continued)

Normal Lung Acinus (Secondary Lobule)

Terminal bronchiole

Septum of acinus

1st order

2nd order — Respiratory bronchioles

3rd order

Alveolar ducts

Alveolar sacs

Centriacinar (Centrilobular) Emphysema

Distended respiratory bronchioles of all orders communicating with one another

Panacinar (Panlobular) Emphysema

All airways and alveoli involved with breakdown of dividing walls

central portions enlarge. Though centriacinar emphysema is often considered to be a diffuse disease process, there is extreme variation in severity from acinus to acinus within the same segment or lobe. In general, more of the acini are affected in the upper lung zones than in the lower zones. Extensive centriacinar emphysema is more common in males than in females, and it is often found in those with histories of heavy smoking and chronic bronchitis. However, minor degrees of centriacinar emphysema are found in the lungs of nonsmokers without chronic bronchitis, especially after the fourth decade of life.

In contrast to centriacinar emphysema, *panacinar* or *panlobular emphysema* (Plate 32) affects the acinus more uniformly with less variability within an individual segment or lobe. Although the panacinar variety somewhat randomly involves the various zones of the lung, there is some tendency for the lower zones to be more severely affected. Panacinar emphysema is the characteristic lesion in alpha$_1$ antitrypsin deficiency (see page 147), in which early involvement of the lower zones is frequent. Progression of the disease brings severe loss of lung parenchyma, including not only alveolar walls but

pulmonary capillaries. As with the centriacinar variety, panacinar emphysema to a mild degree is a common finding after the fifth decade of life. Most persons with morphologic emphysema will not have symptoms or functional abnormalities associated with the process.

In severe chronic obstructive airway disease, both centriacinar and panacinar emphysema are ordinarily found, together with chronic bronchitic changes in the airways.

When alveolar wall destruction is restricted to the periphery of the acinus, most often in regions just beneath the visceral pleura, the disorder is designated *paraseptal emphysema.* This form appears

to be the structural basis for episodes of spontaneous pneumothorax in young adults and may be severe enough locally to form an isolated bulla. Otherwise there are no symptoms, and there is little, if any, functional derangement in association with this form of emphysema; hence it should not be considered further in the context of COPD.

Radiographic and Pathologic Correlations

Chronic Bronchitis. There are no well-documented signs of chronic bronchitis on the plain chest radiograph, although thickening of bronchial walls is often seen as parallel or tapering

(Continued)

Centriacinar (Centrilobular) Emphysema

Magnified section. Distended, inter-communicating, saclike spaces in central area of acini

Chronic Obstructive Pulmonary Disease
(Continued)

Microscopic section. Distention of airspaces with rupture of alveolar walls

Gross specimen. Involvement tends to be most marked in upper part of lung

shadows, referred to as "tramlines." Also frequently seen is a generalized increase in lung markings at the bases. If bronchography is performed to rule out the possibility of bronchiectasis, the ducts of the hypertrophied submucosal glands may fill with contrast medium to produce "beading" or "pitting," which is best seen along the inferior margin of the larger bronchi. In addition, occlusion of small bronchi by mucous plugs results in a square-ended cutoff of the contrast medium.

Emphysema. The frequency with which radiographic abnormalities are detected depends on the stringency of the criteria accepted as representative of emphysema. If the presence of hyperinflation is taken to indicate emphysema, many patients without abnormalities or with only minimal emphysema will be included. If the presence of bullous changes is deemed necessary, a large number of those with severe emphysema will be excluded. Of the four radiographic criteria that have been evaluated systematically—attenuation of the pulmonary vasculature peripherally, flattening and/or eversion of the diaphragm as seen on both PA and lateral projections, irregular radiolucency of lung

fields, and an increase in the retrosternal space on the lateral projection—the extent of diaphragmatic flattening and retrosternal space enlargement have correlated best with the severity of emphysema as assessed at subsequent postmortem examination. It is probable that the so-called typical radiographic changes of emphysema are most easily seen when panacinar emphysema predominates and that moderate centriacinar changes are associated with few radiographic abnormalities.

Pathophysiology

Whether bronchitis or emphysema predominates, by the time a patient with COPD begins to

have symptoms, obstruction to airflow is readily demonstrable. The most easily measured indexes of obstruction are taken from the volume-time plot of a forced expiratory vital capacity maneuver, using an ordinary water-filled spirometer coupled to a rotating drum kymograph (Plate 33). The forced expiratory volume in one second (FEV_1) is low both as a percentage of the reading predicted for a given sex, age and height category and as a percentage of the patient's own forced vital capacity. The forced expiratory time (*i.e.,* the total time required to forcefully exhale the entire vital capacity) is invariably prolonged. The mean flow rate over the middle
(Continued)

Panacinar (Panlobular) Emphysema

Gross section of lung.
Dilated, saccular airspaces.
In cases of disease due
to α_1-antitrypsin deficiency,
lower part of lung tends
to be more affected

Chronic Obstructive Pulmonary Disease
(*Continued*)

Magnified
section.
Diffuse
involvement
of all
portions
of acini

half of the vital capacity ($FEF_{25-75\%}$) is frequently more severely diminished than is the FEV_1, especially in cases of moderate obstruction; the reason for this increased sensitivity of the $FEF_{25-75\%}$ in moderate obstruction is seen more clearly in maximal expiratory flow-volume (MEFV) curves (center left-hand graph, Plate 33). This display of instantaneous flow rate vs volume is no more than a replot of the forced expiratory spirogram.

Even in normal subjects, flow rates over the lower three-fourths of the vital capacity are limited by the mechanical properties of the lungs and airways rather than by the amount of driving pressure the subject can generate. In contrast, peak flow rates are effort-dependent and governed by the force-velocity relationships of skeletal muscle (*i.e.*, greater driving pressures always give higher flow rates). The FEV_1 includes some effort dependency, whereas the $FEF_{25-75\%}$ is more an indicator of flow limitation imposed by the lungs and airways. Determinants of the maximal expiratory flow rates represent a complex and dynamic interplay among intrinsic airway caliber, elastic recoil properties of

the lung, and expiratory collapse of intrathoracic airways during the forced exhalation. In patients with COPD, abnormalities of all three factors usually come into play to limit flow rates.

The normal MEFV curve in relation to normal tidal breathing depicts the functional reserve normally present. In contrast, a patient with severe obstructive airway disease may breathe tidally along his MEFV curve, indicating that there is no functional reserve at all. Higher flow rates can be achieved only by breathing at higher lung volumes, well above functional residual capacity.

With both chronic bronchitis and emphysema, so-called static lung volumes are often normal. The

center right-hand panel of Plate 33 depicts the normal lung volumes and those often found in COPD. The functional residual capacity (FRC) is the lung volume at the end of a quiet exhalation and, in normal subjects, is the volume at which the inward recoil of the lung is equal and opposite to the outward recoil of the *relaxed* chest wall (see page 54). An elevated FRC in COPD can be attributed to loss of the static elastic recoil properties of the lung and/or to initiation of inspiration before the static balance volume is reached. Total lung capacity (TLC) is determined by pressures exerted by the diaphragm and muscles of the chest wall in relation

(*Continued*)

Chronic Obstructive Pulmonary Disease
(Continued)

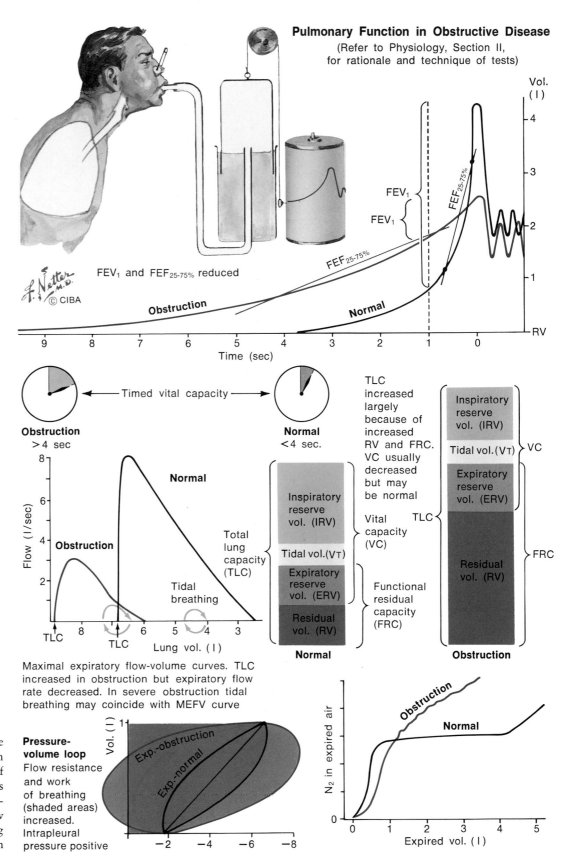

Pulmonary Function in Obstructive Disease
(Refer to Physiology, Section II, for rationale and technique of tests)

FEV$_1$ and FEF$_{25-75\%}$ reduced

Maximal expiratory flow-volume curves. TLC increased in obstruction but expiratory flow rate decreased. In severe obstruction tidal breathing may coincide with MEFV curve

Pressure-volume loop Flow resistance and work of breathing (shaded areas) increased. Intrapleural pressure positive on expiration

Single breath O$_2$ test

to the static elastic recoil properties of both the chest wall and lung. When TLC is elevated in COPD, almost invariably a significant degree of emphysema is present. Residual volume (RV) is elevated when either chronic bronchitis or emphysema predominates: airway closure, severe flow limitation with fatigue, or limits on breath-holding time may account for the elevation of RV. With increasing age RV increases, lung elastic recoil decreases, and airway closing occurs at progressively higher lung volumes. Since the TLC does not change as a function of aging, the vital capacity (VC) falls. Thus values for VC, RV and FRC must be considered in relation to predicted values for a given age (as well as sex and height) in order to identify them as normal.

There is often a discrepancy between the VC exhaled slowly and that which can be exhaled forcefully in COPD. In the event of discrepancy, the slow VC is invariably greater than the forced VC; the difference has been attributed to "trapped gas" secondary to dynamic collapse of airways during the forced maneuver. Another form of "trapped gas" is expressed by the frequent difference between

FRC measured by dilution or equilibration techniques (*e.g.*, helium or nitrogen washout, respectively) and FRC measured plethysmographically by the Boyle's law technique. The latter gives the total intrathoracic gas volume, and the former techniques measure only those lung regions with reasonable turnover rates. Hence, if there is a disparity, the plethysmographic values are always higher. However, should the equilibration or washout procedure be sufficiently prolonged, the values will equal those found plethysmographically. Thus the gas is not truly trapped; rather, the disparity represents a lung region or regions with extremely low turnover rates.

Regional nonhomogeneity of turnover or washout rates can be tested quickly by having the patient take a single inspiration of 100% oxygen. The washout of nitrogen during the subsequent exhalation is usually plotted in relation to expired volume (lower right-hand graph of Plate 33). In contrast to normal subjects in whom the concentration of nitrogen increases very little after the first 0.8 liter is exhaled and before closing volume is reached, patients with COPD have a constantly rising nitrogen concentration. The latter indicates that regions receiving little of the inspired oxygen are emptying later in expiration.

(Continued)

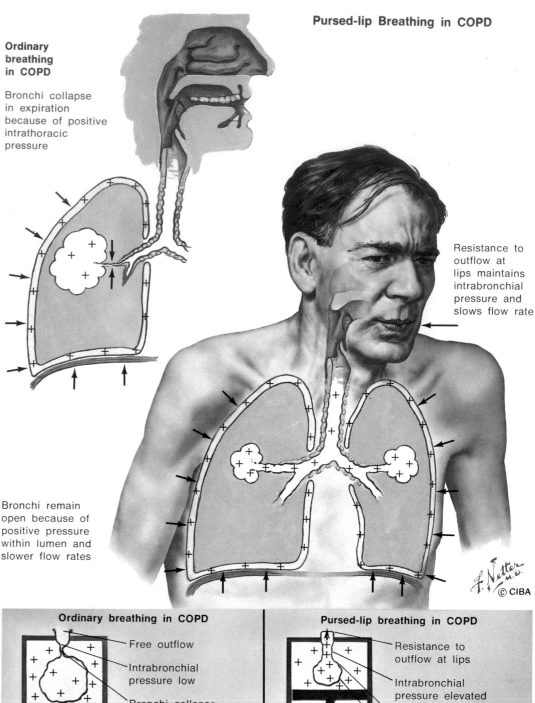

Ordinary breathing in COPD

Bronchi collapse in expiration because of positive intrathoracic pressure

Chronic Obstructive Pulmonary Disease
(Continued)

Resistance to outflow at lips maintains intrabronchial pressure and slows flow rate

Bronchi remain open because of positive pressure within lumen and slower flow rates

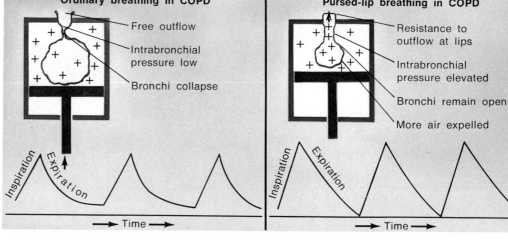

Ordinary breathing in COPD

Free outflow

Intrabronchial pressure low

Bronchi collapse

Inspiration / Expiration

Time

Pursed-lip breathing in COPD

Resistance to outflow at lips

Intrabronchial pressure elevated

Bronchi remain open

More air expelled

Inspiration / Expiration

Time

In addition to the easily demonstrable obstructive abnormalities during forced exhalation, there are significant alterations in the pressure-flow relationships during ordinary breathing in COPD. As mentioned above, the patient with severe COPD often exhales at his *maximal* expiratory flow rates during ordinary breathing. The result is that intrapleural pressures often become *positive* during exhalation (lower left-hand graphs of Plates 33 and 34). This contrasts strikingly with exhalation in normal subjects, in whom the cessation of inspiratory muscle activity is followed by return to FRC by means of the elastic recoil of the system. Positive intrapleural pressures during exhalation are likely to produce collapse of large intrathoracic airways. Pursing of lips during exhalation prevents collapse of airways by elevating intraairway pressures and through slowing of flow rates (Plate 34). Pursed-lip breathing provides some immediate alleviation of discomfort, probably by preventing tracheobronchial collapse rather than through any effect on alveolar ventilation, distribution of inspired gas or diminution of the mechanical load on the respiratory muscles.

Narrowing of airways, even without dynamic collapse, occurs with both chronic bronchitis and emphysema. The functional *sine qua non* of emphysema is a loss of the elastic recoil properties of the lung, and this loss accounts for narrowing of airways through loss of radial support. In addition to providing radial support of airways, the elastic recoil pressure of the lungs serves as the driving pressure across flow-limiting segments of the airways during maximal expiratory flow maneuvers. Elastic recoil loss results in increased resistance to submaximal airflow and decreased driving pressure for maximal expiratory flow. The degree of emphysema can be assessed in the pulmonary

function laboratory by measuring the intraesophageal pressure as an estimate of pleural pressure in relation to lung volume. Transpulmonary pressure (mouth vs intraesophageal) at points of zero flow is plotted against lung volume to give a pressure-volume curve of the lungs (Plate 35). In contrast to normal subjects, those patients suffering from emphysema show a pressure-volume curve of the lungs that is shifted up and to the left. At any lung volume there is a decreased elastic recoil pressure, and the static compliance (*i.e.*, the change in volume divided by the change in pressure) is always increased.

(Continued)

Effect of Emphysema on Compliance and Diffusing Capacity (DL$_{CO}$)

Normal
(or chronic bronchitis)

Capillaries

Airspace

Elastic (recoil) pressure (Pel)

f. Netter
© CIBA

Emphysema

Decreased alveolar surface area
Decreased elastic recoil
Increased alveolar gas volume
Fewer capillaries

↓

Increased compliance ($\Delta V / \Delta P$)
Impaired diffusion
Increased lung volume

Chronic Obstructive Pulmonary Disease
(Continued)

TLC as % of that predicted

Emphysema
ΔV
ΔP
Normal
ΔV
ΔP
Max.

Elastic (recoil) pressure (Pel)

In emphysema, pressure-volume curve unit shifts to left as recoil decreases and volume increases, and compliance ($\Delta V / \Delta P$) is increased

In emphysema DL$_{CO}$ decreases as elastic recoil (Pel) decreases

Normal

DL$_{CO}$ as % of that predicted

Emphysema

Pel as % of that predicted

Normal diffusing capacity for CO (DL$_{CO}$) is an indication that emphysema is not yet severe

In emphysema, the lung's capacity to transfer oxygen is reduced. Because of the complexity of measuring a diffusing capacity for oxygen, it is usually the transfer of small concentrations of carbon monoxide that is measured—*i.e.,* the so-called *diffusing capacity for carbon monoxide* (DL$_{CO}$) (Plate 35). The regional distribution of inspired gas in relation to blood flow, the area and thickness of the alveolar-capillary membrane, the number of perfused pulmonary capillaries, and the mean transit time of red blood cells through the capillaries all influence the DL$_{CO}$; not surprisingly, therefore, it is strikingly decreased in severe emphysema. Perhaps it is more of a surprise that chronic bronchitis has relatively little effect on the DL$_{CO}$. Abnormalities in the DL$_{CO}$ correlate reasonably well with the loss of elastic recoil. Both elastic recoil and DL$_{CO}$ measurements have been used to assess the extent of emphysema in patients with COPD.

Cor Pulmonale. In cor pulmonale (Plate 36) the pulmonary vascular bed normally has an impressive reserve which accommodates large increases in cardiac output with minimal elevations of pulmonary

artery pressures. In COPD there is a decrease in the total cross-sectional area of the pulmonary vascular bed due to anatomic changes in the arteries, constriction of smooth muscle in response to alveolar hypoxia and, to the extent that emphysema is present, a loss of pulmonary capillaries. Therefore, the pressures that must be generated by the right ventricle are elevated, and dilatation and hypertrophy of the right ventricle result. Overt right ventricular failure often occurs in association with endobronchial infections, which leads to worsening hypoxemia and hypercapnia. Such episodes are more frequent in patients in whom bronchitis is dominant.

The patient with cor pulmonale is cyanotic and has distended neck veins that do not collapse with inspiration, hepatic engorgement with a tender and enlarged liver, and pitting edema of the extremities. The heart may or may not appear enlarged on a PA chest radiograph, but pulmonary vessels are prominent. Physical examination usually discloses a palpable right ventricular heave and an audible early diastolic gallop that is accentuated by inspiration. On occasion, there is dilatation of the tricuspid ring with secondary tricuspid insufficiency; this disappears with effective treatment. The hematocrit often exceeds 55% and reflects an
(Continued)

Cor Pulmonale Due to COPD

Elevation of pulmonary artery pressure { Systolic / Diastolic }

Reduction of pulmonary arterial bed (loss of vessels plus reflex hypoxic vaso-constriction)

Normal readings < 25 < 10

Venous distention

X-ray film showing typical enlarged pulmonary artery shadows and outflow tract of right ventricle

Hypertrophy and dilatation of right ventricle, leading to hypertrophy and dilatation of right atrium and to tricuspid insufficiency terminally

Bulge of septum to left may impair left ventricular filling (reverse Bernheim phenomenon)

Enlargement of liver (passive congestion)

Normal   Cor pulmonale

Hematocrit increased

Peripheral edema

Electrocardiogram indicative of right ventricular hypertrophy

Chronic Obstructive Pulmonary Disease
(Continued)

increase in red blood cell mass as a compensatory mechanism for chronic hypoxemia. Although there is an increase in blood viscosity with erythrocytosis, the actual contribution of this factor to pulmonary hypertension remains unclear.

The electrocardiogram may show changes of right ventricular hypertrophy. However, as a rule the cardiogram is nonspecifically abnormal, and the history and physical examination are most important factors in establishing the diagnosis.

Left ventricular dysfunction has frequently been demonstrated in COPD with cor pulmonale. One proposed mechanism for this finding is shown in Plate 36: bulging of the intraventricular septum into the left ventricle, which interferes with diastolic filling. However, a direct effect of hypoxemia on left ventricular function may be a more likely contributory factor.

The primary therapeutic principles are to improve oxygenation and ventilation through treatment of infection and to achieve drainage and dilatation of the bronchi. With improved oxygenation and ventilation, the pulmonary hypertension

abates, the load on the right ventricle decreases, and a return of ventricular compensation occurs. Use of mechanical ventilators and administration of oxygen are measures to buy time while allowing the primary therapeutic interventions to work. Cardiotonic and diuretic regimens clearly play a secondary role in the treatment of cor pulmonale in COPD.

Epidemiology and Pathogenesis of COPD

By using questionnaires for large populations and by applying the definition given previously, chronic bronchitis has been found in approximately 20% of adult males. Undoubtedly, if the airways of

those without rigidly defined chronic bronchitis were examined for signs of disease, a higher incidence of abnormalities would be found. It should also be pointed out that many more persons have chronic bronchitis than will ever develop disabling COPD. Cigarette smoking, atmospheric pollution, occupational exposures and recurrent bronchial infections have been implicated as pathogenetic factors. Cigarette smoking is by far the most important of these factors. Experimental animal studies show that cigarette smoke impairs ciliary movement, causes bronchorrhea, alters the structure and function of alveolar macrophages and leads
(Continued)

Small Airway Disease and Relation to Smoking

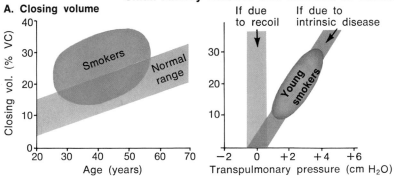

A. Closing volume

Closing vol. (% VC) vs *Age (years)* — Smokers; Normal range

Transpulmonary pressure (cm H_2O) — If due to recoil; If due to intrinsic disease; young smokers

If elastic recoil of lung is impaired, closing volume should occur at about same trans-pulmonary (esophagus-to-mouth) pressure regardless of lung volume (blue column). In young smokers, however, closing volume occurs at higher pressures, indicating that it is due to intrinsic airway disease (pink oblique column)

Closing volume increases with age, but some smokers have closing volume higher than predicted for age

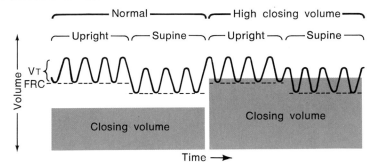

High closing volume may encroach on end-tidal volume (FRC). Some lung areas are closed during breathing, resulting in elevated A-aDO_2. In supine position, end-tidal level is lower, more lung areas are closed during tidal breathing, and A-aDO_2 is further elevated. Smokers show much higher A-aDO_2 than nonsmokers when supine

Normal — Upright — Supine — High closing volume — Upright — Supine
V_T / FRC / Volume / Closing volume / Time →

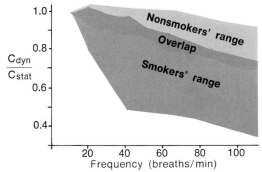

B. Frequency dependence of compliance

$\frac{C_{dyn}}{C_{stat}}$ vs Frequency (breaths/min) — Nonsmokers' range; Overlap; Smokers' range

Normally C_{dyn}/C_{stat} declines only slightly as frequency increases. In some smokers decline is rapid

C. Max. exp. flow-vol. curve; breathing air

Flow l/sec vs Lung vol. (l), TLC ... RV — Normal; Small airway disease; $\dot{V}_{max. 50}$; $\dot{V}_{max. 25}$

In small airway disease $\dot{V}_{max. 50}$ and $\dot{V}_{max. 25}$ may be reduced

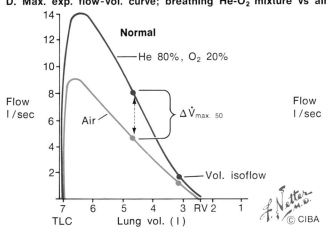

D. Max. exp. flow-vol. curve; breathing He-O_2 mixture vs air

Normal — Flow l/sec vs Lung vol. (l); He 80%, O_2 20%; Air; $\Delta \dot{V}_{max. 50}$; Vol. isoflow

Small airway disease — Flow l/sec vs Lung vol. (l); He 80%, O_2 20%; Air; $\Delta \dot{V}_{max. 50}$ decreased; Vol. isoflow

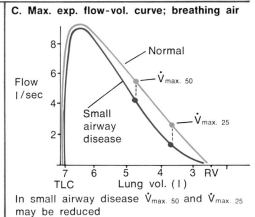

Chronic Obstructive Pulmonary Disease
(Continued)

to hypertrophy and hyperplasia of the mucus-secreting glands. Massive exposure to smoke can cause emphysema.

Smoking and Small Airway Disease. In 1968 Bates proposed that small airway obstruction might be the earliest lesion in the pathogenetic progression to fully developed chronic bronchitis and emphysema. In accord with Bates' proposal, evidence has rapidly accumulated that even asymptomatic cigarette smokers under 30 years of age often have functional changes suggestive of small airway obstruction. Since small airways, because of their large total cross-sectional areas, contribute very little to overall airflow resistance, more sensitive tests must be used to detect mild obstruction (see pages 267 and 268). There are four categories of tests: (A) tests that are volume-dependent, (B) tests that are frequency-dependent, (C) tests that indicate impairment of maximal expiratory airflow rates, and (D) tests that compare maximal expiratory flow rates with air to those with a combination of 80% helium and 20% oxygen (Plate 37). In order for the abnormalities

revealed by the tests to be interpreted as indicating isolated small airway obstruction, there must be *normal airway resistance, normal FEV_1* and *normal elastic recoil properties of the lung.*

A. Airway closure is the volume-dependent phenomenon. The volume at which airways begin to close is called the *closing volume* (Plate 37, A). It is usually measured by taking from residual volume a full inspiratory vital capacity of 100% oxygen and monitoring the relationship between nitrogen concentration and volume during the subsequent exhalation to residual volume (Plate 38, A). The sharp increase in nitrogen concentration as residual volume is approached is thought to indicate the

onset of airway closure in dependent portions of the lung. The reasoning is as follows: the effect of gravity on the lung is such that apical alveoli are more distended than basal alveoli at all volumes below TLC. Therefore, the ventilation-to-volume ratio is much less for apical than for basal alveoli. After a single breath of oxygen, then, apical alveoli have a greater nitrogen concentration than do basal alveoli. The sharp increase in exhaled nitrogen concentration results from emptying of apical regions after basal units have closed.

The closing volume becomes higher with advancing age in nonsmokers, presumably because
(Continued)

Reversibility of Small Airway Disease Due to Smoking

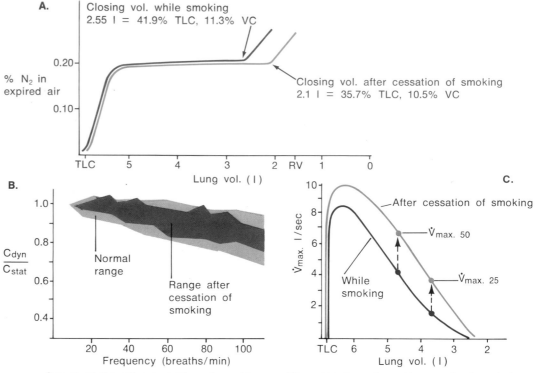

A.

Closing vol. while smoking
2.55 l = 41.9% TLC, 11.3% VC

Closing vol. after cessation of smoking
2.1 l = 35.7% TLC, 10.5% VC

% N₂ in expired air

Lung vol. (l)

B.

$\dfrac{C_{dyn}}{C_{stat}}$

Normal range

Range after cessation of smoking

Frequency (breaths/min)

2 to 8 weeks after cessation of smoking
C_{dyn}/C_{stat} returned to normal range

C.

$\dot{V}_{max.}$ l/sec

After cessation of smoking

$\dot{V}_{max.\ 50}$

$\dot{V}_{max.\ 25}$

While smoking

Lung vol. (l)

After cessation of smoking maximal expiratory
flow rates (air) at 50% and 25% VC increased

Chronic Obstructive Pulmonary Disease
(Continued)

Vulnerability of Small Airway Disease to Viral Infections

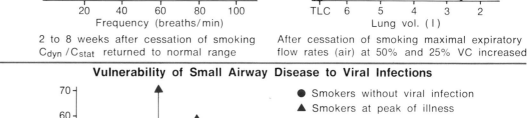

Closing vol. (% TLC)

● Smokers without viral infection
▲ Smokers at peak of illness
● Nonsmokers

Normal range

Six out of nine smokers showed increased closing volumes at peak of their illness and returned to normal at 3 to 6 weeks

Age (years)

Breathing air, smokers showed no change in mean maximal expiratory flow rates during illness

$\dot{V}_{max.}$ l/sec

not ill

ill

% VC

Breathing He-O₂ mixture, however, they showed decreases in expiratory flows at 20% and 40% of VC

$\dot{V}_{max.}$ l/sec

not ill

ill

40% VC

20% VC

% VC

of progressive loss of elastic recoil properties of the lung. Some smokers have higher closing volumes than predicted for their age. In young smokers, this finding is due to intrinsic airway disease rather than to loss of elastic recoil; in smokers past the fifth decade, the higher closing volume is associated with accelerated loss of elastic recoil, which suggests the onset of significant emphysema. The immediate consequences of an elevated closing volume on the alveolar-arterial oxygen difference (A-aDo₂) and the effect of posture are shown in Plate 37.

B. *Frequency dependence* of compliance indicates nonuniform behavior of the lungs at higher breathing rates, a phenomenon often found in young asymptomatic cigarette smokers. Functional consequences of frequency-dependent behavior are seen mainly as an increase in the A-aDo₂ during the hyperpnea of exercise.

C. *Maximal expiratory flow rates* in the vital capacity may be decreased in smokers. At lower lung volumes the relative contribution of small airways to flow-resistance increases, and if small airway

caliber is compromised, abnormalities in flow rates are more likely to be seen at these volumes.

D. Although airflow rates may not be compromised in some smokers, there may be a smaller than normal increase in maximal expiratory *flow rates* when the lungs are filled with an *He 80%–O₂ 20% mixture,* which has a density approximately one-third that of air. Flow limitation normally occurs in *larger airways* where the total cross-sectional area is small and the Reynolds numbers are large, so that a highly *density-dependent* flow pattern of turbulence and convective acceleration predominates. Therefore, the flow rates with He 80%–O₂ 20% are greater. However, if the flow

limitation occurs predominantly in *small airways,* where the total cross-sectional area—although compromised—remains large, the Reynolds numbers are small and a *density-independent* laminar flow pattern predominates. Hence flow is less dependent on gas density.

These four categories of tests may not measure the same abnormality; some smokers may show abnormalities in one or two of the tests and not in the remainder, whereas other smokers may demonstrate different patterns of abnormality. The relationship between structure and function remains to be defined, and the relationship of such "early" and
(Continued)

Hypothesis of the Role of α_1-Antitrypsin

A. α_1-Antitrypsin present in sufficient amount

Circulating granulocyte

Proteolytic enzyme (trypsin)

α_1-Antitrypsin

Granulocyte engulfing and digesting bacteria and/or particulate matter

Granulocyte lysed, releasing proteolytic enzymes

Proteolytic enzymes inactivated by α_1-antitrypsin

Airway

Blood-vessel

Alveolus

Chronic Obstructive Pulmonary Disease
(Continued)

B. α_1-Antitrypsin deficient

Granulocyte lysed, releasing proteolytic enzymes

Proteolytic enzymes attack lung parenchyma; alveolar walls and respiratory bronchioles weakened, resulting in panacinar emphysema

Emphysema with α_1-antitrypsin deficiency tends to be more marked at base, probably due to gravity-induced increase in perfusion and sequestration of granulocytes

subtle abnormalities to the future development of chronic disabling obstructive airway disease is still uncertain.

Whatever the structural basis for or the prognostic value of the abnormalities, their *reversibility with smoking cessation* has been demonstrated in young subjects (Plate 38; A, B and C), although it is doubtful that smoking cessation in older subjects would give the same result. Perhaps of more immediate concern is the fact that changes suggestive of transitory development or worsening of small airway obstruction occur with mild *viral respiratory infections* (Plate 38). The role, if any, of such infections in the pathogenesis of COPD is not clear, but smokers are liable to more severe and prolonged illnesses, and are more likely to develop transitory bronchitis, than are nonsmokers during viral respiratory infections.

Alpha₁ Antitrypsin. Serum levels of alpha₁ antitrypsin are either deficient or absent in some patients with early onset of emphysema (Plate 39), associated with particular genotypes. Acid starch gel and immunoelectrophoresis of the serum are used to characterize the protease inhibitor (Pi)

types. Most people in the normal population have alpha₁ antitrypsin levels in excess of 250 mg/100 ml of serum, along with two M genes, designated as Pi type MM. There are several genes associated with alterations in serum alpha₁ antitrypsin levels, but the most common ones associated with emphysema are the Z and S genes. Individuals who are homozygous ZZ or SS have serum levels of alpha₁ antitrypsin of less than 50 mg/100 ml and develop severe panacinar emphysema at an early age in males and females equally; the panacinar process predominates at the lung bases. The MZ and MS heterozygotes have intermediate levels of serum alpha₁ antitrypsin; hence the genetic expression is

that of an autosomal codominant allele. There is controversy over whether the heterozygous state is associated with lung function abnormalities. Published studies are in direct conflict on this point, and further data are needed to be certain. This matter is of some importance, since the heterozygous state is apparently common, with the incidence estimates varying between 4 and 12% of the population.

The precise way in which antitrypsin deficiency produces emphysema is unclear. In addition to inhibiting trypsin, alpha₁ antitrypsin effectively inhibits elastase and collagenase, as well as several

(Continued)

Chronic Obstructive Pulmonary Disease
(*Continued*)

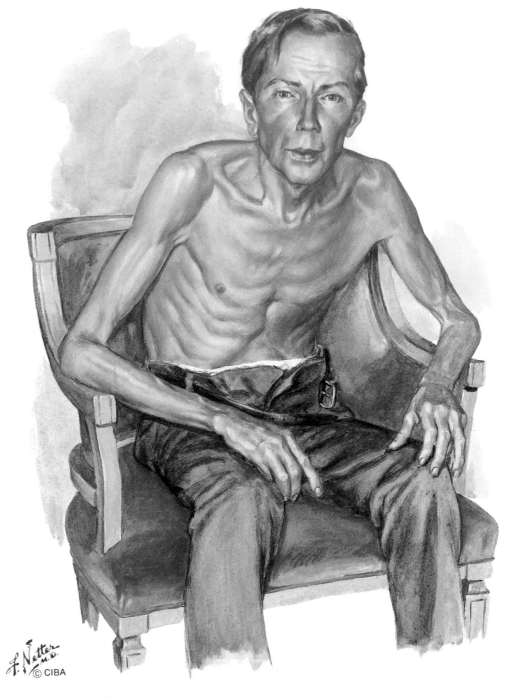

other enzymes. Alpha₁ antitrypsin is an acute-phase reactant, and the serum levels rise in association with many inflammatory reactions and with estrogen administration in all except homozygotes. It has been proposed, with some supporting experimental evidence, that the structural integrity of lung elastin and collagen depends upon this antienzyme, which protects the lung from proteases released from leukocytes. Proteases released by lysed leukocytes in the alveoli may be uninhibited, and consequently free to damage the alveolar walls themselves.

Clinical Syndromes

The clinical presentation of COPD ranges in severity from simple chronic bronchitis without disability to the severely disabled state with chronic respiratory failure. This variation does not indicate a spectrum from the simple to the severe, since the progression from one to the other is not a certainty. Clearly, most patients who come to a physician for treatment have far advanced disease and will ultimately be found to have undergone significant

pathologic changes of both chronic bronchitis and emphysema. To the extent that emphysema contributes to the disability, there is little hope for improvement, since the damage is irreversible. To the extent that bronchitis produces the obstruction and disability, there is reason to expect improvement, although not reversibility. Two polar types of fully developed COPD will be described, with the realization that the majority of patients will have features of both types.

Predominance of Emphysema. The patient with a predominance of emphysema often gives a long history of exertional dyspnea with minimal cough productive of only small amounts of mucoid sputum. On physical examination, the patient appears distressed and is obviously using accessory muscles of respiration, which serve to lift the sternum in an anterior-superior direction with each inspiration (Plate 40). There is tachypnea, with relatively prolonged expiration through pursed lips, or expiration is begun with a grunting sound. While sitting, the patient often leans forward, extending his arms to brace himself. The neck veins

may be distended during expiration, yet they briskly collapse with inspiration. The body build is asthenic, with evidence of weight loss. The lower intercostal spaces retract with each inspiration; by palpation, the lower lateral chest wall can be felt to move inward. The percussion note is hyperresonant, and the breath sounds on auscultation are found to be diminished, with faint, high-pitched rhonchi heard toward the end of expiration (Plate 42). The cardiac impulse, if at all visible, is seen only in the xiphoid and subxiphoid regions, and cardiac dullness is either absent or severely reduced. Palpation frequently reveals a sustained forward and downward right ventricular impulse in the subxiphoid region; an S gallop rhythm, accentuated during inspiration, is commonly heard.

The arterial Po₂ is often in the mid 70 mm Hg range, and the Pco₂ is low to normal. Because of the maintained increase in minute volume and the maintenance of arterial Po₂ sufficient to nearly saturate hemoglobin, patients with this condition have been referred to as "pink puffers" (Plate 40).
(Continued)

Chronic Obstructive Pulmonary Disease
(Continued)

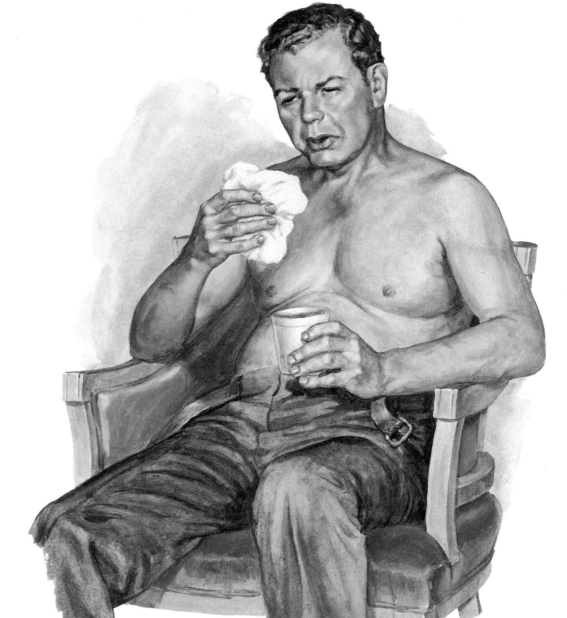

The TLC and RV are invariably increased, the vital capacity is low, and the maximal expiratory flow rates are diminished. Elastic recoil properties of the lung are severely impaired and, in direct proportion to this impairment, the $D_{L_{CO}}$ is correspondingly lowered.

It is fortunate that the patient with predominance of emphysema is less prone to episodes of bronchitis, with an increase in the output of sputum, than is the patient with a predominance of bronchitis, since such relapses frequently lead to respiratory failure and death. In the absence of these episodes, the clinical course is characterized by marked, progressive dyspnea for which little can be done. At postmortem examination, extensive and severe emphysema will be noted, predominantly of the panacinar variety.

Predominance of Bronchitis. The patient with a predominance of bronchitis (Plates 41 and 42) usually has an impressive history of cough and sputum production for many years, along with a history of heavy cigarette smoking. Initially, the cough is present only in winter months, and the

patient is likely to seek medical attention, if at all, only during the more severe of his repeated attacks of purulent bronchitis. Over the years the cough becomes continuous, and episodes of illness increase in frequency, duration and severity. After the patient begins to experience exertional dyspnea, he often seeks medical help, when he will be found to have a severe degree of obstruction. Occasionally such a patient will not seek out a physician until after the onset of peripheral edema secondary to overt right ventricular failure (Plate 36).

The patient with a predominance of bronchitis is ordinarily overweight and cyanotic. There is often no apparent distress at rest; the respiratory rate is normal or only slightly increased; no accessory muscle usage is apparent. The chest percussion note is normally resonant and, on auscultation, one can usually hear coarse rhonchi and wheezes, which change in location and intensity after a deep and productive cough.

The minute volume is either normal or only slightly increased. Failure to increase minute volume in the face of significant proportions of wasted

ventilation and blood flow results in severely deranged arterial blood gas levels, with chronic arterial P_{CO_2} values in the high 40 to low 50 mm Hg range. The lowered P_{O_2} produces desaturation of hemoglobin, serves to stimulate erythropoiesis, and brings on hypoxic pulmonary vasoconstriction. Desaturation and erythrocytosis combine to produce the cyanosis, and hypoxic pulmonary vasoconstriction accentuates the right-sided heart failure. Because of cyanosis and edema secondary to heart failure, patients with this condition have been referred to as "blue bloaters" (Plate 41).

The TLC is often normal, and the RV is moderately elevated. The VC is mildly diminished. Maximal expiratory flow rates are invariably low. Lung elastic recoil properties are normal or only slightly impaired; the $D_{L_{CO}}$ is either normal or minimally decreased.

Despite well-planned management, these patients may experience many episodes of respiratory failure; however, recovery will usually occur with proper therapy. Ultimately, at autopsy, the lungs
(Continued)

Roentgenograms in Chronic Obstructive Pulmonary Disease (COPD)

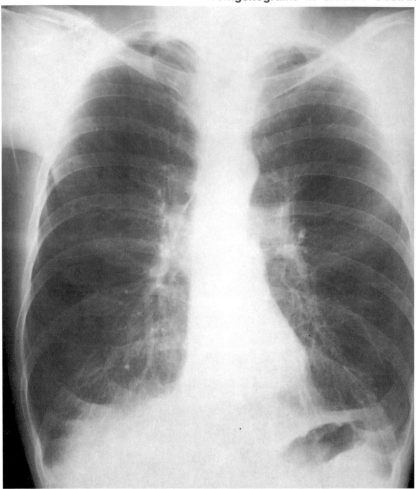

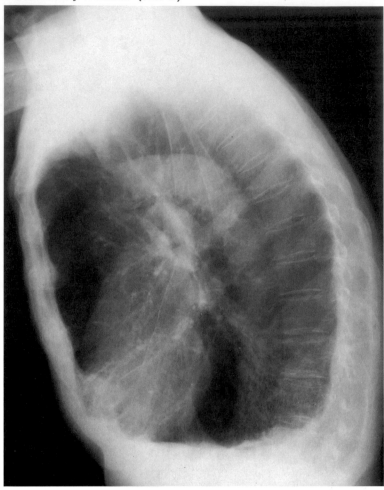

A. Hyperinflation of lungs; depression of diaphragm with its insertion to ribs evident; peripheral attenuation of pulmonary vessels; heart shadow small relative to lungs. Corresponds to "Pink Puffer"

B. Lateral projection of same case as in "A." Diaphragm not only depressed but actually concave downward. Retrosternal clear space greatly enlarged

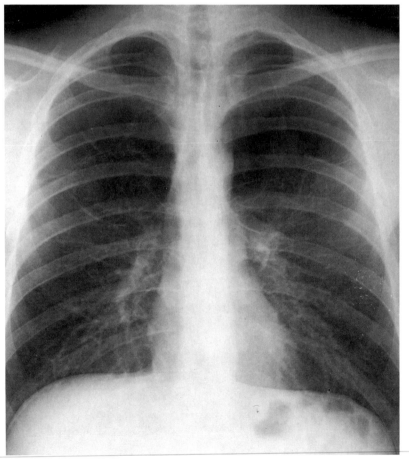

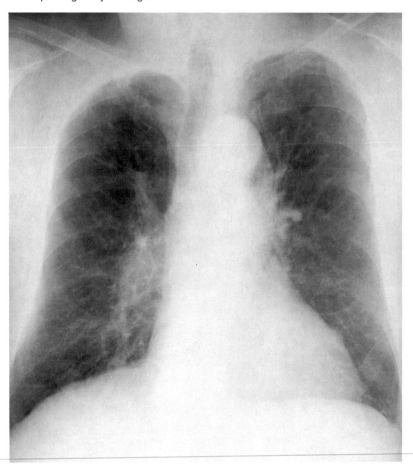

C. Bilateral giant apical bullae

D. No hyperinflation; increased bronchovascular markings, especially at bases; diaphragm well rounded. Patient had chronic CO_2 retention, cor pulmonale, and multiple previous episodes of respiratory failure. Corresponds to "Blue Bloater"

General Measures in Management of Chronic Obstructive Pulmonary Disease

A. Avoidance of respiratory irritants

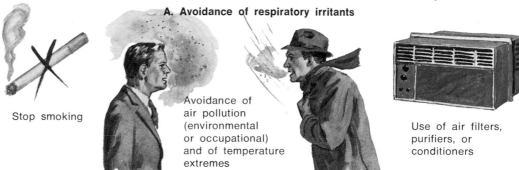

Stop smoking

Avoidance of air pollution (environmental or occupational) and of temperature extremes

Use of air filters, purifiers, or conditioners

B. Exercise

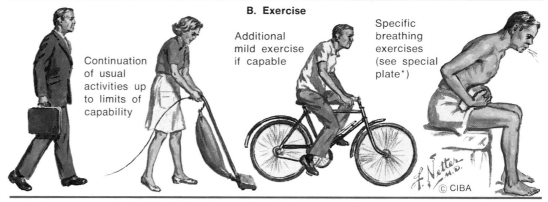

Continuation of usual activities up to limits of capability

Additional mild exercise if capable

Specific breathing exercises (see special plate*)

C. Precautions against infection

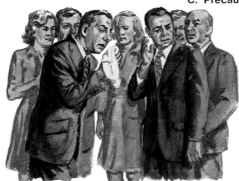
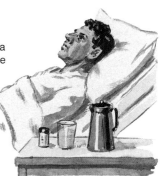

Avoidance of crowds and persons with respiratory infections. Use of influenza and pneumococcal vaccine important

Prompt treatment of respiratory infections with antibiotics, bed rest, and other indicated measures

D. Adequate hydration

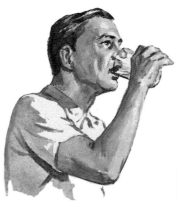

At least 3 liters/24 hr

E. Adequate nutrition

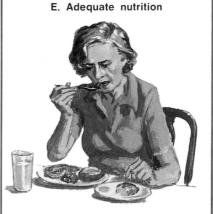

Frequent small meals, bedtime snacks, etc.

F. Practice of pursed-lip breathing

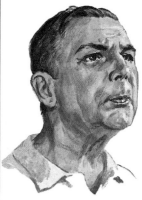

(see special plate†)

Chronic Obstructive Pulmonary Disease
(Continued)

will be found to have severe bronchitic changes in both large and small airways and only moderate emphysema, mainly of the centriacinar variety.

Management

General Measures. Whether emphysema or chronic bronchitis predominates in a patient with COPD, several general measures can be taken to avoid exacerbations and to improve the patient's sense of well-being (Plate 43). Although there may be little, if any, improvement in lung function following smoking cessation in the patient with severe COPD, it is essential to stop smoking to prevent further damage to the lungs and airways. Air pollution from general environmental or occupational exposure should be avoided insofar as possible. Beyond question, episodes of major air pollution produce exacerbations in COPD. During such periods, patients should remain indoors with internal environmental control (*e.g.,* air filters or air conditioners) or arrange to leave the area until the pollution has cleared.

The role of regular physical exercise in management remains controversial, yet the bulk of evidence favors the notion that a regular exercise pro-

*See Section IV, Plate 34, page 142
†See Section V, Plate 21, page 288

gram enhances the sense of well-being and increases toleration of physical activity rather than improves any measurable aspect of lung function. Since improvement in exercise tolerance appears to be relatively task-specific, the exercises prescribed should be activities from which the patient derives some enjoyment and usefulness. Continuation of usual activities such as walking and stair climbing, on a regular basis, is probably of more benefit to the patient than daily routines of treadmill walking, stationary bicycling or use of portable gymnastic equipment.

As endobronchial infections are usually precipitated by episodes of respiratory insufficiency, such

infections should be avoided if at all possible and treated promptly if they do occur. All patients with COPD should be vaccinated in the early fall against anticipated influenza strains. Although it is not possible to completely eliminate exposure to the many causative agents, patients should keep away from large crowds and persons with obvious respiratory infections. Prompt treatment of endobronchial infections is essential in order to keep the illness brief and comparatively mild. Even with sputum cultures, which often grow *Streptococcus pneumoniae* and *Hemophilus influenzae,* broadspectrum antibiotic administration still remains *(Continued)*

Specific Measures in Management of Chronic Obstructive Pulmonary Disease

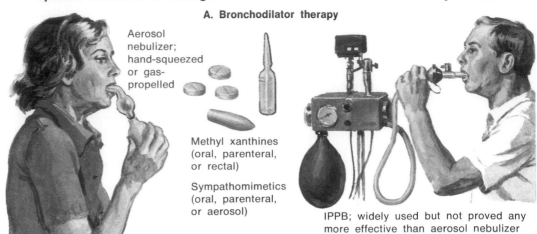

A. Bronchodilator therapy

Aerosol nebulizer; hand-squeezed or gas-propelled

Methyl xanthines (oral, parenteral, or rectal)

Sympathomimetics (oral, parenteral, or aerosol)

IPPB; widely used but not proved any more effective than aerosol nebulizer

B. Clearance of secretions

Postural drainage

Bronchoscopic suction and/or lavage

Nasotracheal suction and/or lavage

For acutely ill patient in hospital

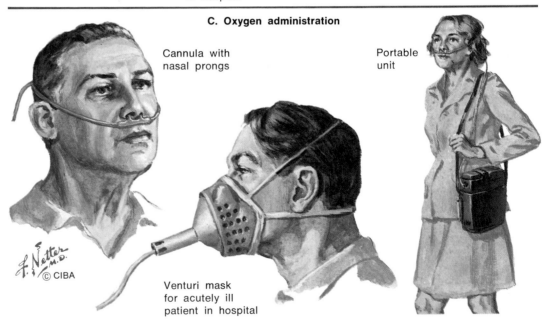

C. Oxygen administration

Cannula with nasal prongs

Portable unit

Venturi mask for acutely ill patient in hospital

Chronic Obstructive Pulmonary Disease
(Continued)

empirical, since the relative roles played by viruses, mycoplasmas and bacteria in these infections are not certain.

As with any debilitating disease associated with progressive weight loss and wasting, patients with a predominance of emphysema must consciously maintain nutrition. Hydration is especially important during episodes of endobronchial infection in order to keep secretions liquefied so they may be easily eliminated. The various expectorants have not been shown to provide any added benefit to bronchopulmonary drainage.

Specific Measures. Several specific measures have been advocated over the years and have traditionally been incorporated into the management of patients with COPD. A recent in-depth review at a combined American Thoracic Society and National Heart and Lung Institute conference revealed an alarming lack of scientific basis for most of the interventions and hence raised unanswered questions concerning efficacy. It is reasonable to ask how some of the measures shown in Plate 44 became the standards of management without scientific justification. The answer probably lies in the

understandably human desire of physicians to intervene vigorously and the beneficial subjective response of patients to daily ritual and physician enthusiasm. However, controlled studies are under way, and conclusive information may be forthcoming. Meanwhile, guidelines must be based upon intuition, *a priori* reasoning and faith.

Bronchodilators administered by any route can be shown to improve airflow rates in many patients with COPD; it is thus reasonable to use them regularly if side-effects are not troublesome. Intermittent positive pressure breathing (IPPB) devices are effective, but expensive generators of bronchodilator aerosols have no greater effect in

patients who can take a deep voluntary breath than less elaborate and less expensive compressor-driven and hand-held nebulizers.

Since it is axiomatic that airways are obstructed by secretions, these should be removed. If cough is relatively ineffective, postural drainage is a useful and inexpensive adjunct (see pages 286 and 287). Direct secretion removal by suction through a bronchoscope or a nasotracheal cannula is usually carried out in hospital during an episode of endobronchial infection (see pages 278 and 279).

Humans are obligate aerobes, and hypoxemia below certain levels calls forth compensatory

(Continued)

Emphysematous Cyst

Cyst does not compress lung
but is expanded by weight
of lung and more intact recoil
properties of dependent portions
of lung. (Principle demonstrated
by "slinky" below)

Chronic Obstructive Pulmonary Disease
(Continued)

A. Slinky suspended; coils more compact at lower portion, especially if supported at bottom (as lung is by diaphragm)

B. If a segment of slinky is weakened, it stretches out and coils become more compact at bottom

C. Weak segment removed and remainder of slinky resuspended. Slinky resumes original coiled pattern (comparable to surgical excision of cyst and reexpansion of lung)

Surface Bullae in Emphysema
Rupture may result in pneumothorax

Paraseptal (plus centrilobular) Emphysema

mechanisms with the potential for biologic backfire; *i.e.,* hypoxic pulmonary arteriolar constriction is a reasonable mechanism for decreasing flow to an underventilated region, but overall hypoxia leads to pulmonary hypertension and the cor pulmonale situation illustrated in Plate 36. Severe hypoxemia requires oxygen therapy. The only substantial controversies in this regard concern the levels of hypoxemia for which oxygen therapy should be given, the levels of improved oxygenation considered therapeutic, and the desirability of continuous or intermittent (*e.g.,* during sleep and with exercise) oxygen therapy. The author's own approach is to give oxygen in COPD only when the arterial Po_2 is at or below the mid 40 mm Hg range, and then to give sufficient oxygen to bring the arterial Po_2 into the mid 50 mm Hg range. These arbitrary guidelines are applied to both hospitalized and ambulatory patients.

The efficacy of breathing exercises (see page 288) also falls into the uncertain category, although it is difficult to see how any harm could come from them. The rationale behind such exercises is as follows: in emphysema the diaphragm is flattened;

contraction therefore results in retraction of the lower intercostal spaces with little, if any, inspiratory expansion of the lungs (see page 47). Contraction of the abdominal muscles during exhalation can be shown to elevate and round up the diaphragm, so that during subsequent inhalation the diaphragm can function effectively as an inspiratory muscle. Thus, the whole sequence is aimed at strengthening the abdominal muscles and at training the patient to use his abdominal muscles for active exhalation.

Management of Bullous Emphysema. Confluent airspaces with diameters in excess of 1 cm are occasionally congenital but most often are found in

association with generalized emphysema or progressive fibrotic processes (Plate 45). Gradual increases in the size of such airspaces (or bullae) result from traction applied by regions with better elastic recoil properties, which then lose volume as the bulla is enlarged. If disability is severe, if the bulla is extremely large, and if it can be demonstrated by either lobar gas sampling or by ventilation and perfusion scans that sufficient function remains in the nonbullous regions, surgical excision of the bulla may lead to functional improvement. Usually, however, improvement is transitory, because other emphysematous regions gradually enlarge into bullae at some time after surgery.

Bronchiectasis

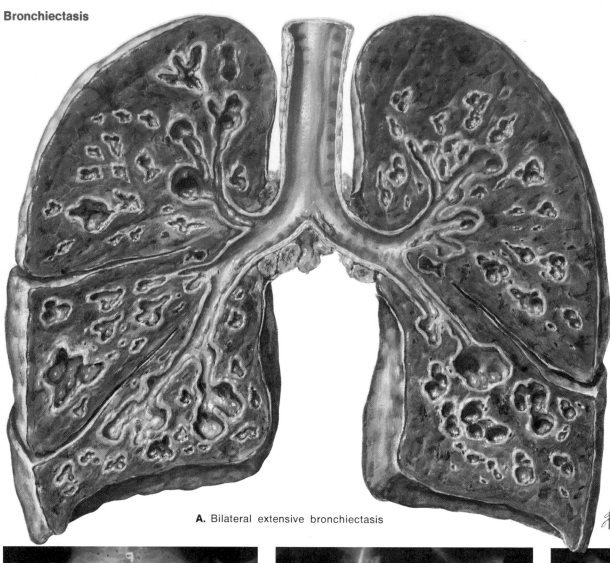

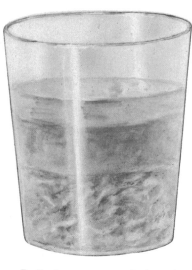

B. Profuse mucopurulent sputum, foul-smelling, settling into layers characteristic of severe bronchiectasis

A. Bilateral extensive bronchiectasis

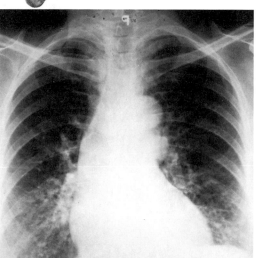

C. PA x-ray film. Peribronchial fibrosis in both lung bases

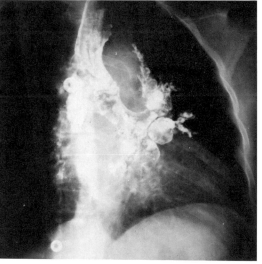

D. Same case as "C": left bronchogram reveals cystic bronchial dilatation

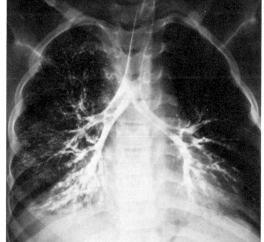

E. Another patient: bronchogram showing less marked bronchial dilatation, mostly in right lung

SECTION IV   PLATE 46

Bronchiectasis

Bronchiectasis is bronchial dilatation due to weakness of the bronchial wall. In the intact patient the condition can be confirmed only by bronchography. The abnormality is permanent and should not be confused with a transient mild cylindrical dilatation which occurs in a pneumonic or atelectatic lung.

The weakness of the bronchial wall may be congenital or acquired as a result of destruction.

Congenital bronchiectasis is sometimes associated with dextrocardia; if there is also sinusitis, the triad is known as Kartagener's syndrome. Congenital bronchiectasis may also be associated with mucoviscidosis (cystic fibrosis; Plates 48 and 49). Frequently the congenital form is cystic in appearance; in rare instances it is found in combination with marked dilatation of the trachea and main bronchi, a condition called tracheobronchomegaly.

Congenital bronchiectasis is usually widespread in both lungs, but it may be limited to one lung or even to one lobe. It tends to be asymptomatic, secondary infection being absent or appearing later in life. Productive cough with purulent sputum is therefore uncommon, and often the only symptom is hemoptysis. Physical signs are likely to be absent, and conventional chest roentgenograms are frequently unremarkable, although sometimes thin-walled annular shadows are barely discernible. The results of a bronchogram may be surprising and striking.

In contrast, *acquired bronchiectasis* is often associated with bronchial obstruction due to such causes as foreign body, tuberculous lymph nodes, tumor or destructive bronchitis (especially in children, whose bronchi are small in caliber).

(Continued)

Bronchiectasis
(Continued)

Bronchiectasis
(continued)

Bronchial dilatation may be the result of inflammatory destruction of the walls, as in tuberculous endobronchial disease. Because tuberculosis occurs in the upper posterior portion of the lungs, this type of bronchiectasis is also located there. Since that area is well drained in the upright position, secondary infection with suppuration is uncommon, and symptoms other than hemoptysis are seldom part of the clinical picture.

Nontuberculous bronchiectasis, on the other hand, tends to occur in dependent portions of the lung. Here drainage is poor, gravity causes secretions to accumulate, infection is frequent, and suppuration is the hallmark. Symptoms include chronic cough, purulent sputum in large amounts, hemoptysis and recurrent pneumonitis. If the disease is extensive, systemic symptoms are also present, including anorexia, weakness, weight loss, mild anemia, dyspnea and retarded development in children. Moist rales are found on examination of the chest; clubbing and signs of malnutrition are common.

The conventional chest x-ray film in acquired bronchiectasis usually shows the streaklike densities of peribronchial inflammation and fibrosis, and less often linear or saccular radiolucencies, sometimes with air-fluid levels, in dependent areas of the lungs. The diagnosis must be confirmed by bronchograms, and mapping of the bronchial tree should be complete if surgical resection is considered. Assessment of the severity of the disease may be aided by a 24 hour sputum collection to determine its volume and character. In moderate or severe acquired bronchiectasis, sputum is copious and tends to separate into several layers on standing. It is usually foul-smelling. Bacteriologic examinations with both aerobic and anaerobic cultures may be helpful in determining the proper antibiotics for medical management; generally penicillin or tetracycline will be the most useful, and prolonged therapy is frequently required. If the patient is treated on an outpatient basis, so that there is no exposure to hospital nosocomial organisms, superinfection is not a significant problem. Single-drug therapy should be used, since there is no evidence that multiple-drug regimens offer any advantages.

Unfortunately, except in patients with extensive bronchiectasis, little diagnostic information is gained by tests of pulmonary function. In these circumstances the vital capacity is low, inert gas distribution is impaired and diffusing capacity is diminished. However, hypoxemia is not proportional to other derangements because there is shunting of bronchial arterial blood into the pulmonary circulation through anastomoses in many segments. When disease is bilateral, split-function studies may reveal that one side is worse than the other, and this information can help in a decision on surgery.

Medical therapy includes the removal of bronchial obstruction, if possible. For this reason

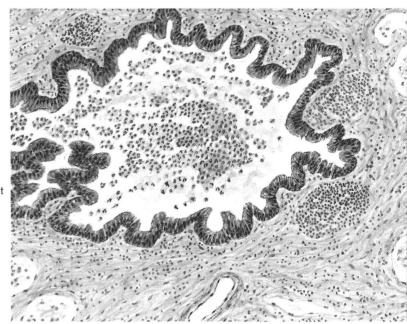

F. Section through dilated bronchus. Epithelium is hyperplastic and lumen contains cellular exudate. Peribronchial area shows replacement by loose connective tissue with many lymphocytes, both disseminated and aggregated into follicles

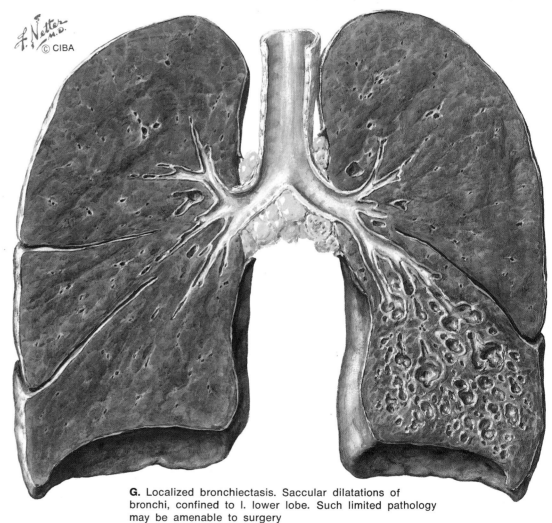

G. Localized bronchiectasis. Saccular dilatations of bronchi, confined to l. lower lobe. Such limited pathology may be amenable to surgery

bronchoscopy is indicated. In older cigarette smokers the procedure is of particular value in ruling out carcinoma. Postural drainage is important for suppurative forms of bronchiectasis, along with antibiotic agents (see pages 286 and 287). Infection should be prevented, and bronchial irritation from such materials as tobacco smoke and industrial gases or fumes eliminated. Improvement in nutrition and hydration requires particular attention.

Surgical resection is indicated for localized disease if it is sufficiently symptomatic. The risk of surgery must be weighed against the expected benefits, taking into account such factors as age,

extent of disease, pulmonary function, and general condition of the patient, including complicating diseases.

Complications include amyloidosis, cor pulmonale and brain abscess. However, these are becoming rare. Indeed, bronchiectasis seems to be less common than it was, probably as a result of improvements in standards of living and the ready availability of antimicrobial agents which have helped to reduce the incidence of severe pulmonary infections. The prognosis of bronchiectasis is good for limited disease amenable to resection, but the uncommon cases of extensive disease remain difficult problems in management.

Cystic Fibrosis of the Pancreas

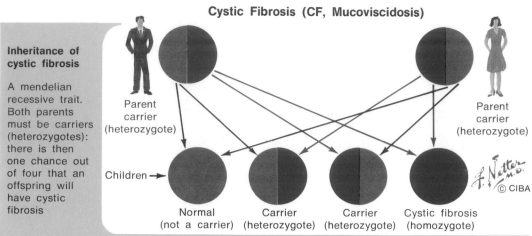

Cystic Fibrosis (CF, Mucoviscidosis)

Inheritance of cystic fibrosis

A mendelian recessive trait. Both parents must be carriers (heterozygotes): there is then one chance out of four that an offspring will have cystic fibrosis

Parent carrier (heterozygote)

Parent carrier (heterozygote)

Children →

Normal (not a carrier) — Carrier (heterozygote) — Carrier (heterozygote) — Cystic fibrosis (homozygote)

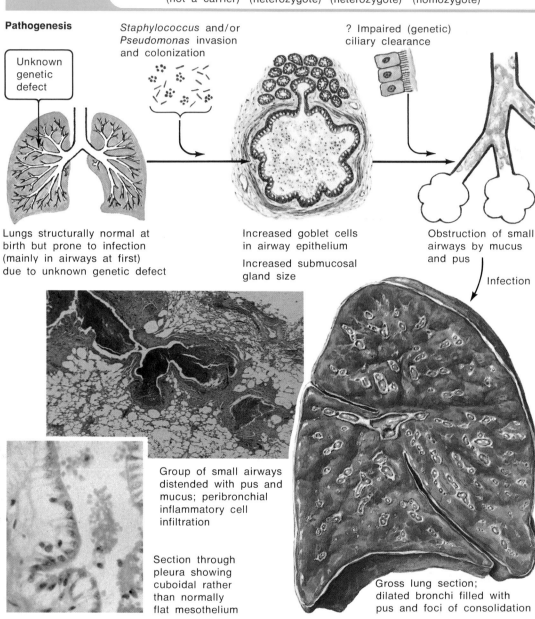

Pathogenesis

Unknown genetic defect

Staphylococcus and/or *Pseudomonas* invasion and colonization

? Impaired (genetic) ciliary clearance

Lungs structurally normal at birth but prone to infection (mainly in airways at first) due to unknown genetic defect

Increased goblet cells in airway epithelium

Increased submucosal gland size

Obstruction of small airways by mucus and pus

Infection

Group of small airways distended with pus and mucus; peribronchial inflammatory cell infiltration

Section through pleura showing cuboidal rather than normally flat mesothelium

Gross lung section; dilated bronchi filled with pus and foci of consolidation

Cystic fibrosis of the pancreas—also known as mucoviscidosis, congenital cystic disease and fibrocystic disease of the pancreas—is one of the most common serious disorders of childhood. The disease also continues into the adult years. It is a multisystem disease, of which the major clinical problems result from damage to the lung and the pancreas.

Incidence. The disease is inherited in an autosomal recessive manner. On this basis, it is assumed that each parent is heterozygous, although there is no clinical or laboratory method of regularly identifying the heterozygote before the disorder appears in the child. The gene frequency is estimated at 1 to 3%, with a disease incidence of 1 per 1000 to 1 per 5000 of the population.

Pathophysiology. Abnormalities are found in chemical content or physical properties of exocrine gland secretions. For example, the sweat is hypertonic with increased concentrations of Na^+ and Cl^-; the viscosity of duodenal liquids is increased; abnormalities of saliva and tears exist; and mucosal gland hypertrophy is prominent in the lung and the intestinal tract. Multiple organ involvement may depend on the presence of abnormal substances in the blood of patients. In the serum of affected children an abnormal "factor" has been found that inhibits ciliary activity in the rabbit trachea, while a "factor" in the sweat of patients interferes with electrolyte transport in the rat parotid duct. Sputum, serum and urine from patients with cystic fibrosis enhance the growth of staphylococci.

An associated defect in some male patients is atresia of the vas deferens, which is responsible for infertility. Since the lesion has been noted at birth, perhaps it represents an associated congenital malformation.

Clinical Manifestations. Most infants in whom cystic fibrosis later develops appear normal at birth, and the disease escapes detection in the nursery. However, when meconium ileus is present in the newborn, the diagnosis of cystic fibrosis is certain. Occasionally, excessive sweating is evident in the neonate, and the sweat electrolyte levels are elevated from birth. Mothers may note a "salty taste" when they kiss their infants. Respiratory infections sometimes develop in the first days of life, with the most consistent feature being hyperinflation of the chest. In addition, failure to gain weight and hypoproteinemia may be evident in the early weeks after birth. Classically, bulky and fatty stools are among the first signs of the deficiency of pancreatic enzymes.

Hypoprothrombinemia from failure to absorb vitamin K can lead to a hemorrhagic diathesis. A sweat test should be performed in all infants who present with vitamin K deficiency. Prolonged obstructive jaundice may be an early manifestation of the disease.

The collection of sweat by iontophoresis for analysis of Na^+ or Cl^-, or measurement of the *(Continued)*

Cystic Fibrosis: Aspects of Diagnosis and Management

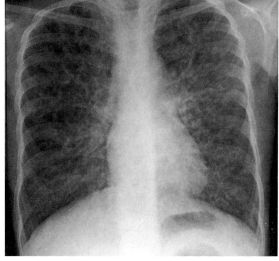

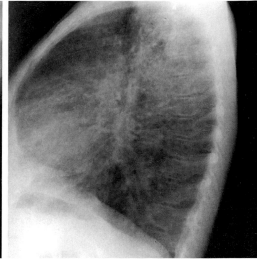

PA and lateral chest x-ray films of a child with cystic fibrosis showing marked hyperinflation with linear and nodular opacities. In mild cases, however, chest x-ray films may be almost normal and thus misleading

Cystic Fibrosis of the Pancreas
(Continued)

Pilocarpine iontophoresis (sweat) test

Not only is intermittent aerosol therapy valuable in hospital care, but patient's family (and, in time, patient) can be taught to use it at home

Postural drainage. Drainage of l. upper lobe apical segment is shown here. Positions for drainage of other segments are similar to those shown for adults in this volume, *q.v.* Infants are lap-held, but older children may use tilted bed as do adults

electrical conductivity which depends on the concentrations of these ions, has come to be the definitive diagnostic test. It is otherwise difficult to collect a sufficient amount of sweat from infants in the first weeks of life for the chemical assays needed. Measurement of the albumin content in meconium has also been used as a screening tool. If an infant has an affected sibling or displays any signs or symptoms suggesting cystic fibrosis, analysis of the sweat is essential before the diagnosis is made.

Treatment. No consensus exists on how vigorously one should treat the asymptomatic infant whose sweat sodium and chloride levels are elevated. Most authorities would agree on the use of a normal diet and the addition of water-soluble vitamins. Prompt identification and treatment of pulmonary infections are imperative, and probably preferable to chemoprophylaxis. However, according to some physicians, even one episode of staphylococcal pneumonia is so harmful that attempts should be made to prevent it by prophylactic daily administration of antibiotics. Pancreatic supplements are recommended as tolerated. (See CIBA COLLECTION, Volume 3/II, page 114, and Volume 3/III, page 142.)

Prognosis. Each year the prognosis for persons with cystic fibrosis improves, in part because of greater recognition and detection of mild cases and in part, doubtless, because of improvements in treatment. Many afflicted individuals have

reached adulthood, and some females have become parents. Sterility is very common in affected males. The severity of the disease varies greatly among siblings; hence, prognostication about the life span of an affected infant is unwise.

For most patients with cystic fibrosis, survival and quality of life depend on the condition of the lungs. These patients are particularly prone to lung infections although, in spite of much investigation, the reason is not understood. In all respects studied, the lungs are anatomically normal at birth. If infections recur, they evidently lead to gland hypertrophy and goblet cell increase—the hallmarks of adult chronic bronchitis. Patients

then produce daily sputum, which is usually purulent, and secondary irreversible structural changes follow. Airway obstruction due to mucus and pus becomes an important factor at this stage, and bronchiectasis and bronchitis are common. Segmental or lobar collapse, with bronchiectasis and lung abscess as sequelae, is less frequent than previously because of improved clinical management. Obliteration of the pleural space may occur late in the disease. Pneumothorax, hemoptysis and aspergillosis are complications seen in adolescence and early adulthood, and death usually occurs from advanced obstructive airway changes and respiratory insufficiency.

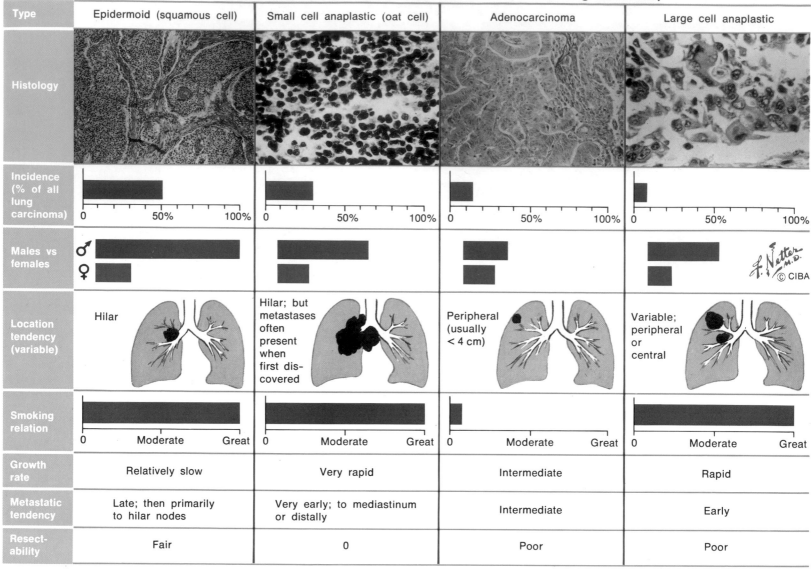

Type	Epidermoid (squamous cell)	Small cell anaplastic (oat cell)	Adenocarcinoma	Large cell anaplastic
Histology				
Incidence (% of all lung carcinoma)	~50%	~25%	~15%	~8%
Males vs females	♂ / ♀			
Location tendency (variable)	Hilar	Hilar; but metastases often present when first discovered	Peripheral (usually < 4 cm)	Variable; peripheral or central
Smoking relation	Great	Great	Slight	Great
Growth rate	Relatively slow	Very rapid	Intermediate	Rapid
Metastatic tendency	Late; then primarily to hilar nodes	Very early; to mediastinum or distally	Intermediate	Early
Resectability	Fair	0	Poor	Poor

Bronchogenic Carcinoma

An estimated 93,000 new cases of primary carcinoma of the lung were diagnosed in the United States in 1976. During the same period, 83,800 people were estimated to have died from this disease. Even more startling than the absolute number of cases is the fact that carcinoma of the lung was considered to be a pathologic rarity at the turn of the century. It now ranks as the most common malignant neoplasm in men and the third most common cancer in women. This apparent explosion in lung cancer incidence and death came to medical attention in the early 1930s when the prevalence of the disease among males was first recognized as a serious public health problem. Between 1947 and 1969 alone there was an increase of 133% in the number of white males reported to have developed cancer of the lung, while the increase of the disease among black males was 233%.

Women remained relatively immune to this disease until around 1960, when the number of lung cancer deaths began to rise. The most ominous implication of this trend is that the incidence of lung cancer continues to grow without there being any indication that definitive solutions are at hand. Once the disease has been contracted, the death rates are appalling. Only 8% of the males and 12% of the females are alive five years after the diagnosis. However, recognition and treatment of the disease while it is still localized increases the overall five year survival to about 18%.

Carcinoma of the lung is a disease of advancing age, the highest incidence being reported in patients between 55 and 75 years old. It is rarely seen before the fourth decade of life. In addition to age, its occurrence is strongly correlated with cigarette smoking, a fact that has been amply documented in the medical literature. Cigarette dose-response curves have been drawn for a number of histologic types of lung cancer and add strength to the epidemiologic observations. If a 20 year latent period is accepted for the interval between the commencement of cigarette smoking and the appearance of lung cancer, the time lag between the upswing of male and female lung cancer rates can be explained. Cigarette smoking became popular among men just before and during World War I. On the other hand, women did not begin to smoke in great numbers until World War II. Approximately 20 years after each of these events, cancer rates began to rise—in the mid-1930s for men and in the early 1960s for women. In addition to cigarettes, there are a number of other well-recognized carcinogenic materials encountered in an occupational setting that affect the lung. They include asbestos, chromium, chloromethyl ether, nickel and arsenic. More carcinogenic agents are sure to be found.

In an attempt to bring some order to the study of primary carcinoma of the lung, histologic tumor typing was organized as a way of correlating pathology with the natural history of the disease. Numerous schemata have been recommended. All suffer from the occurrence of overlapping forms and the uncertainty of borderline diagnoses.

Modern methods of diagnosis include both noninvasive and surgical procedures. Although history and physical examination are the obvious starting points, a chest x-ray examination often gives the first indication of the presence of a pulmonary neoplasm. Special radiographic techniques, such as tomography, may help to differentiate a benign from a malignant lesion. Sputum examination following Papanicolaou staining is frequently helpful in making the diagnosis and occasionally definitive in the histologic typing of a lung tumor. The same stain may be used to advantage on material obtained by rigid or fiberoptic bronchoscopy, either of which permits washing and brushing of the lesion. Direct biopsy of the lesion may be obtained through a bronchoscope. Mediastinoscopy and mediastinotomy are often employed to examine and biopsy the mediastinal lymph nodes for evidence of malignant invasion. Finally, thoracotomy may be required in order to obtain a tissue specimen or remove a suspicious lesion for diagnosis.

Bronchogenic Carcinoma: Epidermoid (Squamous Cell) Type

Low power (H and E); nests of tumor cells separated by fibrous bands. Keratin (horn) pearls present

High power; nuclear pleomorphism and individual cell keratinization (pink)

Tumor typically located near hilus, projecting into bronchi

Broncho-scopic view

Cytologic smear from sputum or bronchoscopic scraping. Cells with dark nuclei and cytoplasm strongly pink because of keratin

Squamous Cell Carcinoma of Lung

Squamous cell carcinoma of the lung is the most common histologic variety of primary pulmonary neoplasm, comprising between 30 and 60% of bronchogenic tumors. The tumor arises from the bronchial epithelium and is thought to represent the end point in a continuum of malignant change. This process probably begins with basal cell hyperplasia and continues through stratification of the epithelium, squamous cell metaplasia and carcinoma *in situ* before invading the surrounding tissues. There is a strong association between cigarette smoking and squamous cell carcinoma of the lung. Although the sex distribution of this type of tumor has always been heavily weighted toward a male predominance, the recent rise in carcinoma of the lung among females appears to be due primarily to an increase in the squamous cell variety, and that may be the result, in part, of increasingly heavy cigarette smoking by women. The mean age at diagnosis is 57 years.

Histologically, squamous cell carcinomas are recognized by intracellular bridging, cell nest formation, keratinization with the presence of horn pearls and whorling of the cellular population. There is more uniformity of recognition of this pattern among pathologists than with any other type of bronchogenic carcinoma. The major mass of the tumor may occur outside the bronchial cartilage and encircle the bronchial lumen.

There is nothing distinctive about the symptoms of tumors with this particular cell type. As with all other carcinomas of the lung, cough and sputum production dominate the clinical picture; hemoptysis, chest pain, pneumonia and dyspnea develop later. Cough is also prominent in smokers, and the onset of a tumor is often missed because this symptom is ignored (see "Small Cell Anaplastic Bronchogenic Carcinoma," page 161).

Since the majority of squamous cell carcinomas are found in the central bronchi, it is not surprising to note that obstructive phenomena are relatively common. Thus, the abnormality most frequently seen radiologically is either a perihilar mass or atelectasis-pneumonia associated with a central shadow. About 13% of squamous cell cancers in the lung will show cavitation on the chest x-ray film, a more frequent finding with this cell type than with any other bronchogenic carcinoma. (Cavitation does not occur in oat cell carcinomas.) Cavitation is either a result of tumor necrosis or secondary to bronchial obstruction with infectious abscess formation. Upper lobe lesions are more likely to cavitate than those in other portions of the lung, but the reasons for this phenomenon are obscure.

Peripheral lesions are the sole radiologic abnormality seen in 24% of patients with squamous

cell carcinomas. These peripheral lesions tend to be larger than those seen in adenocarcinoma. A particular type of peripheral lesion in the apical portion of the lung usually caused by squamous cell tumors may produce Pancoast's syndrome (Plate 55).

Diagnosis of squamous cell carcinoma rests on the demonstration of typical histologic changes in biopsy material or on sputum cytology. Bronchoscopy with biopsy and bronchial washing will confirm the diagnosis in about 65% of cases because of the central location of most tumors.

The tumor has a tendency not to metastasize until late in its course and, if left untreated, has

the longest patient survival of any of the bronchogenic carcinomas. In peripheral lesions without apparent metastasis, surgical extirpation will result in a five year survival rate in excess of 50%. Once metastasis has taken place, however, total surgical resection becomes more difficult and survival rates drop off precipitously. If the tumor cannot be resected, between 0 and 5% of patients will be alive five years after diagnosis.

Although there have been sporadic reports of cure with radiation therapy alone, a surgical approach to this disease is much more rewarding. Chemotherapy has been disappointing in the treatment of squamous cell carcinoma of the lung.

**Bronchogenic Carcinoma;
Large Cell Anaplastic Type**

Tumors are variable
in location

Large Cell Anaplastic Carcinoma

Large cell anaplastic carcinoma
in middle of r. upper lobe with
extensive involvement of hilar
and carinal nodes. Distortion of
trachea and widening of carina

Tumor composed of large multinucleated
cells without evidence of differentiation
toward gland formation or squamous
epithelium. These cells produce mucin
(stained red). Some tumors may be composed
of large clear cells containing glycogen

As its name implies, this type of primary bronchogenic tumor has lost almost all vestiges of cellular differentiation. From the standpoint of classification, it is diagnosed by a process of exclusion. Thus, if there are none of the characteristic histologic findings of squamous cell carcinoma or adenocarcinoma, the tumor must be noted as anaplastic, and, if the cells are generally larger than leukocytes, the diagnosis of large cell carcinoma may be entertained. These cells are pleomorphic and contain large, darkly staining nuclei with prominent nucleoli. Mitoses are common, and the variation in cell size may be accompanied by a range of cell shapes from polygonal to oval or spindle-shaped. Giant cell and clear cell varieties of the tumor have also been described.

Although some reports state that this type of tumor comprises as much as 40% of all bronchogenic neoplasms, no clear-cut pattern of clinical or radiologic presentation distinguishes it from other malignant lung tumors. There is a moderate tendency for the first abnormality found by x-ray examination to be a large peripherally located lesion. Whereas peripheral adenocarcinomas are generally less than 4 cm in diameter at the time of diagnosis, these anaplastic carcinomas are usually larger. The edges of the mass are often indistinct. Conversely, the tumor may be centrally located in up to 40% of cases.

As with other types of lung cancer, the point of origin of large cell anaplastic carcinoma will greatly influence the symptomatic presentation of the disease. Peripheral lesions are silent for longer periods than central lesions, although they may involve the chest wall, causing pain and pleural effusions. As a rule, however, the tumor causes cough, sputum production, hemoptysis and,

when it occurs in a major airway, obstructive pneumonia.

Diagnostic procedures such as sputum cytology and bronchoscopy with bronchial biopsy are highly successful in diagnosing this type of tumor preoperatively. Although the specific cell type usually cannot be determined from cytologic specimens, malignant cells may be found in almost 80% of adequate sputum specimens. Bronchial biopsy is most likely to be diagnostic in centrally situated lesions.

Both by histologic criteria and by clinical observation, these tumors are extremely malignant. There is early invasion of blood vessels and lym

phatics with subsequent widespread dissemination. It is, therefore, somewhat surprising to find that the results of surgical resection of the tumor are definitely better than those for oat cell carcinoma and equal to or better than those for adenocarcinoma. On the other hand, results of surgical resection are decidedly worse than in cases of squamous cell carcinoma. Once the tumor has metastasized, surgical therapy is limited to palliative procedures designed to relieve obstructive pneumonitis or prevent the reaccumulation of pleural effusion. Neither radiation therapy nor chemotherapy has been very successful in prolonging life.

Bronchogenic Carcinoma; Small Cell Anaplastic (Oat Cell) Type

Tumor with metastasis to hilar and carinal nodes and collapse of r. upper lobe

Small Cell Anaplastic Bronchogenic Carcinoma

Small cell anaplastic carcinoma of the lung is the most aggressively malignant of the bronchogenic tumors. There are several histologic subgroups of this cancer, although they are all characterized by a cell size of 6 to 8 microns in diameter, an extremely high nuclear to cytoplasmic ratio and hyperchromatism of the nuclei. A very sparse stroma is present in the tumor mass, with cells densely packed in a medullary configuration. When almost no cytoplasm is present and the cells are compressed into an ovoid form, the neoplasm is called an *oat cell carcinoma*. The cells are occasionally mistaken for lymphocytes, which they closely resemble. Recent studies of oat cell carcinomas suggest that they might be derived from an embryologic precursor in the neural crest. This view has been supported by the observation of neurosecretory granules within the cells, which might account for the unusually high occurrence of paraneoplastic syndromes associated with this type of tumor. Such conditions as ACTH secretion, inappropriate ADH secretion and carcinomatous neuromyopathies are discussed more fully on pages 166 to 167.

Clinically, small cell anaplastic tumors produce symptoms similar to those seen in other bronchogenic carcinomas. The most frequent presenting symptom is cough. However, since the incidence of this type of tumor is linearly related to the intensity of cigarette smoking, cough has often been present for many years and is changed only in severity or productivity by the appearance of the cancer. Chest pain, dyspnea, episodes of pneumonia, hemoptysis and localized wheezing are all fairly common symptoms which bring the patient to medical attention. Spread is so rapid that metastatic lesions themselves may produce the presenting symptoms, as they are often widespread by the time the diagnosis is made.

The chest x-ray film is likely to be helpful in diagnosis, as there is a tendency toward particular patterns of presentation. Since most small cell anaplastic tumors originate in the large bronchi, it is not surprising that hilar or perihilar masses are often seen on radiologic examination. Obstructive pneumonitis is also frequently seen because of the rapid growth and critical position of the tumor. Since these tumors metastasize early by the lymphatic route, mediastinal widening often accompanies the presence of a hilar mass. Even when the primary site of the tumor is in a peripheral portion of the lung—as occurs in about 29% of cases—a small (less than 4 cm) mass can be accompanied by extensive mediastinal widening.

The diagnosis must be confirmed by histologic or cytologic means. In a large percentage of cases

Masses of small cells with hyperchromatic round to oval nuclei and scant cytoplasm

Biopsy specimen. Cells elongated (oatlike)

Intrapulmonary lymphatic spread of neoplasm

this may be accomplished by bronchoscopy because of the central position of most small cell tumors. When three adequate sputum specimens are available for cytologic examination, a diagnosis of malignancy can be made in over 90% of cases, although the specific cell type is often not apparent by this method.

If the natural history of the disease is examined, it is found to differ significantly from other types of bronchogenic carcinoma. Lymphatic spread occurs so early in the course of the disease that it is useless to speak of localized small cell carcinoma of the lung. Involved lymph nodes are noted so consistently at surgery that most physicians have

abandoned this method of therapy. Likewise, careful examination of the bone marrow, even early in the disease, will yield a positive result for tumor cells in as many as 47% of patients. The mean survival time for untreated patients with small cell carcinoma of the lung is seven weeks after diagnosis, death generally being due to metastatic disease. Radiation therapy, too, is of limited value because of the disseminated nature of the illness. Recent reports of chemotherapeutic advances, using cyclophosphamide, bleomycin, doxorubicin and vincristine, have been encouraging in that they have prolonged mean survival to 35 weeks. However, the prognosis with this disease remains grim.

Although it is not possible to distinguish different histologic types of bronchogenic carcinoma from gross specimens or radiographs alone, a peripherally located tumor < 4 cm in diameter is most likely to be adenocarcinoma

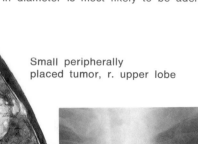

Small peripherally placed tumor, r. upper lobe

Adenocarcinoma of Lung

Glandular configuration and mucin production are the features that distinguish adenocarcinoma histologically from other types of bronchogenic carcinoma. The structure of the glands may be either typically acinar, with mucin filling the lumina, or papillary, consisting of columnar or cuboidal cells cast into irregular fingerlike projections. Mucin may be either extracellular or intracellular in location. At least one of these histologic criteria must be met in order to establish the diagnosis of adenocarcinoma.

Adenocarcinoma of the lung has approximately the same age distribution as do the other bronchogenic malignancies, the mean age at diagnosis being 53.3 years. More than 90% of these tumors occur between the ages of 40 and 69 years, with a slight male predominance. However, this type comprises almost 50% of all bronchogenic carcinomas in females, since the incidence of squamous cell and oat cell tumors in women is relatively low.

A peculiar feature of adenocarcinoma of the lung is its propensity to occur in the peripheral regions of the pulmonary parenchyma. The fact that approximately two-thirds of these tumors are found peripherally has important implications for symptomatology, diagnosis and therapy. Since most of the primary growth occurs away from the large airways, obstructive symptoms are rare and the tumor tends to be clinically silent. Frequently, a mass is found on routine x-ray examination of the chest. When symptoms finally do occur, they include cough, hemoptysis, chest pain and weight loss.

Radiologically, the most common presentation is a solitary peripheral pulmonary nodule, close to the pleural surface and often less than 4 cm in diameter. The remaining one-third of adenocarcinomas originate in a centrally placed bronchus, and may produce the same signs and symptoms observed in other lung cancers. No matter where the primary site of the tumor is located, a striking feature of adenocarcinoma of the lung is its tendency to be associated with parenchymal scars. Thus, the sudden enlargement of a previously stable abnormality in a chest roentgenogram is

Varied histology of adenocarcinoma

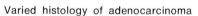

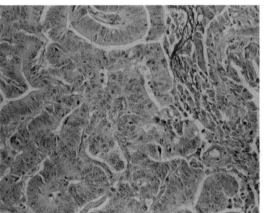

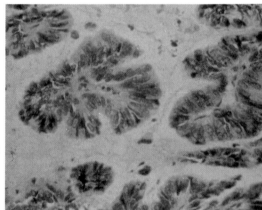

Tumor cells form glandlike structures with or without mucin secretion

Tumor cells may also form papillary structures

highly suggestive of bronchogenic adenocarcinoma. Since so many of these tumors are inaccessible to visualization and direct bronchoscopic biopsy, the correct preoperative diagnosis is made in less than 50% of cases. It is possible that newer diagnostic techniques such as fiberoptic bronchoscopy with brush biopsy under fluoroscopic guidance will increase this percentage in the future. However, current reports indicate that rigid bronchoscopic biopsy is positive in only 15% and bronchial washings are positive in only 25% of cases.

One would expect that a surgical approach to adenocarcinoma of the lung would be highly successful as a result of its usual peripheral location, and its occurrence as a solitary nodule. However, the unfortunate experience of most observers is that, while resection is possible in a high proportion of cases, the five year survival rate is still less than 10%. This is due to the fact that metastasis occurs relatively early in the course of the disease, although not as early as in oat cell carcinoma. The finding of positive lymph nodes in the surgical specimen indicates a poor prognosis for long-term survival. Neither radiation therapy nor chemotherapeutic regimens have as yet increased the five year survival rate above 5 to 10% of affected patients.

Pancoast's Syndrome

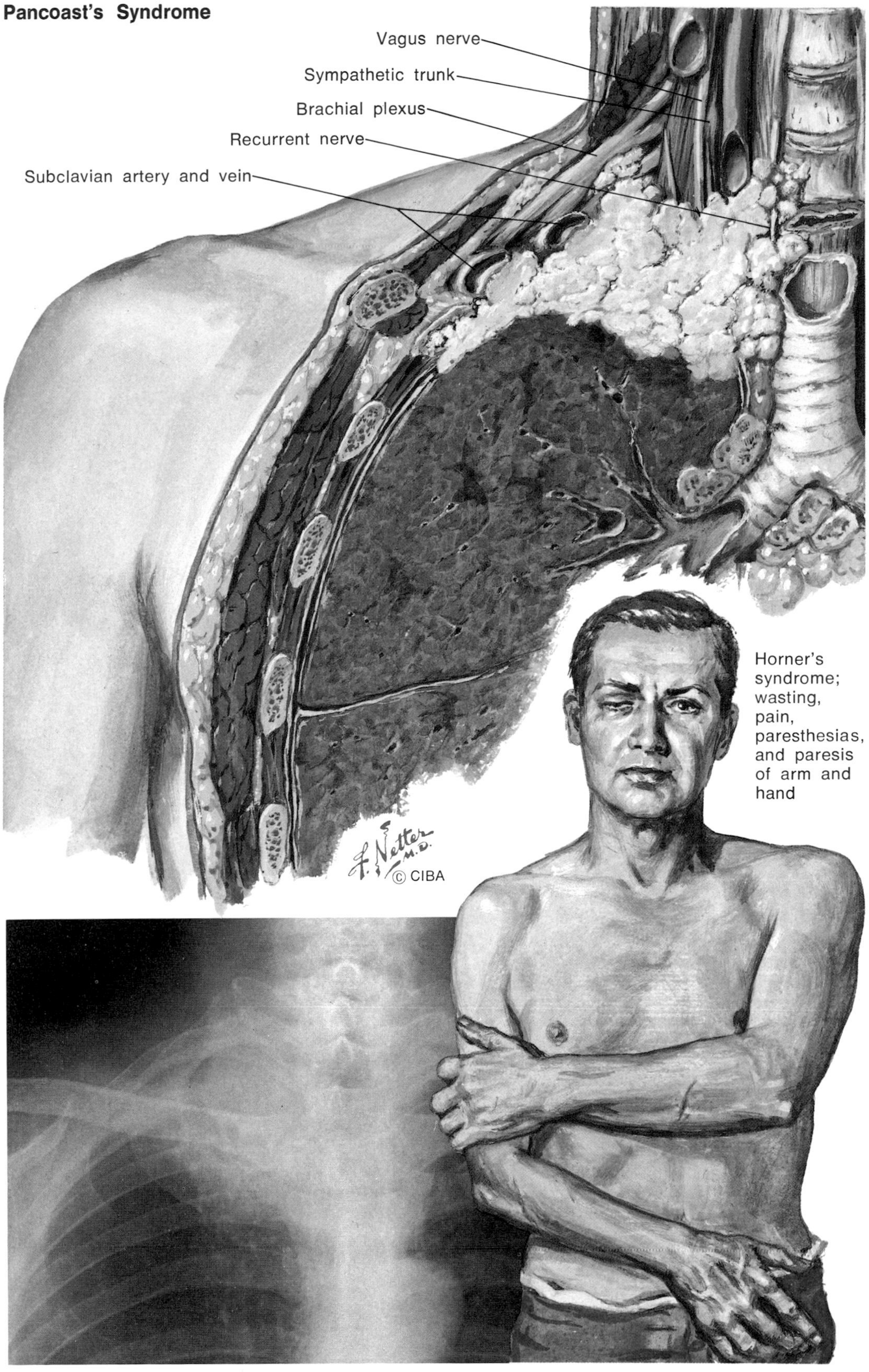

Vagus nerve
Sympathetic trunk
Brachial plexus
Recurrent nerve
Subclavian artery and vein

Horner's syndrome; wasting, pain, paresthesias, and paresis of arm and hand

Pancoast's Syndrome

One of the less common presentations of bronchogenic carcinoma is Pancoast's syndrome. This clinical entity is influenced more by the anatomic location of the tumor than by its specific histology. Although approximately two-thirds of the tumors are epidermoid (squamous cell) in nature, all cell types of bronchogenic carcinoma and many metastatic tumors have been reported to cause the syndrome.

Pancoast's original description of this symptom complex as a "superior sulcus tumor" actually does not correspond to any recognized anatomic location. It would be preferable to designate it as a "thoracic inlet tumor." Nonetheless, as the tumor crowds outward from the pulmonary parenchymal apex, it begins to encroach upon other important anatomic structures. The chest wall is invaded, and the subpleural lymphatics become involved. Posteriorly, just beneath the pleura, the tumor may spread by contiguity to the sympathetic nerve trunks, including the stellate ganglion. This results in loss of sympathetic tone and leads to the appearance of Horner's syndrome, which consists of miosis, mild ptosis, enophthalmos and flushing, with loss of sweating on the affected side of the face. As the tumor increases in size, it involves the upper ribs, producing intractable shoulder pain. Frequently the bone damage is visible on a plain x-ray film of the chest. Similarly, the upper thoracic vertebrae may become involved by the contiguous spread of the tumor. The subclavian artery and vein may also be compressed, producing paresthesias of the arm and hand. Usually, however, the latter symptoms are the result of destruction of the inferior trunk of the brachial plexus, comprising the C8 and T1 contribution to innervation of the upper limb. This nerve destruction will cause pain in an ulnar distribution and may lead to wasting of the small muscles of the hand.

Although one might reasonably assume that the spread of tumor to the chest wall and adjacent structures would prevent effective therapy, this

does not seem to be uniformly the case. In fact, these tumors have responded to preoperative irradiation followed by radical resection somewhat more favorably than lung cancers in other locations, perhaps because most thoracic inlet tumors are well-differentiated epidermoid carcinomas which metastasize late in their course. Preoperative irradiation appears to localize the tumor and may allow removal of the entire tumor mass by *en bloc* resection. This involves removal of part of the chest wall, including the first three ribs, parts of the upper thoracic vertebrae, the lower trunk of the brachial plexus and portions of the sympathetic chain, along with the upper lobe of the lung.

It is obvious that this type of radical approach is taken only as a result of the previous finding of 100% mortality with other modes of therapy. The survival with combined preoperative radiotherapy and radical surgery has been reported to be as high as 35%.

Rarely, this symptom complex may be caused by diseases other than bronchogenic carcinoma, including metastatic lesions from other organs or inflammatory diseases such as tuberculosis. Most physicians and surgeons, therefore, will insist on histologic confirmation of the diagnosis prior to the initiation of therapy, usually by percutaneous needle aspiration of the tumor.

Superior Vena Cava Syndrome

Bronchogenic carcinoma occasionally compromises the return of blood through the superior vena cava to the right atrium, producing a distinct set of symptoms and findings known as the superior vena cava syndrome. Patients complain of a feeling of fullness in the head and neck, headache, blurring of vision, and dyspnea, particularly when recumbent. The physician will note plethora of the face, edema of the head and neck, especially around the loose tissues of the eyelids, and a striking prominence of the superficial veins over the entire upper body. Edema may be seen in the upper portions of the torso, causing enlargement of the breasts. The veins of the upper parts of the body fail to collapse even when elevated far above the right atrium, as when the patient raises his arm above his head.

The syndrome is caused by obstruction of the superior vena cava, either by external compression or by direct invasion of the vessel by tumor. Since the vessel is a right-sided structure, in most cases the syndrome accompanies tumors of the right lung. This vessel is particularly vulnerable because of the lymphatic system, which drains the entire right lung and the lower portion of the left lung through nodes surrounding the superior vena cava. In addition, the vessel lies between the sternum and the right main stem bronchus and thus can be compressed by any malignant process in the central airways of the right lung.

The most common tumor causing this process is oat cell (small cell, undifferentiated) carcinoma of the lung. However, other bronchogenic tumors such as squamous cell, adenocarcinoma and undifferentiated carcinoma may produce the syndrome. Also, lymphomas and metastatic carcinomas from elsewhere have been reported as etiologic factors. Rarely, the process is the result of fibrosing mediastinitis, which may be caused by such nonmalignant diseases as histoplasmosis. A few cases of idiopathic fibrosing mediastinitis followed by the superior vena cava syndrome have been reported. Although the older literature implicates tuberculosis and syphilitic aortic aneurysm as frequent causes, modern treatment has virtually eliminated these diseases from consideration. Thus, an estimated 97% of cases of superior vena caval obstruction are due to malignant disease in the chest.

The syndrome's severity depends on the completeness of venous occlusion, which itself depends on the patency of the azygos system. If blockage occurs above the entry of the azygos vein into the vena cava, symptoms and signs are relatively mild, since this large vessel is a competent and accessible collateral channel for blood returning to the heart from the head and neck. Under these circumstances, the blood courses through the external jugular veins into the superficial thoracic veins, then into the perforating branches of the internal mammary and intercostal veins, and thence into the azygos vein, from which it enters the patent portion of the superior vena cava.

If the superior vena cava is obstructed below the entry point of the azygos vein, signs and symptoms are much more severe. Since venous blood must then be rerouted through the veins of the

Superior Vena Cava Syndrome

Obstruction of superior vena cava by cancerous invasion of mediastinal lymph nodes, with distention of brachiocephalic (innominate), jugular, and subclavian veins and tributaries

Edema and rubor of face, neck, and upper chest. Arm veins fail to empty on elevation

lower abdominal wall, back and groin, the final pathway is through the femoral and iliac veins and so back to the heart by way of the inferior vena cava. All available vessels in the internal mammary, vertebral and lateral thoracic systems are recruited for this purpose. Still, significant pressure must be developed to open the collateral channels. The result is florid evidence of increased blood volume and capillary leakage in the head and upper torso.

The diagnosis is made primarily on clinical grounds, and should be supplemented by the finding of characteristic mediastinal widening on a chest x-ray film. As there is a real danger of life-threatening hemorrhage during confirmatory biopsy procedures, many physicians prefer to start therapy without proof of the malignant nature of the disease. However, after symptoms abate, a tissue diagnosis should be obtained if at all possible.

The most effective and time-honored therapy for the superior vena cava syndrome is irradiation. Appearance of the superior vena cava syndrome in patients with malignant disease is an absolute contraindication to surgery with curative intent. By the very nature of its presentation, this syndrome implies that the disease has spread beyond the confines of its original focus and cannot be successfully extirpated.

Lymphangitic Spread of Cancer in Lung

Lymphangitic Spread and Cavitation of Lung Cancer

Lymphangitic Spread

The spread of carcinoma within the lungs may occur through the lymphatic vessels in addition to the more common hematogenous route. This pathologic entity produces distinctive radiologic and clinical patterns, which frequently permit the accurate prediction of histologic findings prior to the patient's death. Although any type of carcinoma may occasionally produce lymphangitic involvement of the lungs, the most common tumors causing this pattern arise from the breast, the bronchus and the gastrointestinal tract.

For many years it was thought that tumor cells tended to spread in a retrograde fashion from the hilar lymph nodes into the pulmonary parenchyma. Several lines of evidence suggest that this view is incorrect. First, the presence of the lymph vessel valves would make such spread exceedingly difficult. Second, malignant involvement of the hilar lymph nodes occurs in only about half the cases of lymphangitic pulmonary disease. Third, unilateral and even unilobar lymphangitic metastases have been observed, particularly in cases of peripheral bronchogenic carcinoma.

It is now postulated that the origin of lymphangitic tumor growth is usually hematogenous deposition of malignant cells in the pulmonary parenchyma. Next, the growth breaks through into the interstitium, with subsequent disruption and invasion of the lymph vessels. These channels then support cordlike extension of tumor toward the hilus and incite the development of fibrous tissue hyperplasia along the bronchovascular pathways. As more and more lymphatics become involved in the process, x-ray examination shows a sunburst pattern of radiopaque densities radiating from the hilar areas. Reticular and nodular patterns are noted as the thickened, tumor-filled vessels overlap and cause conglomerate densities. Characteristically, the lungs become less compliant, due in part to the extra tissue bulk of the lungs and in part to the impaired drainage of interstitial fluid, leading to dyspnea. Hypoxemia is commonly observed, probably as a result of both altered ventilation-perfusion relationships and true alveolar-capillary block. Although the occurrence of lymphangitic spread of carcinoma generally signals a rapidly fatal course, a few reports of extended survival have appeared in the literature.

Cavitation of Lung Cancer

Cavitation of cancers within the lung may occur in both primary bronchogenic and metastatic lesions. Certain cell types are particularly susceptible to this complication, while some essentially never develop cavitation. Of the primary bronchogenic tumors, cavitation occurs most fre-

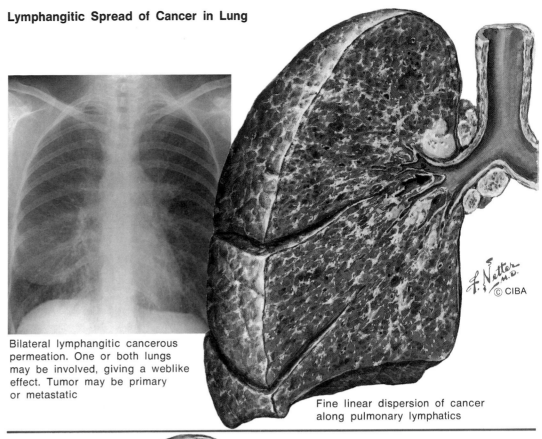

Bilateral lymphangitic cancerous permeation. One or both lungs may be involved, giving a weblike effect. Tumor may be primary or metastatic

Fine linear dispersion of cancer along pulmonary lymphatics

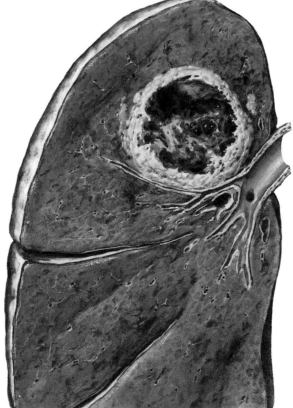

Cavitation of Lung Cancer

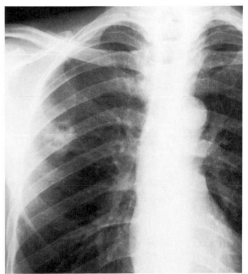

Carcinoma in peripheral zone of r. upper lobe with cavitation

quently in squamous cell carcinoma. It is seen less often in adenocarcinoma of the lung, rarely in large cell undifferentiated tumors, and almost never in small cell anaplastic lesions. Cavitation of pulmonary metastases is well documented in Hodgkin's disease, colon carcinoma and various sarcomas.

There are two major reasons for the occurrence of cavitation in lung tumors. In one instance, the central portion of the tumor becomes necrotic as a result of diminution in blood supply. The necrotic contents then liquefy and drain through the tracheobronchial tree, leaving an air-filled space surrounded by viable tumor. In the other circum-

stance, the endobronchial lesion blocks the lumen and leads to parenchymal infection, which then forms a true lung abscess. Partial or complete drainage of the abscess results in a cavitary lesion, with or without an associated air-fluid level on a chest roentgenogram. Rarely, transitional cell epithelioma of the bladder has produced cavitary metastases in the lungs.

Cavitary carcinomas are most frequent in the upper lung zones, and tend to have thick walls with nodular central borders. Cavitation within a malignant lung lesion is not necessarily a sign of unresectability, since it may occur before distant metastasis has taken place.

Nonmetastatic Extrapulmonary Manifestations of Bronchogenic Carcinoma

Aside from the obvious destructive effects of metastatic bronchogenic carcinoma, a number of more subtle humoral effects are being recognized with increasing regularity.

Endocrine Manifestations

Corticotropin. Several types of carcinoma are associated with the ectopic production of corticotropin (ACTH). These include primary lung carcinoma, thymoma, pancreatic carcinoma, medullary thyroid carcinoma and bronchial carcinoid tumors. Of all these, oat cell carcinoma of the lung most commonly produces ACTH. It has been reported that as many as 12% of patients dying of lung cancer have hyperplasia of the adrenal glands at autopsy. As a result of the elaboration of this hormone by the tumor, the adrenal glands secrete excessive quantities of 17-hydroxysteroids and 17-ketosteroids, leading to an atypical type of Cushing's syndrome. The usual clinical picture in oat cell carcinoma–induced ACTH production is one of a cachectic middle-aged male with muscular weakness, facial edema and severe hypokalemic alkalosis. Hyperglycemia, hypertension and increased pigmentation are also commonly seen, and electrolyte disturbances are prominent. This contrasts sharply with the usual pattern of Cushing's syndrome due to primary pituitary or adrenal causes, in which a young female presents with truncal obesity, moon facies, buffalo hump, diabetes mellitus and hypertension; electrolyte disturbances are generally mild.

A further difference is that there is seldom any suppression of hormonal activity following administration of dexamethasone when oat cell carcinoma is the cause of the syndrome. Although adrenalectomy and metyrapone have been used to control these symptoms associated with lung carcinoma, results are disappointing, and death usually occurs within two months of diagnosis.

Antidiuretic Hormone. Oat cell carcinoma is the most common cause of inappropriate antidiuretic hormone (ADH) secretion, although it has also been reported with other types of lung tumors, gastrointestinal tract tumors, thymomas and lymphosarcomas. The minimal criteria necessary to make this diagnosis include hyponatremia, decreased serum osmolality, high urine sodium content and urine osmolality higher than that of the serum. In addition, there must be no other renal, adrenal or cardiac disease sufficient to account for the defect. Clinically, the patient develops headache, irritability, nausea, vomiting, mental confusion and muscular weakness as the serum sodium level falls below normal. When it drops below approximately 115 mEq/liter, the patient may develop life-threatening seizure activity. The treatment for this syndrome is restriction of water intake, which will tend to raise serum levels of sodium above the dangerously low values. Surgical removal of the tumor mass to relieve the symptoms is not feasible if oat cell carcinoma is the cause.

Endocrine Manifestations of Bronchogenic Carcinoma

A. Corticotropic effects

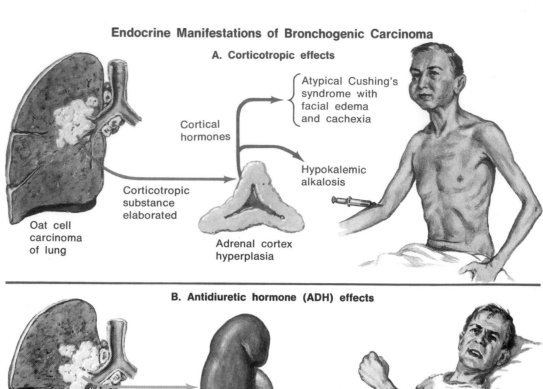

B. Antidiuretic hormone (ADH) effects

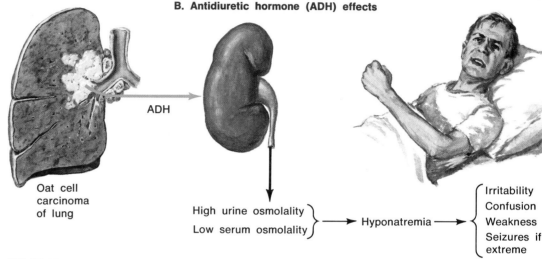

C. Parathormonelike effects   D. Gonadotropin effects

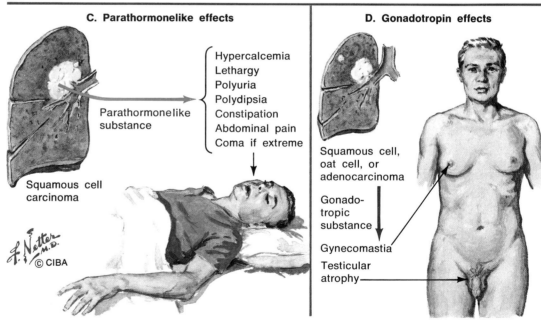

Parathormone. The major cause of hypercalcemia in patients with carcinoma of the lung is metastatic disease to the bone. However, a number of patients with no demonstrable bony lesions have been found to develop hypercalcemia. Analysis of tumor tissue from these patients has led to the extraction of a polypeptide molecule with parathormonelike qualities. The tumors that most commonly produce this hormone are squamous cell carcinomas of the lung. Clinically, the symptoms depend entirely on the serum calcium levels reached during the course of the illness. If the levels are only slightly elevated, no symptoms may be noted. Moderate hypercalcemia may lead to lethargy, polyuria, polydipsia, constipation and abdominal pain. At very high serum calcium levels the patient may become comatose. This syndrome sometimes regresses when the tumor mass is surgically removed.

Gonadotropins. Several cell types of bronchogenic carcinoma have been associated with the elaboration and release of gonadotropinlike substances. Squamous cell carcinoma, oat cell carcinoma and adenocarcinoma of the lung have all been implicated in this unusual syndrome. Its clinical manifestations are gynecomastia and testicular atrophy.

(Continued)

Nonmetastatic Extrapulmonary Manifestations of Bronchogenic Carcinoma
(Continued)

Other Endocrine Syndromes. Also occasionally associated with bronchogenic carcinoma are the carcinoid syndrome, insulin secretion, growth hormone secretion and calcitonin secretion.

Neuromuscular Syndromes

A variety of neuromyopathic disorders are associated with carcinoma of the lung. The existence of these syndromes was not recognized until the late 1940s when attention was called to the sensory neuropathy associated with bronchogenic carcinoma. This late recognition is probably due to the common occurrence of metastatic spread of lung tumors to the central nervous system and the willingness of physicians to assign symptomatic causality to this mechanism. However, careful investigation showed that neurologic abnormalities could occur in the absence of metastasis. In over half the cases the tumors are oat cell carcinomas, although all types of bronchogenic carcinoma have been implicated. There are no recognized humoral mechanisms causing the neural or myopathic changes, but the clinical syndromes evoked by these tumors can affect virtually all points along the neuromuscular pathway with devastating results, including a destructive myopathy resembling polymyositis, sensory and motor neuropathies, and a myasthenialike weakness known as the Lambert-Eaton syndrome.

There are several points that should allow clinical differentiation between myasthenia gravis and the Lambert-Eaton syndrome. In the latter disorder, weakness is most marked in the proximal muscles, particularly in the pelvic girdle region. This often causes difficulty in rising from a sitting position. Unlike myasthenia gravis, the Lambert-Eaton syndrome hardly ever involves the ocular muscles. Furthermore, repetitive exercising of muscle groups in the Lambert-Eaton syndrome tends to make them stronger, whereas in myasthenia gravis continued activity makes them weaker. The electromyographic tracing in the Lambert-Eaton syndrome is quite different from the tracing seen in true myasthenia gravis, and demonstrates this diagnostic response to repeated contraction.

Within the central nervous system, degenerative changes associated with carcinoma of the lung may occur in the spinal cord, causing sensory loss if the posterior column is compromised or muscular weakness if the anterior horn cells are involved, or paraplegia if the entire cord is affected.

A syndrome of subacute cerebellar degeneration is occasionally associated with nonmetastatic bronchogenic carcinoma. This syndrome is marked by severe ataxia, vertigo and dysarthria. The disease progresses rapidly, completely incapacitating the patient. Even if the primary tumor can be controlled, there is little hope of reversing these neurologic changes.

Other forms of encephalopathy can also occur with lung cancer, sometimes leading to cerebral cortical degeneration and dementia. Rarely, the dementia will predate clinical recognition of the lung tumor by as much as three years.

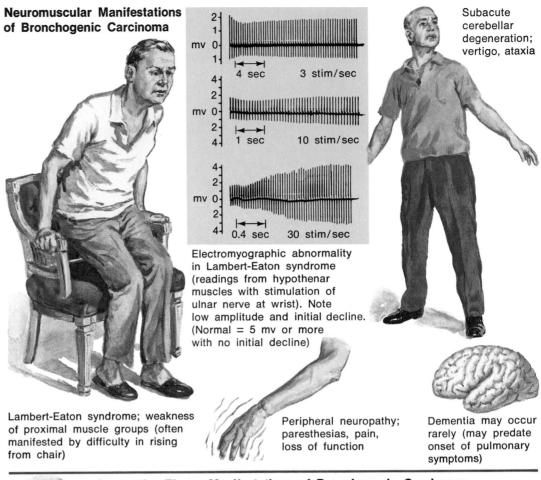

Neuromuscular Manifestations of Bronchogenic Carcinoma

Electromyographic abnormality in Lambert-Eaton syndrome (readings from hypothenar muscles with stimulation of ulnar nerve at wrist). Note low amplitude and initial decline. (Normal = 5 mv or more with no initial decline)

4 sec   3 stim/sec
1 sec   10 stim/sec
0.4 sec   30 stim/sec

Subacute cerebellar degeneration; vertigo, ataxia

Lambert-Eaton syndrome; weakness of proximal muscle groups (often manifested by difficulty in rising from chair)

Peripheral neuropathy; paresthesias, pain, loss of function

Dementia may occur rarely (may predate onset of pulmonary symptoms)

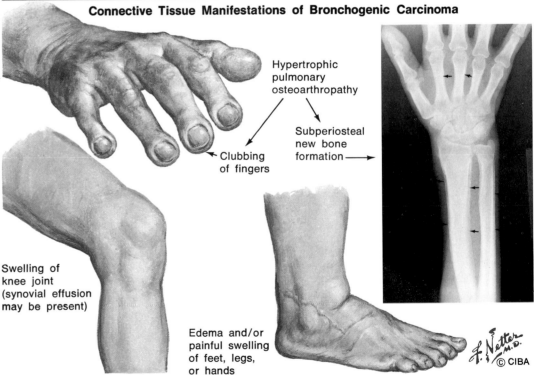

Connective Tissue Manifestations of Bronchogenic Carcinoma

Hypertrophic pulmonary osteoarthropathy

Clubbing of fingers

Subperiosteal new bone formation

Swelling of knee joint (synovial effusion may be present)

Edema and/or painful swelling of feet, legs, or hands

Connective Tissue Manifestations

Hypertrophic pulmonary osteoarthropathy is ordinarily associated with squamous cell bronchogenic carcinoma. Instances have also been described as resulting from adenocarcinoma of the lung, as well as from several noncarcinomatous intrathoracic diseases. The syndrome consists of clubbing of the digits, edema and tender swelling of the distal portions of the limbs, periarticular inflammation with occasional synovial effusions, and subperiosteal new bone formation. Clubbing of the digits is characterized by softening of the nail beds and loss of the angle between the nail

itself and the soft tissue at its proximal edge. Although clubbing is an essential feature of hypertrophic pulmonary osteoarthropathy, it may occur as an isolated physical finding and, as such, is much less likely to indicate squamous cell carcinoma of the lung. However, when all the criteria of the syndrome are met, a thorough search for carcinoma should be undertaken. The symptoms usually respond rapidly to removal of the tumor. If this is not possible, vagotomy may produce regression of the swelling and pain.

Less common extrathoracic manifestations of carcinoma of the lung include anemia, migratory thrombophlebitis and acanthosis nigricans.

Metastatic Malignancy to Lung

Metastases to the lung are a common clinical and radiologic finding, and approximately 30% of all cases of malignant disease will eventually spread there. Diagnosis is seldom a problem when the patient has a known primary tumor, but in the absence of such a lesion metastases to the lung may present a difficult clinical problem.

Metastases in the lung may take almost any roentgenographic pattern, but certain generalizations can be made: (1) Metastases are much more likely to be multiple than solitary. (2) Most hematogenous metastases are sharply circumscribed, with smooth edges, in contradistinction to the often poorly defined edges of primary pulmonary carcinoma. (3) Cavitation is unusual in secondary malignancy, but can occur. (4) Some metastatic tumors involving the lung may have unusual manifestations—*i.e.,* patchy alveolar infiltrates or linear interstitial lung disease (lymphangitic spread).

Solitary pulmonary metastases do occur, and often create a clinical problem. If the patient has a known primary malignancy, a single metastasis is generally suspected, but a second primary neoplasm of the lung is always a distinct possibility. An inflammatory lesion, especially a granuloma, also occasionally masquerades as a metastasis and must be considered in the differential diagnosis of a sharply circumscribed nodule in the lung.

If no other malignancy is known, the major consideration is to differentiate a solitary metastasis from a primary lung carcinoma. In the absence of clinical findings that might suggest another site of origin, even in the absence of positive sputum cytology to indicate primary lung malignancy, it is usually more appropriate to approach a solitary lesion as a primary lung carcinoma, rather than make an extended search for a primary tumor elsewhere.

Certain tumors are more prone to produce solitary metastases than others. Sarcomas of the soft tissue or bone, and carcinoma of the breast, colon and kidney are common offenders.

Multiple, smoothly circumscribed nodules in the lung are almost certainly metastatic neoplasms. Occasionally, an unusual entity such as rheumatoid lung disease, Wegener's granulomatosis or fungus infection (histoplasmosis or coccidioidomycosis) may present as multiple nodules and can be mistaken for the much more prevalent pulmonary metastatic disease.

Multinodular lung metastases may be of varying sizes, from small and miliary to very large,

Metastatic Carcinoma to Lung

Common sites of origin | Most common patterns (but any pattern may occur) | Radiologic patterns of lung metastases

Salivary glands
Thyroid gland
Breast
Kidney
Bowel
Uterus, ovaries, chorionic carcinoma
Bladder
Prostate

"Cannonball" (multinodular) pattern
"Snowstorm" pattern
Solitary nodule

"cannonball" dimensions. Many small nodules have been described as a "snowstorm" pattern. Primary tumors that generally metastasize in this fashion are carcinoma of the thyroid or breast and, somewhat less commonly, carcinoma of the bladder or prostate.

Multiple large (cannonball) nodules are often the result of spread from primary carcinomas of the kidney, testis, colon, breast and salivary gland, and from some bone or soft tissue sarcomas.

Metastatic malignancy sometimes presents as multiple poorly defined nodules; carcinoma of the breast and choriocarcinoma of the ovary are com-

mon neoplasms that metastasize in this way. Breast carcinoma and pulmonary lymphoma may also metastasize to produce a large area of diffuse alveolar consolidation resembling pneumonia, distinguishable from the latter by its chronicity.

Cavitation is not common in metastatic tumors but, when it does occur, it should suggest squamous cell tumors of the head, neck or cervix. Rarely, metastases of adenocarcinoma of the colon and transitional cell epithelioma of the bladder also cavitate.

Calcification in metastatic malignancy is extremely unusual, and almost always indicates a chondrosarcoma or an osteosarcoma.

Alveolar Cell Carcinoma

A distinctive type of primary carcinoma of the lung is seen in the distal portions of the pulmonary parenchyma. This has been called alveolar cell carcinoma, bronchioloalveolar carcinoma or bronchiolar carcinoma.

The neoplasm differs from bronchogenic carcinoma in that the major bulk of the tumor is seen in the alveoli rather than the bronchi. Tall columnar epithelium, resembling mucus-secreting cells of the distal bronchioles, invades the alveolar stroma and causes thickening of the alveolar walls. These cells tend to pile up, and they reveal a papillary or saw-toothed pattern on histologic examination. Few mitotic figures are seen within the tumor, and the individual cells may look quite normal. Often it is only the pattern of stromal invasion that differentiates this tumor from exuberant reparative growth at the edge of a pulmonary parenchymal scar. For years it was felt that, because of its cellular components and its propensity to produce mucin, this type of tumor was simply an adenocarcinoma of the lung. However, the fact that it spreads distally into the alveoli rather than proximally to the bronchi, and fails to metastasize early by a hematogenous route, sets it apart from the usual adenocarcinoma.

Alveolar cell carcinomas account for about 3% of all primary neoplasms of the lung. Unlike bronchogenic carcinomas, they have an almost equal sex distribution, and cigarette consumption does not appear to be an important factor in their genesis. However, there is an increased incidence of this malignancy among patients with previous pulmonary scarring, as in scleroderma.

There is good evidence that alveolar cell carcinomas have a unifocal point of origin within the lung and then spread by the bronchial route to implant on other portions of the respiratory epithelium. Growth of the primary tumor mass may be indolent, and bronchial spread probably occurs late in the course of the disease. In the early, unifocal stage the patient has no symptoms at all, or complains only of mild cough. X-ray films may show a nonspecific peripheral coin lesion, occasionally producing puckering of the pleura. The lesion often grows very slowly and can be relatively stable for as long as 5 to 10 years. Surgical excision of the mass at this stage is frequently curative.

Two other radiologic presentations are seen in the disease, and both imply dissemination of the malignancy. When this occurs locally, an entire lobe may become consolidated, and the x-ray picture is indistinguishable from that in lobar pneumonia.

Alternatively, radiologic evidence of bronchogenic spread of the tumor may be seen as a multinodular pattern, resembling hematogenous metastases from another organ. However, the infiltrates are less sharply circumscribed and have the rosette shape expected of an alveolar-filling disease. Although this pattern may also be confused with that of miliary tuberculosis, the tumor nodules tend to be larger than the infectious foci and may be confined to one lung.

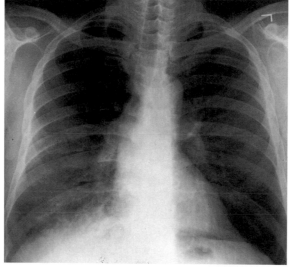

Alveolar cell carcinoma involving r. middle and lower lobes with diffuse pneumonialike appearance

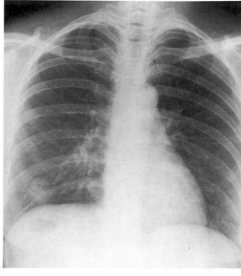

Alveolar cell carcinoma presenting as a solitary nodule in r. lower lobe

Hypothesis of pathogenesis

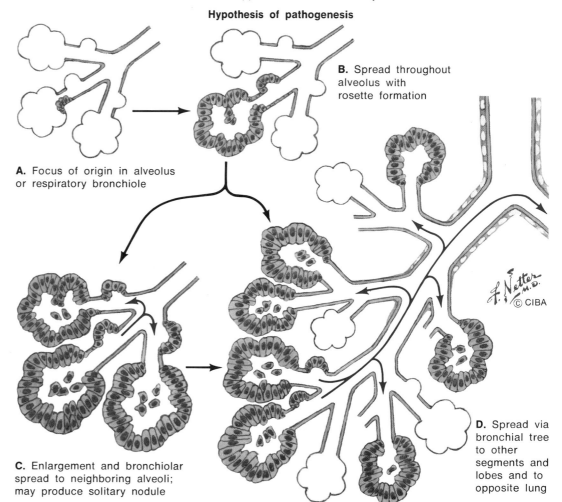

A. Focus of origin in alveolus or respiratory bronchiole

B. Spread throughout alveolus with rosette formation

C. Enlargement and bronchiolar spread to neighboring alveoli; may produce solitary nodule

D. Spread via bronchial tree to other segments and lobes and to opposite lung

Cytologic examination of the sputum leads to the correct diagnosis in only about one-third of the cases. This record is somewhat surprising in view of the copious production of secretions. It can be explained by the fact that the exfoliated cells often have a strikingly normal appearance. The nuclei are small and contain more prominent nucleoli than do normal cells. Multinucleated cells are sometimes seen, and cell clumping is generally present. Firm diagnosis of the disease rests on histologic examination of tissue obtained by transbronchial or open lung biopsy.

Once dissemination of the disease has occurred, surgical intervention is useless. Neither irradiation nor currently available chemotherapy has been found to be useful in treating the disease.

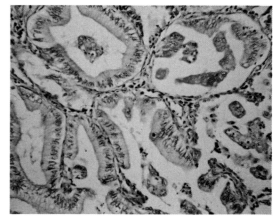

Alveoli lined by and containing tumor cells

Bronchial Adenoma

Bronchial adenomas are primary neoplasms of the lung which comprise between 1 and 5% of all bronchial tumors. They have been traditionally divided into carcinoid and salivary gland subtypes, although there is evidence to suggest that they arise from different cellular precursors and have quite different histologic appearances.

Carcinoid tumors account for 90% of bronchial adenomas. They are slow-growing neoplasms and possess a low grade of malignancy. It is thought that they are derived from Kulchitsky cells, which originate from the embryologic neural crest. This type of cell was first recognized in the gastrointestinal tract by its clear ability to reduce silver salts in various tissue stains. These staining characteristics are related to the production and storage of 5-hydroxytryptamine and 5-hydroxytryptophan within the cells, a fact that helps explain some of the unusual symptomatology occasionally seen with these tumors.

Bronchial carcinoid tumors have an equal sex distribution and tend to occur earlier in life than bronchogenic carcinoma, the mean age at diagnosis being 47 years. They have a strong predilection for the central airways, arising most commonly in the main stem or segmental bronchi. As a result of this location, about 90% of the tumors are accessible to bronchoscopic visualization; they appear as pale yellow or pink abnormalities in the bronchial mucosa. They may occur either as polypoid protrusions into the bronchial lumen or as sessile growths with wide distribution in the submucosa. Either type may project through the bronchial cartilage and assume a dumbbell shape, the so-called "iceberg" tumor.

On microscopic examination, the tumors generally show cellular uniformity with a low ratio of cytoplasm to nuclear material. Very rarely are mitoses seen in the specimens. Tumor tissue occurs in trabeculae, surrounding a highly vascular stroma in which tubular structures are occasionally formed. It has recently been pointed out that the carcinoid tumors found in peripheral portions of the lung are much more pleomorphic in appearance than those of central origin. In the peripheral tumors the cells are more disorganized, and more mitoses are also present.

Approximately 50% of patients with bronchial carcinoid tumors are asymptomatic, and the disease is found on routine chest x-ray examination. When symptoms do occur, they are related to the vascularity of the tumor and its central endobronchial location. Thus, the usual complaints are cough and hemoptysis. As the tumor enlarges, partial or complete bronchial obstruction may occur and cause wheezing, atelectasis or pneumonia. The full carcinoid syndrome, consisting of cutaneous flushing, telangiectasia, abdominal pain, diarrhea, wheezing and cardiac valvular damage, is rarely seen with bronchial carcinoid tumors; this syndrome is much more likely to result from abdominal carcinoid tumors, and is due to their greater content of serotonin or its precursor, 5-hydroxytryptophan.

In a small number of bronchial carcinoid tumors, spread of the disease takes place by vascular invasion or lymph node metastasis. Before spread of the tumor has occurred, local resection

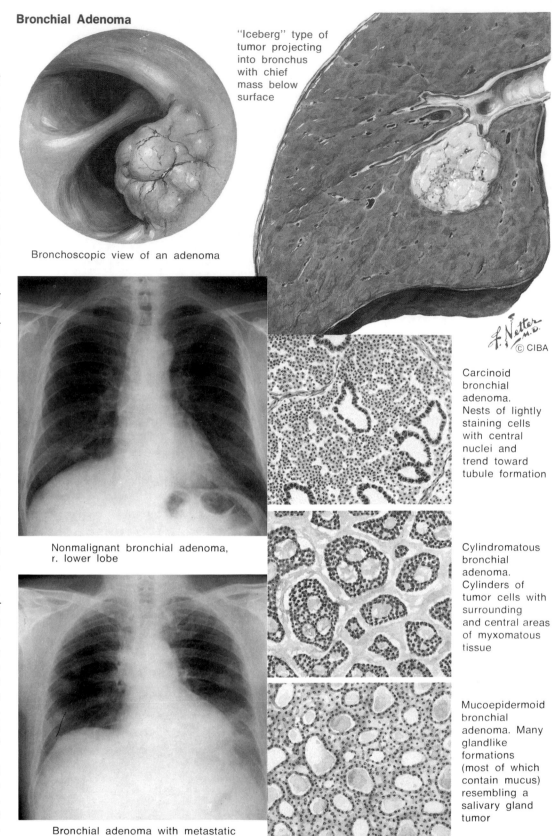

Bronchoscopic view of an adenoma

"Iceberg" type of tumor projecting into bronchus with chief mass below surface

Nonmalignant bronchial adenoma, r. lower lobe

Bronchial adenoma with metastatic nodules in both lungs

Carcinoid bronchial adenoma. Nests of lightly staining cells with central nuclei and trend toward tubule formation

Cylindromatous bronchial adenoma. Cylinders of tumor cells with surrounding and central areas of myxomatous tissue

Mucoepidermoid bronchial adenoma. Many glandlike formations (most of which contain mucus) resembling a salivary gland tumor

of the lesion is curative. However, even after dissemination the progress of the disease is slow and patients may survive for long periods.

Salivary gland tumors are the second kind of bronchial adenoma. They are much less prevalent than the carcinoid variety, and are separated into three subgroups. The most common of the salivary gland bronchial adenomas is the adenocystic carcinoma, otherwise known as *cylindroma*. It consists of trabeculae of cylindrically arranged stellate cells. The lumina of the cylinders of tumor are packed with eosinophilic material, giving the appearance of glandular growth. The tumors' point of origin is ordinarily in the trachea or very large

airways. These tumors tend to be more malignant than the carcinoid variety, invade the local tissues more aggressively, and metastasize earlier. However, the pulmonary parenchymal metastases are usually slow-growing, and it is not uncommon to see a patient with metastatic cylindroma survive 10 to 15 years following detection of the tumor. Treatment of this type of tumor, however, is uniformly unrewarding.

The other two subgroups of the salivary gland type of bronchial adenomas are seen even less often than the cylindromas and deserve only passing mention. They include *mucoepidermoid adenoma* and an extremely rare *pleomorphic* type.

Benign Tumors of Lung

Benign tumors of the lung are rare pathologic entities. They account for less than 10% of all so-called coin lesions in the chest. Occurring as either endobronchial or parenchymal masses, they may cause a wide variety of symptoms and radiographic abnormalities despite their benign nature. As a rule they are found on routine chest x-ray films as well-circumscribed peripheral pulmonary masses. In this location these tumors seldom produce symptoms, but they are frequently confused with primary or metastatic malignancies of the lung. Endobronchial lesions, on the other hand, may not be seen as distinct x-ray shadows but they may induce cough, sputum production, hemoptysis or localized wheezing. If the mass within the bronchus enlarges enough to cause complete obstruction, atelectasis or postobstructive pneumonia may result.

The most common variety of benign pulmonary neoplasm is the *hamartoma.* It consists of normal tissue elements arranged in an abnormal chaotic pattern. For unknown reasons, hamartomas are found four times as often in males as in females. Although it is assumed that they are present from embryologic life onward, they are often found on the roentgenogram after a previous film was normal. Hamartomas are usually located peripherally, and are sharply demarcated round or lobulated structures. About half of them contain calcium, which is best demonstrated by tomography. The pattern of calcification (finely stippled densities present throughout the lesion) is characteristic but not pathognomonic of hamartomas. Other benign lesions such as granulomas may also display this type of calcium deposition. In the absence of such a distinctive assurance of benignity, the differential diagnosis of calcification must include primary malignancies of the lung, and resection of the lesion must be considered, particularly when it is noted that hamartomas as well as malignant tumors may increase in size during a period of preoperative observation. At surgery, the nodule is found to be covered by a thin fibrous capsule which frequently allows simple enucleation. Grossly, hamartomas appear bluish white in color and may have cystic spaces within the mass. Microscopically, they consist mostly of cartilage but also contain fibrous connective tissue, fat and smooth muscle. Once the lesion is removed, it does not recur.

Fibromas are found either in the parenchyma or within a bronchus. They are usually small, dense lesions which do not contain calcium and therefore cannot be differentiated clinically from carcinoma. For this reason they should be removed surgically. Occasionally it is possible to remove an endobronchial fibroma through a bronchoscope.

Chondromas are rare tumors, especially when the criteria for diagnosis are strict and only lesions containing a predominance of cartilage are included. Small chondromas are frequently endobronchial, while the larger ones are usually parenchymal. Endobronchial chondromas may possess a pedicle which allows them to move. Grossly, they are sharply demarcated from normal lung tissue, being covered by a fibrous capsule. The cut

Benign Tumors of Lung

A. Hamartoma

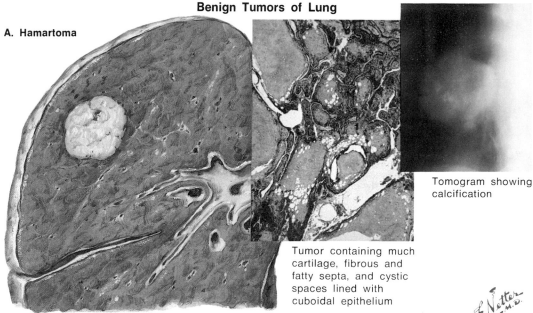

Tomogram showing calcification

Tumor containing much cartilage, fibrous and fatty septa, and cystic spaces lined with cuboidal epithelium

Sharply circumscribed growth with calcified areas

B. Fibroma

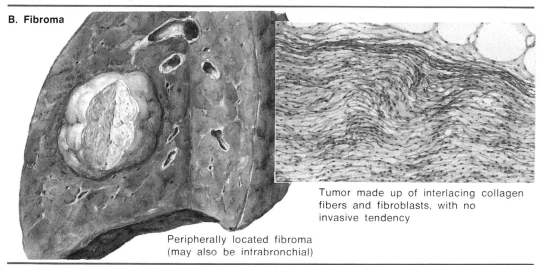

Tumor made up of interlacing collagen fibers and fibroblasts, with no invasive tendency

Peripherally located fibroma (may also be intrabronchial)

C. Chondroma

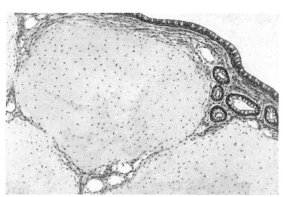
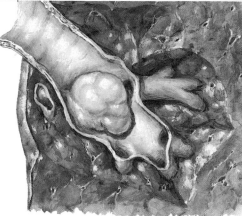

Tumor composed almost entirely of cartilage and covered by bronchial epithelium

Smooth, lobulated growth in a main bronchus

surface may vary in color from white to bluish, depending on the type of cartilage present. Fibrous strands, which may be infiltrated with small blood vessels, sometimes separate the cartilage into bundles. Spicules of true bone formation may be found within the tumor.

Lipomas are very rare endobronchial tumors composed of fatty tissue and related to fibromas. Occasionally they will penetrate the bronchial wall and grow into the pulmonary parenchyma.

Leiomyomas consist of smooth muscle cells interlaced with fibrous tissue. They may occur singly, or in diffuse nodules scattered throughout the tracheobronchial tree.

Vascular tumors such as arteriovenous fistulas, cavernous hemangiomas and endotheliomas of the lung are very rare. Symptoms are sometimes caused by the large volume of blood shunted through the lung by way of patent vascular channels. Arteriovenous fistulas are often associated with hereditary telangiectasia, and in view of their frequently multicentric origin, angiography should be performed prior to surgery.

Mesotheliomas may be malignant (Plate 65) or benign. Benign mesotheliomas usually originate from the visceral pleura and are localized, rather than diffuse, lesions. They are often accompanied by hypertrophic pulmonary osteoarthropathy.

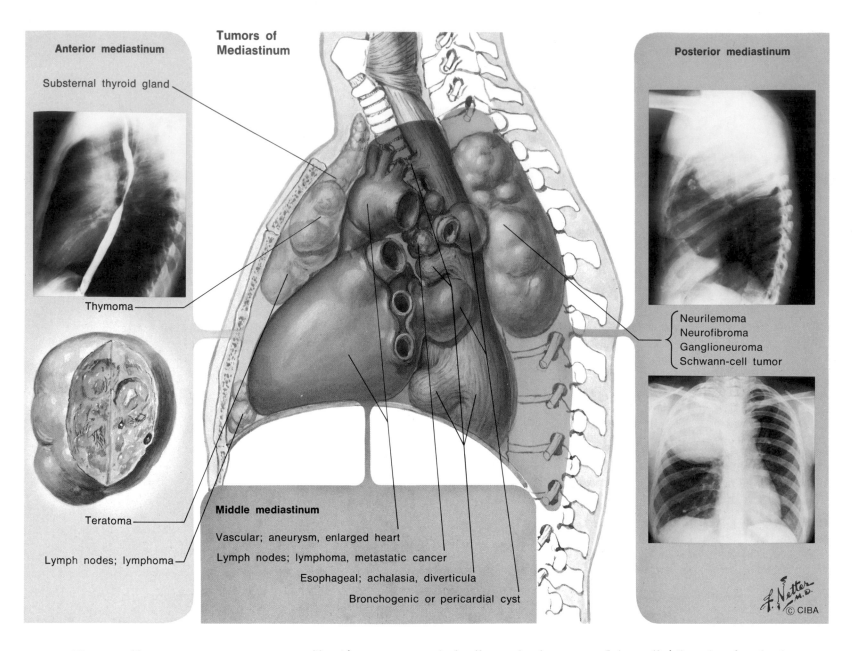

Tumors of Mediastinum

Anterior mediastinum

Substernal thyroid gland

Thymoma

Teratoma

Lymph nodes; lymphoma

Middle mediastinum

Vascular; aneurysm, enlarged heart

Lymph nodes; lymphoma, metastatic cancer

Esophageal; achalasia, diverticula

Bronchogenic or pericardial cyst

Posterior mediastinum

Neurilemoma
Neurofibroma
Ganglioneuroma
Schwann-cell tumor

Mediastinal Masses

Specific mediastinal tumors have a predilection for particular areas of the chest. Nonetheless, all types of masses have been reported in all mediastinal compartments.

Thymomas account for a large proportion of all mediastinal tumors; 50% of thymomas are malignant. They generally occur at the junction of the heart and great vessels, and protrude to either side of the mediastinum. Symptoms caused by local growth include retrosternal pain, cough and fever. Myasthenia gravis occurs in 50% of cases; conversely, 15% of patients with myasthenia gravis have thymomas.

The *thyroid gland* occasionally extends below the sternum and appears as a mediastinal mass. The mass often displaces the trachea and causes an irritative cough or choking sensation. The diagnosis may be made by radionuclide scan of the thyroid. However, if a presumptive thyroid gland fails to concentrate iodine, the mass must be diagnosed surgically.

Parathyroid glands infrequently cause masses within the anterior mediastinum. They are usually cardiophrenic functional and cause signs and symptoms of hyperparathyroidism.

Teratoid tumors are germinal cell growths that occur in benign (dermoid cyst) and malignant (teratoma) forms. They may become huge, compressing normal mediastinal and thoracic structures. Radiologically, the benign tumors are often seen to contain opacities such as a tooth, mandible or other bone. Teratomas are either solid or cystic, and contain elements of ectoderm, mesoderm and endoderm. Endoderm predominates in malignant teratomas; ectoderm is characteristic of the benign variety.

Lymph nodes occur in all parts of the mediastinum but mainly in the anterior and middle compartments. Both infectious and malignant processes can lead to lymph node enlargement along the mammary chain. In the middle mediastinum, 90% of lymph node masses are malignant as a result of metastatic tumor spread from other organs or primary lymphoma. Among benign causes of middle mediastinal lymphadenopathy are infectious diseases such as primary tuberculosis and histoplasmosis.

Most *aortic aneurysms* are arteriosclerotic in origin, but traumatic aneurysms are also frequent; syphilitic aneurysms are not common today. Although most aortic aneurysms are asymptomatic, prior to rupture they are in intimate contact with structures that may cause symptoms if disturbed.

Vascular dilatation such as pulmonary artery enlargement can also appear as a middle mediastinal mass. It is usually bilateral, and on the chest x-ray film the shadow is contiguous with the hilar areas.

Esophageal lesions occasionally produce middle mediastinal masses. Benign neoplasms of the esophageal wall—leiomyomas or enterogenous cysts, for example—must attain great size before they cause symptoms, and thus are more likely to be seen on a plain chest x-ray film than are malignant tumors.

Bronchogenic cysts occur most commonly at the tracheobronchial bifurcation and thus are seen in the middle mediastinum on x-ray examination. They are fluid-filled cysts lined with bronchial epithelium. They may become infected and cause pain. Rupture into the tracheobronchial tree produces an air-fluid level within the cyst cavity.

Pericardial cysts occur at the anterior cardiophrenic angle, more often on the right than on the left. They seldom become infected, and are problems only in differential diagnosis.

The majority of masses in the posterior mediastinum are neurogenic tumors. *Neurilemomas* and *neurofibromas* arise from peripheral nerves.

Schwannomas are malignant lesions arising from sheath cells of the peripheral nerves.

Benign ganglioneuromas arise from the sympathetic nerve fibers and are more common in children than in adults. Malignant tumors of this cell origin include the ganglioneuroblastoma and the sympathicoblastoma.

Malignant Mesothelioma

Diffuse pleural mesotheliomas are primary malignant tumors of the visceral or parietal pleura. There is strong evidence to suggest that this is an occupationally related disorder, since most patients with these tumors have had significant exposure to asbestos (see page 211). In a small number of cases (less than 5%) no exposure to asbestos can be discovered.

The tumors are of two histologic varieties, an epithelial type and a fibrous type. Epithelial tumors have a tubular structure with lining cells projecting into the central spaces in a papillary fashion. Fibrous tumors have a solid appearance microscopically and are composed of spindle-shaped cells with oval, vesicular nuclei. Somewhat less than half of all pleural mesotheliomas contain elements of both histologic types.

The illness most frequently occurs from 30 to 50 years after the initial exposure to asbestos. The mean age at onset of symptoms is around 60 years. The initial symptoms are notoriously vague and are often disregarded by the physician; the patient may complain of fatigue, diffuse unilateral chest pain or mild breathlessness which occurs only on moderate exercise. As the disease progresses, pain becomes the overriding complaint, frequently interfering with sleep.

Chest x-ray examination often suggests the diagnosis, even though the radiologic picture is far from pathognomonic. Unilateral pleural thickening is commonly noted on the x-ray film with a nodular appearance and an association with pleural effusions of varying sizes. Despite moderate or even large collections of fluid, the mediastinum frequently shifts *toward* the side affected, and the intercostal spaces narrow. As the disease progresses, the effusion begins to increase in size and produce respiratory embarrassment.

Thoracentesis reveals bloody fluid in fewer than half the patients. Approximately an equal number produce a serous effusion, and occasionally no fluid can be aspirated because of symphysis of the malignant pleural surfaces. Examination of the fluid alone is rarely diagnostic for mesothelioma, although definitely malignant cells are sometimes seen. The reported incidence of high levels of hyaluronic acid in the fluid has been difficult to confirm. Needle biopsy of the pleura, performed at the same time as thoracentesis, provides specimens diagnostic of the disease in about 25% of cases. The most frequent mistake in examination of this tissue is to misdiagnose the process as adenocarcinoma. Larger biopsy specimens obtained during limited thoracotomy lead to increasing diagnostic accuracy. Histologic examination of biopsy or autopsy material is the only method of arriving at the diagnosis with certainty.

Once the disease begins to progress, dyspnea and pain become the predominating symptoms. Dyspnea can be relieved, at first, by removal of the pleural fluid, and this may require drainage of 1 to 2 liters of liquid per week. Eventually the volume of fluid obtained at each procedure will decrease even in the absence of other therapeutic maneuvers. This is apparently a result of obliteration of the pleural space by growth of the tumor.

Thoracic pain results from infiltration of the tumor into the chest wall, with involvement of

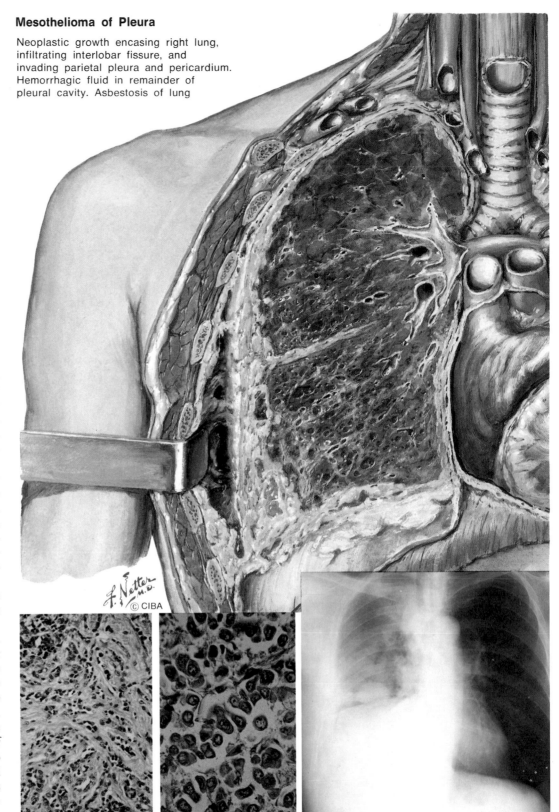

Mesothelioma of Pleura

Neoplastic growth encasing right lung, infiltrating interlobar fissure, and invading parietal pleura and pericardium. Hemorrhagic fluid in remainder of pleural cavity. Asbestosis of lung

Fibrosarcomatous type of tumor

Epithelial cell type of tumor

Mottled shadow over r. lung area with effusion. In advanced cases, lung may be totally obscured

the intercostal nerves and ribs. Tumor growth also spreads to the mediastinum by contiguity and begins to envelop the pericardium, great vessels and nerves. Surgical sites and biopsy needle tracts are consistently invaded by tumor. Palpable tumor masses are felt through the chest wall in the later stages of the disease. The chest pain responds very poorly to therapy, including narcotic analgesics and even intercostal nerve blocks.

While the pleural space and mediastinum are being invaded, the lung itself is being compressed and destroyed. Contraction of the entire hemithorax occurs, shifting the mediastinum toward the side of the disease and raising the involved

diaphragm. Bronchial cleansing deteriorates, leading to recurrent pulmonary infections.

In addition to contiguous spread of the tumor, dissemination takes place by several other routes. Fluid may leak into the contralateral hemithorax by way of the posterior or inferior mediastinum or may filter through the foramina of the diaphragm into the abdomen. Hematogenous spread frequently involves the liver, adrenals and kidneys.

Death is usually caused by infection, vascular compromise or pulmonary embolus. Treatment—whether surgery, radiotherapy or chemotherapy—has not affected survival; the average life expectancy after diagnosis is one to two years.

The Pneumonias

Pneumonia is a pulmonary disease characterized by replacement of air in alveoli and alveolar ducts with an inflammatory exudate, and/or by inflammatory cell infiltration of the alveolar walls and interstitial spaces. Although most pneumonias are caused by infectious agents, other types occasionally occur: (1) *lipid pneumonia* due to aspiration of mineral oil, etc.; (2) *chemical pneumonitis* caused by inhalation of metal-containing or other chemical fumes (*e.g.,* beryllium—page 213); (3) *extrinsic allergic alveolitis* from inhalation of dust containing an allergen (*e.g.,* spores of thermophilic actinomycetes, as in the sugar cane industry—page 216); (4) *idiosyncratic pulmonary reactions to drugs* (*e.g.,* nitrofurantoins, busulfan, methotrexate); (5) *x-irradiation pneumonia;* (6) *unusual pneumonias of unknown cause* (*e.g.,* desquamative interstitial pneumonia, eosinophilic pneumonia).

The pneumonias of infectious origin are emphasized in the plates that follow. The microorganisms involved (see table) range from relatively large agents (bacteria, fungi) to extremely small, obligate intracellular pathogens (viruses).

Infectious Agents Causing Pneumonia

Class	Etiologic Agent	Type of Pneumonia
Bacteria	Streptococcus pneumoniae	Bacterial pneumonias
	Streptococcus pyogenes	
	Staphylococcus aureus	
	Klebsiella pneumoniae	
	Pseudomonas aeruginosa	
	Escherichia coli	
	Yersinia pestis	
	"Legionnaires'" bacillus	"Legionnaires' disease"
	Peptostreptococcus, Peptococcus	Aspiration (anaerobic)
	Bacteroides	pneumonia
	Fusobacterium	
	Veillonella	
Actinomycetes	Actinomyces israelii	Pulmonary actinomycosis
	Nocardia asteroides	Pulmonary nocardiosis
Fungi	Coccidioides immitis	Coccidioidomycosis
	Histoplasma capsulatum	Histoplasmosis
	Blastomyces dermatitidis	Blastomycosis
	Aspergillus	Aspergillosis
	Phycomycetes	Mucormycosis
Rickettsia	Coxiella burnetii	Q fever
Chlamydia	Chlamydia psittaci	Psittacosis Ornithosis
Mycoplasma	Mycoplasma pneumoniae	Mycoplasmal pneumonia
Viruses	Influenza virus, adenovirus, respiratory syncytial virus, etc.	Viral pneumonia
Protozoa	Pneumocystis carinii	Pneumocystis pneumonia (plasma cell pneumonia)

Pneumococcal Pneumonia

Pneumococcal (*Streptococcus pneumoniae*) pneumonia is the most common type of bacterial pneumonia. It is an acute infection of the lung, occurring as either *lobar pneumonia* or *bronchopneumonia*. It is prevalent in the winter or early spring, usually following by several days a viral infection of the upper respiratory tract. Patients with hypogammaglobulinemia or multiple myeloma appear particularly susceptible. During the respiratory infection season, 40% or more of the population are asymptomatic carriers of pneumococci in the upper airway. Thus, isolation of this organism from the pharynx does not necessarily prove that it is responsible for a given pneumonia.

Etiology. The pneumococcus is a lancet-shaped, gram-positive diplococcus that sometimes grows in short chains. Its polysaccharide capsule enables it to resist phagocytosis; mutants lacking a capsule are avirulent. On the basis of reactions of specific antisera with antigenic determinants on the capsule, pneumococci have been divided into over 80 different serotypes. In the past, when the treatment of pneumococcal pneumonia required type-specific antiserum, definition of the exact pneumococcal serotype was mandatory. In the presence of homologous antiserum, swelling of the capsule (quellung reaction) occurs, rendering it readily visible under the microscope (Plate 67). The quellung reaction can be elicited in sputum samples (if abundant organisms are present), or pneumococci can be isolated in pure culture by inoculation in a mouse, where they—but not other bacteria—cause bacteremia and rapid death. In the antibiotic era the routine definition of serotypes is no longer necessary.

Pneumococci grow on blood agar as dome-shaped colonies with surrounding alpha hemolysis. Colonial morphology provides presumptive identification if the colony is large and mucoid (*e.g.,* type 3) or is button-shaped, with a central depression due to autolysis. Pneumococci can be distinguished from commensal alpha hemolytic streptococci by the optochin (Taxos P) test; growth of the former, but not of the latter, is inhibited by optochin.

(Continued)

Pneumococcal
Pneumonia

A. Lobar
pneumonia;
r. upper lobe.
Mixed red and
gray hepatization
(transition stage).
Pleural fibrinous
exudate

Pneumococcal Pneumonia
(Continued)

Pathogenesis and Pathology. Following a viral upper respiratory infection, there is an increase in the volume of nasopharyngeal secretions and the number of potentially pathogenic microorganisms in them. Aspiration of these secretions is facilitated by alterations in the defense barriers of the respiratory tract produced by the preceding infection. Bacteria are carried by the thin secretions into the alveoli where the initial response to bacterial invasion is an outpouring of edema fluid. This fluid serves to transport organisms to other alveoli through the pores of Kohn and terminal bronchioles; this is the edema zone at the outer margin of the spreading lesion. Within this zone is an area *(zone of early consolidation)* where, following the edema stage, polymorphonuclear leukocytes and erythrocytes have entered. More central is a *zone of advanced consolidation* where the alveoli are packed with leukocytes actively phagocytizing and killing pneumococci. Finally, when bacteria have been eliminated, macrophages enter and replace the granulocytes forming the innermost (oldest) part of the lesion, the *zone of resolution*. The gross appearance of "red hepatization" corresponds to the peripheral areas of edema and hemorrhage; "gray hepatization" corresponds to the histologic zone of advanced consolidation in the older, more central portion of the lesion.

Clinical Features. Characteristically, the onset of pneumococcal pneumonia is abrupt and heralded by a shaking chill, which is followed by fever (101° to 105°F). Chest pain on deep breathing, due to pleural involvement by the peripherally located initial area of consolidation, develops shortly thereafter, or may be an initial symptom. Cough then becomes prominent, and is typically productive of bloody or "rusty" sputum, consistent with the early hemorrhagic character of the alveolar exudate. Marked weakness and malaise accompany the febrile course.

Tachycardia and tachypnea are marked; respirations are grunting and shallow because of splinting of the involved lungs; the patient appears acutely ill. Herpes labialis (fever blisters) is frequently present. An inspiratory lag of one side of the chest may suggest the site of the pneumonia. Examination may not reveal signs of consolidation in early pneumonia, or signs may be obscured by

B. R. upper lobe and segment of r. lower lobe pneumonia

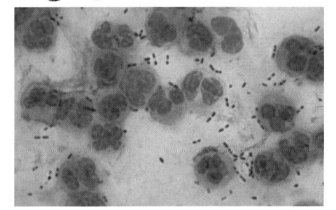

C. Purulent sputum with pneumococci (Gram's stain)

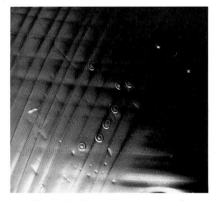

D. Colonies of pneumococci growing on agar plate

splinting. Dullness on percussion, bronchial breath sounds, increased tactile fremitus, and fine crackling rales are observed when extensive consolidation has occurred. A pleural friction rub is frequently audible. Abdominal distention often develops.

The total leukocyte count is usually elevated (15,000 to 40,000/mm³), and there is a marked shift to the left in morphologic appearance. Gram-stained smear of the sputum shows abundant polymorphonuclear leukocytes and large numbers of gram-positive diplococci. Pneumococcal pneumonia generally involves only one lobe, or one segment of a lobe; the most

common sites are the lower lobes or the right middle lobe.

Treatment. Administration of penicillin produces striking improvement, often within 24 hours, but fever may persist for several days. (Recent reports indicate the emergence in South America of pathogenic strains of pneumococci resistant to penicillin and to other antibiotics as well.) As resolution occurs, bronchial breath sounds and fine crepitations are replaced by coarse sticky rales. Radiologic examination of the chest reveals clearing over the next few weeks, but complete resolution may not come for some additional *(Continued)*

Pneumococcal Pneumonia (continued)

E. Pathologic changes in zones of the pneumonic lesion

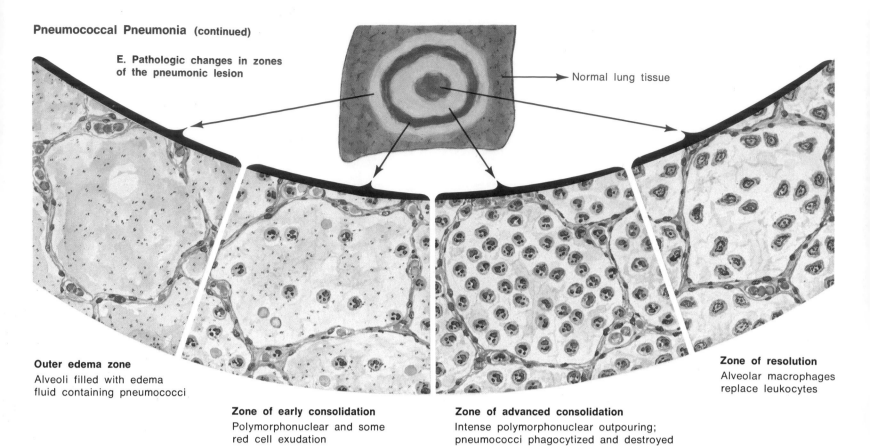

Normal lung tissue

Outer edema zone
Alveoli filled with edema fluid containing pneumococci

Zone of early consolidation
Polymorphonuclear and some red cell exudation

Zone of advanced consolidation
Intense polymorphonuclear outpouring; pneumococci phagocytized and destroyed

Zone of resolution
Alveolar macrophages replace leukocytes

Pneumococcal Pneumonia
(Continued)

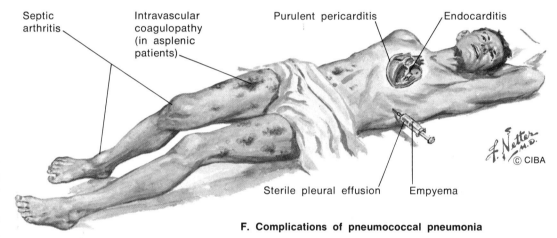

Septic arthritis

Intravascular coagulopathy (in asplenic patients)

Purulent pericarditis

Endocarditis

Sterile pleural effusion

Empyema

F. Complications of pneumococcal pneumonia

time. Failure of resolution should suggest the possibility of bronchial obstruction due to a tumor, although in occasional patients (particularly with involvement of the right upper lobe) radiologic clearing is delayed in the absence of any endobronchial abnormality.

Complications. Complications may occur early in pneumococcal pneumonia or at any time during the course of the disease (Plate 68). *Small sterile pleural effusions* result from inflammation of the pleura overlying the involved area of the lung. In occasional patients, particularly alcoholics who may not have sought early medical attention, the effusion contains organisms, and *frank empyema* ensues. Thoracentesis is needed to establish the diagnosis, and drainage of the empyema is required to control infection and prevent subsequent restrictive pulmonary disease. Extension of infection to the pericardium (by contiguity from the pleural space or via bacteremia) results in *purulent pericarditis.* Although this complication has become relatively rare since the introduction of antibiotics, it is so serious that it should be carefully excluded as a possibility. *Lung abscess* is extremely rare as a complication of pneumococcal pneumonia, but when it does occur, it may be caused by type 3 pneumococci (which have a thick antiphagocytic capsule); more probably there is bacterial superinfection (*Staphylococcus aureus,* or *Klebsiella*), or underlying bronchial obstruction.

About one-third of patients with pneumococcal pneumonia have bacteremia. Metastatic infections are occasionally established, of which *pneumococcal meningitis* is the most frequent. One must

carefully exclude this possibility in any confused or obtunded patient with this type of bacterial pneumonia, since about 10% of patients with pneumococcal meningitis have an initiating pulmonary focus of infection. *Acute bacterial endocarditis,* usually localized on the aortic valve, is now a rare consequence of pneumococcal pneumonia because of the use of antimicrobial drugs. *Pneumococcal arthritis* and *pneumococcal peritonitis* are other septic complications. Fulminant pneumococcal bacteremia, often associated with *disseminated intravascular coagulation,* may occur in patients who have had splenectomy or are congenitally asplenic. The risk appears to be greatest in infants and young children, particularly those with underlying disease affecting reticuloendothelial function.

Prevention. The mortality from bacteremic pneumococcal pneumonia in the elderly and in patients with certain underlying diseases remains high despite the availability of penicillin. In type 3 pneumococcal pneumonia and bacteremia, mortality remains in excess of 50%. Since over 60% of pneumococcal bacteremias in adults are caused by

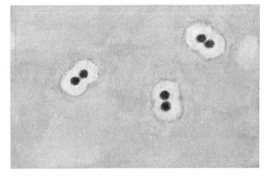

G. Quellung reaction. Swelling of bacterial capsule when exposed to antibody

only six types (1, 3, 4, 7, 8, 12), and 70% of those in children are also caused by either type 1 or just five more (6, 14, 18, 19, 23), attention has been directed toward development of a multivalent polysaccharide vaccine for immunization. Splenectomized patients, patients with sickle cell disease, patients with certain chronic diseases (cirrhosis, nephrotic syndrome) and the elderly are high-risk groups for which such immunization is indicated; a 14-valent polysaccharide vaccine is now licensed for use in the United States.

Klebsiella (Friedländer's) Pneumonia

About 0.5 to 5.0% of bacterial pneumonias acquired in the community are caused by *Klebsiella pneumoniae*. This organism, formerly known as Friedländer's bacillus, causes either "primary" or "secondary" pneumonia. In the former case, it is the initial bacterial pathogen when the patient seeks medical attention; in the latter event, it is a superinfecting organism complicating an existing pulmonary infection or an opportunistic invader in a debilitated or compromised host *(e.g., a tracheostomized patient on ventilatory assistance).*

Etiology. K. pneumoniae is an encapsulated aerobic gram-negative bacillus, somewhat larger than other coliform organisms. It forms large, glistening, mucoid colonies on solid media. About 1 to 6% of normal individuals are oropharyngeal carriers, and this percentage increases strikingly—up to 23%—in hospitalized patients. Aspiration of the causative organisms in such patients in the presence of compromised pulmonary defenses (weak epiglottal reflex, alveolar macrophage activity) initiates a secondary *Klebsiella* pneumonia.

Pathology. The histologic picture conforms in general to that of pneumococcal pneumonia, with a zone of peripheral edema and a more central one of consolidation. However, *Klebsiella* pneumonia differs from the pneumococcal variety in three respects: (1) the larger number of organisms present; (2) the necrotizing nature of the process, as evidenced by destruction of alveolar walls and abscess formation; (3) the occurrence of organization with extensive fibroblastic proliferation during resolution.

Klebsiella pneumonia is described classically as a dense lobar consolidation, most commonly involving the right upper lobe. It may, however, be segmental in distribution, and frequently involves the lower lobes, especially when occurring in its secondary form.

Extensive consolidation of an entire lobe occurs in primary *Klebsiella* pneumonia. In due course destructive changes predominate, producing abscesses, shrinkage of the lobe and scarring.

Clinical Features. Primary *Klebsiella* pneumonia occurs more frequently in older males who are alcoholics and to a lesser extent in patients with chronic bronchopulmonary disease and diabetes mellitus. The onset is usually abrupt, with rigors, pleuritic chest pain and productive cough. The sputum has a characteristic appearance: a viscid, homogeneous mixture of blood and mucus, resembling currant jelly or tomato juice.

On examination, the patient is found to be acutely ill, febrile, dyspneic and cyanotic. Auscultation usually reveals evidence of consolidation of one or two lobes, but early in the disease breath sounds may be diminished.

Empyema may complicate primary *Klebsiella* pneumonia; other sequelae such as purulent pericarditis and meningitis are much less common. The most frequent complication, occurring in as many as half the cases, is abscess formation; this may be evident radiologically within several days of onset of the pneumonia and can progress rapidly if appropriate treatment is not given.

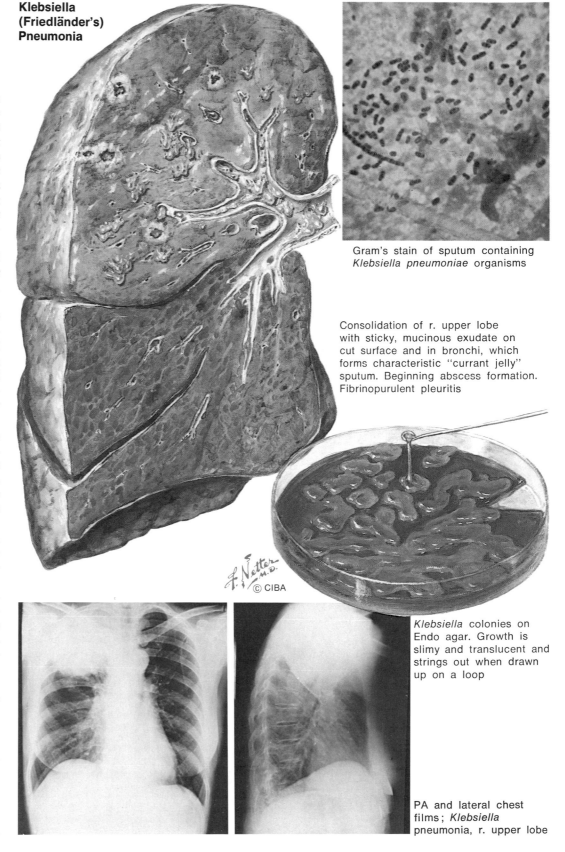

Klebsiella (Friedländer's) Pneumonia

Gram's stain of sputum containing *Klebsiella pneumoniae* organisms

Consolidation of r. upper lobe with sticky, mucinous exudate on cut surface and in bronchi, which forms characteristic "currant jelly" sputum. Beginning abscess formation. Fibrinopurulent pleuritis

Klebsiella colonies on Endo agar. Growth is slimy and translucent and strings out when drawn up on a loop

PA and lateral chest films; *Klebsiella* pneumonia, r. upper lobe

In an occasional patient the infection begins gradually and runs a subacute course. Failure to make the proper diagnosis and to use appropriate antibiotic therapy may allow the disease to smolder and progress. The result is a scarred upper lobe containing several cavities, mimicking chronic cavitary tuberculosis.

Leukocytosis is a usual feature of *Klebsiella* pneumonia, but marked leukopenia may occur and indicates a poor prognosis. Abundant granulocytes and large, plump, gram-negative bacilli are seen on a smear of sputum or tracheal aspirate. Occasionally a wide capsule about the organism is seen with Gram's stain.

The radiologic picture of *Klebsiella* pneumonia can be quite varied. The classic finding is uniformly dense consolidation of an upper lobe (usually the right upper lobe), with bulging of the fissure. However, a conclusive diagnosis of this or any pneumonia cannot be made on radiologic grounds alone, but only after bacteriologic study.

Over 80% of *Klebsiella* strains are susceptible to the cephalosporins, chloramphenicol, gentamicin or tobramycin. Treatment of the seriously ill patient requires initial use of two antibiotics. Prior to the antibiotic era, mortality from *Klebsiella* pneumonia ranged from 50 to 100%; mortality currently remains close to 50%.

Staphylococcus Aureus Pneumonia

Less than 5% of all bacterial pneumonias are caused by *S. aureus,* but the incidence increases considerably during influenza epidemics. The appearance of community-acquired staphyloccocal pneumonia is a very good indication of an influenza outbreak. About half the population are intermittent or persistent carriers of *S. aureus* in the anterior nares or nasopharynx. Isolation of the organism from these locations has no significance in regard to the etiology of any particular lower respiratory tract infection.

Etiology. Staphylococci on stained smear appear as clusters or as individual gram-positive cocci. Individual cocci are larger than streptococci. The two principal species, *S. aureus* and *S. epidermidis,* grow as small opaque colonies on blood agar. The former are usually yellow or cream-colored, whereas the latter are chalk white. Most strains of staphylococci pathogenic to man are *S. aureus;* for this reason distinguishing between the two species is important. Because differentiation on the basis of colony color is difficult and because some pathogenic strains do not produce pigment, reliance is placed on the *coagulase test.* A colony of staphylococci is suspended in broth containing diluted rabbit plasma. *S. aureus* (but not *S. epidermidis*) produces an extracellular enzyme, coagulase, which causes the plasma to clot in four hours. All strains that elaborate coagulase are defined as *S. aureus* even if they fail to produce pigment.

Pathogenesis and Pathology. *S. aureus* enters the lung by either of two routes. The more common is through the tracheobronchial tree, producing primary (bronchogenic) staphylococcal pneumonia. This form of pneumonia is most often seen in infants, in adults with influenza, or in debilitated hospitalized patients receiving antibiotics, corticosteroids or ventilatory assistance. *S. aureus* was the etiologic agent in the majority of cases of nosocomial (hospital-acquired) pneumonia in the 1950s; the gram-negative bacilli (*e.g., Klebsiella, Pseudomonas, E. coli*) have now supplanted *S. aureus* in this regard. The other access route is via the bloodstream, resulting in secondary (hematogenous) staphylococcal pneumonia. This occurs in patients with right-sided *S. aureus* endocarditis or in patients with prolonged staphylococcal bacteremia from a primary focus elsewhere.

Tissue necrosis and abscess formation are characteristic of staphylococcal pneumonia. The pleural space is often involved with development of empyema. Destruction of lung parenchyma may cause a sudden pneumothorax or pyopneumothorax, particularly in infants. The healing process may produce air-filled pulmonary cysts (pneumatoceles), which must be distinguished from thin-walled abscesses on chest x-ray films.

Clinical Features. Chills, high fever, dyspnea, pleuritic chest pain and cough productive of purulent or bloody sputum, occurring in the settings previously described, are features of this form of pulmonary infection. When staphylococcal pneumonia complicates influenza, there is usually a sudden worsening of the patient's condition, accompanied by high fever, tachypnea, cyanosis and the production of purulent sputum contain-

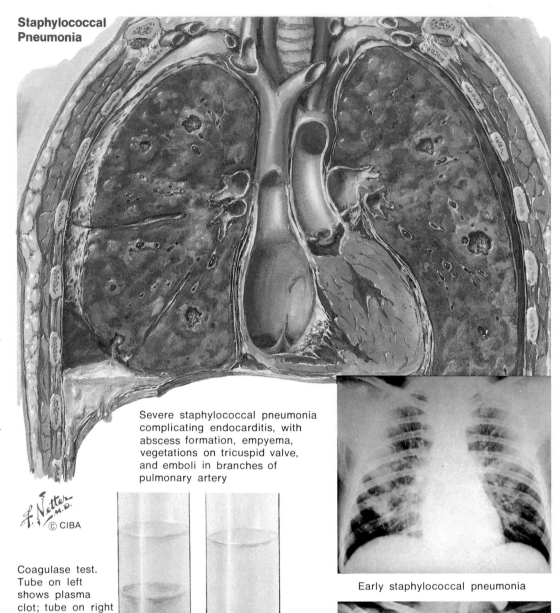

Staphylococcal Pneumonia

Severe staphylococcal pneumonia complicating endocarditis, with abscess formation, empyema, vegetations on tricuspid valve, and emboli in branches of pulmonary artery

Coagulase test. Tube on left shows plasma clot; tube on right is control

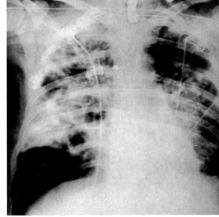

Early staphylococcal pneumonia

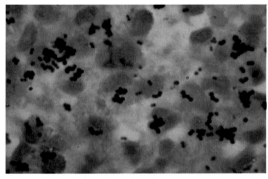

Staphylococci and polymorphonuclear leukocytes in sputum (Gram's stain)

Late staphylococcal pneumonia with abscesses and pneumothorax

ing abundant granulocytes and large gram-positive cocci.

Clinical Findings and Treatment. Physical examination discloses coarse and medium rales scattered over both lung fields. Signs of lobar consolidation are often not present; empyema, pyopneumothorax or pneumothorax may be evident.

Staphylococcal bacteremic pneumonia is characterized by high fever, hemoptysis, pleuritic pain and a chest x-ray appearance of multiple peripheral rounded densities, which rapidly cavitate. (This process occurs particularly in narcotic addicts with tricuspid or pulmonary valve en-

docarditis.) Chest roentgenograms show many foci of patchy consolidation involving multiple lobes. In swift progression multiple cavities, empyema and a pneumothorax can develop.

Empyemas should be drained by chest tube. Antibiotic therapy consists in the use of a penicillinase-resistant semisynthetic penicillin (oxacillin, nafcillin) or a cephalosporin compound (cephalothin), since currently about 80% of *S. aureus* isolates are resistant to penicillin G. In the penicillin-allergic patient, vancomycin is the principal alternative drug. The mortality is 10 to 20% with current therapy and even higher in debilitated older patients and infants.

Influenza Virus and Its Epidemiology

Viral Pneumonias

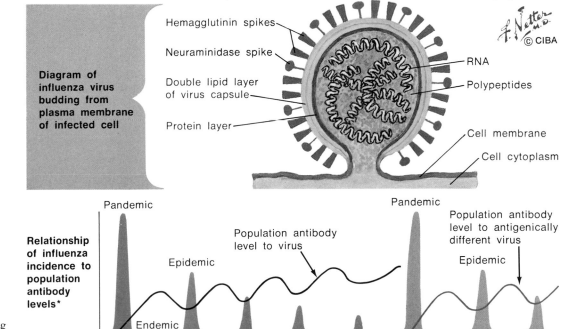

Electron microscopic appearance of influenza A$_2$ virus; filaments and spherical forms (x 10,000)

Virus viewed in section at much higher magnification (x 300,000)

Influenza virus invasion of chorioallantoic membrane cell of chick embryo. **A.** Attachment to cell membrane. **B.** Fusion of viral envelope with cell membrane. **C.** Penetration into cell cytoplasm

Diagram of influenza virus budding from plasma membrane of infected cell

Hemagglutinin spikes

Neuraminidase spike

Double lipid layer of virus capsule

Protein layer

RNA

Polypeptides

Cell membrane

Cell cytoplasm

Relationship of influenza incidence to population antibody levels*

*Modified after Kilbourne

Pandemic

Epidemic

Endemic

Population antibody level to virus

Pandemic

Population antibody level to antigenically different virus

Epidemic

Incidence of influenza

Incidence of influenza

Time (years)

Introduction of immunologically specific virus

New antigenically different virus mutation appears

Many viral agents cause pneumonia, including viruses that produce respiratory diseases in healthy individuals (influenza and parainfluenza viruses, adenovirus, respiratory syncytial virus, coxsackie virus, echovirus) and viruses that usually cause pneumonia only in a compromised host (herpes simplex virus, cytomegalovirus). Viruses associated with exanthematous diseases (measles, varicella-zoster) may produce pneumonia in normal or immunosuppressed hosts. Influenza is unique in its capacity to produce pandemics involving millions of individuals.

Influenza

Influenza is an acute, highly contagious viral infection of the respiratory tract. Viral proliferation occurs in the upper respiratory tract and trachea. In most patients the illness is benign, but it may be complicated by (1) primary influenza viral pneumonia; (2) secondary bacterial

pneumonia; (3) combined influenza viral pneumonia and bacterial pneumonia.

Etiology. The influenza virus is spherical, but filamentous forms also occur. It is covered with two types of protruding antigens (glycoprotein spikes), hemagglutinin and neuraminidase. Beneath these components is a lipid membrane which has budded from the plasma membrane of the host cell and contains host-derived lipid and carbohydrate. Immediately below the lipid layer is a protein membrane surrounding the nucleocapsid. The viral RNA genome is unusual in that it is composed of five to seven separate subunits, enabling the virus to undergo genetic

interchange. Thus, if a cell is simultaneously infected by two subtypes of influenza, their genes can be reassembled to produce additional hybrid variants.

Influenza viruses comprise three species (A, B, C), based on their nucleocapsid and membrane protein antigens.

The initial stage of infection involves attachment of the antigenic spikes of the virus to specific receptors on the host cell surface. Since identical receptors are present on red blood cells (RBC), agglutination of RBC is a rapid method for titration of influenza virus. The hemagglutinin binds

(Continued)

Viral Pneumonias
(Continued)

have occurred to unleash the major influenza outbreaks (see table). The pandemic of 1957 was caused by a species that had undergone decided changes in these coat proteins from the species responsible for the epidemic of 1947, while a further less marked change led to the 1968 pandemic. Significant antigenic shifts in one or both surface antigens occur about every 10 years.

Minor antigenic variations of the virus also occur between epidemics. After a pandemic caused by a new A_2 species, the mean population antibody level rises, and over the next several years the incidence of influenza attributable to this species remains low. As the antibody level falls in the population and as a new minor antigenic variant appears, a mild epidemic occurs. The antibody level in the population then rises again. Succeeding minor variants are followed by smaller and smaller outbreaks as the antibody level increases. By the end of a decade the selective pressure exerted by high antibody levels has eliminated all minor variants of the A_2 species. Thus the stage is set for selection of a markedly different antigenic variant capable of initiating a major pandemic.

Clinical Manifestations. The onset of influenza is usually abrupt, with high fever, headache, myalgias and severe prostration. Upper respiratory symptoms (dry cough, nasal discharge, "scratchy" throat) are common. The disease runs its usually benign course in three to five days.

The important complications of influenza result from spread to the lung. Uncommonly, mild segmental viral pneumonia occurs. Extensive pneumonia rarely develops, but in epidemic influenza large numbers of patients with severe pneumonia are seen.

Complications of Influenza. Primary influenza viral pneumonia, combined influenza viral and bacterial pneumonia, and influenza complicated by secondary bacterial pneumonia are the principal and potentially lethal complications of influenza. They occur more frequently in the aged, in patients with preexisting cardiac and pulmonary disease, and late in pregnancy, but may occur in otherwise healthy adults.

Primary influenza viral pneumonia is a generally serious disease with a high mortality, developing within one to three days of the onset of influenza. Symptoms are high fever, dyspnea and cyanosis. There may be no sputum, or the sputum may be bloody. Diffuse rales, wheezes and generally decreased breath sounds are characteristic, but signs of consolidation are absent. Bacterial pathogens and polymorphonuclear leukocytes are absent from tracheal secretions. Chest x-ray films show diffuse reticulonodular infiltrates that are more prominent in the midlung fields. Respiratory failure and vascular collapse supervene in the majority of cases.

Influenza complicated by secondary bacterial pneumonia has a latent period of three to six days between the onset of influenza and the appearance of the respiratory infection. The infection may be segmental or lobar in distribution, or may appear as a patchy bronchopneumonia. The sputum contains abundant neutrophils and bacteria, of which the principal invaders are *Streptococcus pneumoniae*, *Staphylococcus aureus* and, to a lesser extent, *Streptococcus pyogenes*, *Klebsiella* species, and *Hemophilus influenzae*.

Combined influenza virus and bacterial pneumonia. The onset of diffuse viral pneumonia is followed shortly by pleuritic pain and purulent sputum, suggesting the superimposition of bacterial pathogens. The radiologic picture usually shows segmental or lobar consolidation or scattered dense areas of bronchopneumonia. The bacteria involved are no different from those found in any secondary bacterial pneumonia.

Other complications, such as acute rhabdomyolysis (and myoglobinuria), myocarditis and toxic encephalopathy (including Reye's syndrome) may develop rarely.

Pathology. The lung in influenza virus pneumonia shows consolidation due to hyperemia and hemorrhagic edema of alveolar walls, accompanied by infiltration by mononuclear cells and neutrophils. Thromboses of alveolar capillaries occur, hyaline membrane formation is extensive,

(Continued)

Changes in Hemagglutinin (H) and Neuraminidase (N) Antigens in Relation to Pandemic Influenza Virus

the virion to the target cell. Once attachment has occurred, the viral envelope fuses with the host cell membrane. After being shorn of its envelope, the nucleocapsid enters the cell. When synthesis of new viral RNA and proteins has taken place, newly formed nucleocapsids migrate to the cell membrane where hemagglutinin and neuraminidase molecules have been incorporated. The nucleocapsid then buds from the surface, enveloped in the altered host membrane.

Epidemiology. Influenza A viruses are more mutable than B and C viruses and are responsible for major outbreaks of disease (see table). Techniques for viral isolation were unavailable in 1918, but circumstantial evidence suggests that the swine influenza virus, or a closely related strain, was responsible for the 1918 pandemic. Human influenza virus was isolated in 1933, and many antigenic variants have been identified since then.

Major shifts in antigenic properties of the hemagglutinin and/or neuraminidase molecules

Year of Emergence	Hemagglutinin	Neuraminidase	Previous Designation	Major Change in	Result
1918	Hswl*	N_1	Swine	?	Pandemic (severe)
1920s	H_0	N_1	A_0	H	No pandemic
1947	H_1	N_1	A_1	H	Pandemic (mild)
1957	H_2	N_2	A_2	N and H	Pandemic (severe)
1968	H_3	N_2	A_2 (Hong Kong)	H	Pandemic (moderate)

*Hemagglutinin of swine influenza type

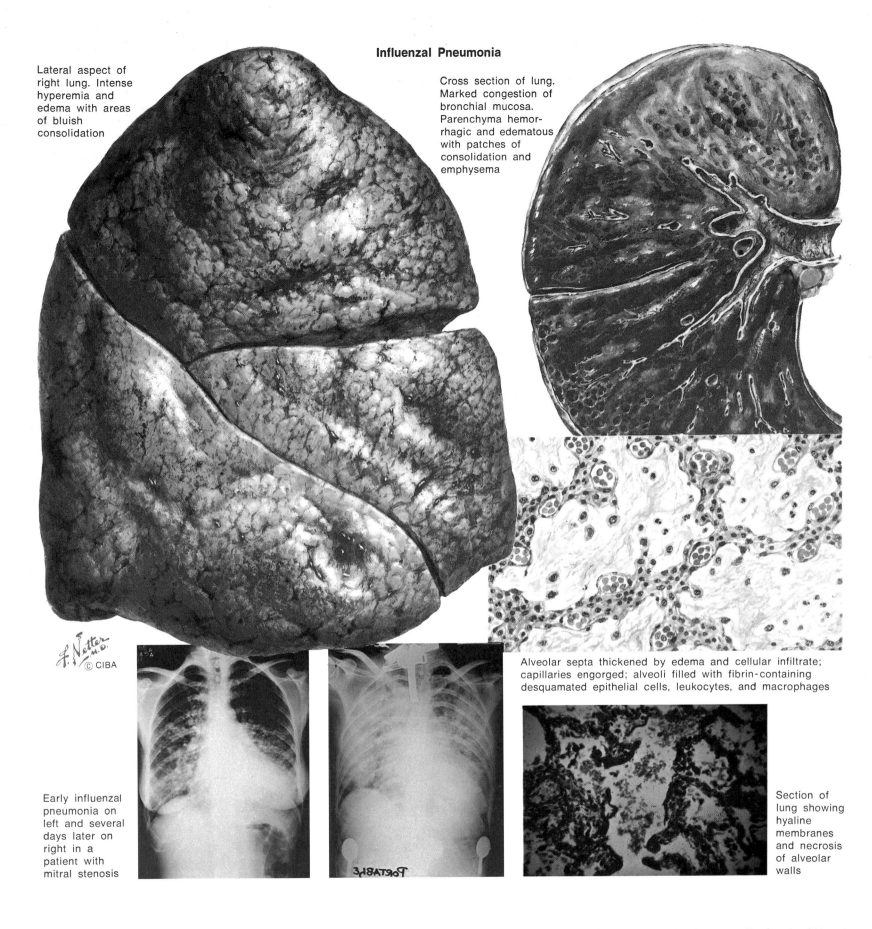

Lateral aspect of right lung. Intense hyperemia and edema with areas of bluish consolidation

Cross section of lung. Marked congestion of bronchial mucosa. Parenchyma hemorrhagic and edematous with patches of consolidation and emphysema

Alveolar septa thickened by edema and cellular infiltrate; capillaries engorged; alveoli filled with fibrin-containing desquamated epithelial cells, leukocytes, and macrophages

Early influenzal pneumonia on left and several days later on right in a patient with mitral stenosis

Section of lung showing hyaline membranes and necrosis of alveolar walls

SECTION IV   PLATE 71

Viral Pneumonias
(Continued)

and focal (fibrinous) necrosis of alveolar lining cells can be seen. Capillary bleeding into alveolar spaces may occur, as well as production of edema fluid.

Diagnosis. The diagnosis of influenza is relatively easy in an epidemic, but difficult in an isolated case when it is necessary either to isolate the virus from sputum or throat washings or to demonstrate a rise in antibody titer. For direct viral isolation, specimens are inoculated into the amniotic sac of chick embryos or into monolayers of monkey kidney cell cultures.

Prevention. Immunization with killed influenza virus vaccine can reduce the incidence of the disease by up to 70%, provided the vaccine strain is antigenically close to the one which is currently predominant. The usual vaccines contain several strains of prevalent influenza A and B viruses. Immunization annually for the fall and winter months is recommended for the elderly and for patients with chronic cardiopulmonary diseases.

Treatment. Specific treatment is lacking. Influenza viral pneumonia requires oxygen therapy, ventilatory assistance, careful monitoring and treatment of bacterial superinfection. Amantadine, a drug which acts by inhibiting influenza A virus penetration or uncoating, has some chemoprophylactic value (if administered before exposure), but no significant therapeutic effect.

Varicella-Zoster (Chickenpox) Pneumonia

Chickenpox is a highly contagious childhood exanthem that usually runs a benign course. Occasional complications include pneumonia, encephalitis, myocarditis, pericarditis, hepatitis, adrenal insufficiency, nephritis and purpura. Pneumonia complicating chickenpox in childhood is almost always bacterial in nature; in contrast, pneumonia occurring during chickenpox (or disseminated herpes zoster) *in the adult* is caused by the varicella-zoster virus.

Etiology and Pathogenesis. The same virus causes chickenpox (varicella) and shingles (herpes zoster). The virus is spread by the respiratory route, viremia ensues and the infecting agent is carried to the skin and other organs. In the rare adult with varicella, the infection can be severe, and diffuse interstitial pneumonia is common.

Herpes zoster is the recurrent form of infection, arising in adults who have had childhood varicella. The virus appears to remain latent in the sensory ganglia of spinal or cranial nerves for many years, but may emerge later, inexplicably, or during the course of immunosuppressive therapy. The vesicular eruption of zoster follows the dermatomal distribution of sensory nerves. Occasionally, widespread cutaneous dissemination takes place following segmental zoster. In the setting of disseminated zoster, zoster viral pneumonia can occur.

Clinical Manifestations. As many as one-third of adults with varicella may develop varicella pneumonia, which may be mild and evidenced primarily by radiologic changes, or severe with a fatal outcome. Pulmonary involvement occurs within five days of the appearance of the rash, which is usually extensive and hemorrhagic with vesicles often present in the oral cavity. The temperature is markedly elevated, and severe dry cough, dyspnea, cyanosis and anterior chest pain develop. Occasionally, blood-tinged sputum is raised. The peripheral white blood cell count may be elevated in about half the patients, but the differential count is normal. Physical findings (*i.e.,* rales and rhonchi) in the lungs are sparse in comparison with the clinical severity of the illness or the extent of radiologic changes. The patient usually recovers in three to seven days.

Radiologic Changes. The characteristic pattern on chest x-ray films is that of widespread nodular densities (larger than those occurring in miliary processes) superimposed on notably increased bronchovascular markings. The nodules sometimes coalesce to form patchy areas of consolidation. The process is most intense about the lung roots and gradually decreases toward the periphery.

Pathology. Pathologic changes in the lungs are similar to those seen in other types of viral pneumonia: proliferation and desquamation of alveolar septal cells, mononuclear cell infiltration of alveolar walls, focal hemorrhage and necrosis.

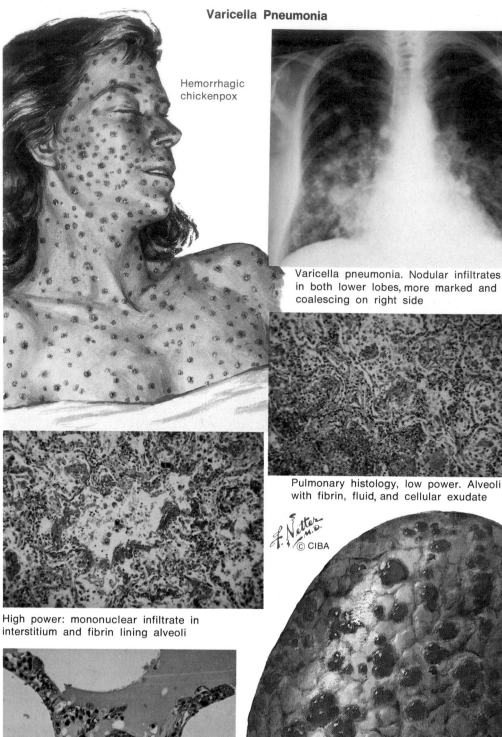

Hemorrhagic chickenpox

Varicella pneumonia. Nodular infiltrates in both lower lobes, more marked and coalescing on right side

Pulmonary histology, low power. Alveoli filled with fibrin, fluid, and cellular exudate

High power: mononuclear infiltrate in interstitium and fibrin lining alveoli

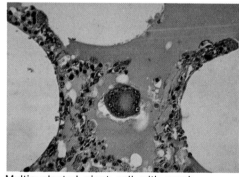

Multinucleated giant cell with much fluid in alveolus

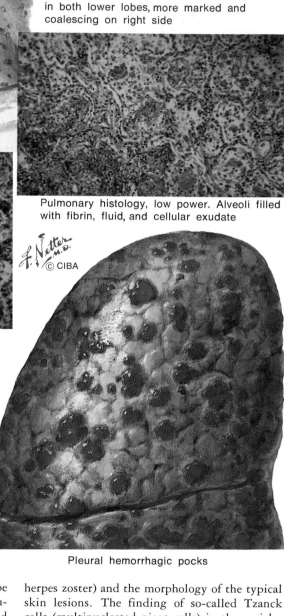

Pleural hemorrhagic pocks

Eosinophilic intranuclear inclusion bodies can be found in macrophages and septal cells. Multinucleated giant cells are present in skin vesicles and in the lung.

In severe varicella, pocks may occur not only on the skin surface but also on serosal surfaces such as pleura, pericardium and peritoneum. Scattered small calcified fibronodular lesions in the lung may be the residue from varicella pneumonia in some patients.

Diagnosis. Varicella pneumonia is diagnosed on the basis of clinical and radiologic features. The diagnosis can usually be made from a history of exposure (to a child with varicella or an adult with herpes zoster) and the morphology of the typical skin lesions. The finding of so-called Tzanck cells (multinucleated giant cells) in the vesicles helps to define the cause as a herpes virus.

Treatment. All adults with varicella should have chest x-ray films taken, and should be promptly hospitalized when indicated. Treatment requires careful observation for rapid progression of any respiratory involvement. Administration of oxygen, mechanical ventilation and careful monitoring for secondary bacterial infection are important aspects of treatment. Corticosteroid therapy has been employed, but generally has not seemed to alter the course of the disease.

Cytomegalovirus Pneumonia

Cytomegalovirus (CMV) is a DNA virus of the herpes group. It is remarkable for its high endemic prevalence (up to 80% of adults show serologic evidence of prior infection), the asymptomatic nature of most infections, the variety of clinical manifestations of active infection, and its capacity for reactivation upon depression of host defense (immunosuppressive therapy, graft-vs-host and host-vs-graft reactions). Congenital CMV infections are manifest during the neonatal period and follow several patterns: (1) fulminating disseminated infection with jaundice, anemia and hepatomegaly (usually with encephalitis and microcephaly), suggesting sepsis or erythroblastosis fetalis; (2) encephalitis with microcephaly, cerebral calcifications, deafness, visual defects and mental retardation; (3) respiratory distress syndrome associated with interstitial pneumonia. In older children and adults CMV causes: (1) heterophil-negative mononucleosis (including the postperfusion syndrome); (2) hepatitis; (3) secondary intestinal infection engrafted on ulcerative or inflammatory bowel disease; (4) aseptic meningitis, meningoencephalitis and Guillain-Barré syndrome; (5) disseminated infection (adrenals, liver, lung, retina) in immunosuppressed patients; and (6) CMV pneumonia in patients who are immunologically compromised.

Clinical Features. CMV pneumonia occurring in immunosuppressed patients commonly represents a mixed infection involving cytomegalovirus and other agents such as *Pneumocystis carinii, Nocardia asteroides* and *Aspergillus*. In many instances cytomegalovirus infection plays only a secondary role or is an incidental finding. However, CMV may be the major or sole cause of pneumonia in an immunocompromised host.

The usual symptoms are nonproductive cough, dyspnea and fever. Fine or medium subcrepitant rales are present in the involved areas, which may be unilateral or bilateral. The arterial PO_2 is reduced. The chest x-ray picture may show a small area of initial involvement, with rapid progression. The abnormalities are primarily those of an interstitial process, but can include airspace involvement.

CMV pneumonia may occur after renal or bone marrow transplantation. The risk of CMV infection of any type is high (50 to 90%) in the recipient of a donor kidney, and the mean incubation period in these circumstances is 50 to 60 days. Either the virus is introduced from an outside source (primary infection) or, more often, a preexisting quiescent infection is activated. The major origin of primary infection is the donated kidney. But transfused blood may also be responsible. Host-vs-graft (kidney) response appears to facilitate infection. In CMV pneumonia following marrow transplantation, the donor marrow is a likely source of the infecting virus.

Pathology. Histologic changes of CMV pneumonia include an interstitial inflammatory infiltrate of mononuclear cells, scattered alveolar hyaline membranes, accumulation of protein-rich fluid in alveoli and patchy alveolar hemorrhages. Intranuclear inclusion bodies are found in alveolar epithelial cells.

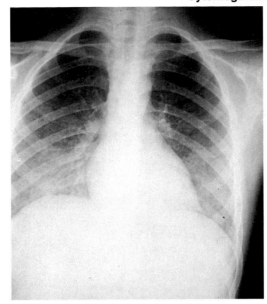

Diffuse densities in both lower lobes

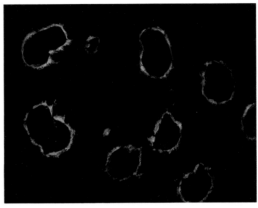

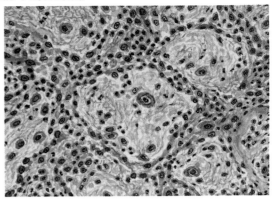

Lung histology in cytomegalovirus pneumonia. Cellular and fibrinous exudate in alveoli and in interstitium plus inclusion-bearing cells and epithelial desquamation

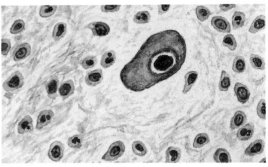

High magnification view of cell with inclusion body and cytomegaly

Cells infected with cytomegalovirus stained by immunofluorescent technique

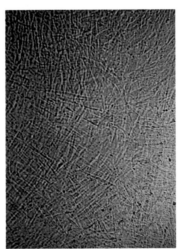

Normal tissue culture (HeLa) cells

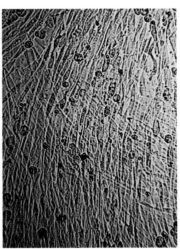

Tissue culture with early rounding of cells due to cytomegalovirus

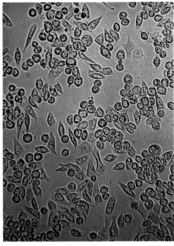

Tissue culture with late cytopathogenic effects due to cytomegalovirus

Diagnosis. Diagnosis of CMV pneumonia requires demonstration of the organism or its histologic effects in the lung. Because of the high incidence of this infection following transplantation, serologic changes or the presence of the virus in buccal swabs or urine is not sufficient to establish it as the main cause of pulmonary changes. Typical intranuclear inclusion–containing cells in bronchial brushings or characteristic histologic changes seen on lung biopsy establish the diagnosis. Confirmatory evidence is provided by immunofluorescent demonstration of the virus or by the finding of antibody in the presence of known virus-infected cells. The virus can be isolated in tissue culture, where infection of a monolayer allows spread between neighboring cells. Infected cells become swollen and rounded, and focal collections of them develop and enlarge.

Clinical Course and Outcome. Since many patients infected with cytomegalovirus are simultaneously infected with organisms other than CMV, the specific clinical course and outcome of this type of pneumonia are not well established. Most of the cases studied have come to autopsy. However, recovery can occur from even severe CMV pneumonia. Effective antiviral chemotherapy is not yet available. Decrease in immunosuppression may be helpful in management.

Legionnaires' Disease
(Pneumonia Due to Legionnaires' Bacillus)

"Legionnaires' disease" (L.D.) is a recently described (but probably previously existent) acute respiratory infection caused by an unusual gram-negative bacillus not known in the past as a cause of illness or yet designated as a species. The disease has occurred either as sporadic cases or as discrete outbreaks of "atypical pneumonia." Since 1964 there have been at least seven outbreaks in the United States attributable to the agent of *legionnaires' disease,* involving over 350 patients. More than 130 sporadic cases have been identified from all parts of the United States. The outbreaks have occurred in the summer, but individual cases have been observed all year round. It is estimated that the bacillus of legionnaires' disease is the cause of about 1% of all cases of pneumonia.

Etiology. A fastidious gram-negative filamentous bacillus (not yet classifiable) has been recovered from the lung or pleural fluid of a few patients with legionnaires' disease. It can be isolated on Mueller-Hinton medium (supplemented with 1% hemoglobin and 1% Isovitalex) in 5% carbon dioxide. It can also be grown by inoculation of guinea pigs or embryonated eggs. The organism is not revealed by tissue Gram's stain, but can be demonstrated in alveoli—particularly within macrophages—in sections stained with the Dieterle silver impregnation method.

Epidemiology. The ecologic niche of the L.D. bacillus is unknown, as is the source for the various outbreaks. The largest and most intensively studied cluster of cases (American Legion Convention, Philadelphia, July 1976) suggested airborne spread of the bacterium. A striking feature in both the sporadic cases and the small epidemics has been the lack of secondary infections among close contacts of patients. In several of the outbreaks construction work (earth-moving) had been going on in the vicinity.

Clinical Features. The disease is most common in middle-aged individuals, but occurs at all ages. Patients often have been heavy smokers. Predisposing factors appear to include chronic renal failure and immunosuppressive therapy. The incubation period is 2 to 20 days. The clinical onset, after a one to two day prodrome of malaise and headache, is abrupt with chills and fever up to 105°F. Cough is prominent but nonproductive. Pleuritic chest pain is common. Extrapulmonary symptoms include abdominal pain, diarrhea, vomiting and confusion (or delirium).

Physical examination reveals an acutely ill, tachypneic patient. Signs of consolidation are present in some patients; localized or diffuse rales are audible.

Routine laboratory studies are not helpful in making an etiologic diagnosis. There is a moderate leukocytosis with a shift to the left. Gram-stained smear of the sputum reveals few polymorphonuclear leukocytes and few, if any, bacteria. Indications of possible renal (proteinuria, microscopic

Legionnaires' Disease

A. Small, blunt, pleomorphic intracellular and extracellular bacilli in lung of patient with Legionnaires' disease as shown by Dieterle silver impregnation stain, × 1500 (after Chandler, et al.)

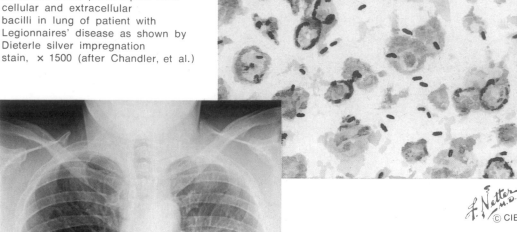

B. Chest x-ray film on fifth day of illness of 58-year-old man with serologically confirmed Legionnaires' disease. L. lower lobe consolidation the only involvement. Clinical improvement within 2 to 3 days of initiation of treatment with erythromycin. Radiologic changes did not completely disappear for 2 months

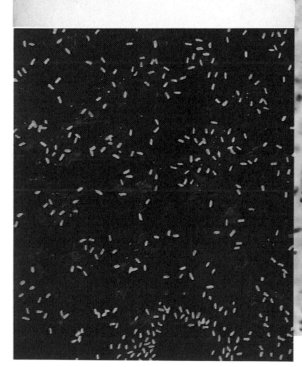

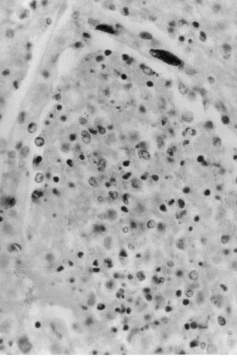

C. Legionnaires' bacilli identified by specific fluorescent antibody stain

D. Histologic section of lung (H and E stain) from fatal case of Legionnaires' disease. Extensive intraalveolar exudate present, containing many large macrophages

hematuria, azotemia) and hepatic (SGOT elevations) involvement may be present.

Radiologic findings in the chest include initial patchy infiltrates going on to lobar or multilobar consolidation in some cases. Small pleural effusions may develop. (Larger effusions may occur in patients receiving corticosteroids.)

Diagnosis. The diagnosis is usually established serologically (indirect fluorescent-antibody test using the L.D. bacillus) by the finding of a fourfold or greater rise in titer between acute and convalescent sera (reaching a minimum titer of 1:64). A single convalescent titer of at least 1:128 is highly suggestive of recent infection. Routine histologic

sections of lung show the picture of lobar pneumonia; macrophages, polymorphonuclear leukocytes and fibrin are abundant. The etiologic agent can be identified in fresh or frozen (or sometimes in deparaffined formalin-fixed) lung biopsy sections by direct fluorescent-antibody staining.

Treatment. The organism of L.D. is susceptible *in vitro* to a large number of antibiotics, although in experimental infections many of these drugs (penicillin, chloramphenicol, gentamicin, tetracycline) do not appear to be effective. On the basis of available clinical evidence and experimental data, erythromycin is the recommended therapy for patients with legionnaires' disease.

Pneumocystis Carinii Pneumonia

Pneumocystis carinii pneumonia (pneumocystosis) is an often fatal, acute, opportunistic pulmonary infection caused by organisms which are of unknown nature but which are generally considered to be protozoan. It occurs in compromised hosts such as (1) premature or malnourished infants, during the period of physiologic hypogammaglobulinemia; (2) infants and young children with severe combined immunodeficiency (Swisstype agammaglobulinemia); (3) patients with neoplastic disease, especially lymphomas and leukemias, frequently while undergoing antimetabolite and corticosteroid therapy; (4) patients who have recently undergone organ transplantation and have received corticosteroid drugs and other immunosuppressive agents. In the first two categories of patients *P. carinii* is usually the sole cause of the pneumonia; in the last two the role of *Pneumocystis* is more variable. It may be the only cause, or it may be a significant element in a mixed infection. Alternatively, *Pneumocystis* may be present but contributes little to the pulmonary picture.

Etiology. The life cycle of the organism in the lungs of infected animals or man includes a trophozoite stage followed by cyst formation. Subsequently eight oval bodies form within the cyst and are released as trophozoites, initiating another cycle.

Clinical Features. The impact of pneumocystosis is confined to the lung. Onset may be insidious over several weeks or abrupt in a two to three day period. Most patients have been receiving corticosteroid drugs, and the dose has often been reduced at the time of infection. Dry cough, fever and dyspnea are the major symptoms. Examination reveals tachypnea and cyanosis with scattered fine crackling rales heard in half the patients. There are no signs of consolidation, and pleural effusions do not occur. A chest x-ray film shows a diffuse bilateral reticulogranular pattern with definite airspace involvement, particulary in the central lung fields. Although an interstitial pattern is present, it is not the main feature.

Untreated, the disease has essentially a 100% mortality; treatment with pentamidine isethionate (and, more recently, trimethoprim-sulfamethoxazole) has reduced the mortality to between 20 and 50%. After institution of treatment, a response is observed in 5 to 10 days, but radiologic improvement may take weeks longer.

Although it is likely that clinical disease usually results from activation of endogenous infection, person-to-person transmission may be responsible for outbreaks among institutionalized children and for clusters of cases in hospitals.

Pathology. Histologic sections of involved lung show an interstitial infiltrate of mononuclear cells and alveolar airspaces filled with foamy eosinophilic material, in which there are no inflammatory cells. The proteinaceous eosinophilic material, with a honeycomb appearance in the alveolar spaces on hematoxylin-eosin staining, is a conglomerate of cystic organisms and trophozoites. With methenamine-silver staining under light microscopy, the cysts show up as round or semilunar black-staining objects (4 to 6

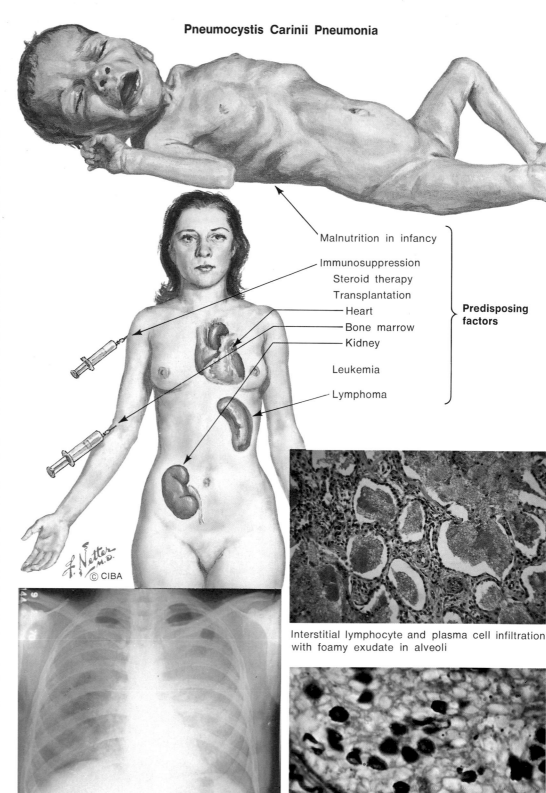

Pneumocystis Carinii Pneumonia

Malnutrition in infancy

Immunosuppression
Steroid therapy
Transplantation
Heart
Bone marrow
Kidney
Leukemia
Lymphoma

} Predisposing factors

Interstitial lymphocyte and plasma cell infiltration with foamy exudate in alveoli

Diffuse bilateral pulmonary infiltrates

Methenamine AgNo₃ stain showing *Pneumocystis* organisms in lung (black spots)

microns in diameter) against a blue backgound. The trophozoites do not stain with methenamine-silver but are seen as clear areas in the foamy material filling the alveoli.

Diagnosis. Bilateral pneumonia in an immunosuppressed host, particularly one receiving corticosteroids, raises the suspicion of *P. carinii* infection. The diagnosis is established by finding the organism in smears or histologic sections. *P. carinii* has not been grown in culture. Occasionally, the diagnosis can be made using secretions obtained by transtracheal aspiration, but usually, bronchial brushing, transbronchial biopsy, needle aspiration lung biopsy or open lung biopsy is

needed. Brushings or biopsy material, stained with Giemsa, methenamine-silver, Papanicolaou or Gram-Weigert stain, may provide the diagnosis before fixed tissue sections are available.

Measurement of immunofluorescent antibody titers is not a very sensitive diagnostic test, because many patients have a high degree of immunosuppression. A titer of 1:20 or higher is considered positive, and a rise in titer from negative to positive levels supports the diagnosis. About 25% of confirmed cases show a positive immunofluorescent antibody titer. However, demonstration of the organism is the only definitive way of establishing its presence in the lung.

Mycoplasmal Pneumonia

In the 1940s, a seemingly new form of segmental or interstitial pneumonia was described; it was labelled *primary atypical pneumonia* (PAP). It often occurred in outbreaks, especially in military camps. Bacterial pathogens were not isolated. This form of pneumonia has since proved to be caused by a variety of different organisms: viruses, rickettsiae (Q fever), chlamydiae (psittacosis) or mycoplasmas.

Although a variety of *Mycoplasma* species have been isolated from man, only *M. pneumoniae* is clearly established as a cause of human respiratory tract disease. Infection with this organism can take varied forms: pharyngitis, tracheobronchitis, pneumonia or asymptomatic infection. *M. pneumoniae* is the cause of at least half the cases of primary atypical pneumonia in young adults and of at least 4 to 9% of all cases of pneumonia (including bacterial) in urban adults requiring hospitalization.

Etiology. Mycoplasmas, formerly called "pleuropneumonialike organisms" (PPLO), are the smallest known free-living organisms. In the late 1940s a filterable agent *(Eaton agent)* from sputum of patients with atypical pneumonia was grown in embryonated eggs and caused pneumonia when inoculated intranasally in cotton rats. The offending pathogen was later grown in tissue culture. In 1962, Chanock and co-workers cultivated the organism on an agar medium and showed that it was a specific *Mycoplasma* species, *M. pneumoniae*. Infection of human volunteers with *M. pneumoniae* grown in the laboratory uniformly produced antibodies to the infecting agent and pneumonia in some subjects.

Mycoplasmas lack a cell wall and do not stain by Gram's method. On solid media the colonies are so minute as to require a hand lens or microscope for detection. They show up best when stained, and exhibit a granular surface with a dark center, providing a distinctive "fried-egg" appearance. Although most *Mycoplasma* species exhibit this "fried-egg" colony morphology, *M. pneumoniae* does not.

Clinical Manifestations. After an incubation period of about three weeks, the pneumonia has an insidious onset with malaise, headache, fever and a dry cough; occasionally there is an abrupt onset with high fever. Although it may be absent or only slight initially, *cough* soon becomes the dominant symptom. *Headache* is also very prominent. Most patients are uncomfortable but do not appear seriously ill.

The appearance of interstitial or patchy subsegmental pneumonia may be striking on chest x-ray films, yet physical findings are often totally absent. Infiltrates are characteristically in a lower lobe, unilateral, and more marked near the hilus. Sometimes upper lobe infiltrates are present, and suggest a diagnosis of tuberculosis. Occasionally, frank segmental or lobar consolidation is evident both radiographically and on examination. Pleural effusions are uncommon. Auscultation may reveal medium or fine subcrepitant rales.

The leukocyte count is usually normal, but in 10 to 25% of patients it may be elevated to 10,000 to 20,000 mm³. Sputum examination shows mainly mononuclear cells, although rarely neutrophils predominate. Normal flora are observed on smear and culture.

The course in the untreated patient is variable, with fever lasting several days to several weeks. Cough, malaise and radiologic changes often persist for three to six weeks. Bacterial superinfection is most unusual.

Rarely, complications occur during or immediately following mycoplasmal pneumonia. Bullous and hemorrhagic myringitis occurs in 2 to 8% of patients with naturally acquired disease. Neurologic manifestations or sequelae (Guillain-Barré syndrome, aseptic meningitis, meningoencephalitis, transverse myelitis) are very uncommon. Skin (Stevens-Johnson syndrome) and cardiac (myocarditis, pleuropericarditis) involvements have occurred but are also unusual features of this infection. Associated cold agglutin-induced hemolytic anemia may occur but is extremely rare; when it does occur, the level of cold agglutinins is usually markedly elevated (titers greater than 1:512), the anemia develops in the second or third week of illness, and jaundice is a feature.

Pathology. Pathologic study of human mycoplasmal pneumonia is limited because of the low mortality of this disease—less than 0.1%. Postmortem examination of the rare fatal case shows patchy or confluent bronchopneumonia, interstitial pneumonia, or acute bronchiolitis and bronchiolitis obliterans. Mononuclear cell infiltration of the peribronchiolar areas and alveolar walls is prominent, as in the viral pneumonias.

Epidemiology. *M. pneumoniae* spreads slowly (over several months) but extensively in families. Discrete localized outbreaks occur in the military and in school populations; the disease is endemic at military bases, and *M. pneumoniae* is responsible for 20 to 40% of cases of PAP among military recruits. Community-wide outbreaks may occur in cycles of four or five years, when the incidence of mycoplasmal pneumonia increases several fold. Unlike the usual bacterial and viral respiratory tract pathogens, this infection has no striking seasonal prevalence. However, more cases occur in the fall and early winter. The disease is most often found in school-age children, adolescents and young adults. It is much less common in the older population, in whom antibodies are usually present. Pharyngitis may be the only manifestation of *M. pneumoniae* infection in some susceptible contacts of patients with mycoplasmal pneumonia. Asymptomatic infection is also quite common. Among secondary cases of *M. pneumoniae* infection in families, 20% are subclinical.

Infection is spread by the respiratory route. The organism appears in throat washings and sputum several days before the onset of clinical infection, and persists for several weeks thereafter. Convalescent carriage may go on for as long as six to eight weeks and, if associated with a persistent cough, may be an important source for spread of infection.

Naturally acquired antibody is associated with a high degree of resistance to challenge with *M. pneumoniae*. Rare second attacks of mycoplasmal pneumonia have occurred in patients with immunodeficiency syndromes, and also in immunocompetent individuals.

Diagnosis. The diagnosis is suggested by the marked headache and cough, and the distinctive radiologic findings. Sputum production is scanty; mononuclear cells or neutrophils may predominate, but no pathogenic bacteria are found. Cold hemagglutinins (at a titer of 1:32 or greater) appear in the blood of 50% of patients by the end of the second week of illness, and their presence provides substantial support for the diagnosis. They occasionally occur during other infections (influenza, adenovirus and cytomegalovirus infections, and infectious mononucleosis), but the titers are usually low. Most cold agglutinins have anti-I specificity, I being an antigen present on erythrocytes of almost all individuals. The anti-I specificity of cold hemagglutinins in *M. pneumoniae* infections is probably due to the sharing of I-type antigenic determinants by *M. pneumoniae* and human red cells. Cold agglutinins are demonstrated by the mixing of serial dilutions of a patient's serum with a fresh suspension of human O-type erythrocytes or the patient's own red cells as antigen. After overnight incubation at 4°C, the presence of agglutination is determined; it is reversible at 37°C, unlike other antibody-mediated reactions of this kind.

Isolation of *M. pneumoniae* from sputum or throat washings provides a definitive diagnosis. The diagnosis can also be established serologically by complement fixation or indirect fluorescent antibody studies on acute and convalescent sera.

Treatment. As would be expected because of their lack of a rigid cell wall, mycoplasmas are resistant to antibiotics whose antibacterial action is at that site (*e.g.*, penicillins, cephalosporins). Consequently, erythromycin and the tetracyclines are the drugs of choice for treatment of mycoplasmal pneumonia. Drug therapy shortens somewhat the duration of fever and malaise, length of hospitalization, and duration of cough and abnormal radiologic findings. However, cough may persist, and continued shedding of organisms for several weeks is not uncommon after short courses of antibiotic treatment.

Mycoplasmal (Eaton Agent) Pneumonia (Primary Atypical Pneumonia)

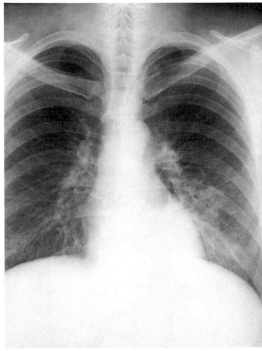

PA chest x-ray film: Patchy perihilar infiltrates chiefly in left lung

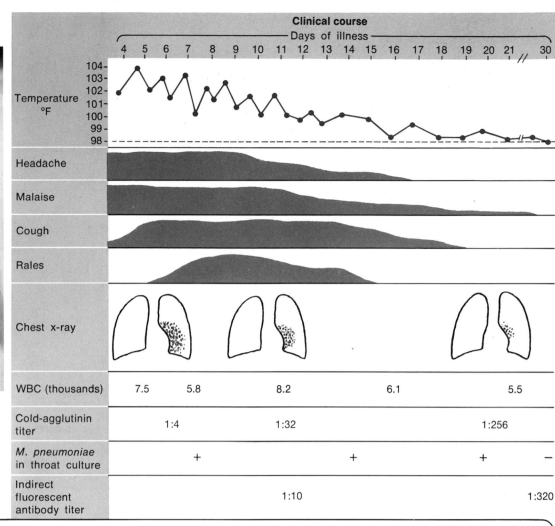

Clinical course						
Days of illness						

WBC (thousands)	7.5	5.8	8.2	6.1	5.5
Cold-agglutinin titer		1:4	1:32		1:256
M. pneumoniae in throat culture		+	+	+	−
Indirect fluorescent antibody titer			1:10		1:320

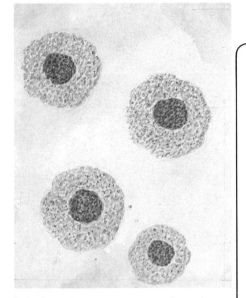

Colonies of mycoplasma growing on agar and stained, showing typical "fried egg" appearance due to penetration of agar by the growth in central area of each colony

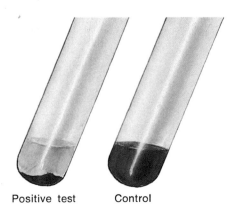

Positive test   Control

Cold-agglutinin test

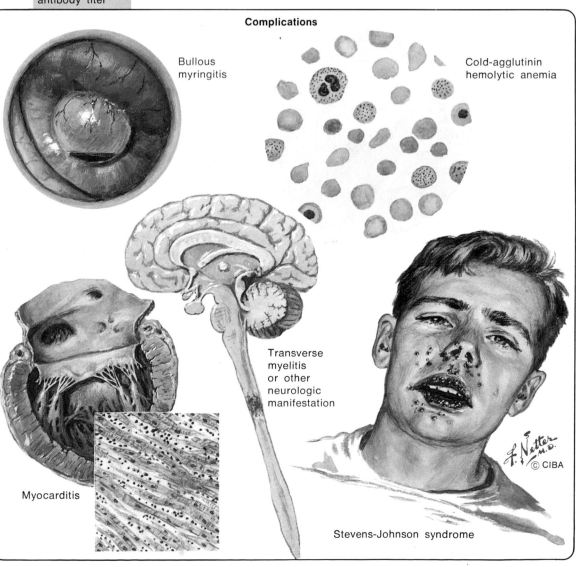

Complications

Bullous myringitis

Cold-agglutinin hemolytic anemia

Transverse myelitis or other neurologic manifestation

Myocarditis

Stevens-Johnson syndrome

Lung Abscess

Lung Abscess

Lung abscess is a localized inflammatory disease, with central necrosis surrounded by pneumonitis, that may be either acute or chronic. Most abscesses are due to aspiration of infected material from the upper airway in a patient who is unconscious or obtunded by alcohol, general anesthesia or drugs, or because of an epileptic seizure. The infectious agents in such cases are often initially anaerobic bacteria, and sometimes the suppuration is putrid. Aspiration of blood, infective material or other substances during tonsillectomy or tooth extraction has also been implicated as a causative factor.

Other causes include infection by specific organisms such as *Klebsiella pneumoniae* (Plate 68), *Staphylococcus aureus* (Plate 69), *Actinomyces bovis* (Plate 79), beta hemolytic *Streptococcus,* and *Amoeba histolytica.* In addition, abscess formation may occur as a result of bronchial obstruction by a foreign body or by actual cavitation within a bronchogenic carcinoma (Plate 57), and in a pulmonary infarct as a result of septic pulmonary embolism.

Lung abscesses are usually single when due to aspiration, but may be multiple when due to a staphylococcus. The locations of aspiration abscesses are highly characteristic because of the factor of gravity, the usual position of the unconscious or obtunded patient (supine), and the anatomy of the bronchial tree. A majority occur on the right side, because the right main stem bronchus is more in line with the trachea than the left. Since the bronchial orifices of the posterior segment of the upper lobe and the superior segment of the lower lobe on the right are posterior, these segments are most commonly involved. On the left side, the orifices of the apical posterior

A. Sagittal section of lung with abscess (cavity in superior segment of lower lobe containing fluid and surrounded by fibrous tissue and pneumonic patches). Also pleural thickening over abscess

B. PA x-ray film showing an abscess cavity with fluid level in superior segment of r. lower lobe

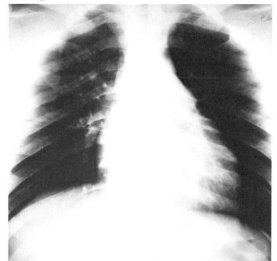

C. Same case as "B": after 2 1/2 months of treatment shows almost complete resolution

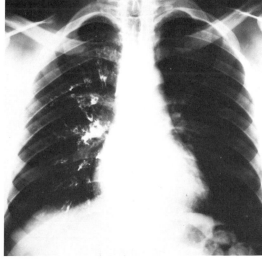

D. Bronchogram, same time as "C," reveals some persistence of cavity

segment of the upper lobe and the superior segment of the lower lobe are most directly in line with the main stem bronchus, so these segments are ordinarily the site of aspiration abscess, although the posterior basal segment of the lower lobe can also be involved.

The abscess usually communicates with a bronchus, and its purulent secretions are expectorated, so that a cavity with an air-fluid level results. If drainage is adequate and pneumonitis subsides, the abscess walls become thin, contract, and collapse. Otherwise, the abscess wall fibroses and persists. Occasionally, an abscess may rupture into the pleural cavity and produce an empyema,

sometimes with a persistent bronchopleural fistula. Rare complications include bronchiectasis, erosion of vessels with resultant hemoptysis, and hematogenous spread with secondary brain abscess.

Onset may be acute or insidious. The latter course is common in aspiration abscess. When onset is acute, symptoms include malaise, anorexia, productive cough, sweats, chills and fever. Sputum is purulent (unless there is no bronchial communication), often blood-streaked and sometimes foul-smelling. In aspiration abscess, prostration and high fever are rare. Pleuritic pain

(Continued)

Lung Abscess
(*Continued*)

Lung Abscess (continued)

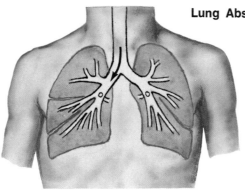

R. main bronchus is more in line with trachea than is the left, so that aspiration is more likely and incidence of abscess is greater on right side

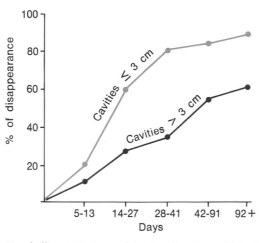

% of disappearance of lung abscess cavities in relation to size and time after beginning of effective antimicrobial therapy

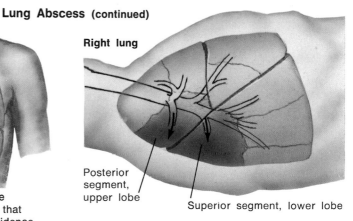

Right lung

Posterior segment, upper lobe

Superior segment, lower lobe

In supine position, posterior segment of r. upper lobe and superior segment of lower lobe are most vulnerable to aspirational abscess due to gravitational influences

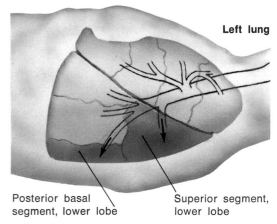

Left lung

Posterior basal segment, lower lobe

Superior segment, lower lobe

Although left lung is less commonly affected, superior and posterior basal segments are most vulnerable on that side

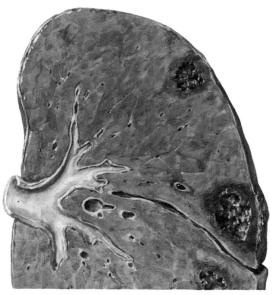

Multiple lung abscesses following septic embolization

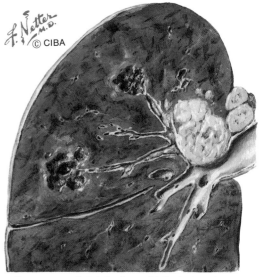

Abscesses distal to bronchial obstruction (in this case by carcinoma)

may be present. Weight loss is common in patients with severe and prolonged disease. Dyspnea occurs only with massive involvement or as a result of complicating disease.

Physical signs include a small area of dullness over the pneumonitis and often suppressed breath sounds with fine or medium moist rales. If the cavity is large, there may be tympany and amphoric breathing. Pallor due to moderate anemia is common, but clubbing occurs only with a chronic abscess of long standing.

The chest x-ray film shows a segmental consolidation and central cavitation, typically with an air-fluid level. Sputum should be examined by smear and culture for both aerobic and anaerobic bacteria. Blood cultures seldom reveal an organism. There is usually a mild to moderate leukocytosis, with an increase in polymorphonuclear cells, often with a rise in nonsegmented forms.

The course of the disease should be followed with chest x-ray films at daily to weekly intervals depending on the severity of the illness. Periodic 24 hour sputum collections, with attention to their volume and character, are necessary, in addition to surveillance of symptoms and signs. Resolution of disease is prompt after institution of appropriate antibiotic therapy. The drug of choice for aspiration abscess is penicillin G, which may be given orally or intramuscularly if the patient is unable to swallow medication.

If there is no clinical response in four to seven days, and if a specific pathogen has not been isolated, tetracycline may be substituted for penicillin. If a specific organism such as *Klebsiella*

or a staphylococcus is isolated, an appropriate antibiotic is given.

Postural drainage (see pages 286 and 287) should be used in addition to symptomatic therapy. Medical measures are continued until the pneumonitis has resolved and the cavity has disappeared or stabilized on serial x-ray films—usually within three to six weeks. If resolution does not occur, an obstructing lesion in the draining bronchus must be considered—particularly carcinoma—and bronchoscopy should be undertaken, along with an appropriate search for malignant cells or tissue. Therapeutic failure with an appropriate antibiotic regimen suggests an in-

correct diagnosis, and other causes of cavitation such as tuberculosis or fungus disease ought to be considered in such cases.

Planography and bronchography may show the persistence of a cavity or bronchiectasis despite the apparent resolution of disease on conventional x-ray films, but this defect is of no clinical significance in the absence of continued symptoms and signs. Because medical therapy is almost invariably successful in uncomplicated cases when the proper antibiotic is used, surgery is not indicated unless there is life-threatening hemoptysis, suspicion of underlying carcinoma, or chronicity of the abscess with persistent illness.

Actinomycosis

Actinomycosis is a noncontagious, chronic, suppurative or granulomatous bacterial infection occurring in man and domestic animals.

Actinomyces israelii, a gram-positive, filamentous, branching, non-spore-forming, anaerobic or microaerophilic, non-acid-fast bacterium, is the usual cause of actinomycosis. This organism, commonly called the ray fungus, is now classified as a true bacterium. There are at least four other gram-positive bacteria that may produce this disease; in decreasing order of importance they are: *Arachnia propionica, Actinomyces naeslundii, Actinomyces viscosus* and *Actinomyces odontolyticus.* These organisms exist as obligatory commensals in the human mouth, throat and gastrointestinal tract. Except for *A. viscosus,* which is facultative, they grow best anaerobically. Carbon dioxide stimulates the growth of most isolates, and the optimum temperature for incubation is 37°C. The organisms exhibit highly variable morphology, but are usually diphtheroid or filamentous, although bacillary and coccoid forms may occur. Branching in the form of V or Y is characteristic, but may be difficult to demonstrate.

Actinomycosis is a cosmopolitan, sporadically occurring endogenous infection. *A. israelii* has not been recovered from exogenous sources such as soil. In the United States, males are more likely to have the disease than females; most patients are in their second to fourth decade, but no age is exempt. Poor oral hygiene is important as a predisposing factor.

Clinical types of actinomycosis and their incidence include: cervicofacial (55%), pulmonary (20%), abdominal (20%) and disseminated (5%). Cervicofacial infection usually follows tooth extraction or other trauma to the oral mucosa and is characterized by a firm indurated mass in the region of the jaw ("lumpy jaw") that often suppurates and gives rise to multiple cutaneous fistulas. *Pulmonary actinomycosis* may result directly from a cervicofacial focus, or from extension through the diaphragm from an intraabdominal lesion. As a rule it is secondary to aspiration of the organism from the mouth, and generally the lower lobes are involved. Initial symptoms include mild fever and cough with purulent sputum. With abscess formation, the sputum may become blood-streaked. If not treated, the infection often spreads to the pleura and through the thoracic wall, causing subsequent empyema, soft tissue abscesses and multiple draining sinuses.

The clinical and roentgenographic signs of pulmonary actinomycosis are similar to those of nocardiosis, tuberculosis and other lung disorders. Abdominal infection most often follows appendectomy or bowel perforation, which may be either traumatic or spontaneous. Abdominal actinomycosis can involve any part of the gastrointestinal tract, but is more common in the cecum and appendix where it is frequently associated with sinus formation. In disseminated actinomycosis virtually any organ may be involved.

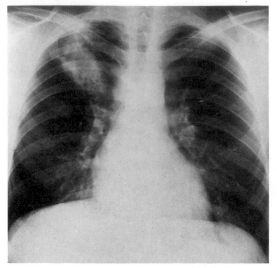

Actinomycosis of upper lobe of right lung simulating tuberculosis

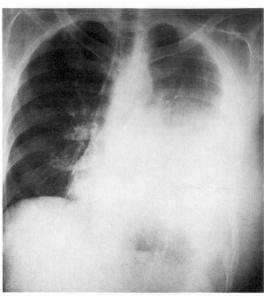

Pneumonia, empyema, and huge soft-tissue abscess of chest wall due to actinomycosis

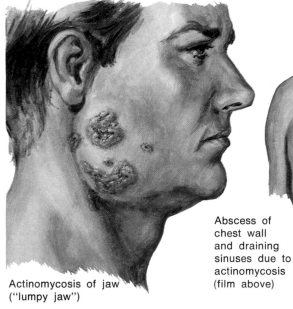

Actinomycosis of jaw ("lumpy jaw")

Abscess of chest wall and draining sinuses due to actinomycosis (film above)

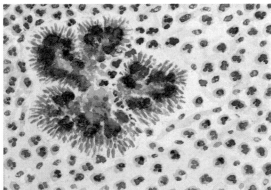

The "ray fungus" as it appears in H and E stained tissue section

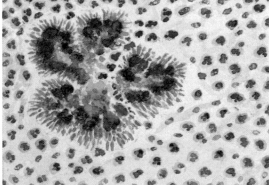

Pus in a Petri dish showing two sulfur granules (small lumps indicated by arrows)

Although the clinical findings are suggestive, actinomycosis is definitively diagnosed only by detecting *A. israelii* or a less common agent in pus from sinuses, empyema fluid, abscesses or other exudates. Pus should be placed in a sterile Petri dish and examined with a hand lens against a dark background for so-called sulfur granules. If present, these granules are yellowish white to white firm flecks that vary in size from a barely visible speck to 5 mm in diameter. Under an oil immersion lens, Gram's stain of the granules reveals delicate gram-positive filaments with coccoid and bacillary forms. Granules and other material should be cultured anaerobically.

Treatment. Penicillin is preferred for treatment of actinomycosis. Most infections heal after two to three months of therapy. If the patient is allergic to penicillin, such other agents as tetracycline, minocycline, erythromycin, lincomycin, clindamycin or chloramphenicol may be used. The benefits of chloramphenicol, lincomycin and clindamycin should be weighed against their potential toxicity. There is no advantage to combined chemotherapy. In the penicillin-allergic patient, tetracycline is probably the drug of choice.

Prognosis is excellent when the disease is diagnosed early and effective antimicrobial therapy is used.

Nocardiosis

Nocardiosis

Nocardiosis is an uncommon, suppurative, bacterial infection of man and animals usually caused by *Nocardia asteroides*. Although the lungs, skin and subcutaneous tissues are ordinarily involved, the disease may spread to other parts of the body, particularly to the central nervous system, with the production of pyogenic brain abscess or, less frequently, meningitis.

N. asteroides is a gram-positive, nonmotile, nonencapsulated, partially acid-fast, filamentous, aerobic organism, in the past considered a fungus but now classified as a highly evolved bacterium. Less commonly, other species of *Nocardia* such as *N. madurae, N. brasiliensis* and *N. caviae* also produce disease in man. All of these agents grow as filaments that fragment to yield bacillary and coccoid forms.

Nocardia species occur worldwide and exist in the soil as saprophytes. Man and such animals as cats, dogs and guinea pigs usually become infected by inhaling the organisms. There is no person-to-person or animal-to-person transmission. Individuals of all ages may be infected, but most cases occur between the third and fifth decades of life. Males contract the disease three to four times as often as females, presumably because of occupational exposure. Although nocardiosis may be an "opportunistic" illness, particularly in patients with lymphoreticular malignancies and in patients with pulmonary alveolar proteinosis, it is also seen in persons without discernible defects in host defense. In occasional cases *Nocardia* can be cultured from the sputum of patients who have no detectable evidence of clinical disease.

The high incidence of primary pulmonary involvement suggests that the respiratory tract is the most common portal of entry, although the organism may enter the body in contaminated food or may be traumatically implanted into the skin and subcutaneous tissue (especially *N. brasiliensis* and *N. madurae*). In the lungs, nocardiosis produces a disease ranging from chronic to fulminating; in other viscera and skin, it causes chronic suppuration, sinuses and abscess formation. From the primary site of infection there may be hematogenous dissemination to almost any organ, but especially to the central nervous system.

Presenting symptoms are often similar to those of tuberculosis and include fever, night sweats, cough productive of purulent sputum, and weight loss. X-ray manifestations of pulmonary nocardiosis can also mimic those of tuberculosis and other pulmonary disorders; there may be upper or lower lobe involvement and marked suppuration of the involved lung. Empyema is common. Initially, the patient may have fever, without localizing manifestations. Fever, headache, stiff neck, nausea and vomiting usually occur in patients with brain abscess and meningitis. Nocardiosis may also show itself as a localized, chronic, suppurating granuloma of subcutaneous tissues and bones, with draining sinuses.

Nocardiosis should be suspected in any patient with an undiagnosed suppurative pneumonia unresponsive to conventional antimicrobial therapy, particularly if there is immunosuppression due to drugs or a complicating disease. However, defini-

Massive pneumonialike lesion, r. upper lobe

Multiple necrotic abscesses in r. upper lobe covered by extensive pleuritis

Nocardia asteroides in culture on Sabouraud's glucose agar. The branching filaments do not appear in yeast phase. In sputum or pus, filaments fragment and may be mistaken for tubercle bacilli since they may be acid-fast

Brain abscess with blood in ventricles and asymmetric lobes due to nocardiosis

Section showing acid-fast organisms in brain tissue

Multiple nocardial abscesses in kidney

tive diagnosis of nocardiosis depends on the isolation of *N. asteroides* or other *Nocardia* species from clinical specimens. Gram's stains of expectorated sputum or pus usually reveal gram-positive, branching, nonseptate, slender filaments or hyphae. Acid-fastness is variable in nocardial species, both in clinical specimens and in culture, but, when observed, it is helpful in distinguishing these organisms from others that are not acid-fast. When fragmented, the organisms may appear in bacillary form on smears of sputum or pus or in tissue sections, and they can easily be confused with various mycobacteria. A mistaken diagnosis of tuberculosis may result.

Treatment. Sulfadiazine is the drug of choice, and treatment is continued for six months after clinical lesions have disappeared. Preferred treatment currently consists of a sulfonamide preparation in combination with either minocycline or ampicillin.

Before sulfonamide therapy was available, about 75% of patients with nocardiosis died. Even with treatment the overall case fatality is still about 50%. If the infection disseminates to the central nervous system, the mortality may be greater than 80%. In patients with localized pulmonary nocardiosis and no underlying disease, the death rate is about 10%.

Histoplasmosis

Histoplasmosis

Ulcerating lesion of tongue due to histoplasmosis. Lesion is identical in appearance to carcinoma of tongue

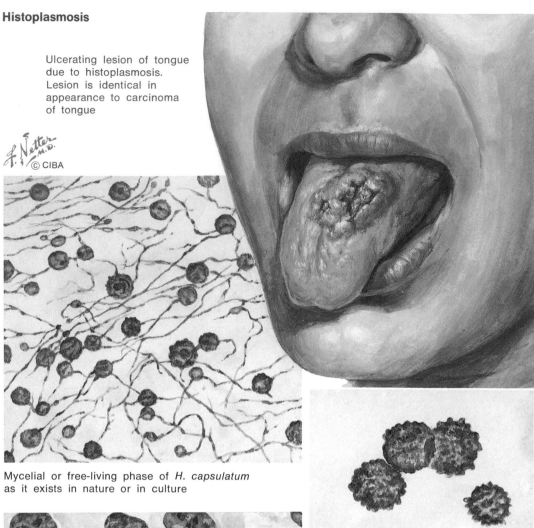

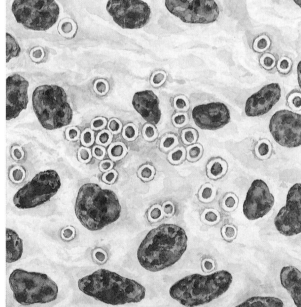

Mycelial or free-living phase of *H. capsulatum* as it exists in nature or in culture

Spores of mycelial phase of *H. capsulatum.* Inhalation of these is source of infection

H. capsulatum in tissue

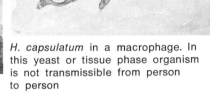

H. capsulatum in a macrophage. In this yeast or tissue phase organism is not transmissible from person to person

Histoplasmosis is caused by inhalation of spores from the free-living biphasic fungus *Histoplasma capsulatum.* The organism exists widely in nature and is found throughout the United States, but is most common in the St. Lawrence and Missouri-Ohio-Mississippi River valleys. It also exists in South and Central America and, indeed, in most of the river valleys throughout the world between the 45th parallel north and the 45th parallel south, with the possible exception of the Nile River. Factors controlling the growth of the fungus in nature appear to be related to the presence of droppings of bats and birds such as chickens, pigeons, blackbirds, starlings, oilbirds (*quacharo,* a South American nocturnal fruit eater) and grackles, all of which seem to provide in their excreta the essential elements for stimulating growth of the fungus. Thus, exposure to soil that has been contaminated with the excreta of bats or birds is the chief way in which the infection is acquired.

Infections with *H. capsulatum* are extremely common; it has been estimated that at any one time some 30 million living Americans have been infected with this organism. In the vast majority of cases the infection is subclinical, and the individual is not aware that it has occurred. In other persons the disease may manifest itself in the form of a flulike syndrome or a mild or severe pneumonia, which is usually self-limited and often undiagnosed. When the pulmonary lesions heal, they often leave the lungs studded with miliary calcific deposits, and this roentgenographic appearance is virtually pathognomonic of a former histoplasmal infection. In a few infected

individuals the pulmonary disease is chronic and progressive and closely simulates cavitary tuberculosis. On even rarer occasions it may disseminate in an acute or chronic manner throughout the body to the bone marrow, skin, liver, spleen, meninges and alimentary tract. When untreated, this form of histoplasmosis is usually fatal.

Other pulmonary manifestations of histoplasmosis may include: (1) a single small pulmonary density with unilateral hilar lymphadenopathy which, when calcified, may be identical in appearance to the primary complex or Ghon complex of primary tuberculosis; (2) a larger localized

(Continued)

Histoplasmosis
(Continued)

Histoplasmosis (continued)

Diffuse pneumonic lesions throughout both lungs, representing acute or epidemic histoplasmosis

Miliary histoplasmosis

Many small parenchymal and hilar areas of calcification in both lungs; classic appearance of healed histoplasmosis

Bilateral infiltrates with cavitation in l. upper lobe. This chronic progressive, cavitary form of histoplasmosis appears identical to tuberculosis
© CIBA

pneumonic infiltrate associated with hilar adenopathy; (3) a single nodule or coin lesion, which may be uncalcified and simulate a bronchogenic carcinoma or contain a central core and concentric rings of calcium identical to those in a tuberculoma; (4) multiple pulmonary nodules simulating metastatic tumor; (5) pleural effusions without parenchymal disease; (6) mediastinal lymphadenopathy without parenchymal lesions, simulating lymphoma; and (7) bilateral hilar adenopathy simulating sarcoidosis.

When the spores from the free-living mycelial phase of *H. capsulatum* gain entry into the body, they convert to the tissue or yeast phase and appear as tiny intracellular, encapsulated organisms. This is the form in which the fungus appears in tissues, sputum and other body excrements. It is not transmissible from person to person, and the illness is therefore noncontagious. Demonstration of the offending organism in body tissue or

excrements by microscopy, and confirmation by culture, are the only absolute ways of establishing a diagnosis.

Serologic tests are often difficult to interpret. Complement fixation titers of 1:8 to 1:16 are of doubtful significance, since false positive reactions in this range are not uncommon. However, high or rising complement fixation titers may be regarded as strong evidence that histoplasmosis (or a similar fungus infection) is present. Nonetheless, serologic studies can never be regarded as establishing more than a presumptive diagnosis. The histoplasmin skin test is essentially worthless for diagnostic purposes; in addition, it has the disadvantage of causing a false positive rise in complement fixation titers, often leading to diagnostic confusion.

Treatment is indicated for the disseminated form of histoplasmosis, for chronic progressive

pulmonary disease and for cases of acute pneumonia that are unusually severe. None of the other forms of histoplasmosis requires specific treatment unless progression of the lesions is demonstrated.

Treatment. Acute pneumonic histoplasmosis, if particularly severe, may be treated with a short course of amphotericin B. The concomitant use of hydrocortisone is helpful in relieving toxicity caused by the disease or by amphotericin B.

In the treatment of chronic progressive histoplasmosis or disseminated disease, amphotericin B should be administered in full doses. Rifampin should probably be given concurrently, since this drug has been shown to exert a synergistic effect when used in combination with amphotericin B in animal and *in vitro* studies. However, clinical trials with this drug combination have not yet been reported.

Coccidioidomycosis

Coccidioides immitis (valley fever fungus) grows in the arid or semiarid soil of North, South and Central America. The organism is biphasic and exists in culture and in nature in a mycelial phase. Its arthrospores are light and fluffy and highly infectious. In the body the fungus converts into a yeastlike spherule which produces endospores. In this form the organism is not transmissible from person to person, but after extrusion from the host's body it will convert back to the infectious vegetative phase if suitable conditions develop. Coccidioidomycosis has been reported in humans and animals in Mexico, Paraguay, Argentina, Venezuela, Peru and Bolivia. In the United States it is endemic in California, Arizona, Nevada, New Mexico, Utah and western and southwestern parts of Texas.

Humans may become infected simply by passing through an endemic area, and it is believed that at any one time some 10 million living Americans in the southwestern United States are infected with the spores of *C. immitis*. Animals, including dogs, cattle, sheep and rodents, are also susceptible to infection; dogs are most susceptible to disseminated disease. For unknown reasons, dark-skinned people manifest more severe disease and are more susceptible to dissemination than are members of light-skinned races.

Infections with *C. immitis* are exceedingly common in endemic areas, but, as with histoplasmosis, clinical illness does not develop in the vast majority of infected individuals; the only evidence of infection is the later development of delayed cutaneous hypersensitivity to coccidioidin. In the southern San Joaquin Valley the incidence of skin reactivity in schoolchildren has been reported to be as high as 90%, although the figure is somewhat lower in more recent studies. The number of infected individuals is believed to be between 35,000 and 100,000 per year.

In spite of the large number of infections which are known to occur, in about two-thirds of these cases no significant clinical illness develops, although an occasional pulmonary granuloma or cavity may be left behind. In the remaining one-third a pneumonitis may arise which is of sufficient severity to be brought to the attention of a physician. Typical symptoms are fever, pleuritic chest pain, cough, general malaise and sometimes erythema nodosum, particularly in females and young children.

The chest x-ray film ordinarily shows single or multiple areas of patchy pneumonitis, either unilateral or bilateral. Hilar or mediastinal adenopathy or pleural effusion may be present. The primary pneumonitis usually clears spontaneously, leaving a residual in the form of a nodule or a cavity in about 5% of the cases. In about 1% of patients the disease may spread to any or all organs of the body including the skin, bones, meninges, liver, spleen, kidneys, adrenals, myocardium and prostate.

An absolute diagnosis can be established only by demonstration of the causative organism, but a positive complement fixation test is highly suggestive of the correct diagnosis, and a high or

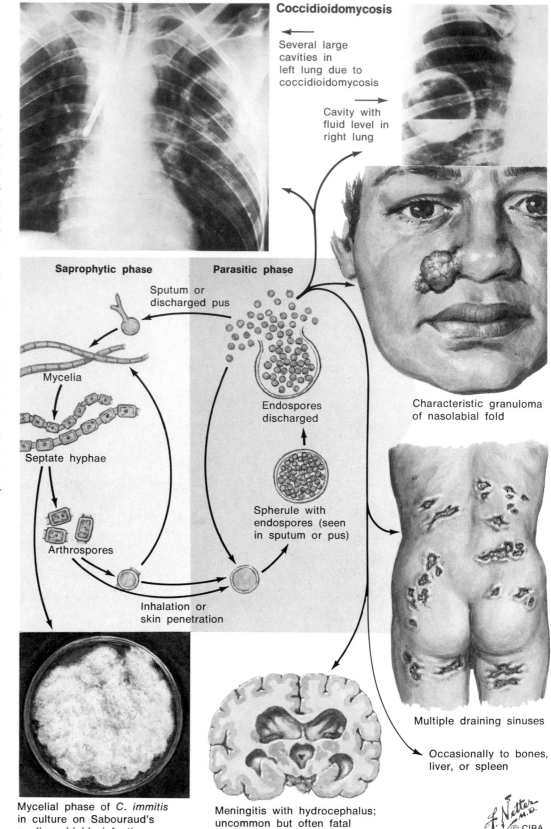

Coccidioidomycosis

Several large cavities in left lung due to coccidioidomycosis

Cavity with fluid level in right lung

Characteristic granuloma of nasolabial fold

Saprophytic phase

Parasitic phase

Sputum or discharged pus

Mycelia

Septate hyphae

Arthrospores

Inhalation or skin penetration

Endospores discharged

Spherule with endospores (seen in sputum or pus)

Multiple draining sinuses

Occasionally to bones, liver, or spleen

Mycelial phase of *C. immitis* in culture on Sabouraud's medium; highly infectious

Meningitis with hydrocephalus; uncommon but often fatal

rising titer (above 1:32) is present in most cases of disseminated infection.

Most patients with primary pulmonary infection will recover spontaneously. However, a definite course of treatment is indicated in infants; debilitated elderly individuals; patients with severe pneumonia in whom there are high antibody titers, especially if they are nonwhites; diabetics; pregnant women; and patients receiving cortisone or other immunosuppressive drugs. Treatment is also advisable in patients with so-called progressive primary disease, particularly those with persistent hilar or mediastinal lymphadenopathy and accompanying rising complement-fixing antibody titers.

Treatment. Amphotericin B is the only drug of established value in the treatment of coccidioidomycosis. The drug is administered intravenously, and dosage varies with the age of the patient. In patients with meningeal involvement it may be necessary to give amphotericin B by the intrathecal, intracisternal or intraventricular route for months or even years.

Corticosteroids are helpful adjuncts to suppress the severe allergic manifestations of the primary infection or the toxic effects of amphotericin B, and there is some evidence that tetracycline is synergistic against *C. immitis* when given in combination with this antifungal agent.

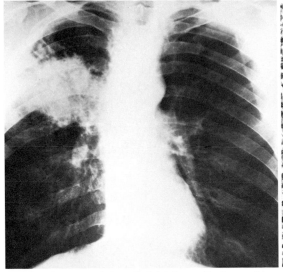

Lesion in upper lobe of right lung. Radiographic pattern may, however, be very diverse

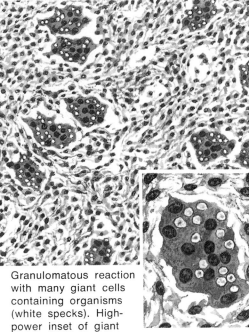

Granulomatous reaction with many giant cells containing organisms (white specks). High-power inset of giant cell with organisms

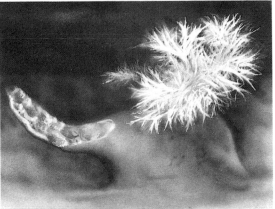

Organism in culture; free-living or infectious phase of *Blastomyces dermatitidis*

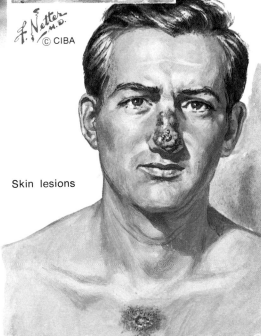

Very high-power view of a budding and nonbudding organism

Skin lesions

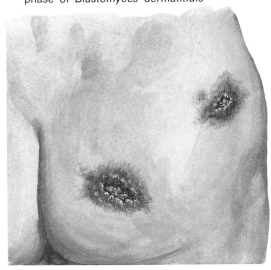

North American Blastomycosis

North American blastomycosis is caused by inhalation of the infective spores of the diphasic fungus *Blastomyces dermatitidis*. The organism exists in soil or on forest vegetation in a *mycelial* or *filamentous* form, which can be cultured on Sabouraud's agar at room temperature. When the spores from the mycelial growth gain entry into the body, either by inhalation or rarely by direct inoculation, the organism converts into a *yeast with single buds;* it can be cultured in this form on blood agar at 37°C. The yeast phase is found in infected tissue, pus, sputum or other body exudates. It is noninfective, and the disease is therefore nontransmissible from person to person. However, on expulsion from the body of the host, the organism can probably change back to its vegetative form under suitable conditions, although attempts to accomplish this conversion experimentally have not been successful.

Blastomycosis usually occurs in individuals whose occupations bring them into close contact with the soil or raw timber. It is found principally in the Mississippi–Ohio River valleys and the South-Central and Middle Atlantic states. However, cases have occurred in all parts of the United States and some provinces of Canada, as well as Mexico, Central America and Africa. Blastomycosis also occurs in animals, and surveys in Arkansas, Mississippi and Kentucky indicate that the infection is more frequent in dogs than in man. There is no evidence to indicate that the infection is transmitted from dogs to man or vice versa. Apparently both acquire the disease from a common source in the soil.

The disease may remain localized in the lungs or disseminate throughout the body, affecting the skin, bones, meninges, brain and genitourinary tract.

Principal symptoms include cough (60%), weight loss (47%), chest pain (44%), fever (38%) and hemoptysis (35%). X-ray manifestations are those of pneumonitis, large and small nodules or masses, cavitation, and diffuse miliary patterns. Lesions may be unilateral or bilateral and involve any or all lobes of the lungs. They may closely simulate a bronchogenic carcinoma in appearance, as well as tuberculosis and other pulmonary disorders.

The diagnosis of blastomycosis is made by demonstrating the presence of the causative or-

ganism in the patient's sputum, gastric contents, prostatic secretions, spinal fluid, urine, other exudates or body tissue. Any diagnosis that does not include the demonstration of *B. dermatitidis* must be considered presumptive. Skin tests are totally unreliable, and complement fixation tests are only infrequently helpful.

Although occasional lesions due to proved blastomycosis have been observed to undergo spontaneous regression and apparent cure, identification of *B. dermatitidis* in any body exudate or tissue is an absolute indication for specific treatment.

Treatment. Amphotericin B given by intravenous injection is the most effective drug available

for the treatment of blastomycosis. Hydroxystilbamidine isethionate (commonly referred to as 2-hydroxystilbamidine) is another agent effective against blastomycosis. However, since the relapse rate is somewhat higher with this drug, its use should probably be restricted to mild infections, or to patients who cannot tolerate amphotericin B.

Rifampin has been shown to exert a definite fungistatic effect on *B. dermatitidis* and a synergistic fungicidal action when used in combination with amphotericin B. Administration of this agent along with customary or smaller amounts of amphotericin B, now represents the probable treatment of choice for blastomycosis.

South American Blastomycosis

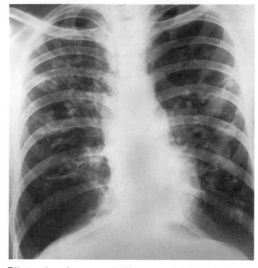

Bilateral pulmonary infiltrates which closely resemble tuberculosis. Pulmonary lesions may range from minimal to very extensive

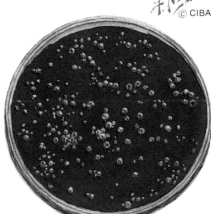

Lesions of lips, nose, and tongue with cervical lymphadenopathy

South American Blastomycosis

South American blastomycosis, known in Latin American countries as paracoccidioidomycosis, is caused by inhalation of the spores of a biphasic fungus, *Paracoccidioides brasiliensis*. Although the lung is probably the main portal of entry into the body, in some instances direct inoculation into skin or mucous membranes seems to have occurred. The organism lives in soil or on vegetable matter in a *mycelial form* and can be cultured in this phase on Sabouraud's glucose agar at room temperature. After gaining entry into the body, the fungus is transformed into a *yeast*, which reproduces itself by the formation of multiple buds. However, organisms with single buds are also observed. The yeast form of the fungus can be cultured on blood agar at 37°C, and when it is extruded from the body of the host, it can revert to the free-living mycelial or vegetative phase under suitable conditions. The yeast, however, is not transmissible from person to person.

The disease was first discovered in Brazil, where the greatest number of cases has been reported, but it has also been found in other countries of Central and South America, including Mexico, Guatemala, Honduras, Panama, Argentina, Bolivia, Colombia, Ecuador, Paraguay, Peru, Uruguay and Venezuela. The true incidence of South American blastomycosis in most of these countries is unknown, but the magnitude of the problem is illustrated by the fact that by 1964, 2,902 cases had been registered at the University of São Paulo, Brazil. Since the disease may have a very long incubation period (30 years or more), cases have been detected in former residents of areas where it is endemic after they have lived for years in Europe or the United States. Under these circumstances the disease has often been confused initially with tuberculosis.

It is probable that the illness indeed behaves like tuberculosis, histoplasmosis and coccidioidomycosis, in that many people are infected but most do not become clinically ill, and in only a few does frank clinical disease develop.

Clinically the disease may manifest itself as a 'flulike syndrome, as a mild or severe pneumonitis, or as progressive pulmonary lesions, which closely simulate pulmonary tuberculosis in behavior and appearance. These lesions may be unilateral, but are more often bilateral and symmetrical. They involve the midlung zones and contain areas of cavitation. A miliary pattern has been described. Residual fibroemphysema is a frequent residual of the pulmonary lesions. Involvement of the lungs has been reported in up to 94% of cases.

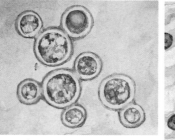

Yeast phase of *P. brasiliensis* in fresh unstained sputum prepared with 10% NaOH, showing double walls with single and multiple budding

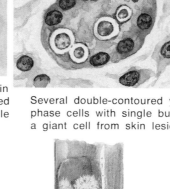

Several double-contoured yeast-phase cells with single buds in a giant cell from skin lesion

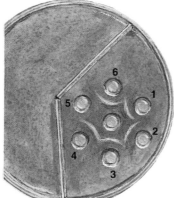

Precipitin test. Antigen in central well, serum from five different patients in peripheral wells showing precipitin bands. Wells 4 and 5 from same patient before and after treatment evidencing response

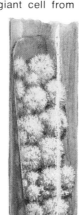

Mycelial colonies of *P. brasiliensis* grown on Sabouraud's medium at room temperature. Downy appearance due to filamentous hyphae with intercalate or terminal chlamydospores

Colonies of yeast form of *P. brasiliensis*, grown on blood agar at 37° C

Lesions of the eyes, nose, mouth, lips, tongue and cervical lymph nodes are common in South American blastomycosis, and dissemination to the skin, bones, adrenal glands, central nervous system and particularly the peritoneum and gastrointestinal tract may occur.

A definite diagnosis depends on demonstration of the causative organism, but serologic tests, particularly precipitin studies and complement fixation tests, are helpful adjuncts to diagnosis and guides to prognosis.

Treatment. Various sulfonamide preparations have long been the cornerstone of treatment of South American blastomycosis. Sulfadiazine, sul-

famerazine, sulfisoxazole, triple sulfonamide preparations, sulfadimethoxine, and sulfamethoxypyridazine are all effective. Of these, sulfisoxazole is probably the sulfonamide of choice because of its low order of toxicity. However, any of these agents must be administered for very long periods (one to three years), and they are considered only suppressive at best. South American blastomycosis responds well to amphotericin B. Probably this drug should be used for all but the most minimal infections, and certainly for all forms of disseminated disease. In particularly resistant cases alternate courses of a sulfonamide and amphotericin B can be employed.

Cryptococcosis

Cryptococcus neoformans, previously known as *Torula histolytica,* is a budding, yeastlike fungus which is the principal cause of cryptococcosis, although on rare occasions other species of cryptococci have been implicated in human disease. Unlike the organisms that cause histoplasmosis, blastomycosis, coccidioidomycosis and sporotrichosis, *Cryptococcus* is a uniphasic fungus which does not exist in a mycelial form. It has a worldwide distribution and has been isolated from soil, milk and fruit juice, as well as from matter contaminated by pigeon excreta.

The organism probably gains entry into the body through the lungs, from which it may disseminate to all organs, including the meninges, bone marrow, skin and kidneys. Mild, subclinical, self-limited infections are undoubtedly quite prevalent, as is also true for histoplasmosis and coccidioidomycosis. Clinical disease can develop in healthy individuals or in those who have some type of immunologic defect from diabetes, leukemia or lymphoma, or from steroid or other immunosuppressive therapy.

Meningeal involvement has been regarded as the most common form of cryptococcosis and has received much attention in the medical literature. In recent years, however, the clinical picture of *pulmonary cryptococcosis* has begun to emerge. Pulmonary lesions are often nodular in appearance and may simulate primary or secondary carcinoma. As a rule the lower lobes are involved, but upper lobe lesions do occur in either a unilateral or a bilateral distribution. If there is meningeal involvement, the physician may be deceived into thinking that the patient has cancer of the lung with central nervous system metastasis. Other pulmonary manifestations of cryptococcosis include cavitation within lung nodules, calcification, pneumonitis, pleural effusions and enlargement of hilar or mediastinal lymph nodes.

Treatment of cryptococcosis is indicated in the following situations: (1) when dissemination from the lungs to any other organ of the body has occurred; (2) when progressive pulmonary lesions are present as demonstrated by serial x-ray examinations or when symptoms are increasing in severity; (3) when stable pulmonary lesions are detected, either symptomatic or asymptomatic, in individuals in whom dissemination is likely to occur (*i.e.,* in those who are immunodeficient from either underlying disease or drug therapy).

Patients with *C. neoformans* in their sputum but without evidence of clinical or radiographic disease do not require treatment other than exclusion of hidden dissemination and careful follow-up observation. The same is true for those with stable

Cryptococcosis (Torulosis)

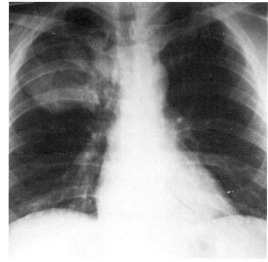

Pulmonary cryptococcosis presenting as a large masslike lesion, easily mistaken for carcinoma

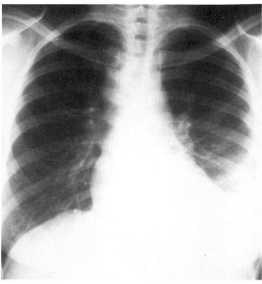

Pulmonary cryptococcosis. Mediastinal lymph nodes enlarged and pleural effusion on left

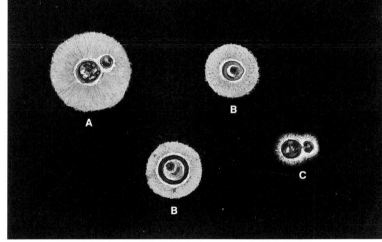

India ink preparation showing *C. neoformans* in spinal fluid

A. Budding organism with thick capsule

B. Nonbudding organisms

C. Unencapsulated form (budding)

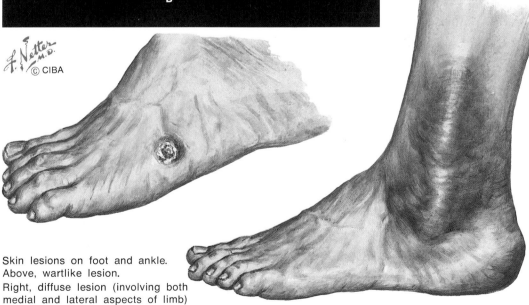

Skin lesions on foot and ankle. Above, wartlike lesion. Right, diffuse lesion (involving both medial and lateral aspects of limb)

asymptomatic pulmonary lesions. Chemotherapy is not considered necessary when an asymptomatic cryptococcal nodule is surgically excised from the lung, provided that a search for occult dissemination proves negative.

Treatment. 1. Amphotericin B administered intravenously is the treatment of choice for systemic infections of cryptococcosis, either pulmonary, disseminated or meningeal.

2. Flucytosine, also known as 5-fluorocytosine, has been shown to be relatively effective against *C. neoformans.* However, when used alone it seems to be definitely inferior to amphotericin B, and a high degree of resistance may emerge during

therapy. When flucytosine is used in combination with amphotericin B, the antifungal effects are increased, and the drug has an additive and perhaps a synergistic action.

3. Recent evidence indicates that tetracycline and rifampin also have a synergistic effect against *C. neoformans* when used in combination with amphotericin B.

4. A newer drug, clotrimazole, has shown activity against *C. neoformans in vitro,* but has not proved effective against systemic infections.

5. At present the preferred treatment in all cases of cryptococcosis appears to be a combination of flucytosine and amphotericin B.

Aspergillosis

Constantly a part of the natural environment, fungi of the genus *Aspergillus* usually coexist with man in harmless symbiosis. In special circumstances, however, some species may play an opportunistic role in producing disease in humans. Of the approximately 300 species of *Aspergillus,* only about 10 have been definitely implicated as pathogens, including *A. fumigatus, A. niger, A. flavus, A. niveus, A. nidulans, A. terreus, A. clavatus, A. restrictus, A. amsteloidami* and *A. versicolor.*

"Aspergillosis" is actually a spectrum of diverse disorders as described here.

Asthma. In atopic individuals, allergy to the spores of various aspergilli may cause classic extrinsic bronchial asthma, which does not differ from asthma caused by hypersensitivity to other allergens.

Hypersensitivity Pneumonitis. Extrinsic allergic alveolitis or hypersensitivity pneumonitis has been described in malt workers exposed to barley dust heavily contaminated by *A. clavatus.* A single case of interstitial lung disease resulted from contact with moldy straw containing *A. versicolor.* The above disorders are similar to farmer's lung and bagassosis (Plates 105 and 106).

Bronchopulmonary Allergic Aspergillosis. This condition, caused primarily by *A. fumigatus,* is also known as asthma and pulmonary eosinophilia; it is common in the United Kingdom but rare in the United States. The symptoms are coughing and wheezing. Sputum is often gelatinous, sometimes bloody, and usually contains aspergilli, which colonize but do not invade the bronchial mucosa. Eosinophilia of the blood, sputum and pulmonary tissues is present. Chest x-ray films usually show transient pulmonary infiltrates and areas of upper lobe collapse or atelectasis due to bronchial occlusion by mucoid impaction. Skin tests are almost invariably positive, and the serum of up to 90% of patients contains precipitins to *Aspergillus.*

Antifungal agents, particularly amphotericin B, are not indicated, since response to steroids is usually prompt. Early treatment is important to prevent the common complications of bronchiectasis, upper lobe contraction, and formation of aspergillomas in dilated bronchi.

Intracavitary Myceliomas. Aspergilli often colonize a preexisting lung cavity and form an intracavity *aspergilloma* or fungus ball. The cavity may be the result of tuberculosis, lung abscess, carcinoma, emphysematous cyst, histoplasmosis, sarcoidosis, bronchiectasis or other conditions. Colonized cavities are almost always in the upper lobes, and x-ray findings are highly characteristic, showing a rounded mass within the dependent portion of the cavity which is capped with a meniscus of air. The mass moves within the cavity as body position is altered. Other fungi or bacteria such as *Candida, Coccidioides, Phycomycetes, Allescheria boydii, Nocardia, Sporotrichum* and possibly *Trichophyton* are rare causes of fungus balls. Aspergillomas are composed of a tangled mass of fungal hyphae, which do not invade the cavitary wall but apparently produce enough irritation in some cases to cause mild or severe hemorrhage.

Aspergillosis

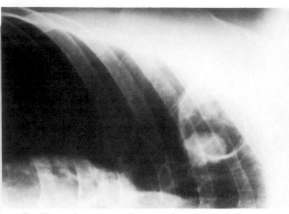

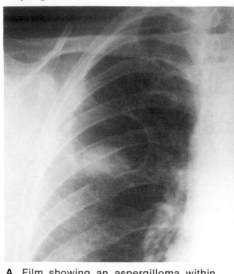

A. Film showing an aspergilloma within a cavity in right lung

B. Film of same patient as in "A" in l. lateral decubitus position, demonstrating shift of fungus ball to dependent portion of cavity

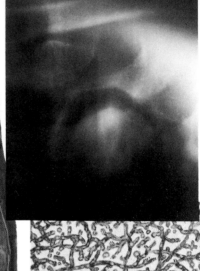

C. Tomogram of an aspergilloma within a cavity in l. upper lobe, demonstrating characteristic radiolucent crescent above fungus ball

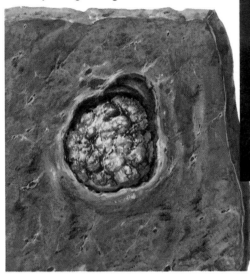

D. Gross appearance of an aspergilloma in a chronic lung cavity

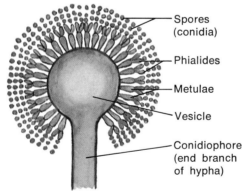

- Spores (conidia)
- Phialides
- Metulae
- Vesicle
- Conidiophore (end branch of hypha)

E. Structure of fruiting form of *Aspergillus niger.* Other species of *Aspergillus* vary in configuration but general structure is similar

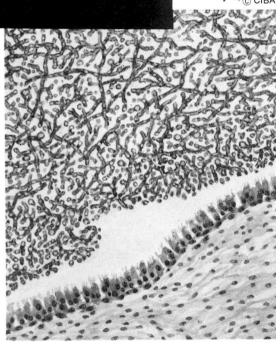

F. Microscopic structure of an aspergilloma composed of a tangled mass of hyphae within a dilated bronchus. No evidence of tissue invasion

Skin tests with *A. fumigatus* extracts are positive in only 22% of patients with aspergillomas, but precipitating antibodies against *Aspergillus* antigens can be shown in virtually all cases.

The need for treatment depends on whether significant bleeding is present. If hemoptysis is mild, occasional or absent, the lesion should simply be observed; if bleeding is severe, frequent or life-endangering, the fungus ball and cavity should be resected. Treatment with amphotericin B intravenously, by aerosol or by endobronchial instillation is of dubious value.

Invasive Aspergillosis. As a rule, the invasive form of aspergillosis occurs in those patients who have impaired immune responses. From the lungs, which are most often involved, generalized dissemination may take place to any site. The course is usually fulminant.

When confined to the lungs, the disease may present as a necrotizing pneumonia, lung abscess(es) or solitary granuloma. Fungus balls may evolve within lung abscesses. Pulmonary manifestations of hematogenous dissemination include miliary microabscesses and hemorrhagic pulmonary infarction. Amphotericin B in combination with flucytosine is probably the treatment of choice. Surgical removal of isolated lesions is sometimes possible.

Dissemination of Tuberculosis

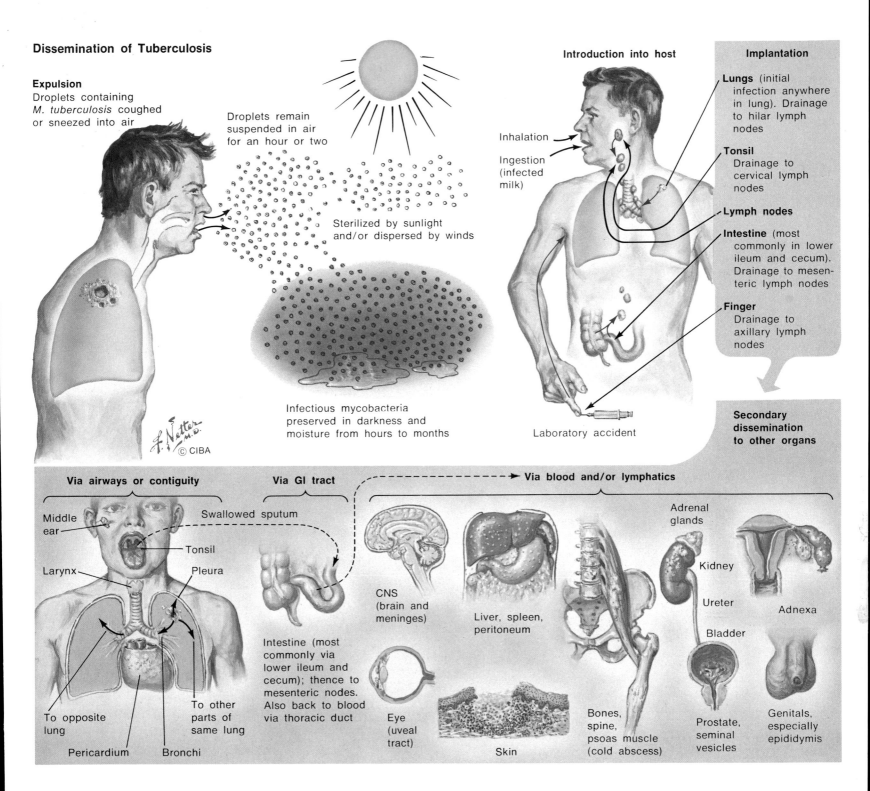

Expulsion
Droplets containing *M. tuberculosis* coughed or sneezed into air

Droplets remain suspended in air for an hour or two

Sterilized by sunlight and/or dispersed by winds

Infectious mycobacteria preserved in darkness and moisture from hours to months

Introduction into host

Inhalation

Ingestion (infected milk)

Laboratory accident

Implantation

Lungs (initial infection anywhere in lung). Drainage to hilar lymph nodes

Tonsil Drainage to cervical lymph nodes

Lymph nodes

Intestine (most commonly in lower ileum and cecum). Drainage to mesenteric lymph nodes

Finger Drainage to axillary lymph nodes

Secondary dissemination to other organs

Via airways or contiguity

Middle ear
Tonsil
Larynx
Pleura
To opposite lung
To other parts of same lung
Pericardium
Bronchi

Via GI tract

Swallowed sputum

Intestine (most commonly via lower ileum and cecum); thence to mesenteric nodes. Also back to blood via thoracic duct

Via blood and/or lymphatics

Adrenal glands
Kidney
Ureter
Adnexa
Bladder
CNS (brain and meninges)
Liver, spleen, peritoneum
Eye (uveal tract)
Skin
Bones, spine, psoas muscle (cold abscess)
Prostate, seminal vesicles
Genitals, especially epididymis

Tuberculosis

Background

Until recent years, tuberculosis was one of the most frequent causes of death throughout the world, including the United States. As recently as 1900, the United States' death rate from tuberculosis was approximately 100 per 100,000 and the new case rate approximately 200 per 100,000 population per year. Virtually everyone who lived to be 30 to 35 years of age became tuberculin-positive.

For reasons only partially understood, the incidence of tuberculosis and the death rate from the disease slowly but steadily decreased prior to the introduction of effective chemotherapy. Socioeconomic conditions were becoming better; initial

infection occurred at a young age, and the highly susceptible died quickly. Thus a population with enhanced antituberculosis immunity was gradually produced. Just before the introduction of specific chemotherapeutic agents for *Mycobacterium tuberculosis* in the 1940s, the death rate in the United States had fallen to approximately 16 per 100,000 and the new case rate to approximately 50 per 100,000. However, the majority of United States adults had still had infective contact with the disease, as evidenced by tuberculin reactivity rates of 50 to 85% in those aged 35 and older who lived in all but strictly rural populations.

In the ensuing 30 years the situation has changed in an almost unbelievable manner. By 1976 the tuberculosis mortality in the United States had fallen to 1.4 per 100,000 and the new case rate to 15.9 per 100,000. The tuberculin reactivity of 35-year-old adults was reduced to 5 to 25% except in a few very crowded and deprived ghetto areas, where the incidence of new cases was still high.

Transmission and Dissemination

Tuberculosis is almost always transmitted through the air from direct, often close personal contact—*i.e.,* persons sleeping or working in the same room, especially in the absence of good ventilation (Plate 88). The source individual is usually unaware of having infectious tuberculosis.

A pulmonary or bronchial focus ulcerates into an airway, causing both an irritative cough and excessive secretions laden with viable *Mycobacterium tuberculosis*. A cough, sneeze or even exhalation discharges *droplet nuclei* into the surrounding air. These minute infectious particles remain airborne for periods ranging from minutes to over an hour, depending upon the presence or absence of ultraviolet light, of moisture and especially of good ventilation. When the droplet nuclei are inhaled by an uninfected person, they may lodge anywhere in the lungs or airways. Most of these organisms die or

(Continued)

Tuberculosis
(Continued)

Evolution of Tubercle

Course modified by:

| Virulence and number of infecting organisms | Natural and acquired immunity of host | Age (newborn, 15 to 30 years, and elderly most susceptible; race, malnutrition, alcoholism, pregnancy | Silicosis, diabetes, other debilitating diseases; gastrectomy | Chemotherapy (adequacy thereof) |

Resolution

Inspissation, encapsulation, fibrosis (healing); after variable time; almost immediately to months

Calcification

Patch of local inflammatory response

Contiguous spread

Reactivation

Caseation

Liquefaction, cavitation, erosion into bronchus

F. Netter M.D. © CIBA

Dissemination in same or to distant organ

Swallowed sputum

Thoracic duct

By contiguity

Via airways

Via GI tract

Via bloodstream

Via lymphatics

are cleared from the tracheobronchial tree by macrophage ingestion and ciliary removal of secretions.

Tubercle bacilli may also enter the body through the gastrointestinal tract when unpasteurized milk taken from tuberculous cattle is consumed, or when bacilli-laden sputum is swallowed. Systematic testing and sacrifice of tuberculin-positive cattle have virtually eliminated the bovine source of tuberculosis infection in the United States and Canada since the 1920s.

Another entryway for tubercle bacilli into the human body is through injured or even intact skin or mucous membranes, although these forms of transmission are rare. The newly arrived mycobacteria that survive this penetration double in numbers about once every 24 hours, until enough are present to produce an inflammatory reaction. Once a focus of tuberculosis has formed, the disease may be disseminated to other parts of the body by the bloodstream, by the lymphatics, by contiguity, by way of the gastrointestinal tract (occasionally from the intestine back to the blood via the thoracic duct) and, finally and most commonly, through the airways.

Pathology

The initial response to the implantation of tubercle bacilli is an inflammatory reaction that is indistinguishable from any acute pneumonia. Within 3 to 10 weeks the process becomes a *tubercle*, a granulomatous form of inflammation

peculiar to tuberculosis and to a limited number of other diseases (Plate 89). It is characterized by histiocytes and Langhans multinucleated giant cells, admixed with and surrounded by lymphoid cells and a variable amount of fibrous tissue, depending on the age of the tubercle (Plate 93).

Influenced by the number and virulence of the organisms inhaled, and especially by the natural or inherent *immunity* of the host, the initial pneumonic foci may be small and limited in scope, or they may be numerous and coalesce into massive acute pneumonic areas. The initial area of inflammation may largely or completely resolve, but more commonly it undergoes necrosis. Tuberculous

necrosis is called *caseation,* as the gross appearance is cheesy. The caseous tissues may liquefy and empty into an airway, to be transmitted to other parts of the same or opposite lung, or into the exhaled air. New areas of pneumonia are likely to arise from this airborne dissemination.

Meanwhile, if the individual has satisfactory inherent and now acquired immunity, pneumonic foci may partially resolve and form fibrous scars; the necrotic centers eventually become organized, and ultimately calcified.

The disease process may improve (resolve, inspissate, dry out or calcify) in some areas and

(Continued)

Tuberculosis
(Continued)

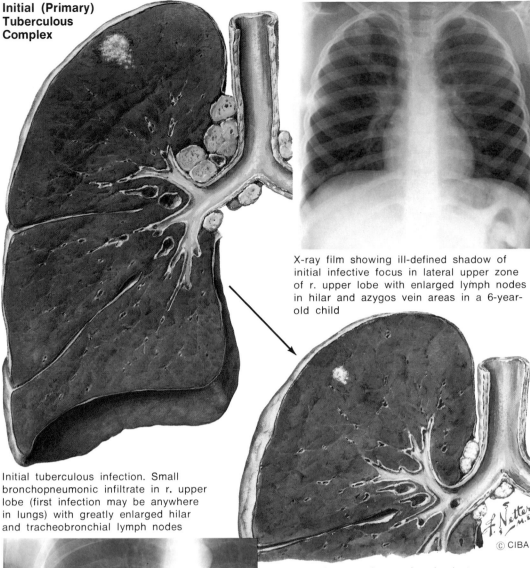

Initial (Primary) Tuberculous Complex

X-ray film showing ill-defined shadow of initial infective focus in lateral upper zone of r. upper lobe with enlarged lymph nodes in hilar and azygos vein areas in a 6-year-old child

Initial tuberculous infection. Small bronchopneumonic infiltrate in r. upper lobe (first infection may be anywhere in lungs) with greatly enlarged hilar and tracheobronchial lymph nodes

In time, pulmonary focus often heals to a fibrosed, calcified "Ghon lesion" and lymph nodes regress and calcify as shown here

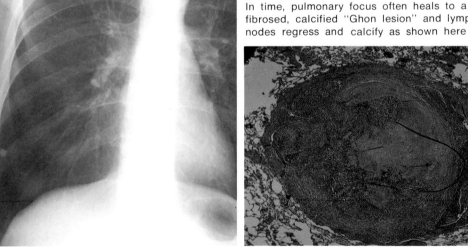

Calcified "Ghon lesion" in lateral portion of r. lower lobe

Section of a very inspissated, dried-out focus with fibrous capsule

worsen (liquefy and disseminate via airways, lymphatics, bloodstream or gastrointestinal tract) in others. Whichever course the untreated process takes at first, it may change direction without apparent cause. The course of tuberculosis is particularly likely to worsen months or years later, coincident with the introduction of some factor inhibitory to antituberculosis immunity—*e.g.*, advancing age, diabetes, silicosis, gastrectomy or chronic alcoholism.

Initial Tuberculous Complex. An initial infection (Plate 90) was originally called a "childhood" infection; later the term was changed to *primary infection* because of evidence that its special features were attributable to its being the first infection in an individual and not to its occurrence in a child *per se.* The initial infection has two components: the inflammatory focus or foci in an organ, and the resultant inflammation that soon appears in the lymph nodes draining the area. By far the most common initial complex occurs in the lung and hilar nodes; in time, the pulmonary focus often heals to a fibrosed, calcified *Ghon lesion,* and the lymph nodes regress and calcify. Other sites for a primary complex include the lower small intestine and mesenteric nodes, the tonsils and posttonsillar nodes, the finger (*e.g.,* of a laboratory technician), and the axillary nodes. It is important to note that the location of the initial parenchymal focus may be anywhere in the lung, but this is not the case with later reactivation.

Depending upon the inherent and acquired immunity of the host and the number and virulence of the invading organisms, hematogenous and to a lesser extent lymphogenous spread occurs to distant parts of the body. These new foci may subside and heal; more often they become quiescent. Occasionally, in the absence of adequate immunity, a hematogenous spread may propagate without check (once called progressive primary infection) and become *miliary tuberculosis,* often associated with *tuberculous meningitis.* The clinical appearance months or years later of active tuberculosis somewhere in the body (*e.g.,* bone, kidney, genitals, adrenals) is thus due to reactivation of the foci

which were seeded during the initial hematogenous dissemination in the absence of adequate antituberculosis immunity. While tuberculosis can spread to any organ, certain organs, such as the myocardium, endocardium, testis, stomach, thyroid and gallbladder, are seldom involved.

A Cautionary Case History. The 19-year-old daughter of a man with newly diagnosed infectious pulmonary tuberculosis was found to be tuberculin-positive after having been a nonreactor one year previously (Plate 91). Her chest roentgenogram was read as normal, and a sputum smear was negative for acid-fast bacilli.

(Continued)

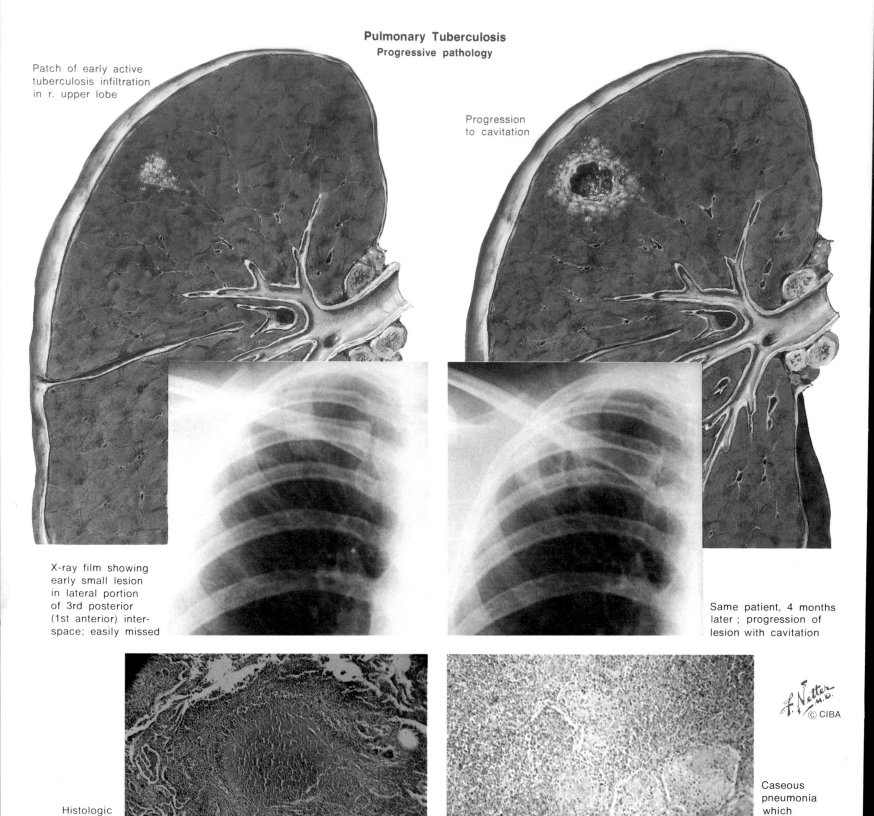

Patch of early active tuberculosis infiltration in r. upper lobe

Progression to cavitation

X-ray film showing early small lesion in lateral portion of 3rd posterior (1st anterior) interspace; easily missed

Same patient, 4 months later ; progression of lesion with cavitation

Histologic section of tubercle beginning to caseate

Caseous pneumonia which may closely simulate any other bacterial pneumonia

SECTION IV   PLATE 91

Tuberculosis
(Continued)

She was placed on 300 mg isoniazid (INH) per day as "prophylactic" treatment because of the skin test conversion, and was not seen again for four months. Meanwhile, the culture of the initial sputum specimen was found to be positive for *M. tuberculosis* susceptible to the common antituberculous drugs. When the woman was located, a fresh chest x-ray film revealed an acute process with a 2 cm diameter cavity in the right upper lobe. Review of the supposedly negative initial film revealed a 0.5 cm diameter soft-looking infiltrate (pneumonia) in the same area. Sputum obtained after four months of chemotherapy produced *M. tuberculosis* resistant to INH.

This case not only demonstrates a common early course of pulmonary tuberculosis, but also represents one of the classic reasons for using more than a single drug to treat active clinical disease (see discussion of treatment).

The location of reactivated (formerly called reinfected) pulmonary tuberculosis, as distinguished from initial infection, is predominantly in the upper posterior parts of the lungs. Since man is upright most of the time, the flow of low-pressure pulmonary artery blood—as distinct from normal-pressure bronchial artery blood from the aorta—is considerably reduced in the upper lung for long periods. On the other hand, ventilation to the various parts of the lung is much less affected by body position. As a consequence, oxygen uptake and carbon dioxide excretion are impaired in the upper as compared with the lower parts of the lungs in the erect position. This situation produces a more oxygenated environment in the upper lungs, which enhances the multiplication of the strongly aerobic *M. tuberculosis*.

(Continued)

Tuberculosis
(Continued)

Pulmonary Tuberculosis:
Extensive cavitary disease

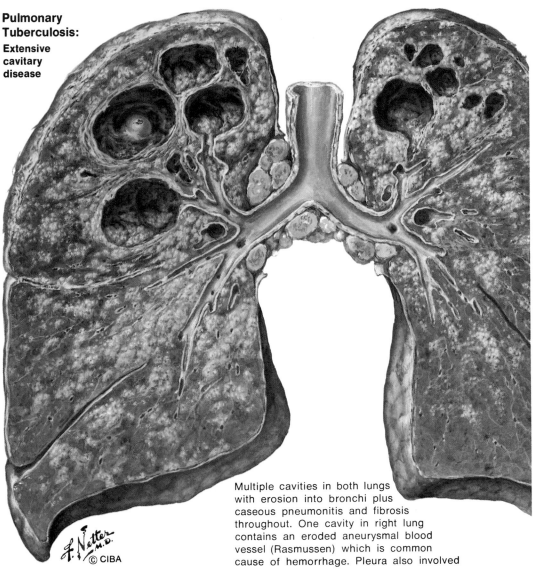

Multiple cavities in both lungs with erosion into bronchi plus caseous pneumonitis and fibrosis throughout. One cavity in right lung contains an eroded aneurysmal blood vessel (Rasmussen) which is common cause of hemorrhage. Pleura also involved

Progressive Tuberculosis. Tuberculosis that progresses to widespread cavitation, pneumonitis and lung fibrosis occasionally results from continuation of an initial infection (Plate 92), but more often represents reactivation of foci that have lain dormant for months or years.

Early symptoms are seldom diagnostic. Easy fatigue, weight loss, low-grade afternoon fever, pleurisy with or without effusion and recurrent deep chest infections are the most suggestive signs, *but they are often absent.* Chronic cough with purulent expectoration, hemoptyses, night sweats and cachexia are the usual hallmarks of advanced disease—familiar in romantic literature.

Miliary Tuberculosis. Miliary tuberculosis (Plate 93)—named from the resemblance of the scattered small lesions seen in the lungs at postmortem examination to millet seed—and tuberculous meningitis were universally fatal prior to the introduction of specific chemotherapy. Even with the best of modern therapy, however, tuberculous meningitis can still cause irreversible brain or cranial nerve damage, despite the fact that the active infection itself is cured. These complications are usually the result of delay in diagnosis and in starting specific treatment.

Tuberculin Test

Once, the tuberculin test was positive in so many people of all ages that it was of little practical use; it is now an extremely valuable diagnostic tool

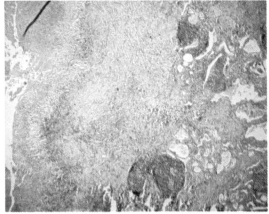

Section through wall of cavity. Cavity is to the left and is bordered by liquefying caseation with degenerating tubercles and collections of lymphoid cells

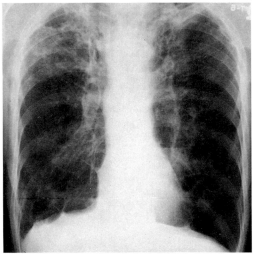

Bilateral advanced fibrocavitary tuberculosis

(Plate 94). Tuberculin is a mixture of numerous proteins and polysaccharides extracted from sterilized cultures of tubercle bacilli. There is some similarity among the proteins extractable from the different types of mycobacteria; consequently, cross-reactivity frequently occurs with so-called atypical mycobacteria, including those capable of causing disease in man.

The current standard tuberculin procedure, the *Mantoux test,* consists of the injection of approximately 0.1 ml of 5 TU tuberculin *intracutaneously* into the forearm, with the needle bevel up to help avoid subcutaneous injection. The result should be a pale elevation measuring 2 to 3 mm in diameter.

The test is read at 48 to 72 hours. The area is examined both directly and from the side and gently palpated or pinched. The margins of visible or palpable *induration* are marked and measured in the transverse plane; redness has no significance. (The induration is due to local cell-mediated delayed hypersensitivity, specifically a response to one or more tuberculoproteins to which the host had been sensitized by prior invasion of the organism.) More than 9 mm of induration is considered positive; 5 to 9 mm is considered suspicious; and less than 5 mm is considered negative. When the reaction is suspicious or negative, the test may be
(Continued)

Tuberculosis
(Continued)

repeated after seven days, when a booster effect may be discerned and a questionable reading converted (reliably) to positive.

Doses of 1 TU and 250 TU (previously called first- and second-strength PPD) are no longer commonly used. A few observers still favor the use of the 250 TU dosage in patients without a definitely positive reaction to 5 TU. The generally accepted opinion at present, however, is that established reactions to 250 TU in subjects nonreactive to the smaller dose will identify too many false positive reactors (in reality indicating probable atypical infection) to balance the few false negative results that may otherwise occur.

The *tine, Heaf* and other *multiple-puncture* tests are useful in surveying large groups rapidly and efficiently for epidemiologic purposes, but are not quite as accurate as the standard Mantoux test. The *Vollmer patch* has long been abandoned as quite unreliable.

Sputum Examination

Proper examination of sputum (Plate 95) is of paramount importance in the diagnosis and treatment of tuberculosis. The specimen should be the first coughed up in the morning from deep in the chest, and it must be transferred promptly to the laboratory. In the past, inability to raise sputum led to the performance of gastric washing to obtain a fasting specimen. Today, when a specimen cannot be coughed up, it can usually be obtained by sputum induction. The subject inhales a heated

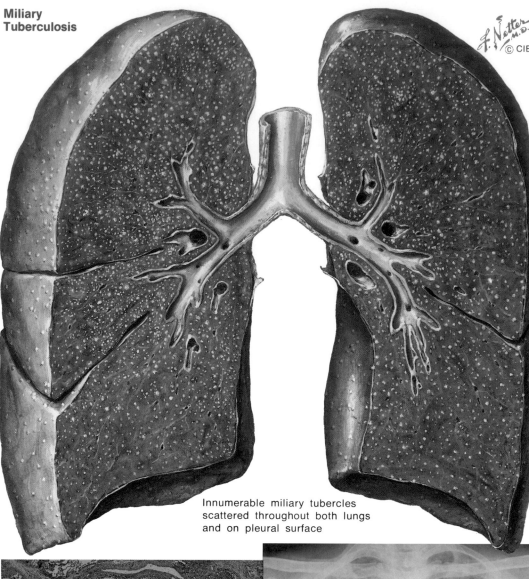

Miliary Tuberculosis

Innumerable miliary tubercles scattered throughout both lungs and on pleural surface

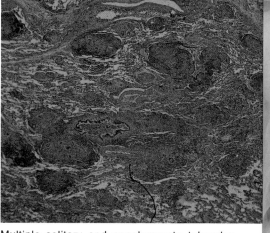

Multiple solitary and conglomerate tubercles composed mostly of epithelioid cells with an occasional giant cell of the Langhans type and surrounded by numerous lymphoid cells

hypertonic saline aerosol for 20 to 30 minutes in the office or clinic, and then is instructed and assisted in coughing up tracheobronchial secretions. Rarely, when this maneuver fails, a specimen may be collected using a bronchoscope.

A smear for microscopic examination for acid-fast bacilli (AFB) is prepared as follows: a fleck of purulent sputum is placed on a glass slide and crushed with another slide; the two are then drawn apart to make smears. To be stained using the *Ziehl-Neelsen* method, the slide is:

(1) flooded with carbolfuchsin,
(2) heated enough to make steam,
(3) rinsed with water,
(4) decolorized with acid alcohol,
(5) rinsed again,
(6) counterstained with methylene blue or malachite green for 30 seconds,
(7) rinsed again, and
(8) dried.

The slide thus prepared is viewed under oil immersion for 10 to 30 minutes, depending upon the viewer's experience; 200 fields should be reviewed. AFB are seen as bright red rods.

In the auramine 0 method, a sputum smear is prepared as above. Auramine 0 stain is added; the slide is heated to make the stain steam; it is then

(Continued)

Tuberculosis
(*Continued*)

Tuberculin Testing

0.1 ml tuberculin (5 TU) injected just under skin surface of forearm. Pale elevation results. Needle bevel directed upward to prevent too deep penetration

Test read in 48 to 72 hr. Extent of induration determined by direct observation and palpation; limits marked. Area of erythema has no significance

Diameter of marked indurated area measured in transverse plane. Reactions over 9 mm in diameter are regarded as positive; those 5 to 9 mm are questionable, and test may be repeated after 7 or more days to obtain booster effect. Less than 5 mm of induration is regarded as negative

allowed to stand at room temperature for 15 minutes. The preparation is counterstained with 0.5% potassium permanganate. The entire slide is scanned using low (25×) power, and doubtful areas are examined under high (60×) power. AFB are usually readily identified as bright yellow fluorescent dots.

Sputum Culture

Culturing for tubercle bacilli (Plate 96) requires careful preparation of the sputum specimen. An aliquot of preferably purulent sputum is shaken in a test tube for 1 minute with an equal quantity of 4% NaOH plus 0.5% N-acetyl-L-cysteine. The intent is to liquefy the mucus present and kill off most of the contaminants. The resultant liquid is then incubated at room temperature for 15 to 20 minutes, although this step also unavoidably kills some of the living tubercle bacilli. The specimen is next centrifuged for 15 minutes, the supernatant is decanted, and the remaining sediment is neutralized with a phosphate buffer (pH 6.8) and then spread over plates or slants of medium. The *slants* usually contain Löwenstein-Jensen (whole egg) or ATS (egg yolk only) medium.

The slants are examined under direct light with the hand lens at weekly intervals for six to eight weeks; growth, which later proves to be luxuriant, ordinarily starts to become evident in three to four weeks. A positive culture is manifested by tiny or conglomerate rough buff-colored colonies. The *plates* are usually filled with 7-H-11 oleic acid (no

egg) translucent agar. This ability to transmit light through the medium permits earlier detection of growth (*i.e.*, after two to three weeks).

Slants or individual quadrants of plates are prepared with various dilutions of antituberculous agents. Comparing the growth on drug-containing media with that on control media permits determination of the sensitivity of individual cultures. When the drug susceptibility tests are run with digested and appropriately diluted sputum specimens (direct test), the results are semiquantitatively precise; this is not the case when these tests are run with an already growing culture (indirect test).

To distinguish atypical from classical mycobacteria colonies, certain color reactions are helpful. *M. kansasii* (photochromogenic) colonies become orange colored after exposure to light for one hour or more, and are then reincubated. Scotochromogens are orange pigmented without exposure to light. *M. intracellulare-avium* colonies are nonpigmented but, like those of all atypical mycobacteria, are niacin-negative in contradistinction to those of *M. tuberculosis*, which are niacin-positive. Some atypical mycobacteria grow out in a few days. All these atypical forms have a tendency to primary multidrug resistance.

(*Continued*)

Tuberculosis; Sputum Examination
(Stained Smear)

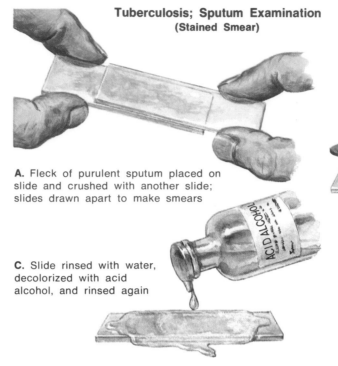

A. Fleck of purulent sputum placed on slide and crushed with another slide; slides drawn apart to make smears

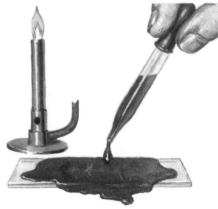

B. Slide flooded with carbolfuchsin and then heated

C. Slide rinsed with water, decolorized with acid alcohol, and rinsed again

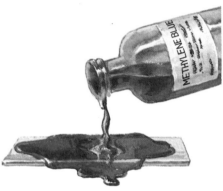

D. Counterstained with methylene blue or malachite green for 30 seconds, rinsed again, and dried

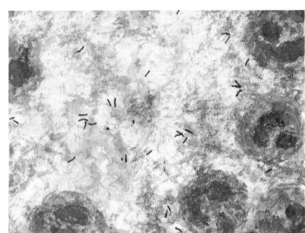

E. Slide of sputum stained with carbolfuchsin (Ziehl-Neelsen method as above), viewed under oil immersion, showing acid-fast bacilli (*M. tuberculosis*) as bright red rods

Tuberculosis
(*Continued*)

Treatment

Treatment of tuberculosis today consists entirely in selecting an appropriate chemotherapeutic regimen and in making sure that the patient follows it. The regimen should begin with two of the three major bactericidal agents or combinations available. These are: (1) isoniazid (INH), (2) rifampin (RFP) and (3) the combination of streptomycin (SM) and pyrazinamide (PZA). Other effective agents currently available include ethambutol (EMB), para-aminosalicylic acid (PAS), cycloserine (CS), ethionamide (ETA), kanamycin (KM), capreomycin (CPM) and thiacetazone (TB-1).

Especially in severe cases, treatment is provided in two phases—an initial intensive phase, often in hospital, for one to three months, and a continuation phase of 12 to 18 months. Intensive regimens that will produce reliable cures in a total of nine or even six months are currently being developed. The rationale for the initial intensive phase of treatment is to reduce the bacterial population as rapidly as possible in order to stop tissue destruction, prevent drug-resistant mutation, and minimize the chance of dissemination within the host and to others. It is also essential to appreciate that only actively dividing tubercle bacilli can be killed by chemotherapy. The rationale for the prolonged continuation phase of treatment is to kill bacilli when they multiply, which they do much less frequently as treatment proceeds. Host immunity can then develop, leading to encapsulation and inactivation of those living bacilli still remaining.

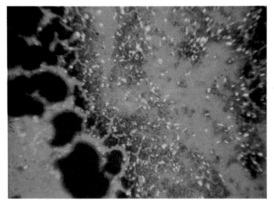

F. *M. tuberculosis* stained with auramine O which causes acid-fast bacilli to fluoresce (× 200)

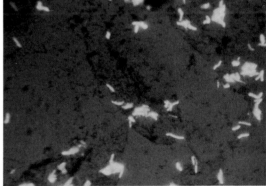

G. Auramine O stain of *M. kansasii* (acid-fast "atypical" mycobacteria) which are much larger than *M. tuberculosis* (× 200)

A commonly used and highly effective regimen for severe tuberculosis is INH-RFP for two to six months, followed by INH-EMB for a total of 12 to 18 months.

Antituberculous drug toxicity is a very significant problem in 5 to 10% of cases, frequently forcing a change in the regimen. This problem and its management should be well understood by the physician before treatment of the tuberculosis begins.

Acquired drug resistance can now be prevented by avoidance of single-drug therapy, by proper regimen selection, and by ensuring patient compliance in drug ingestion. When resistance has occurred,

use of multidrug programs is essential; the appropriate drug regimen should be determined by quantitative susceptibility testing in a reliable laboratory.

Primary drug resistance is an infrequent problem in most of the United States—*i.e.*, in 3% of patients or less. This term refers to the presence of drug-resistant bacilli in cultures obtained prior to the institution of therapy. When primary resistance is suspected, the possibility of inaccurate information or of infection with atypical mycobacteria should always be borne in mind. Except in very crowded and deprived areas with a high rate of

(*Continued*)

Sputum Culture

| Concentration and decontamination | Equal amounts of 4% NaOH plus 0.5% *N* acetyl-L-cysteine added to sputum, shaken for 1 minute and incubated at room temperature for 15 to 20 minutes. This kills most contaminants but also kills some *M. tuberculosis* | Specimen centrifuged for 15 minutes and supernatant decanted | Sediment diluted with 0.5 ml water or albumin, neutralized with phosphate buffer (pH 6.8), then spread over plates or slants of medium |

Tuberculosis
(Continued)

M. tuberculosis on slant of Löwenstein-Jensen opaque, egg-containing medium. Colonies non-pigmented or buff colored and rough

M. kansasii colonies on Löwenstein-Jensen medium. Orange pigmentation appears only after exposure to light

M. tuberculosis colonies on 7-H-11 oleic acid agar translucent medium, which allows earlier reading. *M. tuberculosis* as well as other pathogenic mycobacteria appear in about 2 weeks and are read weekly for total of 8 weeks

Drug susceptibility testing
(for selected patients)

INH 0.2   EMB 5.0   INH 1.0   EMB 10.0

RFP 0.2   Control   RFP 0.5   Control

Direct. Medium in each of 3 quadrants contains a different drug; 4th is control. Diluted sediment is spread evenly over all; 3 or 4 plates required as each drug is tested in 2 or 3 concentrations. INH 0.2 and 1.0; EMB 5.0, 10.0, and 15.0; RFP 0.2, 0.5, and 1.0; and SM 2.0 and 10.0 mg are most frequently tested

Indirect. Organisms are first cultured and then measured aliquots of culture are spread over quadrants containing different drugs in varying concentrations as well as control

INH = isoniazid, EMB = ethambutol,
RFP = rifampin, SM = streptomycin

tuberculosis and an established risk of primary resistance, however, drug susceptibility tests are no longer considered routinely necessary before treatment is started. Nevertheless, where suspicion of this problem is high, treatment with three agents or more may be started while the outcome of susceptibility tests is awaited.

Rest as part of the treatment program is indicated only for subjects who are febrile or easily fatigued. *Pulmonary resection* is indicated for uncontrolled hemoptysis, total destruction of one lung, severe symptomatic bronchiectasis and certain undiagnosed lesions. *Collapse therapy* is no longer used.

Hospitalization for isolation is not necessary, except in the first few days or weeks of treatment or for patients who are clinically quite ill. It is now eminently clear that patients given appropriate and well-planned chemotherapy become noninfectious within a few days. The overriding issue, however, is making sure that the medication prescribed is actually taken. Various techniques for accomplishing this essential goal have been developed. Perhaps the most reliable is supervised therapy administered by a nurse specialist in a clinic, office or even the home. All antituberculous agents may, and probably should, be prescribed in single daily doses, although most of them will be effective when taken as infrequently as twice or three times a week, especially in the continuation phase of treatment. A week's supply of medication, or certainly no more than enough for a month, is given to outpatients; a tablet count of the amount remaining at each revisit is then made. Other monitoring systems have been devised such as automatic dose dispensers and record-keepers. Unscheduled urine tests for drug content may be made. Patients found not to be

cooperating may have to be placed in hospital for brief periods of reevaluation and education. Enforced isolation of patients for the protection of the general population, and the laws and personnel needed to enforce this isolation, should ideally be available in all communities with a sizeable tuberculosis problem.

INH alone, on a daily basis for one year, is indicated as prophylaxis for subjects with tuberculous infection demonstrated by a positive tuberculin test without any evidence of manifest disease: namely, a negative chest x-ray film, urinalysis and physical examination. The indication for preventive treatment is strong when the risks of progression or

reactivation are great. The principal risk factors include a recent tuberculin conversion or the coexistence of some immunity-suppressing condition such as diabetes, silicosis, advanced age, debilitation, chronic alcoholism or gastrectomy. No drug other than INH has so far been proved reliable for these purposes.

If given before infection occurs, *BCG vaccination* is a safe and effective method for preventing tuberculosis from progressing once infection does take place. Nevertheless, it is applicable only when the incidence of the disease is very high, and its use renders ineffectual the later case-finding assistance of a positive or converted tuberculin skin test.

Silicosis

Silicosis is widespread because free silica is useful in many industries. In essentially pure form, it is used in ceramic manufacture (flint), as a building material (sandstone) and as an abrasive (sand); in mixed form it is widely used in production of construction materials, including cement. The common denominator in all cases of silicosis is the inhalation of high concentrations of crystalline silica. Respirable particles are less than 10 microns in diameter; those that reach the alveolar spaces and are deposited there usually have a diameter of 1 to 3 microns.

Pathology. The pathologic pattern of silicosis is related to the number of respirable free silica particles deposited within the lungs. The nodules are the result of a process in which macrophages, which ingest the particles, are killed by intracellular liberation of enzymes. The materials thus produced attract other macrophages and fibroblasts to form a fibrous nodule with an acellular center. Cellular reaction at the periphery gives a distinctive onionskin appearance on microscopy. These nodules are usually situated near the bronchiolar entrance to the alveoli or at the acinus.

In complicated forms of silicosis there is aggregation of the nodules, forming large masses. In the more slowly progressive forms of complicated silicosis associated with lower inspired concentrations of free silica, these masses are usually located within contracted upper lobes and are frequently accompanied by bullous changes in both the upper and lower lobes.

Roentgenographic Appearance. The pathologic changes of simple and complicated silicosis can be readily seen on x-ray films (see illustration).

Clinical Signs. In complicated disease, with massive changes and structural distortion, the patient has dyspnea on effort, obstructed breathing, cough and expectoration, and reduced exercise tolerance. There is increased susceptibility to secondary infection. The massive changes are often related to mycobacterial disease. Heart disease secondary to pulmonary hypertension may complicate advanced silicosis. The disease progresses most rapidly in the diffuse type associated with heavy deposition of particles.

Course, Treatment and Prognosis. Silicosis is a progressive disease that can run a very rapid course in individuals in whom diffuse reactions develop after heavy exposure without protection. In individuals with so-called acute silicosis, death may occur within one to three years. In accelerated silicosis, in which disabling disease occurs after an average of 10 years of exposure, progression is common, with rapid changes in course. In both groups, positive serologic reactions for antinuclear factor are common, as are clinical manifestations of autoimmune connective tissue disorders including scleroderma, rheumatoid arthritis and systemic lupus erythematosus. In individuals whose exposure has lasted more than 20 years, a protracted course is the rule. There is no specific treatment for silicosis. The prognosis in all cases is unfavorable. It is particularly poor for persons who develop lesions within 10 years of their first continuous exposure.

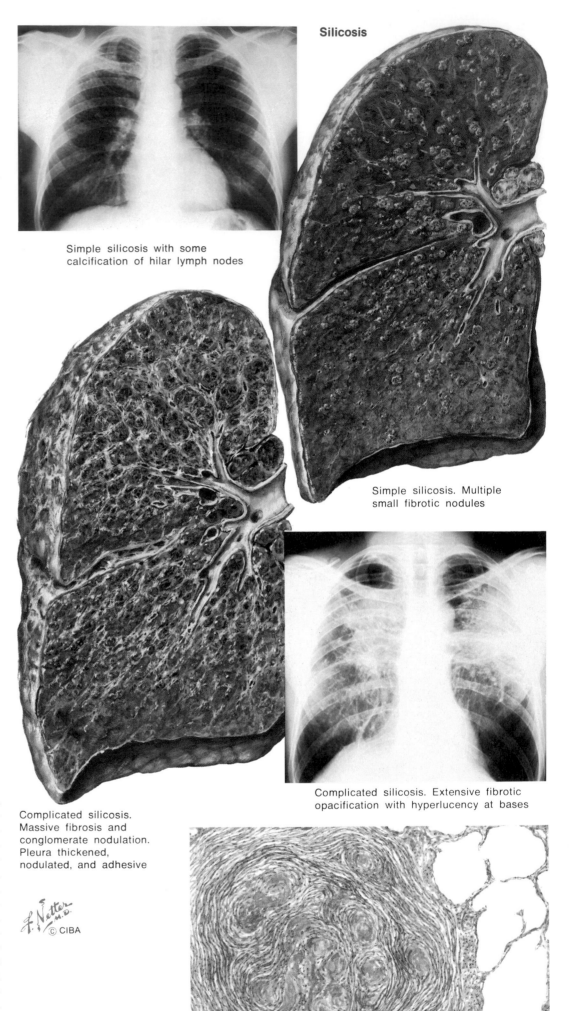

Silicosis

Simple silicosis with some calcification of hilar lymph nodes

Simple silicosis. Multiple small fibrotic nodules

Complicated silicosis. Extensive fibrotic opacification with hyperlucency at bases

Complicated silicosis. Massive fibrosis and conglomerate nodulation. Pleura thickened, nodulated, and adhesive

Typical silicotic nodule. Concentric ("onionskin") arrangement of collagen fibers, some of which are hyalinized

Silicotuberculosis and Rheumatoid Pneumoconiosis

Documentation is incomplete on the role of exposure to free silica when tuberculosis is acquired by persons who handle this material. However, even without roentgenographic evidence of silicosis, the predisposition of silicotic patients to tuberculosis is beyond question. Although tuberculosis as a complication of chronic nodular simple silicosis is less common today than in the past, and bacteriologic proof may be difficult to obtain, this is not the case in patients with rapidly developing silicosis. In patients with fatal "acute" silicosis, mycobacterial infection is almost always present.

In less fulminating, though accelerated, silicosis, mycobacterial infections are found in 25% of cases, but either typical or atypical organisms may be responsible for the disease. In two recent series, it was found that as many as 33% and 50% of the complicated cases were produced by atypical mycobacteria. The common atypical organism in a series from the United States Gulf Coast was *Mycobacterium kansasii*. In a district of the upper Midwest of the United States, *M. intracellulare* (Battey bacillus) was the prevailing bacillus.

Silicomycobacterial lesions may be cavitary, although these heal in the usual manner in response to antituberculosis chemotherapy. However, massive fibrotic lesions with variable amounts of cavitation are also commonly encountered. Treatment almost always converts the sputum, but the massive lesions progress and are associated with the early appearance of end-stage phenomena such as respiratory insufficiency, pulmonary hypertension and cor pulmonale. In accelerated silicosis, the distribution of lesions complicated by tuberculosis varies from that typically found in silicosis, and predominantly lower lobe involvement is not unusual.

The combination of massive changes associated with nodular deposits may make it difficult to distinguish silicotic from tuberculous nodules on roentgenogram. The two forms are easier to distinguish after chemotherapy has been effective and the sputum has become negative for mycobacteria. At that time, simple tuberculous lesions will usually resolve, and the fixed foci will represent either silicotic nodules or larger silicotuberculous lesions, which often progress because of altered cellular immunity.

Autoimmunity and Caplan's Nodules

Caplan noted that coal miners with rheumatoid arthritis or diathesis who are exposed to respirable free silica may develop nodular pulmonary lesions that form more rapidly than chronic silicotic foci, and which resemble sites of metastatic cancer as seen on chest x-ray films. He and his co-workers also demonstrated that disseminated simple

Silicotuberculosis

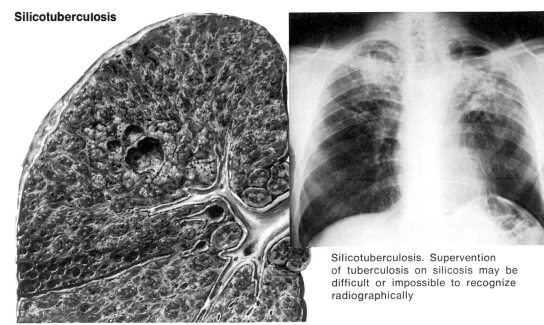

Silicotuberculosis. Supervention of tuberculosis on silicosis may be difficult or impossible to recognize radiographically

Tuberculosis with cavitation superimposed on silicosis

Caplan's Syndrome (Rheumatoid Pneumoconiosis)

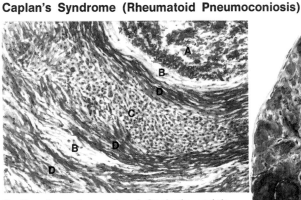

Section through margin of Caplan's nodule. A = necrotic central area, B = clefts, C = zone of fibroblasts and inflammatory cells, D = collagen

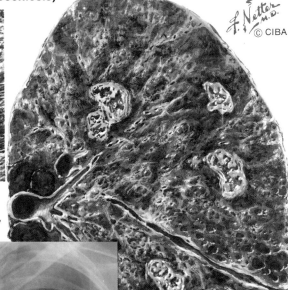

Caplan's nodules of various sizes in lung with silicotic nodules and coal dust deposits

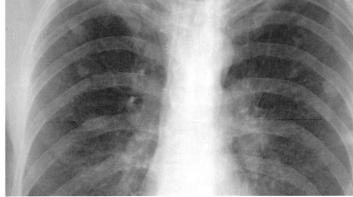

Caplan's nodules in both lungs with some evidence of diffuse fibrosis

silicotic foci can be transformed and enlarged in patients with rheumatoid disease. These changes are usually accompanied by general malaise and aggravation of joint symptoms associated with rheumatoid arthritis. The "Caplan's nodules" contain silica and other dusts if exposure is mixed, and show characteristic rheumatoid reactions, with palisading inflammatory cells surrounding a zone of central necrosis. The diagnosis of rheumatoid pneumoconiosis is usually based upon clinical findings and serologic changes.

Miners exposed to silica appear more likely to develop progressive systemic sclerosis, a type of autoimmune connective tissue disease, which is ordinarily more common in women than in men. Sandblasters with accelerated silicosis have shown an increased incidence of antinuclear factor in the bloodstream, as high as 45%. In this group of patients the incidence of autoimmune connective tissue disorders approaches 10%. In addition to rheumatoid arthritis and diffuse scleroderma, systemic lupus erythematosus and localized scleroderma complicating silicosis have been identified as well. These complicated varieties of silicosis usually have an accelerated course but, except when associated with generalized scleroderma, have sometimes been suppressed or stabilized by adrenocorticoid drugs.

Coal Worker's Pneumoconiosis (CWP)

Pneumoconiosis occurring in coal miners has attracted great attention since the period before World War II, when it was noted that the disease was on the increase in the great industrial countries. The new frequency of the illness was related to the introduction of mechanical methods employing high-energy sources to speed up production. Investigations showed that coal pneumoconiosis was not restricted to miners but also occurred in workers on the surface, such as coal trimmers, who were exposed to pure and even washed coal. In subsurface coal mining, intense dust concentrations are produced. Protection by external air supply is not provided, however, because of practical problems and the low fibrogenic effect of the dust, which is largely composed of carbon particles.

Coal worker's pneumoconiosis results from the inhalation of respirable dust that first settles within the alveoli and later accumulates near the respiratory bronchioles. There, coal macules form with limited scarring, leading to disease of the respiratory bronchioles and focal emphysema. (If scarring is excessive, it may be related to increased silica content.) Simple and nodular types of pneumoconiosis are reflected on chest x-ray films by nodular densities varying in size from 1 to 10 mm in diameter. This pattern is rarely associated with exertional dyspnea. In nonsmokers the simple disease may be asymptomatic. Cigarette smoking is the usual cause of increased cough and expectoration, but in coal miners with many years of exposure specific industrial bronchitis related to dust inhalation can contribute to the bronchial symptoms. Progression to higher grades of simple or complicated disease is not uncommon in those who continue to work in the mines, but it is rare in ex-miners. Recent studies indicate that 10% of miners develop pneumoconiosis and that 0.5% go on to develop complicated disease, usually progressive massive fibrosis.

In the simple form of the disease, pulmonary function changes are seldom found and are usually limited to an increase in residual volume. In several studies, however, individuals with fine p nodules (less than 1.5 mm in diameter) on the average have shown reduction of pulmonary diffusing capacity.

The situation is altered with the development of complicated disease, which is associated with important clinical changes. The masses formed in this stage of pneumoconiosis are composed of black material bordered by fibrous capsules; the lesions lie within scarred and contracted upper lobes in which the airways are obstructed and distorted (progressive massive fibrosis), leading to demonstrable emphysema and reduced prominence of the preexisting simple nodular pattern. These changes are quite evident on roentgenogram. Effort dyspnea is an important symptom in complicated pneumoconiosis, and coughing and expectoration, often of black sputum from excavated massive densities, are increased. The functional changes in complicated disease, which usually appear after many years, include a small vital

Slightly magnified detail of lung showing indurated coal nodules

Whole lung thin section with massive black deposits as well as smaller nodules, necrotic areas, and emphysematous changes

Microscopic section through a coal nodule. There are large amounts of coal dust, both intracellular and extracellular, with irregularly arranged collagen fibers near an artery (fibrosis)

Chest x-ray film of retired coal miner showing massive upper lobe lesions, sometimes referred to as "angel wings"; also associated nodular disease

capacity and increased residual volume, with reduced airflow rates and pulmonary diffusing capacity. There is a disturbance of gas exchange, resulting in low oxygen tension at rest, which becomes worse during exercise. Severe ventilatory failure and right-sided heart failure secondary to pulmonary hypertension have been reported but are far less common than in silicosis.

Although tuberculosis was commonly associated with pneumoconiosis of miners in the past, the incidence of this complication is no longer excessive. Studies in the United Kingdom and the United States show no increased incidence of cancer in coal workers with pneumoconiosis or

industrial bronchitis. Clearly, the complicated form of CWP is disabling, and a decision must be made to remove workers from the mining environment after roentgenograms show excessive reaction to dust. Changes visible on the chest x-ray film are, in general, proportional to the amount of dust inhaled and thus provide an approximate basis for judgment concerning disposition of workers.

There is no treatment for the pneumoconiosis, but complicating diseases such as bronchitis, rheumatoid arthritis, tuberculosis and secondary infections can be given specific or symptomatic treatment.

Asbestosis

Asbestosis

The term *asbestos* refers to a group of fibrous silicates whose unusual properties of durability and resistance to heat have been known since antiquity. Exposure to asbestos varies in different occupations, and there is, undeniably, widespread contact with asbestos in pure or mixed form by workers in mines and mills and by consumers. Respirable particles are usually quite long and may be more than 50 microns in length. The most important factor influencing where fibers are deposited after inhalation is their diameter; when this is small (about 0.5 micron), particles will remain suspended within the airways and drift in the direction of the airflow to deposit in the airspaces. Because of their length, these fibers commonly impact within the respiratory bronchioles, and pathologic studies show that some of the earliest cellular and fibrotic lesions occur in that location.

The development of pulmonary fibrosis, the characteristic lesion of asbestosis, is related to the fiber concentration in the inspired air. The fibrosis is interstitial and involves the dependent portions of the lungs where asbestos bodies are usually found. (Asbestos bodies are asbestos fibers that have become encased in a brown proteinaceous sheath rich in iron.) As the disease progresses, obliterative changes may take place; in late stages, great thickening and cellular fibrosis surrounding the airspaces create the roentgenologic appearance of honeycomb lung. Advanced asbestosis is often associated with bronchogenic carcinoma, which in the majority of cases arises in scar tissue, is peripheral in location, and is an adenocarcinoma. Multiple primary tumors of this type have been encountered in patients with asbestosis. In addition to the peripheral form, squamous cell carcinomas of the larger bronchi also occur. The combination of exposure to asbestos and the practice of cigarette smoking probably accounts for the variety and forms of lung cancer encountered, and greatly increases the risk of its development, even in the absence of pulmonary fibrosis.

Since 1960 the occurrence of pleural and peritoneal mesothelioma (Plate 65) following relatively short periods of exposure to asbestos has been frequently noted. Some of these contacts were not industrial but occurred in family members who had secondary exposure, or in children who played near asbestos mine sites. The fatal tumor may arise as far into the future as 20 to 40 years after exposure has ended.

Fibrous and calcified pleural plaques also occur frequently in individuals exposed to lower concentrations of asbestos fiber, but it is unusual for calcification to occur less than 20 years after the initial exposure. Follow-up of patients with pleural plaques has not been carried out for a sufficient time to establish the relationship to mesothelioma.

Clinical manifestations of these structural changes are clear cut. The principal symptom of pulmonary asbestosis is shortness of breath on effort. Physical examination of affected individuals demonstrates rales at the lung bases and, often,

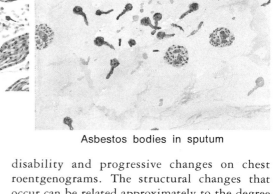

Oblique chest x-ray film. Calcified pleural plaques and irregular densities, chiefly in lower part of lungs

Extensive fibrosis with emphysematous changes and great pleural thickening: visceral, parietal, and diaphragmatic. Lower lobe predominantly involved

Pleural plaques in pulmonary asbestosis

Section of moderately advanced asbestosis with extensive fibrosis and distorted alveoli. Asbestos bodies (some fragmented) in airspaces and interstitium. Also a few asbestos fibers

Asbestos bodies in sputum

clubbing of the fingers. In the early stages of the disease, the pulmonary infiltrations may not be obvious on x-ray films, and clinical signs and pulmonary functional changes may be present before definite roentgenographic changes are detected. Early pulmonary function changes are of diagnostic value in asbestosis. Reduction in vital capacity is important and indicates the presence of group disease when an entire shift of workers exposed to asbestos shows this change. Spirometric tests may show reduced airflow proportional to lung volume.

Course. The disease is progressive and is characterized by increasing exertional dyspnea,

disability and progressive changes on chest roentgenograms. The structural changes that occur can be related approximately to the degree of exposure to respirable asbestos fibers. Early changes on the chest film may appear after only 10 years of exposure, but most commonly appear after 20 years of work with the mineral. From then on, serial chest films will demonstrate the progressive pulmonary reactions and pleural thickening. The respiratory disability of asbestosis is severe, progressive and irreversible. There is no treatment that will affect the pulmonary fibrosis, and the ultimate outlook is poor for the worker with established disease.

Reactions Produced by Metals and Mixed Dusts

Inhalation of very fine metal particles is common in industrial processes. The material inhaled may be pure metal or one of its compounds, or part of a mixture of dusts.

Inhalation of metal iron oxide particles by arc welders results in a benign pneumoconiosis with little or no fibrosis, called *pulmonary siderosis*. This material has minimal fibrogenic effect and, although these workers are exposed to high concentrations of particles, the reaction is simply due to the bronchoalveolar dust clearance mechanisms becoming overwhelmed with retained particles and accumulated dust-laden phagocytes. The iron oxide gives a red coloration to the lungs, when examined grossly, but histologic studies demonstrate little fibrosis. Nodular deposits are often seen on chest roentgenograms and may resemble the simple lesions of silicosis. In arc welder's siderosis there are no associated clinical symptoms or defects of pulmonary function; disability is not excessive, and neither is the incidence of lung cancer increased. The working life of arc welders is not reduced.

Because of the great variety in industrial processes, workers are often exposed to *mixed dusts*. Welders and foundry workers are commonly exposed to a mixture containing iron oxide, carbon and free silica. Pneumoconiosis usually appears after long exposure, often more than 20 years in duration. The patterns of disease seen on chest roentgenograms are similar to those noted in silicosis, varying from simple nodular to massive changes. Characteristic irregular and linear patterns are often seen as well. Pathologic examination of the lungs shows mixed-dust retention, with black deposits corresponding to retained carbon. The appearance is dominated by the red deposits of iron oxide in both the diffuse and massive lesions. Tuberculosis is said to be a common complication of mixed-dust fibrosis. The prime symptom of the advanced and complicated disease is shortness of breath on exertion, leading to disability and shortened life span.

Tungsten workers are subject to pulmonary fibrosis. They are exposed to very fine particles of tungsten, which is combined with carbon under the influence of cobalt to form the hard metal needed for the manufacture of precision industrial equipment. Exposure to metallic fumes can produce an obstructive syndrome. This is often associated with pruritus, which may be the result of individual idiosyncrasy or hypersensitivity. Diffuse pulmonary disease is not uncommon and usually appears after 10 years of exposure. A fine pattern of infiltration within the upper lung zones is seen on the chest roentgenogram. The earliest symptom is an unproductive cough, followed by shortness of breath on exertion associated with tachypnea, rales and clubbing. Ultimately, a severe restrictive disorder develops, followed by pulmonary hypertension and cor pulmonale. Pathologic study reveals infiltration and thickening of the alveolar walls, with metaplasia of the epithelium. Phagocytic and multinucleated cells may be seen in the alveolar spaces and cellular infiltration of the alveolar walls. Crystals believed

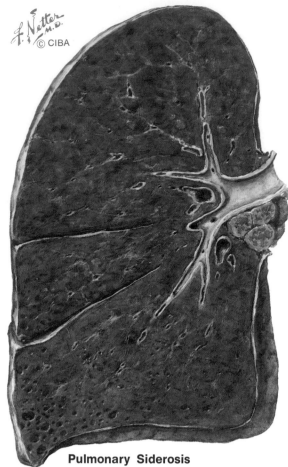

Pulmonary Siderosis

Iron dust inhalation is believed to be relatively benign, producing little change other than brick-red discoloration unless mixed with other dusts (chiefly silica, silicates, and/or carbon). The mild fibrosis, nodulation, and emphysema shown are probably due to such admixture

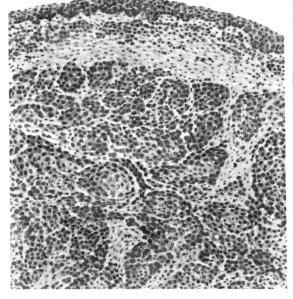

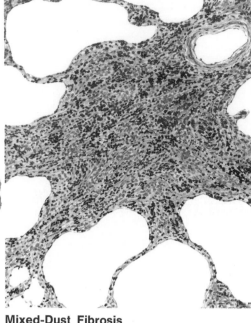

Mixed-Dust Fibrosis

Fibrosis surrounding deposits of iron oxide, carbon, and silica, found in sandblasters, steel dressers, oxyacetylene cutters, and welders long exposed to such mixed dusts

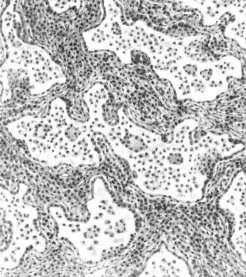

Tungsten Inhalation Effects

Cellular infiltration and increased collagen in lung interstitium. Alveoli show epithelial metaplasia and contain cellular exudate with some multinucleated cells

Nickel Inhalation Effects

Squamous cell carcinoma with overlying metaplastic bronchial mucosa, believed attributable to this metal

to represent retained tungsten and carbide have been observed by means of electron microscopy. Experimental work has not shown that tungsten carbide can reproduce these lesions in the absence of cobalt, which suggests that cobalt is responsible for both the disease of the airways and the lesions within the smaller airspaces.

Other metals have been involved with several varieties of pulmonary disease. The association of *chromates* with perforation of the nasal septum and bronchogenic carcinoma has been noted in the past. The same results may follow continuous exposure to *nickel* when it is treated with carbon monoxide to form nickel carbonyl, although the

possibility that arsenic may be contributory in these circumstances has not yet been disproved.

The toxicity of nickel stirred popular interest in 1976 because of unexplained death from acute pulmonary disease among individuals attending a convention in Philadelphia. In the fatal cases, an excess of nickel within the tissues was reported, and for a time the investigation was directed to the possibility that nickel fumes emitted from decomposing copying paper may have been responsible for this "epidemic." Laboratory studies disproved this hypothesis and established a bacterial cause for what is now considered a distinct entity named "legionnaires' disease" (Plate 74).

Special Metals

Cadmium and beryllium are metals producing important pathologic reactions within the lungs.

Cadmium-associated pulmonary disease follows the inhalation of fumes produced by the smelting of ores or the application of heat to mixtures of metals. The usual respiratory reaction is acute and occurs within three to four hours. Upper respiratory irritation and general symptoms of illness are followed by dyspnea, hemoptysis, cyanosis, and subsequent tachypnea and rales. The appearance of the chest x-ray film in severe cases is that of pulmonary edema, which may be followed by atelectasis. In fatal cases the lungs show edema, congestion and hemorrhage; necrotic lesions are found in the cortex of the kidneys, and degenerative changes have been demonstrated in the testes. The effects of chronic exposure to cadmium upon the human lung have not been adequately studied.

Beryllium is extensively used in the production of metal alloys and in the electronics and aerospace industries. It is a light substance, having great tensile strength and offering little resistance to the passage of x-rays. These positive features could be more widely applied in an industrial setting were it not for beryllium's toxic effects; its compounds, for example, were used in the manufacture of fluorescent lighting tubes until 1949, when recognition of beryllium toxicity led to its replacement.

Toxic effects are most evident in the skin and lungs. Skin reactions include papular and vesicular rashes, ulcers and granulomas, and may be caused by sensitivity to beryllium compounds. Beryllium can also become widely distributed throughout the body and persists in bone and liver. Conjunctivitis has also been noted.

The acute respiratory reaction to beryllium is more severe than that accompanying the usual metal fume fever. There may be swelling and ulceration of nasal mucosa, with progression to septal perforation. Tracheitis, bronchitis and chemical pneumonia, which has the roentgenographic appearance of pulmonary edema, are the principal features. Since there is no specific therapeutic agent, only symptomatic management can be provided for the acute respiratory insufficiency present. About 90% of patients recover from the acute reaction but some of them develop chronic disease.

Chronic beryllium disease has usually appeared in those who have been involved in the manufacture of fluorescent lighting fixtures, and the effective dose required to cause the chronic form of the disease can be very small.

It is possible for chronic beryllium disease to develop without a symptomatic acute phase. Latent periods of 10 to 15 years have occurred after the earliest exposure; sometimes the typical chronic granulomatous form appears long after the worker has broken his contact with beryllium. The course of chronic disease is usually slowly progressive, with a terminal phase of interstitial fibrosis and cor pulmonale. The principal symptoms are dyspnea, dry cough and, in some cases, associated skin lesions. Rales and rhonchi are heard during the physical examination. Com-

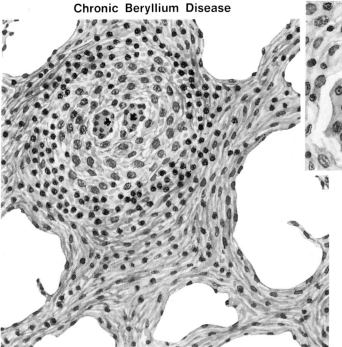

Acute effect of cadmium inhalation; metaplasia of alveolar epithelium. Acute inflammation of the tracheobronchial tree and upper respiratory tract may also occur

Renal effects of chronic cadmium poisoning. PAS-positive cast material in tubules

Cadmium Inhalation Effects

Bullous emphysema with consolidation at base possibly attributable to chronic cadmium inhalation

Chronic Beryllium Disease

Granuloma with interstitial fibrosis resembling sarcoidosis: central deposition of endothelioid cells, some multinucleated, with surrounding cuff of lymphocytes and fibrous tissue. Skin and other tissues may show similar lesions. High-power inset above shows detail of giant cells containing Schaumann bodies

plicating pneumothorax and evidence of pulmonary hypertension with right heart failure are not unusual. The slow progression is accompanied by hypoxemia and occasional clubbing of the fingers; it may run its course over 15 to 20 years. The appearance of the chest x-ray film cannot be used to distinguish chronic beryllium disease from sarcoidosis, which also manifests hilar adenopathy and bilateral infiltration. However, in the former condition tuberculin sensitivity is preserved, and peripheral adenopathy is not marked. Pulmonary function studies show reduced lung volumes, low compliance and diffusing capacity, and a reduced arterial oxygen tension.

A specific patch test for beryllium is positive in most patients with chronic beryllium disease; an acute inflammatory reaction appears within two or three days, followed by granuloma formation. Examination of biopsy specimens for beryllium content is of questionable value because test results may be negative in disease and positive in normal individuals exposed to the mineral, which accumulates in liver and bone before excretion. If exposure is recent, beryllium may be found in the urine. A temporary suppressive effect can be obtained with corticosteroid agents, but the disease will ultimately result in terminal pulmonary fibrosis and respiratory failure.

Various Mineral Pneumoconioses

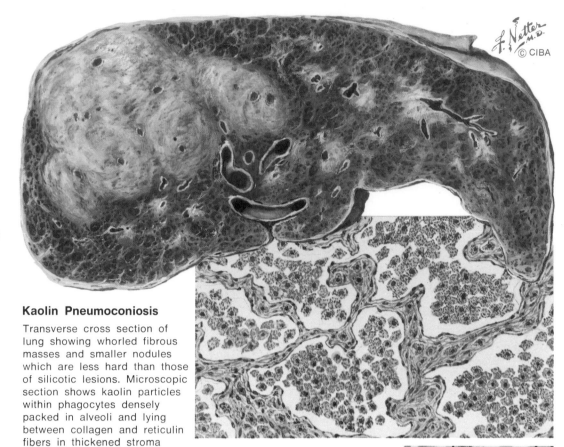

Kaolin Pneumoconiosis

Transverse cross section of lung showing whorled fibrous masses and smaller nodules which are less hard than those of silicotic lesions. Microscopic section shows kaolin particles within phagocytes densely packed in alveoli and lying between collagen and reticulin fibers in thickened stroma

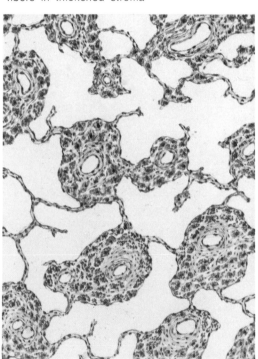

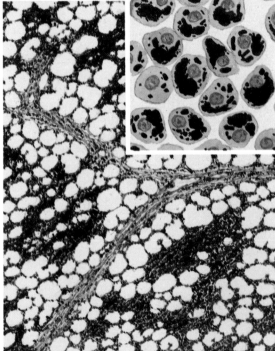

Fuller's Earth Pneumoconiosis. Masses of brown pigment within macrophages, chiefly perivascular. Scant tissue reaction

Graphite Pneumoconiosis. Black deposits and extensive fibrosis. High-power inset shows graphite clumps in alveolar macrophages

Besides the pneumoconioses produced by free silica, asbestos and coal, tissue reactions with sometimes serious clinical effects can also be incited by other dusts.

One variety of pneumoconiosis that produces the same clinical picture as coal worker's pneumoconiosis (CWP) is caused by the inhalation of respirable particles (less than 10 microns in diameter) of *graphite*. Graphite is carbon which contains variable amounts of quartz impurities. The silica content of the graphite is usually low and probably makes a minor contribution to the typical tissue reaction in this disease. Graphite is milled after mining and used in the manufacture of steel and electrotyping, and in the production of electrodes. It also serves as a lubricant and has a familiar use in ordinary pencils. The structural patterns of disease produced are those characteristic of either a simple nodular pneumoconiosis or a complicated massive reaction. The pathologic evidence of the simple variety is a carbon macule with limited fibrosis next to the respiratory bronchioles and associated emphysema of the center of the respiratory lobule. However, in complicated pneumoconiosis, which is less common, the masses may excavate. Severe cases of pneumoconiosis may be complicated by right ventricular hypertrophy.

Nonfibrous silicates can also produce diffuse pulmonary disease. One, *fuller's earth*, is calcium montmorillonite, an aluminum silicate containing iron and magnesium. This material is obtained by quarrying, and the dust is used as absorbent clay. Formerly, it was used in fulling, which is the extraction of grease from wool, but today it is an important agent in the refining of oils.

Marked dust retention has been observed in men who have had long exposure to fuller's earth, but the degree of fibrosis has usually been limited. However, in several cases progressive massive fibrosis has been described, although contamination with quartz could account for the high fibrogenic effect of this dust.

Another industrially important nonfibrous silicate is *kaolin*, or china clay. This hydrated aluminum silicate is obtained by quarrying and then washing the material containing the specific dust from the quarry walls. Subsequent treatment involves drying, milling, bagging and loading. In these dangerous phases of the operation the worker is exposed to excessive concentrations of respirable dust. Prolonged exposure to heavy dust or to dust with too great an admixture of quartz accounts for the rare appearance of the characteristic pneumoconiosis. Kaolin containing less than 1% quartz is classed as a nuisance particulate with a TLV (threshold limiting value) of 50 MPPCF (million particles per cubic foot), or 15 mg/m³.

Another clay frequently associated with complicated silicosis is *bentonite* (85% sodium montmorillonite), which is found mixed with sandstone and shale in nature. The mixture may contain more than 15% free silica, with an excess of cristobalite.

Toxic Gases

Acute respiratory disorders produced by the inhalation of irritant gases are not infrequent and are usually the result of accidental exposure involving single workers or groups of workers. In rare instances, larger numbers of persons are injured in community disasters. The situation is aggravated when the individual or group is trapped without access to protective devices. Excessive concentrations of the offending material are then inhaled, and the development of acute respiratory disorders is likely; in addition, chronic disease may follow. The toxic materials, such as hydrogen sulfide (H_2S), sulfur dioxide (SO_2), and polymers of nitrogen dioxides (NO_2, N_2O_4), may be end products of industrial processes. In other instances, inhaled materials may be components of the industrial process itself, such as chlorine (Cl_2) and phosgene ($COCl_2$) in industrial chlorination, and SO_2 and ammonia (NH_3) in refrigeration.

Effects of Gases. Irritant gases are usually classified according to whether their primary effect is on the upper or the lower part of the respiratory tract. *Soluble gases* that irritate the conjunctivae and upper respiratory tract will cause the victim to seek rapid escape from exposure. Such immediate reaction is well illustrated by the response of individuals who sense leaks of NH_3, SO_2 and Cl_2. If the exposure is brief, there may be only simple irritation of the upper respiratory tract, with cough and expectoration. However, if the person is trapped, excessive concentrations of gas are inhaled into the airways and alveolar spaces, with damage to bronchial mucosa and alveolocapillary membranes. Injury to the lower respiratory tissues can lead to severe dyspnea, wheezing and orthopnea, followed by fever and purulent expectoration, which indicate secondary infection. Chest roentgenograms may demonstrate the changes of pulmonary edema and later of bronchopneumonia, which can lead to early death after overwhelming exposure.

Insoluble gases such as $COCl_2$ and the nitrogen dioxides have only mild effects upon the upper airways. Thus they may be unwittingly inhaled to an excessive degree, producing severe alveolar injury by chemical transformation to their corresponding acids. Acute pulmonary edema and secondary pneumonia are the results of heavy exposure. The pneumonia will respond to chemotherapy, and chronic pulmonary disease may not develop; this is usually the case after successful treatment for exposure to $COCl_2$. (The course of events after inhalation of the nitrogen dioxides is unique and will be described later.)

Irritant Gas Effects on Lungs

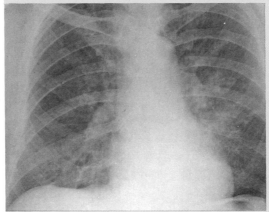

Ammonia fumes exposure. X-ray film compatible with pulmonary edema within a few hours of exposure

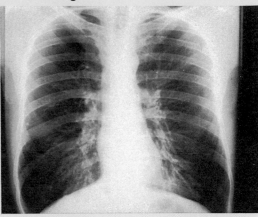

Ammonia fumes exposure. Six months later, diffuse emphysematous changes
© CIBA

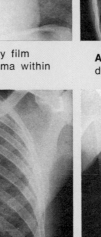

Chlorine gas poisoning. Acute effect, diffuse pulmonary edema

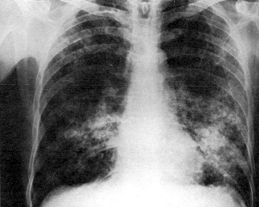

Nitrogen dioxide exposure. Fine and coarse nodular infiltrates, confluent in some areas

Pulmonary function tests carried out in individuals with mild upper respiratory irritation provide normal results. Tests of patients who respond to treatment for lower respiratory injury and who are capable of forced expiration may demonstrate transient reduction of ventilatory volumes, airflow rates, pulmonary diffusing capacity and arterial oxygen tension.

Course. If there are no destructive changes, response to appropriate treatment with oxygen and antibiotics, after acute exposure, will be satisfactory. If there is severe damage to the airways and the terminal airspaces from prolonged and heavy exposure to NH_3 and SO_2, cough and expectoration will persist. The chest x-ray film will show persistent abnormalities and infiltrations during recurrences of pneumonia. Pulmonary function studies will demonstrate reduced vital capacity and definite evidence of airway obstruction. These findings are consistent with chronic purulent bronchitis and bronchiectasis and indicate that the prognosis is poor.

An unusual course of events often follows heavy inhalation of the nitrogen dioxides, such as the gases produced by the oxygenation of fresh corn in a closed silo (silo filler's disease), or after exposure to the combustion of nitrogen and oxygen at very high temperatures in enclosed tanks. An early phase of pulmonary edema is common, and may be fatal. If the worker survives, a second bout of dyspnea may occur about two weeks later. In both phases the chest roentgenogram shows widespread involvement of the lungs, similar to the butterfly pattern of pulmonary edema but more

nodular in character. Bronchiolitis fibrosa obliterans, with polypoid clumps of cells in respiratory bronchioles and alveoli, is responsible for the second stage. The disorder is usually reversible, but the disease can become chronic, progressing with disturbances of ventilation, lung volume and alveolocapillary gas exchange; eventually it can lead to a fatal termination.

Chest symptoms disappear in those cases of irritant gas exposure in which the damage is completely resolved; this has been the rule in survivors of exposure to Cl_2 and $COCl_2$ who have received modern chemotherapy. Chronic bronchitis or bronchiectasis is related to the corrosive action of the soluble products of agents such as NH_3 and SO_2: exposure often leads to reduction in exercise tolerance, paralleled by abnormalities of pulmonary function with reduced vital capacity, airflow rates, and often pulmonary diffusing capacity. Arterial oxygen tensions are lowered, and are likely to fall further during exercise. Progressive changes of emphysema or fibrotic lung disease may be noted on the chest x-ray films. Nevertheless, chemotherapy for complicating pyogenic infections is ordinarily effective and is enhanced by the proper use of postural drainage.

Patients with chronic pulmonary disease following irritant gas exposure cannot return to their previous employment and have difficulty performing sustained physical work. Their life span is usually reduced, and they face an increased risk of complications such as amyloidosis from chronic infection and cor pulmonale secondary to diffuse pulmonary disease and pulmonary hypertension.

Hypersensitivity Pneumonitis Due to Inhalation of Organic Dusts

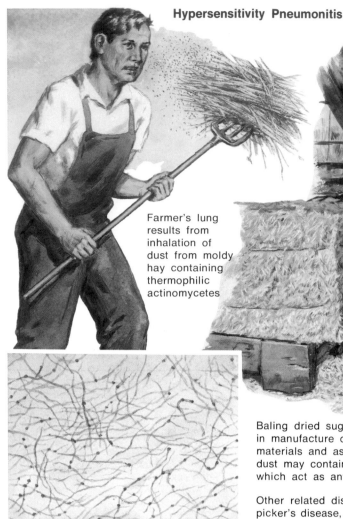

Farmer's lung results from inhalation of dust from moldy hay containing thermophilic actinomycetes

Baling dried sugar cane or "bagasse," widely used in manufacture of paper, wallboard, and building materials and as chicken litter. When moldy, dust may contain spores of thermophilic organisms which act as antigens in causation of bagassosis

Other related diseases in this group are mushroom picker's disease, pigeon breeder's disease, budgerigar (parakeet) fancier's disease, malt worker's lung, sequoiosis, maple bark disease, wheat thresher's lung, thatched roof disease, air conditioner disease (due to moldy dust or water from air conditioners), and fog fever of cattle

Slide culture of *Thermoactinomyces saccharii,* a thermophilic actinomycete which is principal source of antigen in causation of bagassosis

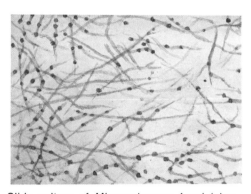

Slide culture of *Micropolyspora faeni* (also known as *T. polyspora),* a thermophilic actinomycete which is a principal source of antigen producing farmer's lung, mushroom picker's disease, and fog fever of cattle

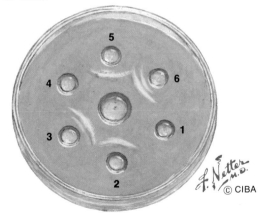

Precipitin reactions in bagassosis. Patient's serum in central well and extracts of bagasse from various sources in peripheral wells. Specimens 1 and 4, from fresh bagasse, show no precipitin bands

Hypersensitivity pneumonias caused by the inhalation of organic dusts containing a variety of microorganisms or animal proteins have only recently emerged as an important segment of pulmonary medicine. Unlike allergic bronchial asthma, these disorders produce infiltrative lesions in the lungs and are not characterized by bronchospasm. In the British literature they are referred to as "extrinsic allergic alveolitis."

Farmer's lung, caused by the inhalation of dust from moldy hay or grain, was the first illness to be recognized as a hypersensitivity pneumonia; later bagassosis, an almost identical disorder due to the inhalation of dust from dried sugar cane fiber (bagasse), was identified as belonging to the same disease category. Many additional illnesses of this type have since been recognized (see table).

In addition to causing acute illness of a pneumonic nature, these conditions may result in chronic pulmonary fibrosis, particularly if the patient has inhaled low doses of antigen over a long period, as has been described in farmer's lung, bagassosis, thatched roof disease and budgerigar fancier's disease. Further, it seems likely that many patients who are found to have idiopathic pulmonary fibrosis are really suffering from some form of chronic hypersensitivity pneumonitis due to other environmental antigens which have not yet been identified.

Known antigens that cause hypersensitivity pneumonitis include animal protein from birds, cows or pigs; spores from various fungi; insects such as the wheat weevil, *Sitophilus granarius;* and a variety of microorganisms known as thermophilic actinomycetes. The latter group of organisms were only recently discovered and their identification and classification are still in progress. It has been determined that they are the principal cause of bagassosis, farmer's lung, mushroom picker's disease, fog fever of cattle, and the illnesses associated with inhalation of mist or dust from contaminated heating and air-conditioning systems. They have been designated as heat-loving or thermophilic, since they show optimum growth in culture at temperatures ranging up to 60°C, and it was the final realization of this temperature requirement that led to their discovery. Originally, these organisms were regarded as fungi; although they show some characteristics of both fungi and bacteria, they have now been classified as bacteria of a high order of development. *Thermoactinomyces saccharii, T. vulgaris* and *Micropolyspora faeni* are apparently the most important disease-producing members of the group, but other types of thermotolerant bacteria may be implicated.

(Continued)

Hypersensitivity Pneumonitis Due to Inhalation of Organic Dusts
(Continued)

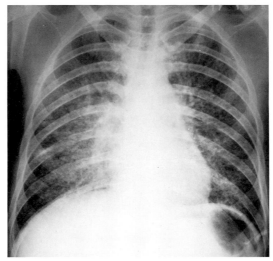

Acute bagassosis: small nodular and miliary densities throughout both lungs. Deposits may be more hazy and homogeneous in some cases

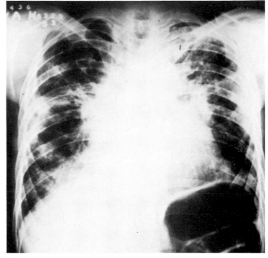

Chronic bagassosis: intense fibrosis and bullous emphysema after many episodes of respiratory illness during 9 years of industrial exposure

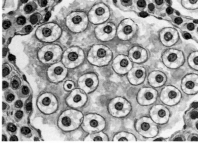

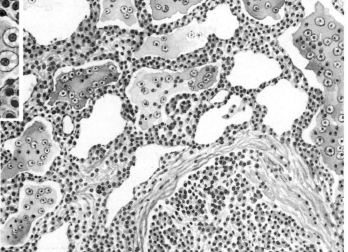

Tissue reaction in bagassosis. Alveolar walls thickened with infiltrate of plasma cells and lymphocytes. Some alveolar spaces contain edema fluid and desquamated histiocytes with vacuolated cytoplasm. High-power section inset above shows macrophages with vacuolated cytoplasm filling alveolar space

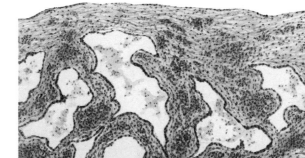

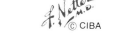

Extensive subpleural and interalveolar fibrosis with inflammatory cell infiltration characteristic of advanced stage of farmer's lung (low-power section)

The blood of patients sensitized to these organisms usually contains antibodies which can be detected by agar gel double diffusion techniques.

Along with farmer's lung, bagassosis has served as an investigational model of other hypersensitivity pneumonias. Discoveries relating to the etiology, pathology and epidemiology of these conditions have fostered a more complete understanding of similar syndromes. The remainder of this discussion will apply specifically to bagassosis, which may be regarded as a model for most of the other hypersensitivity pneumonias.

Bagassosis. Bagassosis is caused by the inhalation of thermophilic actinomycetes, and possibly other organisms, present in the dust from bagasse. This material is the fibrous residue of sugar cane from which the juice has been extracted. The organisms do not produce injury by tissue invasion, but invoke an allergic or hypersensitivity reaction in the lungs, which manifests itself as an interstitial granulomatous pneumonia. Bagasse fiber or dust itself is innocuous, and workers who handle freshly produced material never develop bagassosis. However, the processing of bagasse requires that it be compressed into bales and stored in the open fields for long periods, where it is exposed to moisture and high temperatures. Under these conditions it becomes contaminated and serves as a culture

medium for the offending organisms. Individuals who are subsequently exposed to the stored material are at high risk of developing bagassosis.

Bagasse had been produced in Louisiana for many years, but initially it was discarded (its very name means "something worthless") or burned as fuel in the boilers of the sugar mills. Eventually, however, its immense industrial value was appreciated, and it became an important ingredient of paper, wallboard and other building materials. Problems of storing and shipping it to manufacturing plants stimulated invention of the baling technique. It was at this point that the disease appeared, occurring almost exclusively in workers

who were heavily exposed to contaminated dust while engaged in bale-breaking and processing the dried fiber for manufacturing purposes.

Bagassosis was first recognized in Louisiana by Blitz, in 1937, and was subsequently detected in workers who had been exposed to exported Louisiana bagasse in Missouri, Texas, Illinois and England. Later, cases were reported in individuals exposed to natively produced bagasse in Italy, India, Peru, Puerto Rico, the Philippines and Spain. That the disease has not been reported from other sugar cane—producing countries can probably be attributed to misdiagnosis, or to the fact
(Continued)

On pathologic examination, the acute disease presents as a granulomatous pneumonia. Accumulations of plasma cells, lymphocytes and histiocytes are seen in the interstitial tissues, while the alveolar spaces contain edema fluid and collection of macrophages with vacuolated cytoplasm known as foam cells. When the illness becomes chronic, the granulomatous changes are replaced by interstitial fibrosis.

Treatment. Treatment involves simply removing the patient from contact with bagasse dust; gradual and eventually complete recovery then usually takes place in a matter of weeks or months.

If contact with the offending antigen is reestablished, the illness almost invariably recurs and the danger of permanent disability increases accordingly. When the illness is severe, recovery may be hastened and symptoms relieved by steroid therapy. Prednisone is usually administered in doses of 60 mg daily for about one week, after which the dosage is gradually decreased over a period of a month or more.

Prevention of bagassosis, and of all other forms of hypersensitivity pneumonitis, can be accomplished by eliminating the offending antigen from the individual's environment.

Hypersensitivity Pneumonitis Due to Inhalation of Organic Dusts
(*Continued*)

Etiologic Agents in Hypersensitivity Pneumonitis

Disease	Exposure	Antigen
Farmer's lung	Moldy hay or grain	*Micropolyspora faeni, Thermoactinomyces vulgaris*
Bagassosis	Stored sugar cane fiber (bagasse)	*T. saccharii* and possibly other organisms
Mushroom picker's disease	Moldy vegetable compost	*M. faeni, T. vulgaris*
Humidifier, air-conditioner or heating system disease	Contaminated forced air system	Thermophilic actinomycetes and other organisms
Fog fever (cattle)	Moldy hay	Same as farmer's lung
Maple bark stripper's disease	Maple tree logs or bark	*Cryptostroma corticale*
Sequoiosis	Redwood sawdust	*Graphium, Pullularia, Aureobasidium pullulans* and other fungi
Suberosis	Moldy cork dust	*Penicillium* species
Paper mill worker's disease	Moldy wood pulp	*Alternaria*
Pulpwood handler's disease	Moldy wood pulp	Same as above
Brewer's or malt worker's lung	Malt or barley dust	*Aspergillus clavatus, A. fumigatus*
Cheese washer's lung	Cheese mold	*P. casei*
Paprika slicer's disease	Moldy paprika pods	*Mucor stolonifer*
Wheat thresher's lung or grain measurer's lung	Wheat flour containing weevils	*Sitophilus granarius*
Pigeon breeder's disease	Pigeon serum and droppings	Avian proteins
Budgerigar fancier's disease	Contact with parakeets	Parakeet proteins
Chicken handler's or feather plucker's disease	Contact with chickens	Chicken proteins
Turkey handler's disease	Contact with turkeys	Turkey proteins
Pituitary snuff disease	Porcine, bovine pituitary gland (Pitressin snuff)	Porcine, bovine proteins
Smallpox handler's lung	Smallpox scabs	Unknown
Thatched roof disease (Papuan or New Guinea lung)	Dried grass and leaves	Unknown
Tobacco grower's disease	Tobacco plants	Unknown
Joiner's disease	Sawdust	Unknown
Tea grower's disease	Tea plants	Unknown
Bible printer's disease	Moldy typesetting water	Unknown
Coptic or mummy disease	Cloth wrappings of mummies	Unknown
Detergent disease (asthmalike symptoms—true pneumonitis not identified)	Enzyme detergents	*Bacillus subtilis*
Furrier's lung	Animal hairs	Unknown
Coffee worker's lung	Coffee beans	Coffee bean dust
Doghouse disease	Moldy straw	*Aspergillus versicolor*
Lycoperdonosis	Puffball spores (*Lycoperdon pyriform*)	Unknown
Sauna-taker's disease	Contaminated sauna bath water	*Pullularia*

that the fiber is not used for manufacturing or is processed by methods other than the baling and storing technique.

The onset of the disease may be acute or insidious, and is characterized by dyspnea, cough, fever, chills, weakness, chest pain, anorexia and rapid loss of weight. Illness may result from contact with bagasse dust for only a few days or after many months; it may be critical in nature or consist of mild transient symptoms after short periods of intermittent exposure.

When bagassosis is acute, the chest roentgenogram shows a variety of patterns, including changes typical of extensive pulmonary edema, diffuse bilateral and symmetrical small nodular deposits suggestive of miliary tuberculosis, and upper or lower lobe lesions, which are most often bilateral but which may be unilateral and simulate bacterial or viral pneumonia. In its chronic form the disease may show x-ray changes of a fine reticular "honeycomb" appearance, or those of intense fibrosis and bullous emphysema.

Pulmonary function testing characteristically shows a restrictive defect manifested by reduced vital capacity and total lung capacity. Gas transfer at the alveolar-capillary level is also impaired, and hypoxemia and hyperventilation are present. A small percentage of patients develop diffuse bronchial obstruction, which may result in permanent and progressive disability.

Cascade of Clotting Factors and Sites of Action of Heparin and Warfarin

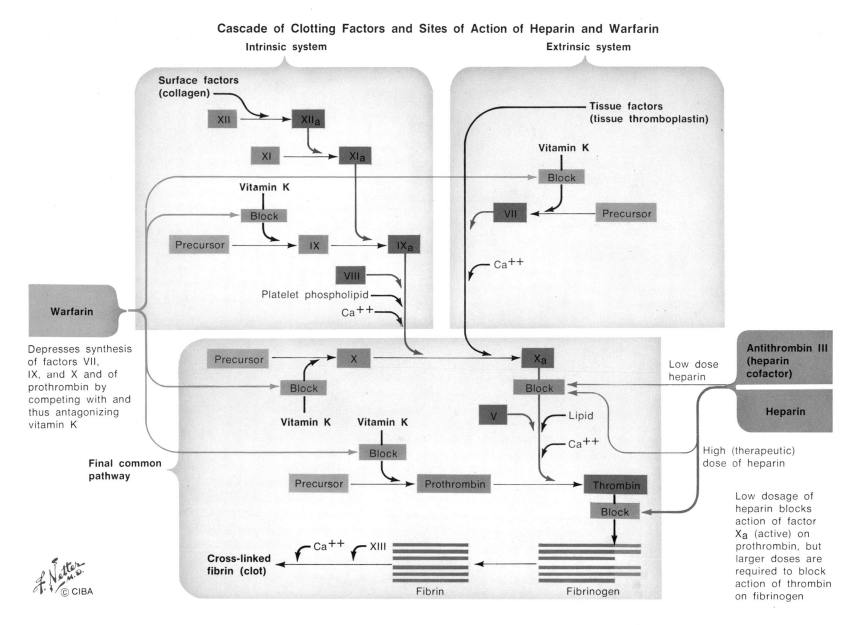

Cascade of Clotting Factors

The coagulation system is an integrated series of sequential reactions in which each proteolytic enzyme converts the succeeding zymogen into an active species, here designated with a subscript a. The cascade is divided into three parts: the intrinsic system, which contains only proteins occurring in the blood plasma; the extrinsic system, involving a tissue lipoprotein; and the final common pathway, identical for both systems.

Intrinsic System. The initiating reaction of the intrinsic system is a conformational change in factor XII following exposure to the collagen-containing basement membrane which underlies the endothelial cell. Once formed, factor XII$_a$, in the absence of Ca^{++} but still adsorbed to the surface, catalyzes the conversion of factor XI to XI$_a$. Recent investigations suggest that prekallikrein and high-molecular-weight kininogen can accelerate factor XII activation as well as its action on factor XI. Factor XI$_a$ can then, in the presence of Ca^{++}, convert factor IX to IX$_a$. Although factor IX by itself can convert factor X to X$_a$, it does so at a slow rate. To effect this transformation rapidly, three cofactors are needed. The first, factor VIII, is a large protein without proteolytic activity itself but which can markedly accelerate

the action of factor IX$_a$ on factor X. The second, phospholipid, contained in the platelet membrane, is not normally available on the platelet surface but is made available by exposure of the platelet to collagen, ADP (adenosine diphosphate) or thrombin. Finally, Ca^{++} is necessary for rapid activation of factor X. Like activation of factor IX, conversion of factor X to factor X$_a$ involves a proteolytic split in the heavier subunit of factor X to yield an active enzyme.

Extrinsic System. Factor VII and tissue thromboplastin, a lipoprotein, combine to form a complex which, in the presence of Ca^{++}, converts factor X to X$_a$. The mechanism of conversion is similar to that in the intrinsic system.

Final Common Pathway. Factor X$_a$ can by itself convert prothrombin to thrombin, but the reaction rate is very slow. Factor V, a glycoprotein, is required to accelerate the reaction. Like factor VIII, factor V has no proteolytic activity but acts as an accelerator of the enzyme X$_a$ and combines with the substrate prothrombin to increase its susceptibility to proteolysis. The entire reaction takes place on a phospholipid surface provided by platelets or tissue thromboplastin. Extrinsic Ca^{++} is essential for binding prothrombin and factor X$_a$ to phospholipid while factor V is a metalloprotein containing endogenous Ca^{++}.

The conversion of prothrombin to thrombin involves several proteolytic splits to eventually yield a two-chain thrombin molecule having a

molecular weight of 32,000. Thrombin hydrolyzes four bonds in fibrinogen, removing two pairs of peptides designated fibrinopeptides A and B. The resulting fibrin monomer spontaneously polymerizes to form the fibrin clot in the presence of Ca^{++} and factor XIII (the fibrin stabilizing factor) which catalyzes a transamination reaction cross-linking fibrin with covalent bonds.

Site of Action of Warfarin. Warfarin is a vitamin K antagonist. Vitamin K participates in the carboxylation of glutamic acid residues in the N terminal portion of factors IX, X and VII and of prothrombin. The formation of gamma carboxyl glutamic acid residues facilitates the binding of Ca^{++} by these proteins and their subsequent attachment to phospholipid. The net effect of warfarin is to block the conversion of precursor protein to zymogen, leading to a decrease in the concentration of factors IX, X and VII, and of prothrombin zymogens, and thus to a decrease in the rate of thrombin formation.

Site of Action of Heparin. Antithrombin III is a naturally occurring alpha globulin that combines with thrombin and factor X$_a$ to inhibit their proteolytic action. Heparin markedly accelerates the rate of inhibition of these enzymes. Only small doses are needed for X$_a$ neutralization, which is sufficient for prophylaxis of postsurgical thromboembolism. For established disease with high thrombin production, large doses are needed.

Clinical Manifestations of Leg Vein Thrombosis

Clinical manifestations of thromboses in the leg veins remain important despite a recently developed diagnostic technique utilizing radioactive fibrinogen (Plate 111). While this development represents a major advance, it does not relieve the physician of the responsibility of making the diagnosis by history and physical examination. In fact, the newer approach to diagnosis is expensive and cannot—on economic grounds—be applied widely without reasonable expectation of a positive diagnosis. Further, this method depends on anticipating the presence of thrombophlebitis in that the physician must give radioactive fibrinogen before the expected development of thrombophlebitis. Thus, the greatest application of this diagnostic method would be in such situations as immediately after surgery, or following burns or other injuries.

History. Thrombophlebitis is usually brought to the patient's attention by pain in the muscles of the affected leg. The pain may be diffuse or localized, and the patient usually does not confuse it with joint pain. Patients may notice that the pain is far worse on dependency and, conversely, completely relieved by elevation. There is often swelling of the affected leg and foot; the extremity may be warm locally, and the patient may be febrile.

Certain circumstances are likely to be associated with thrombophlebitis, and the physician should review these points with the patient. An initial event may be dependency of the leg for several hours. Obesity apparently makes the patient more susceptible to thrombophlebitis. Chronic illness, particularly carcinoma and most particularly carcinoma of the pancreas, enhances the possibility of this complication. Use of oral contraceptives increases the incidence of thrombophlebitis.

Physical Examination. The patient should first be examined in the standing position. The presence of varicose veins should be noted since they increase the patient's susceptibility to thrombophlebitis. Enhancement of the pain by dependency may provide a useful diagnostic clue. The patient is then examined in the recumbent position. A valuable method of detecting unilateral thrombophlebitis is to evaluate the tissue consistency of the affected leg as compared with that of its neighbor. The comparison is made as illustrated by ballottement of the tissues of the leg with the entire hand. Once the physician becomes experienced in this maneuver, clear-cut differences in the resistance of the tissues can be noted. The examination should be preceded by palpation of the calves for tenderness, with the patient's leg slightly flexed, as shown. Generalized tenderness of the calf or thigh may be found. In addition, there may be tenderness along the major veins of the calf or thigh and superficial point tenderness of small segments of veins involved with thrombophlebitis. The finding of superficial phlebitis is most important in that the potential for complicating thromboembolism is much less when a segment of vein is tender and a thrombus can be felt, but there is little or no tenderness elsewhere. The area of thrombosis may appear red because of inflammation spreading to the skin. Homans' sign is difficult to evaluate. The problem is that the tenderness may be bilateral. Elderly people, par-

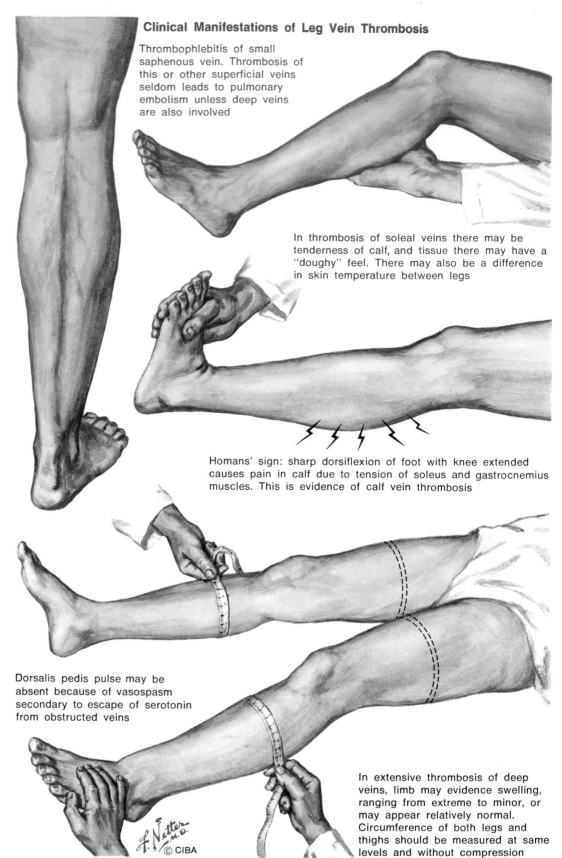

Clinical Manifestations of Leg Vein Thrombosis

Thrombophlebitis of small saphenous vein. Thrombosis of this or other superficial veins seldom leads to pulmonary embolism unless deep veins are also involved

In thrombosis of soleal veins there may be tenderness of calf, and tissue there may have a "doughy" feel. There may also be a difference in skin temperature between legs

Homans' sign: sharp dorsiflexion of foot with knee extended causes pain in calf due to tension of soleus and gastrocnemius muscles. This is evidence of calf vein thrombosis

Dorsalis pedis pulse may be absent because of vasospasm secondary to escape of serotonin from obstructed veins

In extensive thrombosis of deep veins, limb may evidence swelling, ranging from extreme to minor, or may appear relatively normal. Circumference of both legs and thighs should be measured at same levels and without compression

ticularly, experience some pain in their calves with dorsiflexion of their feet.

One of the main techniques for diagnosing and following a patient is that of comparative circumferential measurements of the legs at several levels. The aim is to look for minor amounts of edema that are not readily apparent. A difference of as little as 0.5 cm may be significant. Normally the patient's dominant leg may be slightly larger than the other leg. This normal increase may be as much as 2 cm at the calf, and more in the thigh.

Finally, a serious complication (phlegmasia cerulea dolens) which may arise is the absence of arterial circulation in the affected leg. This repre-

sents a medical emergency in that the reflex reduction of arterial circulation, as a relatively infrequent complication of thrombophlebitis, may lead to gangrene of the tissues of the foot. The diagnosis is made by observation of the deepening blue color of the extremity as well as the lack of arterial pulses and coldness of the distal part of the extremity, in contrast to the usual warm state in uncomplicated thrombophlebitis. The diagnosis is crucial because the arterial circulation can be restored promptly through use of a differential spinal block. This technique allows blockade of the sympathetic innervation of the blood vessels without blocking motor and sensory pathways to the leg.

Fibrin Degradation Products (FDP) in Diagnosis of Pulmonary Embolism

Source of Thrombus. Most clots that eventually result in pulmonary embolism begin in the soleal or calf veins. The first step in the diagnosis of pulmonary embolism is to diagnose deep vein thrombi. Unfortunately, thrombosis of deep veins is not only relatively insensitive to clinical diagnosis (50% of the thrombi are asymptomatic), but tests are also falsely positive in about 50% of cases. The diagnosis can be confirmed by venography (phlebography).

Recently, fibrinogen leg scanning has been shown to have a 90% correlation with venography (Plate 110). For fibrinogen leg scanning, radiolabeled fibrinogen, after injection, is incorporated into the thrombus, which is then detected by measuring the increase of overlying surface radioactivity (Plate 111). Lysis of the clot can also be followed by a decrease in surface radioactivity. Unfortunately, the small surface area of the thrombi in leg veins prevents the levels of the products of fibrinolysis in the blood from exceeding normal concentrations.

Two tests for assaying products of thrombin action, using soluble fibrin and fibrinopeptides, are under evaluation and show promise in the diagnosis of venous thromboembolism.

Pulmonary Embolism. When a leg vein thrombus is embolized to the lung capillaries, the resulting increased surface area occupied by the fibrin allows enhanced fibrinolysis and raises the levels of fibrin degradation products (FDP). The concentration of FDP is then much greater than normal and, in the absence of liver disease or disseminated intravascular coagulation, may reach diagnostically useful elevations.

Biochemistry of Fibrinogen Proteolysis. Thrombin attacks only four bonds in the fibrinogen molecule (molecular weight 340,000), splitting off two moles of fibrinopeptide from the N terminal end of the A alpha and B beta chains. In contrast, plasmin attacks a total of 80 bonds in fibrinogen (or fibrin), giving rise to FDP of various types in the bloodstream. One can classify these peptide products into several categories. The first acts to hydrolyze bonds primarily in the C terminal end of the alpha chain and eventually yields a product designated as fragment X (molecular weight 240,000). This fragment retains its fibrinopeptides and is still clottable by thrombin, although more slowly than the native molecule. It therefore remains with the clot when thrombin is added to plasma and is not present in serum. Each molecule of X is then further degraded by plasma to one molecule of Y (molecular weight 150,000) and one molecule of D (molecular weight 80,000). Fragment Y is not clottable by thrombin and, indeed, antagonizes the proteolytic activity of thrombin. It is consequently a powerful anticoagulant that prevents coagulation of fibrinogen. Fragment D is not clottable by thrombin. However, it functions as an "antimetabolite" of fibrin, being incorporated in the fibrin polymer but in the process slowing the polymerization and resulting in a structurally

Fibrin Degradation Products (FDP) in Diagnosis of Pulmonary Emboli

Clot disseminated to lung

Because of small surface area, thrombi in leg veins offer little exposure to plasmin. Effects are therefore not diagnostically significant for leg thrombosis

Large surface area of lung emboli in pulmonary capillaries offers great exposure to plasmin, and test may therefore be of diagnostic value

Plasmin of circulating blood splits fibrinogen (and fibrin) into a number of fragments

Thrombin

Gives rise to fibrinogen degradation products (FDP) in circulating blood

FDP may then be quantitated immunologically because their antigenic reaction is similar to that of fibrinogen (latex agglutination, tanned red cell, or other tests)

Patient's blood allowed to clot, thus removing free fibrinogen from serum

disordered clot. Thus, it also functions as an anticoagulant. Fragment Y is then further degraded into a second molecule of D and a molecule of E (molecular weight 50,000).

Detection of Fibrin Degradation Products. The assay measures nonclottable FDP (Y, D and E). After the addition of excess thrombin to make sure that all fibrinogen is clotted and of plasmin inhibitor to prevent any *in vitro* fibrinolysis, the resulting serum is used for FDP determination.

There are several methods for quantitation of FDP. In one of the most popular, latex particles coated with antibodies against fragments D and E are added to the serum. Any FDP will clump the

particles, and the highest dilution at which clumping occurs gives a measure of FDP concentration. The normal concentration is less than or equal to $5\mu g/ml$. Elevations of up to $40\mu g/ml$ occur in liver dysfunction. Concentrations in excess of $40\mu g/ml$ have been reported in pulmonary embolism and disseminated intravascular coagulation. The latter condition usually exhibits profound coagulation abnormalities. Pulmonary embolism, however, usually shows elevated FDP without the clotting abnormalities, since fibrinolysis occurs only in the pulmonary capillary bed. Further evaluation of the usefulness of FDP determinations in pulmonary embolism is now in progress.

Phlebography for Diagnosis of Leg Vein Thrombosis (Venography)

Water-soluble contrast medium injected into distal vein of lower extremity. Tourniquet applied just tightly enough to occlude superficial veins and drive solution into deep veins. Exposures made at ½ minute and 1 minute

34 inch cassette

Lower Extremity Phlebography (Venography)

Phlebogram showing patency of most of deep venous system with thrombus in common femoral vein

Failure of filling of deep venous system due to thrombus below. Common femoral vein filled via superficial collaterals

Pulmonary embolism is a major cause of morbidity and mortality in hospitalized patients, and lower limb phlebothrombosis is the major source of pulmonary embolism. Thus, in addition to establishing the diagnosis of pulmonary embolism by radionuclide or angiographic criteria, it is important to demonstrate the presence or absence of phlebothrombosis in the lower limbs. Phlebography (venography) is the definitive method to establish this diagnosis as well as for (1) diagnosis of chronic edema and venous stasis, (2) study of varicose veins, and (3) evaluation of a postphlebitic syndrome. However, the principal indication for lower limb phlebography is suspected deep venous thrombosis.

Less invasive diagnostic techniques are correspondingly less accurate. Clinical diagnosis alone has an accuracy of approximately 50%. Impedance plethysmography and the Doppler method (Plates 112 and 113) are 60 to 90% accurate, and radioactive ^{125}I-fibrinogen uptake (Plate 111) has an accuracy of approximately 85%. Properly performed lower limb phlebography has an accuracy approaching 100% and is highly reliable and safe.

In the technique described by Rogoff and De-Weese, 40 to 50 ml of water-soluble contrast material are injected into a foot vein, with the patient semierect. A tourniquet is placed just tightly enough about the ankle to drive the contrast material into the deep venous system. An initial radiograph is made following the injection. The tourniquet is then removed; the patient flexes the sole of the involved extremity 3 to 10 times, and a second radiograph is made.

In the technique described by Rabinov and Paulin and generally now favored, 100 to 150 ml of water-soluble contrast material are injected without a tourniquet. Again the patient is semierect, with the involved leg non-weight-bearing. Progress of the contrast material is followed fluoroscopically and by appropriate spot films and overhead radiographs. The patient does not exercise the leg.

Anatomically, the venous system of the lower extremity can be divided into four types of veins:

(1) deep veins, which run parallel to the arteries and are paired in the lower leg and single in the thigh; (2) superficial veins, located in the subcutaneous tissues; (3) deep muscle veins; (4) communicating veins, which connect the superficial and the deep veins.

The diagnosis of deep venous thrombosis is made by demonstrating an intraluminal defect outlined by contrast material from either one or both sides. The defect must persist in at least two radiographs in different projections. Other presumptive evidence includes nonfilling of the entire deep venous system or portions of it, and diversion of flow in the presence of nonfilling of the deep venous system.

Any complications are primarily systemic side-effects from administration of intravenous contrast material. Most side-effects are minor allergic reactions (e.g., hives) but, on occasion, serious anaphylactic reactions can occur.

Local effects may occur if there is extravasation of contrast material about the injection site. This primarily causes pain, but skin necrosis sometimes takes place. Some authors feel that phlebography itself may initiate deep venous thrombosis or at least a clinical syndrome resembling it. Rapid performance of the examination and careful drainage of contrast material from the involved leg help to prevent this complication.

Fibrinogen Scan for Thrombosis

The ^{125}I-fibrinogen test is based on the fact that when labeled fibrinogen is injected into an individual, it circulates with endogenous plasma fibrinogen and is incorporated with it into newly forming thrombi. It can be detected as an accumulation of radioactivity over peripheral venous channels when a thrombus exists. The test is best applied prospectively in the patient who is at risk of developing venous thrombosis and who is to be monitored for days or even weeks. A suspicion of current thrombotic disease may also warrant the study, particularly if the clinical situation permits a delay of several days before definitive evidence is obtained.

Human fibrinogen is purified from the plasma of carefully selected donors who have been shown to be free of hepatitis antigen and antibody by *in vitro* tests and by clinical follow-up of plasma recipients. After separation from other plasma proteins, the fibrinogen is tagged with iodine 125. A dose of 100 microcuries of radioactivity is effective and safe for a single study lasting from 7 to 10 days. If necessary, the test can be repeated for prolonged monitoring. The potential for transmitting hepatitis has been virtually eliminated by careful and stringent control in screening potential donors. Uptake of the ^{125}I tag by the thyroid is prevented by thyroid blockade with cold iodide before and after injection of the radiopharmaceutical. Patients allergic to iodides cannot be pretreated and therefore cannot undergo the test.

The labeled fibrinogen is administered intravenously via the antecubital vein or any suitable peripheral vein. In the prospective monitoring of patients scheduled for elective surgery, the baseline can be established preoperatively. If extensive blood loss is anticipated, the test may be started in the final operative stages or just after surgery. Patients bedridden for prolonged periods can be injected repeatedly at 7 to 10 day intervals without increasing the risk of complication or decreasing the usefulness of the reagent. Surface counting is performed over the precordium and over the major deep veins of the thighs and calves of both legs. Positions on the leg are marked with indelible ink at 2 inch intervals, starting at the medial aspect of the thigh just below the inguinal ligament to just above the knee, then on the posterior or medioposterior aspect of the calf to just above the ankle.

Counts are always obtained with the patient supine and, when possible, with the legs elevated to reduce venous pooling and to accommodate the probe on the posterior aspects of the calf. Counts obtained in each position on the legs are calculated as a percentage of the precordial count, and the values obtained for the initial measurement are considered as baseline for subsequent observations. The "percent increase index" reflects local accumulations of radioactivity and is calculated by the percentage change from heart counts at any given position. Such changes are then compared with the baseline values in the same position, the corresponding position of the opposite leg on the same day, and the adjacent position on the same leg on the same day. Increases greater than 20% on two successive days are usually considered suggestive of active thrombosis.

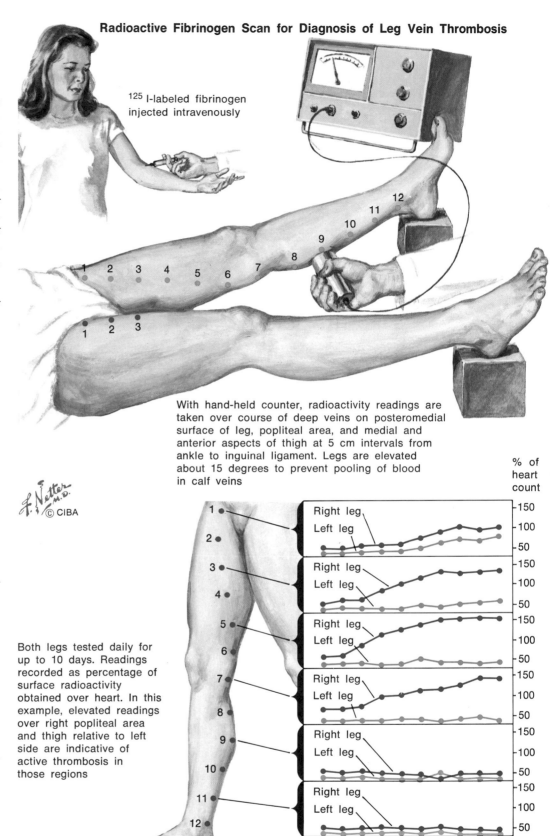

Radioactive Fibrinogen Scan for Diagnosis of Leg Vein Thrombosis

^{125}I-labeled fibrinogen injected intravenously

With hand-held counter, radioactivity readings are taken over course of deep veins on posteromedial surface of leg, popliteal area, and medial and anterior aspects of thigh at 5 cm intervals from ankle to inguinal ligament. Legs are elevated about 15 degrees to prevent pooling of blood in calf veins

F. Netter M.D. © CIBA

Both legs tested daily for up to 10 days. Readings recorded as percentage of surface radioactivity obtained over heart. In this example, elevated readings over right popliteal area and thigh relative to left side are indicative of active thrombosis in those regions

% of heart count

Days after injection

The validity of the radiolabeled fibrinogen test has been checked against results obtained by phlebography (Plate 110), performed after abnormal uptake of radioactivity or after completion of a negative study. It seems that 75 to 90% of the ^{125}I-fibrinogen tests accurately reflect the presence or absence of deep vein thrombosis, with the rest divided into false positive and false negative results. A false positive result, defined as a positive scan associated with a normal phlebogram, may be related to a hematoma, ruptured Baker's cyst, cellulitis, phlebitis, a surgical wound or torn muscle.

Because of the proximity of the urinary bladder and the large iliac and femoral vessels, thrombi above the inguinal ligament generally cannot be reliably detected by the ^{125}I-fibrinogen test. The unexplained appearance of high radioactivity over all regions of both legs and over the precordium suggests that an additional radiopharmaceutical has been administered—*e.g.,* technetium 99m for the performance of a lung scan. A false negative result, defined as a negative test associated with an abnormal phlebogram, could stem from a small thrombus localized to a single valve cusp, healed or inactive thrombotic disease, or effective anticoagulant therapy. Inadequate treatment could reasonably be assumed if uptake of the radiolabel occurred despite anticoagulant medication.

Ultrasonography and Plethysmography

When acute deep venous thrombosis is suspected in a patient, there are two common laboratory methods of verifying the diagnosis. One of them uses the ultrasonic velocity detector and the other employs plethysmographic techniques to assess quantitatively the degree to which the rate of venous outflow has been reduced by the thrombosis. Both tests are noninvasive and may be used at the patient's bedside to verify with great accuracy venous occlusion of the major deep veins of the lower leg. A great advantage of these relatively new tests is that, if necessary, they may be used repetitively to follow the patient's clinical course.

Ultrasonography. For a complete examination utilizing the Doppler effect, the probe is placed over the following veins in this order: (1) common femoral vein, (2) midsuperficial femoral vein, (3) posterior tibial vein and (4) popliteal vein. Evaluation of flow in the first three veins is done with the patient in the supine position. The popliteal vein is best examined with the patient in the prone position and the feet supported by pillows.

The procedure is carried out systematically by examining venous flow dynamics from comparable veins; that is, the right common femoral vein is examined first, the left common femoral vein next, and so on. This sequence is very important because often subtle differences in venous flow between identical sites of the two limbs can be of diagnostic significance.

The vein is located by first identifying its companion artery. In the case of the common femoral vein, it is identified by moving the transducer slightly medially after the characteristic pulsatile velocity signal from the artery has been found. With the superficial femoral, popliteal and posterior tibial veins, the flow velocity signals are heard simultaneously with those from arterial flow because of their proximity to one another.

The venous flow pattern is largely dominated by respiration. For example, at the level of the common femoral and superficial femoral veins, flow normally goes to zero at the end of inspiration, when intraabdominal pressure exceeds the pressure in the iliac veins and inferior vena cava. These phasic changes with respiration are not so prominent in the popliteal and posterior tibial veins. It may be necessary to augment flow (increase its velocity) by compressing the limb distal to the probe. For instance, with the probe over the midsuperficial femoral or popliteal vein, flow is augmented by compressing the calf. In the case of the posterior tibial vein at the ankle, augmentation is carried out by forcefully squeezing the foot.

With acute venous obstruction, changes occur that are of diagnostic importance: if the vein being examined is occluded, there will be no spontaneous or augmented flow signals heard from the involved

vein. If the vein examined is open but is distal (toward the foot) to the area of venous thrombosis, flow may be detected, but it loses its phasic quality and becomes continuous (not influenced by respiration).

The technique is accurate in experienced hands for detecting occlusion of the major deep veins (posterior tibial, popliteal, femoral and iliac). It will not detect small thrombi confined to the soleal plexus of veins.

In practice, the pocket-sized Doppler instrument is used with stethoscope earphones as the examiner listens to the flow changes. It is possible to record the velocity changes, but this measure-

ment is not necessary for routine use. Strip chart recordings are helpful for demonstrating the flow changes graphically and for teaching purposes.

Plethysmography. The two types of plethysmography in common use to measure venous outflow are the mercury strain gauge and the impedance method. The mercury strain gauge directly measures the volume change of the calf, which can then be expressed as flow in terms of milliliters/100 ml of tissue/minute. With the impedance plethysmograph, the volume change of the calf is expressed as a percentage change of the baseline impedance.

(Continued)

Ultrasound in Diagnosis of Acute Venous Thrombosis

Normal
Phasic flow

Inspirations

Thrombosis
Continuous flow

A. For common femoral vein

CF

SF

Placement points of ultrasonic stethoscope for common femoral (CF) and superficial femoral (SF) veins

B. For posterior tibial vein

Normal
Augmentation

Foot compression — Calf compression — Release

Thrombosis

No augmentation

Normal
Augmentation

Calf compression

Thrombosis

No augmentation

C. For popliteal vein

Plethysmography in Diagnosis of Leg Vein Thrombosis

Ultrasonography and Plethysmography
(Continued)

In practice, the tests are carried out in a nearly identical manner. A large cuff is placed about the thigh and rapidly inflated to 50 mm Hg; this temporarily obstructs venous outflow. After the limb volume has stabilized, the cuff is suddenly deflated and the maximal rate at which the calf volume empties (maximal venous outflow) can be calculated from the initial portion of the downslope. With the strain gauge method, a maximal venous outflow of less than 25 ml/100 ml/minute is abnormal. A change in the impedance of less than 1%/second is highly suggestive of acute venous thrombosis.

Comparison of Tests. These two diagnostic methods, ultrasonography and plethysmography, used either singly or in combination, have their greatest application in evaluating patients who develop symptoms and/or signs suggesting deep venous thrombosis. When the thrombi involve the major deep veins, accuracy of the tests should approach 95%. The basis for errors is the presence of thrombi inaccessible to the methods—*i.e.*, in the soleus plexus, or in the tibial or peroneal veins, where they do not produce enough total venous occlusion to interfere with venous outflow. False positive results are obtained when the test is improperly performed or there are coexisting conditions that interfere with venous flow.

In patients with symptoms and signs suggesting acute venous occlusion, about one-half will have normal veins. This fact has been verified by several studies in which venography has been the diagnostic method of choice for evaluating patients suspected of harboring venous thrombi in the deep venous system.

While venography remains the best diagnostic method for assessing deep venous thrombosis, it has serious drawbacks: (1) it is painful; (2) it is costly; (3) it is not easily repeated to follow the course of disease; and (4) the complications—while their incidence is low—may be serious, such as chemical phlebitis.

In clinical practice, a positive test with either ultrasound or plethysmography is adequate to make the diagnosis of venous thrombosis and to institute anticoagulant therapy. It is not necessary to perform venography unless there is either some question as to the test results or a need for critical anatomic information for the medical or surgical management of the patient. Any equivocal test can be repeated on a daily basis if necessary to validate the initial observations.

The more troublesome patients are those with symptoms or signs although tests are normal. This finding means one of three things: either (1) the thrombi are in the muscular veins of the calf; or (2) the thrombi are not occlusive to the extent of interfering with venous flow; or (3) there is some other cause for the problem. The noninvasive tests

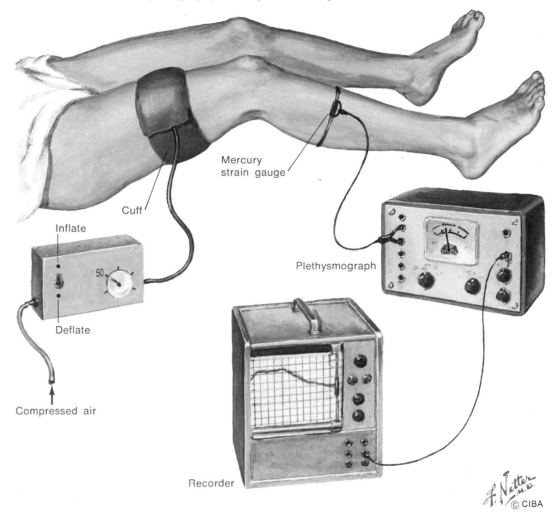

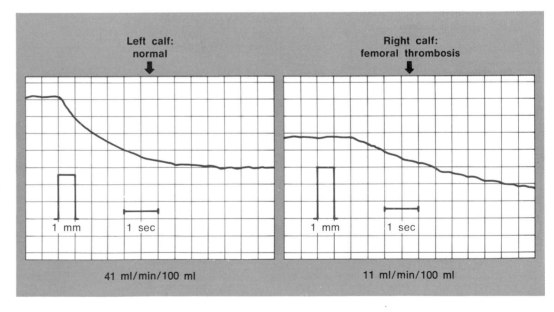

Left calf: normal

1 mm   1 sec

41 ml/min/100 ml

Right calf: femoral thrombosis

1 mm   1 sec

11 ml/min/100 ml

must be repeated to be sure that the initial impression was correct. Thrombi which remain confined to the muscular veins rarely cause problems, but they can propagate into the major deep veins, producing more serious difficulties. In this event the noninvasive tests will become positive and therapy should be instituted.

A very important fact to remember is that whenever the physician is concerned and wants an immediate, conclusive answer, venography can be performed. In most cases the noninvasive tests described here can be used to screen symptomatic patients and obviate the need for an invasive procedure. The noninvasive methods have proved useful

as an integral part of the workup of patients with acute venous occlusion.

Finally, the two noninvasive tests described should be considered in relation to the other commonly used method, the ^{125}I-labeled fibrinogen scan (Plate 111). It is designed to detect very early thrombi in the muscular veins of the calf. Its greatest utility is in the evaluation of prophylactic methods devised to prevent venous thrombosis. It is less sensitive to thrombi located above the knee, where ultrasonography and plethysmography have their greatest utility. Further, since the fibrinogen must be given before thrombosis occurs, it is of little value in patients with established occlusion.

Pulmonary Embolism

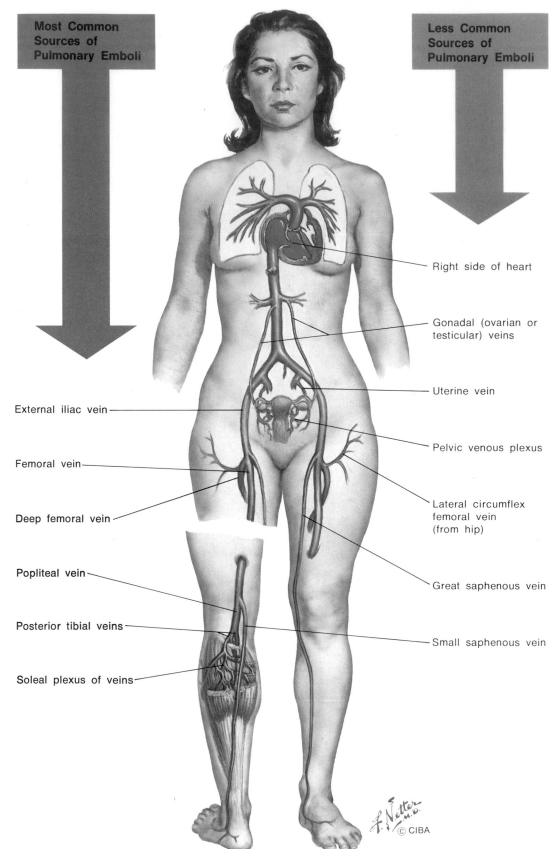

Most Common Sources of Pulmonary Emboli

Less Common Sources of Pulmonary Emboli

Right side of heart

Gonadal (ovarian or testicular) veins

Uterine vein

Pelvic venous plexus

External iliac vein

Femoral vein

Deep femoral vein

Lateral circumflex femoral vein (from hip)

Popliteal vein

Great saphenous vein

Posterior tibial veins

Soleal plexus of veins

Small saphenous vein

The lungs are natural filters for venous clots that are larger in diameter than the formed elements of the blood. Ordinarily, the lung can cope easily with the small clots because of its fibrinolytic mechanisms. However, large thrombi or a shower of small clots may overwhelm the ability of the lung to fragment and dissolve them.

Sources of Emboli

The source of clots is generally the deep veins of the legs and pelvis—*i.e.,* a femoral, popliteal or iliac vein. Most often, clots in a thigh vein originate as an extension of a clot in a deep calf vein. Superficial thrombophlebitis in the legs or thighs rarely gives rise to emboli but may signal a deep venous thrombosis. It is the loose propagating thrombus in the deep veins that constitutes the hazard of pulmonary embolization. When broken loose, the clot is carried to the lungs through the venous stream and right heart. Clots from the peripheral veins ultimately lodge in pulmonary arteries and, depending on their size and location, may either fragment further or remain fixed *in situ*.

Quite often no definite source for the pulmonary emboli can be found. Superficial thrombophlebitis, which may be associated with deep venous thrombosis, occurs in less than one-third of patients with pulmonary embolism. Signs of deep venous thrombosis in the calf or thigh are difficult to detect until the venous circulation is extensively compromised (Plate 108). When careful examination fails to implicate veins of the extremities, it is usual to suspect thrombosis of less accessible deep veins, particularly the pelvic veins in women who have had complicated obstetric manipulations, pelvic inflammatory disease or septic abortion associated with suppurative pelvic thrombophlebitis.

Local or systemic disorders that predispose to venous thrombosis in the legs are also potential precursors of pulmonary emboli (Plate 115). Paramount among these is venous stasis. Even in a normal person, a prolonged ride with flexed knees in an automobile or airplane may lead to venous stasis and thrombosis in the legs. Older people are more vulnerable than the young, especially if venous valves in the legs are incompetent or the venous circulation is sluggish because of heart failure. Prolonged bed rest in patients with slowed circulation is a common cause. Patients who have undergone major abdominal surgery are prime candidates for venous thrombosis and pulmonary embolization.

Polycythemia and increased blood coagulability are less likely to be predisposing causes. Least common is direct injury to vessel walls.

Oral contraceptives predispose to venous thrombosis and pulmonary emboli. Although the precise basis for this relationship is unclear, the association is well established.

It must be emphasized that small pulmonary emboli (Plate 116) are probably common occurrences during a normal lifetime, but they are handled quietly by the lungs. During pregnancy, tissue fragments are frequent in the uterine veins, en route to the lungs. These too cause no problem.

(Continued)

Predisposing Factors for Pulmonary Embolism

Venous stasis

Prolonged bed rest

Prolonged sitting

Heart failure

Local disorders; varicosities, phlebitis

Coagulation disorders

Oral contraceptives

Polycythemia

γ spike   Alb.

β α2 α1

Multiple myeloma

Trauma

Fractures; also soft-tissue (vessel) injury

Post-operative or post-partum

Hip operations

Extensive pelvic or abdominal operations

Phlegmasia alba dolens (milk-leg)

Pulmonary Embolism
(Continued)

However, when the emboli are sufficiently large or numerous, or cause infarction, or involve the pleura, they become clinically evident.

Clinical Manifestations

A massive embolus that either lodges in the main pulmonary artery or overrides both branches to the point of compromising the bulk of the pulmonary blood flow is a disaster that elicits circulatory collapse and acute cor pulmonale (Plates 117 and 119). This form of pulmonary embolization is a dire emergency, but it is difficult to distinguish from an acute myocardial infarction. The chances of detecting it depend on the physician's suspicion that the patient is predisposed to pulmonary embolization. Once clinical suspicion has been raised, support for the diagnosis is provided by the classic S_1-Q_3 pattern in the electrocardiogram. Almost as convincing is a fresh "P pulmonale" pattern, a new right axis shift, or a new pattern of incomplete right bundle-branch block.

Much less dramatic but equally distinctive clinically is pulmonary infarction secondary to pulmonary embolization (Plate 118). This type of presentation is seen more frequently than the massive embolus, but it is still relatively uncommon; *i.e.,* it occurs after less than 10% of pulmonary emboli. The evidence for pulmonary infarction is acute onset of pleural pain, hemoptysis, breathlessness, pleural effusion or pleural friction rub.

Far more prevalent than the previous two categories is pulmonary embolization *without* infarction (Plate 116). The clinical manifestations of pulmonary embolization *per se* are generally subtle: unexplained tachypnea and dyspnea, anxiety, vague substernal pressure and occasionally syncope. In a patient predisposed by bed rest, surgery, or local thrombophlebitis, these symptoms constitute strong evidence for a pulmonary embolus even though the physical examination is unrewarding, the ECG indeterminate, and the chest x-ray film normal.

The roentgenographic appearance depends on the size and number of emboli, whether they have produced pulmonary infarction, and whether the infarcted area reaches the pleural surface to cause pleuritis and pleural effusion. A massive embolus located at the origin of a major pulmonary artery causes hypoperfusion of the ipsilateral lung manifested by a decrease in vascular markings. Increase in size of a major hilar vessel or an abrupt cutoff, the "knuckle sign," is strong supportive evidence when present. If not distinctly oligemic, areas of the lung will often show unduly small vessels.

Sometimes the only indication of a large embolus is an unusually high diaphragm on the affected side or the presence of a pulmonary infiltrate, a consequence of infarction, hemorrhage or atelectasis. An ipsilateral pleural effusion may also be the only sign of an otherwise unsuspected pulmonary infarction. All this x-ray evidence takes on

(Continued)

Embolism of Lesser Degree Without Infarction

Multiple small emboli of lungs

Sudden onset of dyspnea and tachycardia in a predisposed individual is cardinal clue

Dyspnea

Auscultation may be normal or few rales and diminished breath sounds may be noted

Tachycardia

F. Netter, M.D.
© CIBA

Angiogram; small emboli (arrows)

Ventilation scan normal

Perfusion scan reveals defects in right lung. Emboli in left lung not visualized

X-ray film often normal; elevation of hemidiaphragm (as above) significant. Areas of atelectasis may be visible

Pulmonary Embolism
(Continued)

a great significance if the individual is predisposed to peripheral or pelvic venous thrombosis and has been identified as a serious candidate for pulmonary embolism. Often nothing abnormal can be seen. Pulmonary angiograms provide the only definitive method of establishing large vessel occlusion and are indicated when the increased risk is clinically justified.

Laboratory Tests

A mainstay in the diagnosis of massive pulmonary embolism is a decrease in arterial oxygen tension, generally in association with reduced arterial carbon dioxide tension. The arterial hypoxemia is a consequence of ventilation-perfusion abnormalities, whereas the hypocapnia is caused by hyperventilation that is presumed to be reflexly induced by the emboli via the J receptors. Hypoventilated areas probably result from interference with surfactant and resulting atelectasis in small areas of lung.

Other blood tests are of much more limited value. Leukocytosis generally accompanies infarction. Appreciable levels of fibrin-degradation products in the blood signify that fibrin thrombi have formed and are undergoing lysis, but they do not localize the site; the value of this test remains to be determined. Other measurements, including concentrations of LDH (lactic dehydrogenase) and bilirubin in serum, have proved to be of little practical value.

A lung scan, using a radioisotope as a marker, is generally done to establish the diagnosis of pulmonary embolism (see pages 95 and 96). Macroaggregated albumin, labeled with iodine 131 or technetium 99, is commonly used for this purpose. The tracer substance is injected intravenously. The radioactive particles, which are of the order of 50 to 100 microns in diameter, are trapped in the microcirculation of the lung. The pattern of distribution of these radioactive particles, detected by an external counter, defines the pattern of pulmonary blood flow. Alternatively, an intravenous injection of labeled xenon (xenon 133) may be used as a tracer. In patients without intrinsic disease of the lungs or airways a perfusion scan may suffice. However, it is considerably more helpful to have ventilation and perfusion scans performed at the same sitting, so that areas of inadequate blood flow may be related to ventilation abnormalities. Most specific in reaching a diagnosis is the finding of multiple perfusion defects in normally ventilated lungs.

Lung scans are practical, simple and safe. They can be repeated as necessary to trace the resolution of defects and to detect fresh emboli. On occasion, perfusion scans are noninformative because of the limitations in current scanning techniques or because occlusion of vascular lumina is incomplete.

Exceedingly helpful in recognizing pulmonary emboli and in preventing recurrence is the detection of a site of venous thrombosis in a leg or thigh (Plate 108). The clinical manifestations of local

(Continued)

Massive Embolization

Pulmonary Embolism
(Continued)

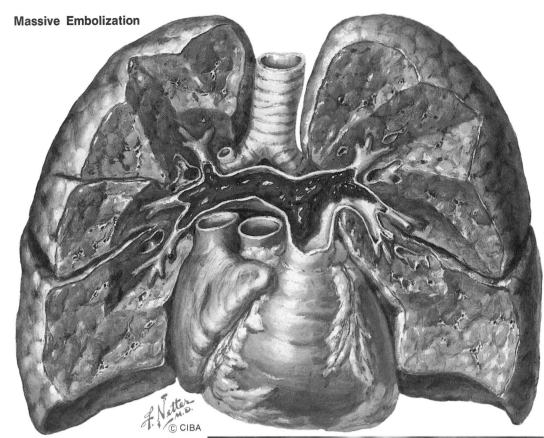

Saddle embolus completely occluding r. pulmonary artery and partially obstructing main and left arteries

X-ray film shows dense shadow of r. pulmonary artery with increased luminescence of peripheral lung fields

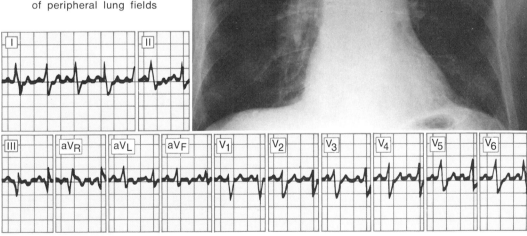

Characteristic electrocardiographic findings in acute pulmonary embolism. Deep S_1; prominent Q_3 with inversion of T_3; depression of S-T segment in lead II (often also in lead I) with staircase ascent of S-T_2; T_2 diphasic or inverted; r. axis deviation; tachycardia

venous thrombosis include swelling and induration of the extremity, with tenderness on pressure along the course of a deep vein. Phlebography (Plate 110), which identifies site(s) of obstruction in the deep venous system of the extremity, is most accurate for diagnosis. Since this technique involves the injection of radiopaque material and x-ray examination, other less cumbersome approaches are being sought. Among the more promising are radioactive fibrinogen (^{125}I) and ultrasound (Plates 111 and 112). Radioactive fibrinogen is most useful in detecting thrombi in the lower leg; it is less accurate in detecting venous thrombi in the thigh and is of no value for the iliac veins. Since the procedure is simple to perform, and since most venous thrombi begin in the calf, it has value as a diagnostic tool. Its major drawback is the risk of infectious hepatitis that it entails.

Prophylaxis and Treatment

Prophylaxis (Plate 120) is concerned with the prevention of clot formation in the deep veins of the legs and with the extension of a clot that can break off and travel to the lungs. This approach involves the use of elastic stockings to direct blood to the deeper veins and increase the velocity of flow, motion of the legs to prevent undue stasis, elevation of legs to promote venous drainage, and frequent shifts in posture.

More aggressive prophylaxis is currently common practice for surgical patients. Small doses of heparin (about 5000 units) may be given intravenously or subcutaneously, starting the day before surgery and continued two to three times per day

for five days to one week postoperatively. This program has proved to be remarkably effective in decreasing the incidence of deep venous thrombosis, even though heparin at this dosage exerts no effect on conventional clotting tests, and is free of bleeding complications.

For seriously ill patients predisposed to emboli, the approach is different. At the first signs of deep venous thrombosis, therapy with heparin, rather than prophylaxis, is begun. The doses required are larger than those used for prophylaxis (5,000 to 10,000 units every four to six hours) and preferably should be administered intravenously. Heparin in these doses prevents propagation of the clot. The

program is continued up to 12 days, including ambulation on the last two days when the signs of thrombosis in the legs have disappeared.

Before the heparin therapy is stopped, warfarin is started in a dosage of 10 to 15 mg/day. This program is continued for one to three months after discharge, prothrombin times being used to control dosage; the prothrombin time is kept at one and one-half to twice normal. Drug interactions can be troublesome during warfarin therapy, and each new medication must be examined for its effect in enhancing or diminishing the action of warfarin (Plates 107 and 121).

(Continued)

Pulmonary Infarction

Pulmonary Embolism
(Continued)

Infarct in
l. lower lobe.
Pleural exudate
over lesion

Causative obstructed vessel.
A few small scattered emboli
without infarction also present
in both lungs

X-ray film shows wedge-shaped opacity
in l. costophrenic region

Pleural pain and breathlessness
suggest infarction; hemoptysis
may also occur

Once embolization has been recognized, medical management is the rule, except in the case of massive embolization, which may require surgical intervention. Surgery is practical only in an institution with a well-trained surgical team that is prepared to intervene promptly. In general, this approach is reserved for a few selected cases with special indications. The role of thrombolytic agents is not yet clear.

Therapeutic doses of heparin are begun as soon as the diagnosis of pulmonary embolism is made. Administration of heparin is continued until evidence of venous thrombosis disappears and there are no fresh signs of embolization. Before the heparin therapy is stopped, the patient is generally instructed to ambulate, wearing elastic stockings, and treatment with warfarin is started.

Surgical intervention (Plate 122) is almost exclusively reserved for the source of emboli in the legs rather than for emboli that have lodged in the lungs. Rarely is an attempt made to remove clots from the veins of the legs. Instead, surgery is usually directed at the inferior vena cava. Either ligation, plication or positioning of an "umbrella" to capture emboli has been used. Each procedure has its complications, and does not always protect the lungs from emboli because of large collateral vessels that serve as alternative routes from the legs to the lungs, and because thrombi may arise in peripheral venous beds that drain elsewhere than into the inferior vena cava.

One clear indication for vena caval ligation is suppurative thrombophlebitis in pelvic veins, followed by septic emboli to the lungs. In such a case

heparin and antibiotics rarely suffice, and ligation of the inferior vena cava and of the left ovarian vein is mandatory.

Small emboli are occasionally dispatched to the lungs for months to years without clinical evidence of acute embolizations. The patients present with evidence of severe pulmonary hypertension and often die in right ventricular failure. The course of patients with multiple pulmonary emboli may be so subtle as to mimic that of patients with primary pulmonary hypertension (Plate 123). At this late stage of disease, therapeutic intervention, using anticoagulants, is often tried but is rarely successful.

Chronic Effects of Pulmonary Embolism (Cor Pulmonale)

Cor pulmonale is defined as enlargement of the right ventricle due to hypertrophy or dilatation. As a complication of pulmonary embolism, it assumes two clinical forms, acute and chronic (see Plate 36 for general features of cor pulmonale).

Acute Cor Pulmonale. The effect of one or more massive emboli is a reduction in the cross-sectional area of the pulmonary vascular tree and an increase in pulmonary vascular resistance to blood flow. If most of the pulmonary vascular tree is blocked,

(Continued)

Chronic Effects of Pulmonary Embolism (Cor Pulmonale)

Pulmonary Embolism
(*Continued*)

X-ray film: cor pulmonale

Hypertrophy of right ventricle; distention and atherosclerosis of pulmonary arteries

Organized embolus of intra-pulmonary artery with beginning recanalization (trichrome stain)

Plaque, cords, and web in a lobar pulmonary artery as result of organization of embolus

ECG. Deep S₁ and high R₃ indicative of r. axis deviation. High R in aV$_R$ and in V₁ plus inverted or diphasic T in V₁ to V₃ evidence of r. ventricular hypertrophy

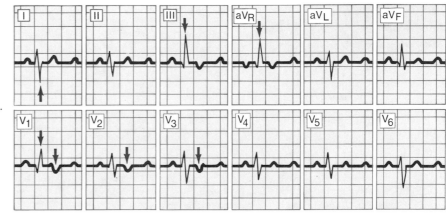

marked pulmonary hypertension occurs followed by dilatation and even failure of the right ventricle. In patients with previously normal lungs, the severity of these changes correlates closely on a lung scan with the extent of perfusion defects. Whether the total hemodynamic effect is attributable to the restricted vascular bed or to associated reflex or humoral vasoconstrictor mechanisms is unclear. While a reflex mechanism seems unlikely on the basis of existing evidence, it is believed that serotonin released from platelets and possibly other pressor substances may play a significant role. Mean pulmonary artery pressure in these circumstances is often greater than 30 mm Hg, or about twice the normal value.

A decrease in cardiac output and a fall in systemic blood pressure accompany the right ventricular enlargement. Preexisting cardiac or lung disease aggravates these changes and may precipitate intractable heart failure.

When pulmonary embolism is extensive enough to produce acute cor pulmonale, it often results in syncope and cardiopulmonary arrest. Profound apprehension, central chest pain and cardiac dysrhythmias — especially atrial flutter — may also occur, and in many patients death follows within a few hours of the embolic episode. The physical findings of acute cor pulmonale include tachycardia, an elevated jugular venous pressure with prominent A wave, shock and cyanosis. Wide splitting of the second heart sound may be present and is often fixed. It disappears with the resolution of the embolus and relief of right ventricular failure. Occasionally a right ventricular gallop can be heard, along with a systolic ejection murmur in the pul-

monary area. There may be a palpable lift over the right ventricle and a loud pulmonary closure sound.

Chest roentgenograms may show little change in cardiac configuration, but cardiomegaly, when present, is due to right ventricular enlargement. Electrocardiographic changes may be transient, but right shift of the QRS axis and complete right bundle-branch block often accompany acute cor pulmonale.

Fortunately, most emboli resolve by a combination of fragmentation and dislodgment of the smaller particles to the periphery and by fibrinolysis. Massive embolism resulting in acute cor

pulmonale requires support of cardiogenic shock, oxygen therapy and usually mechanical ventilation, and anticoagulant or thrombolytic agents. Rarely, when all other measures fail, surgical embolectomy is performed.

Chronic Cor Pulmonale. In the absence of intrinsic lung disease, chronic cor pulmonale from occlusion of the pulmonary vascular bed is most often due to recurrent pulmonary emboli and rarely to an episode of unresolved pulmonary embolism. In some patients there is little question that repeated embolization has taken place; in others evidence of pulmonary vascular occlusion
(*Continued*)

Pulmonary Embolism
(Continued)

Medical Prophylaxis and Therapy for Thromboembolic Disease

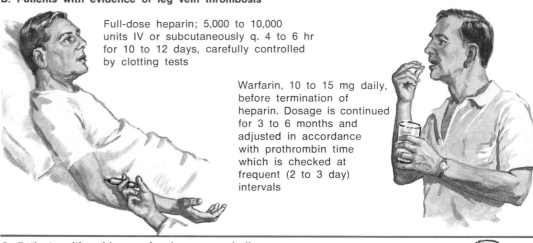

A. Prophylaxis

Early ambulation postoperatively; elastic stockings or wrappings, especially if stasis is present

Leg exercises and elevation; frequent changes of position

Low-dose heparin; 5,000 units subcutaneously b.i.d. or t.i.d. beginning 24 hr preoperatively and continuing 5 to 7 days postoperatively

B. Patients with evidence of leg vein thrombosis

Full-dose heparin; 5,000 to 10,000 units IV or subcutaneously q. 4 to 6 hr for 10 to 12 days, carefully controlled by clotting tests

Warfarin, 10 to 15 mg daily, before termination of heparin. Dosage is continued for 3 to 6 months and adjusted in accordance with prothrombin time which is checked at frequent (2 to 3 day) intervals

C. Patients with evidence of pulmonary emboli

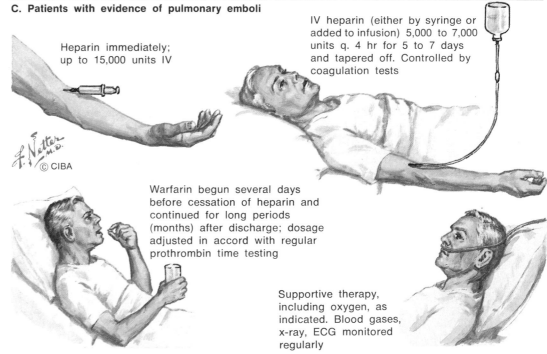

Heparin immediately; up to 15,000 units IV

IV heparin (either by syringe or added to infusion) 5,000 to 7,000 units q. 4 hr for 5 to 7 days and tapered off. Controlled by coagulation tests

Warfarin begun several days before cessation of heparin and continued for long periods (months) after discharge; dosage adjusted in accord with regular prothrombin time testing

Supportive therapy, including oxygen, as indicated. Blood gases, x-ray, ECG monitored regularly

from this cause is uncovered only at autopsy. Progressive pulmonary hypertension develops, with pulmonary arterial pressures sometimes reaching systemic levels. With the passage of time, the right ventricle responds by muscular hypertrophy, which gives way to preterminal dilatation when the ventricle can no longer compensate for the load placed on it. At right heart catheterization, these changes are reflected in pulmonary arterial hypertension, with a normal pulmonary wedge pressure and increasing right ventricular systolic and end-diastolic pressures. When cardiac output can no longer increase with exercise, right heart failure follows and, unlike the usual episodic course of chronic obstructive lung disease, is usually unremitting and progressive. At autopsy the distal pulmonary arterial tree is found to be extensively curtailed by organized thrombi that are widely disseminated throughout the lungs.

A history of pulmonary embolism heightens the suspicion that widespread occlusion of the pulmonary vascular bed has occurred. Diffuse obliteration and generalized narrowing of pulmonary resistance vessels also occur in primary pulmonary hypertension after the continued ingestion of certain anorexigenic drugs, and as a complication of a generalized connective tissue disorder.

In these patients with severe pulmonary hypertension, dyspnea and tachypnea, fatigue and syncopal episodes or precordial pain during exertion are usually found in some combination. On physical examination, an impulse may be felt over the main pulmonary artery, and there is splitting of the second heart sound with accentuation of the pulmonary component. An ejection click and a

systolic or diastolic murmur may be present in the pulmonary valve area. Subsequently, evidence of right ventricular hypertrophy is found, with a prominent A wave in the jugular venous pulse and a right ventricular heave and fourth heart sound. As failure develops, a right ventricular gallop can be heard, and there is evidence of tricuspid valve insufficiency along with the peripheral consequences of an ineffectively functioning right ventricle. Transient arrhythmias may occur, and sudden death is likely.

Chest roentgenograms usually show an enlarged heart with right ventricular and right atrial prominence. The main pulmonary artery shadow

is increasingly enlarged as hypertension becomes more severe, while the peripheral lung fields are oligemic and lack vascular markings. Evidence of right axis deviation appears on the electrocardiogram, with evidence of right ventricular hypertrophy in the precordial leads. There is usually indication of right atrial enlargement, and, when changes are severe, inversion of right precordial T waves is commonly present. Right heart catheterization and radioisotope lung scans provide definitive evidence of the disease process. No curative treatment has been found, although anticoagulant and thrombolytic agents may be tried.

Tests for Monitoring Anticoagulant Therapy

Principles of Tests for Monitoring Anticoagulant Therapy

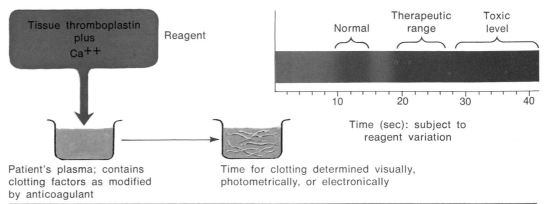

A. Prothrombin time (PT); more sensitive to warfarin effect

Tissue thromboplastin plus Ca++ — Reagent

Patient's plasma; contains clotting factors as modified by anticoagulant

Time for clotting determined visually, photometrically, or electronically

Time (sec): subject to reagent variation

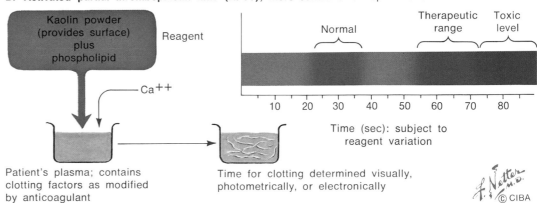

B. Activated partial thromboplastin time (APTT); more sensitive to heparin effect

Kaolin powder (provides surface) plus phospholipid — Reagent

Ca++

Patient's plasma; contains clotting factors as modified by anticoagulant

Time for clotting determined visually, photometrically, or electronically

Time (sec): subject to reagent variation

Methods of Testing

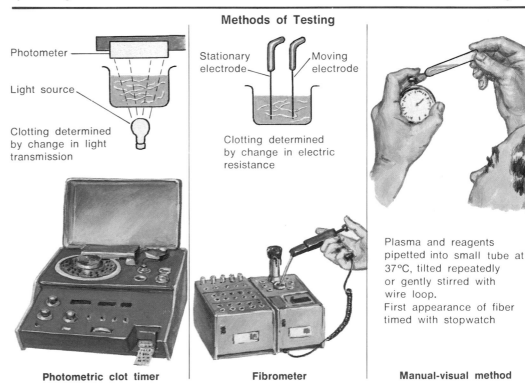

Photometer, Light source. Clotting determined by change in light transmission

Stationary electrode, Moving electrode. Clotting determined by change in electric resistance

Plasma and reagents pipetted into small tube at 37°C, tilted repeatedly or gently stirred with wire loop. First appearance of fiber timed with stopwatch

Photometric clot timer | **Fibrometer** | **Manual-visual method**

Monitoring Warfarin Effect. The administration of warfarin antagonizes the effect of vitamin K on the postribosomal carboxylation of the glutamic acid residues of factors IX, X and VII and of prothrombin. The result is a decrease in synthesis of these coagulation proteins and a slowing of the rate of thrombin formation. All but factor IX are reflected in the prothrombin time (PT). The PT measures the extrinsic system plus the final common pathway. The test is performed by adding tissue thromboplastin and Ca^{++} to plasma anticoagulated with citrate.

The rate of clotting can be measured manually, by the use of the semiautomatic fibrometer, or the automated photometric clot timer (see below). The normal time is 12 ± 1 seconds. The slow step in the reaction series is factor VII-induced activation of factor X. For this reason the test is most sensitive to factor VII levels. The substrate of the reaction is prothrombin, and this is the protein to which the PT is least sensitive. Consequently, after warfarin administration, factor VII (with a half-life of six hours) declines rapidly, leading to prolongation of the PT. This may occur when the prothrombin concentration (half-life = 40 hours) is still within normal limits. The therapeutic range (1.5 to 2 × control) is, therefore, valid only for long-term anticoagulation; during the early phases of anticoagulation the PT may not reflect the antithrombotic effect.

Attainment of the long-term therapeutic range (more than five days) after anticoagulation reflects a steady state of factors II, VII and X (and, by analogy, factor IX) of 10 to 20% of the normal levels, which signifies a safe therapeutic range. A PT greater than twice normal indicates that less than 10% of vitamin K-dependent factors remains—a toxic dose of warfarin—and predisposes to increased bleeding.

Monitoring Heparin Effect. The administration of heparin potentiates the action of antithrombin III, leading to neutralization of thrombin, factor X_a and other serine proteases (factor IX_a and factor XI_a). The test used to monitor heparin action is an overall measurement of coagulation, namely, the activated partial thromboplastin time (APTT); it measures the intrinsic coagulation system and the final common pathway. The test uses kaolin powder, which provides a surface to activate factor XII to XII_a. Phospholipid is added, being necessary for reactions that involve the activation of factor X by factor VIII and IX_a and the activation of prothrombin to thrombin by factors V and X_a. The normal APTT is 30 ± 4 seconds. The slow steps of this sequence are those involving factors XII and XI. Since kaolin rapidly activates factor XII, factor XI activation of factor IX is probably rate-limiting. Since heparin inhibits factor XI_a as well as later steps, the APTT is a convenient way to monitor heparin action.

Before widespread use of the APTT, the whole blood glass clotting time was used to measure heparin action. From both experimental and clinical observations, it was found that when the clotting time was prolonged to two to three times the control level by administration of heparin, the extension of and embolization from preformed clots was prevented. The APTT was found to correlate well with the clotting time, and the therapeutic time for the APTT was the equivalent of two to three times the clotting time. However, the APTT has an error of about 8% compared to the error in the clotting time of over 30%. Moreover, the APTT takes 30 to 90 seconds to perform compared to 15 to 60 minutes for clotting time. Finally, the APTT can be auto-

mated and thus has become the procedure of choice for monitoring heparin action.

Testing Methods. Three methods of testing applicable to PT and APTT are illustrated. The earliest, the manual method, requires much experience and considerable observer time, has a subjective end point, and is limited by observer fatigue. The second method, using the semiautomatic fibrometer, gives an objective end point but requires constant attention. The third, the automated method, which is used increasingly, allows unattended operation after pipetting of the plasma samples and can be incorporated into a computer-operated information system.

Surgical Defenses Against Massive Pulmonary Embolism

The great majority of patients with venous thromboembolic disease are satisfactorily managed by medical measures. Sometimes, however, if anticoagulant therapy is contraindicated or pulmonary embolization occurs despite adequate systemic anticoagulation, surgical management is indicated.

Surgical treatment consists in venous interruption—either complete or partial. The rationale is to prevent pulmonary embolism by trapping the thrombus in the peripheral venous system so that it cannot migrate to embolize the lung. With improved knowledge of the origins of fatal pulmonary emboli, venous interruption in the extremities has given way to more logical proximal entrapment at the level of the inferior vena cava.

A variety of both open surgical and transvenous techniques for partial or complete caval interruption have been developed.

Vena caval ligation is usually performed through an extraperitoneal right flank incision. The inferior vena cava is ligated just distal to the right renal vein to prevent forming a pocket in which thrombi might develop above the ligature. The addition of bilateral spermatic or ovarian vein ligation is generally believed to increase protection; such ligations are performed as an adjunct to caval occlusion. Ligation of a vein in which there is distal venous thrombosis is likely to result in propagation of a thrombus to the ligature site. The incidence of significant lower extremity venous insufficiency subsequent to vena caval ligation varies, depending largely on preexisting venous disease in the extremities rather than on caval ligation *per se*. Still, important stasis symptoms occur in a relatively large percentage of patients with ligation (21%) compared to that effected in partial interruption (7%). For this reason, alternative procedures have been devised in an attempt to prevent fatal embolism without causing total interruption of caval blood flow.

Partial caval interruption was first suggested by Adams and DeWeese, who developed a vena caval filter by traversing the lumen of the cava with multiple sutures of silk forming a grid to trap emboli. Caval plication, using suture, metallic staples and various externally applied plastic (Teflon) clips, has largely replaced ligation and suture grids. Although complete caval occlusion may occur as the consequence of thrombosis or trapped emboli below the filter, the results are no worse than with ligation. Patients in whom complete caval occlusion does not occur enjoy the potential protection of the filter without the sequelae of caval ligation. Both ligation and plication are associated with about a 5% incidence of nonfatal pulmonary embolism and less than 1% fatal embolism. There is a threefold increase in late postphlebitic lower extremity complications following ligation compared to plication.

All of the procedures described require general or spinal anesthesia for their performance. While many patients safely tolerate surgical intervention, its routine use in desperately ill patients can result

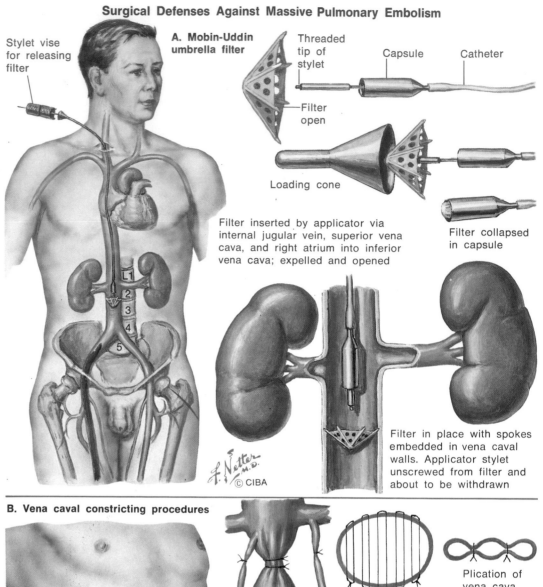

Surgical Defenses Against Massive Pulmonary Embolism

A. Mobin-Uddin umbrella filter

Stylet vise for releasing filter

Threaded tip of stylet · Capsule · Catheter

Filter open

Loading cone

Filter collapsed in capsule

Filter inserted by applicator via internal jugular vein, superior vena cava, and right atrium into inferior vena cava; expelled and opened

Filter in place with spokes embedded in vena caval walls. Applicator stylet unscrewed from filter and about to be withdrawn

B. Vena caval constricting procedures

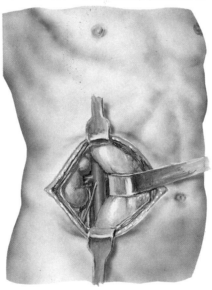

Retroperitoneal dissection approach to inferior vena cava. Peritoneum and contents reflected medially

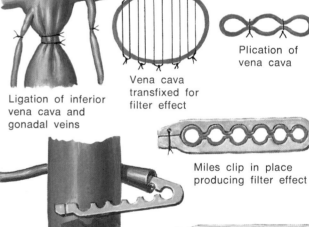

Ligation of inferior vena cava and gonadal veins

Vena cava transfixed for filter effect

Plication of vena cava

Miles clip in place producing filter effect

Miles Teflon clip being applied with aid of catheter encircling vena cava

Adams-DeWeese filter in place

in an increased mortality which may equal that for pulmonary embolism. A relatively low-risk transvenous method of caval interruption therefore has great appeal.

The *Mobin-Uddin umbrella filter* was first reported in 1969 as a new simplified method of caval interruption which could be effected under local anesthesia through a small incision in the neck, thus avoiding a major surgical intervention. The prosthesis consists of six spokes of stainless steel radiating from a central hub and covered on both sides by a thin sheet of silicone rubber. The umbrella is introduced via the right internal jugular vein, folded in a capsule attached to a guide wire

housed in a long catheter. The capsule is advanced under fluoroscopic control into the inferior vena cava to a point below the renal veins. The folded umbrella is opened fully on ejection from the capsule with the guide wire. As the umbrella opens, the pointed ends of the radiating spokes penetrate the caval wall, anchoring the prosthesis in place. The guide wire is unscrewed from the umbrella hub; the catheter, capsule and guide wire are removed, and the cervical venotomy site is repaired. Late complications are rare. Most complications occur during implantation or shortly afterward as the result of misplacement or migration of the filter.

Extravascular Sources of Pulmonary Emboli

A wide range of tissue elements and foreign substances may gain access to the systemic veins and give rise to pulmonary emboli. They may be *solid* fragments of tissue, parasites, blood clots or particulate substances. They may be *liquid* droplets of fat, oil or plastics. They may be *gaseous* — air or nitrogen. They may be sterile or septic. They can reach the venous circulation directly through intravenous injection or be sucked into patent venous radicles as a result of trauma, surgical procedures or other maneuvers.

The effect of embolism is related to the extent and rapidity of the process. In most instances the emboli under consideration are asymptomatic. If embolism is massive and rapid, complete or partial obstruction of the pulmonary blood flow may lead to serious hemodynamic and respiratory insufficiency and death. Less frequently, emboli cause irreversible anatomic changes in small pulmonary blood vessels and result in pulmonary hypertension and cor pulmonale.

Fat Embolism. The most common cause of fat embolism is trauma to bones, particularly the long bones of the legs. Fat embolism may also be associated with air emboli in decompression sickness (caisson disease). Microscopically, the fat emboli can be demonstrated with fat stains such as Sudan III or IV or oil red O. With these stains they appear as red-orange droplets, several microns in diameter, filling the small arteries and alveolar capillaries. With routine stains they appear as optically clear spaces in the vascular lumina. Clinically, fat embolism is often associated with acute respiratory failure (adult respiratory distress syndrome). Cutaneous and conjunctival petechial hemorrhages and embolism of retinal vessels are found in about half the cases.

Bone marrow embolism is also a frequent complication of severe bone trauma or fracture.

Formed-blood aggregates are sources of emboli in blood transfusion and have given rise to the use of line filters of 10 to 40 Å in diameter.

Amniotic Fluid Embolism. This relatively rare condition is caused by the massive leakage of amniotic fluid into the uterine veins. The amniotic fluid reaches the uterine venous circulation either as a result of vigorous uterine contraction after rupture of the membranes or through tears or surgical incisions in the myometrium or endocervix. Clinically, the condition is characterized by sudden dyspnea, cyanosis, systemic hypotension and death during or immediately after delivery. The mechanism of death is not clear since the emboli consist of a suspension of epithelial squames, lanugo and cellular debris, usually occluding a few small blood vessels. Death has been attributed to either anaphylactoid reaction to the amniotic fluid or disseminated intravascular coagulation due to activation of the clotting mechanism by amniotic fluid thromboplastin.

Air Embolism. Air may be sucked into veins during attempts at abortion, following chest injury as a result of a motor vehicle accident, during the induction of artificial pneumothorax or pneumoperitoneum, and in a number of other

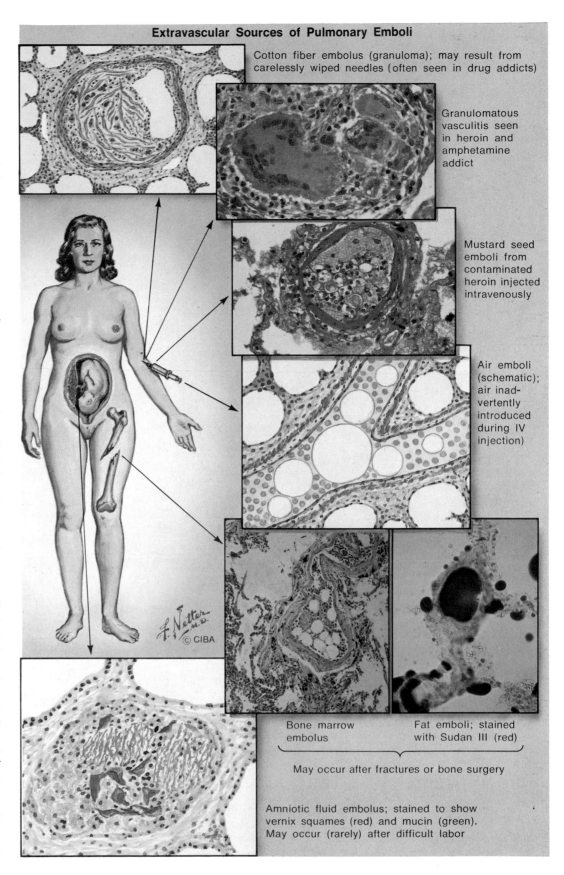

Extravascular Sources of Pulmonary Emboli

Cotton fiber embolus (granuloma); may result from carelessly wiped needles (often seen in drug addicts)

Granulomatous vasculitis seen in heroin and amphetamine addict

Mustard seed emboli from contaminated heroin injected intravenously

Air emboli (schematic); air inadvertently introduced during IV injection)

Bone marrow embolus

Fat emboli; stained with Sudan III (red)

May occur after fractures or bone surgery

Amniotic fluid embolus; stained to show vernix squames (red) and mucin (green). May occur (rarely) after difficult labor

circumstances. The effects of air embolism depend on the amount of air that reaches the circulation and the rapidity of its entry. The volume of air necessary to cause death in man is usually more than 100 ml. In debilitated persons a smaller volume of air may be fatal. Death is due to blockage by an air trap in the outflow tract of the right ventricle, but small air bubbles can be seen in small pulmonary blood vessels.

Foreign Body Embolism. A wide variety of organic or inorganic substances may enter the venous circulation and reach the lungs. This type of embolism has become common in certain groups addicted to narcotic drugs. The drugs are rarely

chemically pure and are frequently adulterated with vegetable seeds, talc and other substances.

As with the other kinds of emboli, the effect of foreign bodies depends to a great extent on the rapidity and extent of embolization. Such particles as fibers or talc are likely to produce an inflammatory response in the wall of small pulmonary arteries, with formation of foreign body granulomas composed of macrophages and multinucleated giant cells. The granuloma may cause partial or total occlusion of the involved blood vessel. If several blood vessels are involved, pulmonary vascular resistance may become elevated and lead to pulmonary hypertension.

Pulmonary Edema

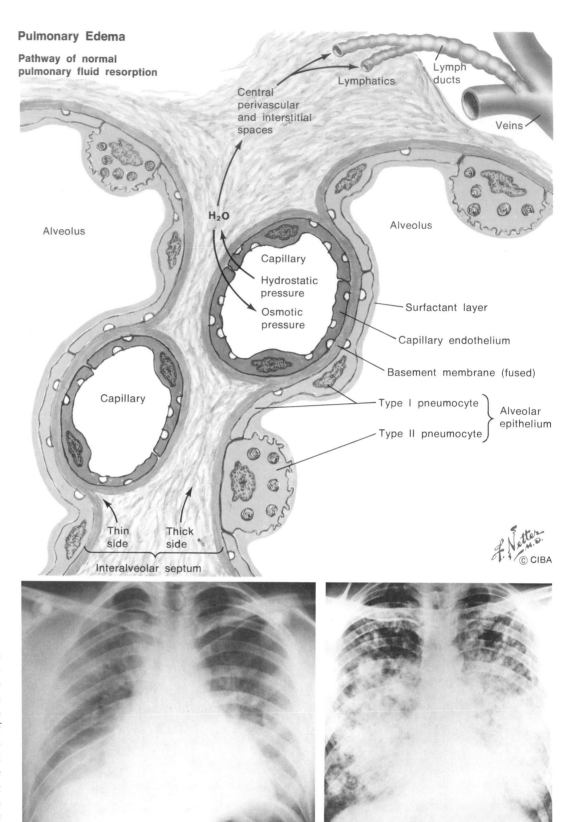

Pulmonary Edema

Pathway of normal pulmonary fluid resorption

Central perivascular and interstitial spaces

Lymphatics

Lymph ducts

Veins

Alveolus

Alveolus

H₂O

Capillary

Hydrostatic pressure

Osmotic pressure

Surfactant layer

Capillary endothelium

Basement membrane (fused)

Type I pneumocyte

Type II pneumocyte

Alveolar epithelium

Capillary

Thin side

Thick side

Interalveolar septum

Pulmonary edema. Hazy opacification chiefly in central lung areas (butterfly pattern)

Advanced pulmonary edema distributed chiefly in lower parts of both lungs

The movement of water in the lungs follows Starling's law of transcapillary exchange. For practical purposes, the endothelial surfaces of the minute vessels are visualized as semipermeable membranes. Water moves across a membrane whenever the balance of forces on the two sides of the membrane is upset. The opposing forces are hydrostatic and osmotic. The hydrostatic and osmotic pressures in the interstitial space are not measurable directly. In contrast, the osmotic pressure of blood in the pulmonary capillaries can be measured directly, and the hydrostatic pressure in the minute vessels of the lungs can be approximated with reasonable assurance.

Water that enters the interstitial space has two routes of egress—it can either continue up the interstitial space to leave the lungs by way of the lymphatics, or enter the alveoli. Since the alveolar aspect of the interstitial space is much less permeable than the endothelial aspect, and since pressures within the interstitial space favor drainage toward lymphatics in the vicinity of terminal bronchioles, interstitial water may increase considerably before alveolar edema appears (interstitial edema without alveolar edema).

For the lungs to function properly in gas exchange, the alveolar surfaces must be kept moist but not flooded. Anatomic arrangements make possible excellent gas exchange when interstitial edema occurs. Each capillary has a thin aspect for

gas exchange and a thick aspect which is organized for the efflux of water. The thick aspect is easily identified in the nonedematous lung because of the distinct interstitial space between the basement membranes of the alveolar and endothelial linings. In contrast, the thin side has no distinct interstitial space since the two basement membranes are fused.

Within the alveolar interstitial space are the "juxtacapillary receptors" originally described by Paintal. These represent specialized, ultrastructural end-organs, which sense swelling of the components of the interstitial space, leading to tachypnea. The lung thus appears to have a specialized system for water exchange involving

the thick side of the alveolar-capillary membrane. The adjacent interstitial space has J receptors, activated by interstitial edema, and pulmonary lymphatics, which operate efficiently to remove excess water when the respiratory rate is increased.

When hydrostatic and oncotic forces are seriously deranged so that water escapes from the interstitium into alveoli, the surfactant lining is lifted and the affected alveoli tend to collapse. Alveolar collapse is spotty at first, so that flooded, atelectatic alveoli alternate with normal alveoli which have retained their surfactant lining. Late in alveolar edema, the alveolar fluid becomes richer

(Continued)

Pulmonary Edema; Some Etiologies and Hypotheses of Mechanisms

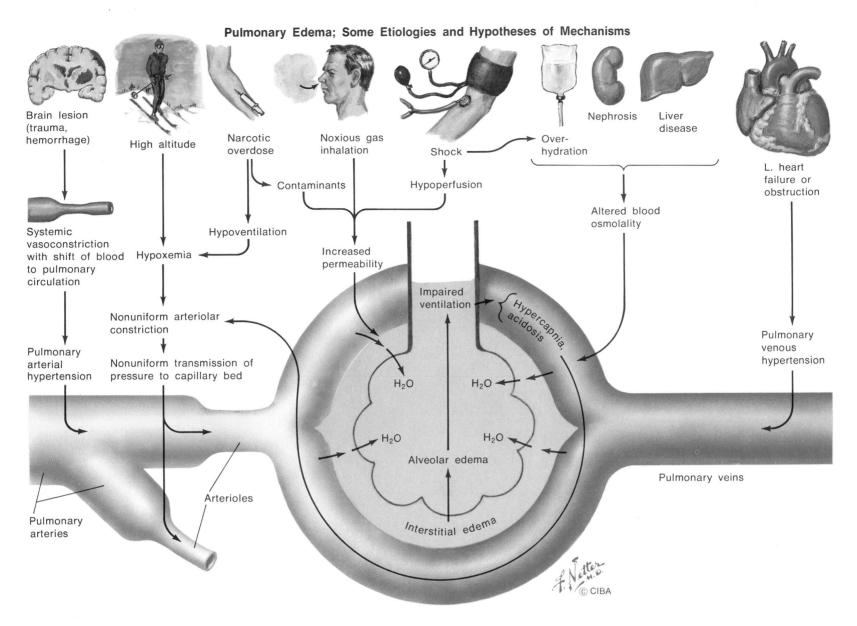

Pulmonary Edema
(*Continued*)

and richer in proteins as alveolar-capillary permeability increases, and red cells also enter the alveoli.

As hydrostatic pressures rise in the pulmonary capillaries (*e.g.,* in acute left ventricular failure), the interendothelial junctions stretch and allow the egress of blood proteins. Once the proteins are in the interstitial space, they modify the oncotic pressure of interstitial fluid. If the leak of proteins into the interstitial space is large, and excess proteins accumulate there, the edema fluid tends to persist. Large proteins in the interstitial space set the stage for pulmonary fibrosis.

These observations have many practical implications for the pathogenesis of pulmonary edema. Any imbalance in the forces governing water exchange, particularly an increase in capillary pressure, or a decrease in capillary oncotic pressure, or both, promotes the movement of water into the pulmonary interstitial space. Interstitial edema regularly precedes alveolar edema. Tachypnea is an important manifestation of interstitial edema, and depression of ventilation can interfere with water removal from the lungs.

Causes and Possible Mechanisms. Pulmonary edema is generally categorized as "hemodynamic" or due to "increased permeability." Among the familiar causes of hemodynamic pulmonary edema are left ventricular failure and mitral valve disease. Pulmonary edema due to increased permeability of the minute vessels of the lungs is much less common. Striking examples of this type are produced by inhalation of phosgene or nitrogen dioxide. Although these extremes illustrate the fundamental differences between the two types, frequently they coexist. For example, large increases in capillary hydrostatic pressures in the lungs not only promote the movement of water into the interstitial space in accord with Starling's law of transcapillary exchange, but also stretch interendothelial "junctions," thereby increasing capillary permeability to both water and proteins.

Overtransfusion edema is a common complication of intravenous administration of fluids. The pulmonary blood volume shares in the overall expansion of total blood volume. Pulmonary edema occurs as hydrostatic pressure increases in the pulmonary capillaries, particularly if the osmotic pressure of the proteins is concomitantly decreased by the protein-free fluids given therapeutically.

The edema of high altitude is probably a variant of hemodynamic pulmonary edema. It presupposes nonuniform arterial and arteriolar constriction throughout the lungs in response to acute hypoxia and to other influences that are poorly understood. Pulmonary capillary beds distal to intensely vasoconstricted vessels are protected from the increase in pulmonary arterial pressure induced by the generalized pulmonary vasoconstriction. In contrast, capillaries that are less protected by precapillary vasoconstriction share the rise in pulmonary arterial pressure and become the site for pulmonary edema.

Brain lesions elicit pulmonary edema that is caused by left ventricular failure. The initiating mechanism for the heart failure is a burst of systemic hypertension following an increase in intracranial pressure.

Two fairly prevalent types of pulmonary edema are suspected of having increased permeability as their major basis: narcotic overdosage and "shock lung" (Plate 136). Narcotic overdose elicits coma and pulmonary edema. The mechanism for the latter is unknown, but acute hypoxia has been ruled out as a cause. In shock lung, pulmonary edema is characteristically intermingled with congestion and atelectasis. The mechanism remains a matter of speculation, but, depending on the clinical circumstances, a bout of pulmonary hypotension in the course of shock, or the liberation of enzymes into the blood, as in acute pancreatitis, may be the cause. At times, overtransfusion and oxygen toxicity in the course of treatment contribute to its development.

Thoracic Cage Injuries

Thoracic cage injuries are treated according to the principles that apply to trauma elsewhere in the body, with certain modifications for specific anatomic features and for disturbed cardiorespiratory dynamics. Thoracic cage injuries are unique in that mild injuries improperly treated may be fatal, whereas massive trauma can be treated by proper measures with excellent results.

A rib fracture is the result of trauma, but pathologic rib fractures may occur in patients with malignant metastases, myeloma and hyperparathyroidism. Simple rib fractures occur primarily in adults and usually involve the upper and lower ribs. Ordinarily the first, eleventh and twelfth ribs are spared. With severe trauma, fractures of any rib, or combination of ribs, with or without dislocations, may occur. The posterior angle is structurally the weakest point, and fractures in this area are likely. However, the fracture usually occurs at the point of impact, often laterally. Such fractures are hard to see on x-ray films.

Crushing injuries may produce multiple eggshell fractures, the sites being dependent on the direction of the compressing forces. For example, impaling the anterior chest on a steering wheel, as in an automobile accident, often fractures the sternum and several ribs anteriorly on both sides. Besides rib fractures, costovertebral dislocations may occur at any level, as may costochondral and chondrosternal separations. Fractures may be transverse or oblique, and the fragments may override, or a pointed fragment may be pushed inward, tearing the pleura and underlying lung.

Penetrating wounds of the chest (gunshot or stab wound) may cause comminuted fractures of a rib, with bone fragments driven into the lung substance. In the elderly patient with atrophic, decalcified ribs, fractures may result from simple trauma, coughing or any severe muscle pull.

Fractures of the rib or sternum or costovertebral separations are diagnosed from movement of fragments, ecchymosis and crepitus, as well as by x-ray examination. Since pain characteristically occurs with inspiration, the patient tends to splint the chest wall and, therefore, hypoventilates. A chest x-ray film is always indicated, not only to identify the number and extent of rib fractures but also to determine whether there is an associated pneumothorax, hemothorax or pleural effusion.

Rib fractures usually heal readily if complications are handled properly. However, the pain associated with the fracture can prevent proper ventilation and coughing, leading to atelectasis, retained secretions and pneumonia, especially in the elderly. Damage to the underlying lung may cause pneumothorax or subcutaneous emphysema. Laceration of the intercostal vessels sometimes causes hemothorax, which can become severe. Multiple rib fractures may produce paradoxical movement of the chest wall, with a flail segment.

Pain from a rib fracture is best treated by intercostal or paravertebral block; this promptly relieves the pain and quiets the labored respiration which may be accentuating paradoxical motion of the chest. The major problem with a block is increased reflex bronchial secretions; these must be removed if patients are to avoid an obstructive type of

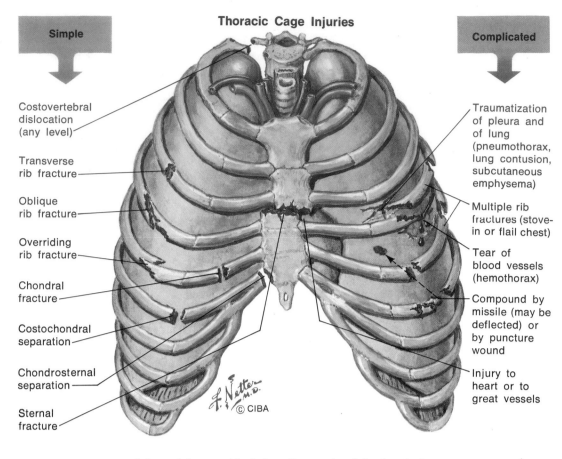

Thoracic Cage Injuries

Simple

- Costovertebral dislocation (any level)
- Transverse rib fracture
- Oblique rib fracture
- Overriding rib fracture
- Chondral fracture
- Costochondral separation
- Chondrosternal separation
- Sternal fracture

Complicated

- Traumatization of pleura and of lung (pneumothorax, lung contusion, subcutaneous emphysema)
- Multiple rib fractures (stove-in or flail chest)
- Tear of blood vessels (hemothorax)
- Compound by missile (may be deflected) or by puncture wound
- Injury to heart or to great vessels

F. Netter M.D. © CIBA

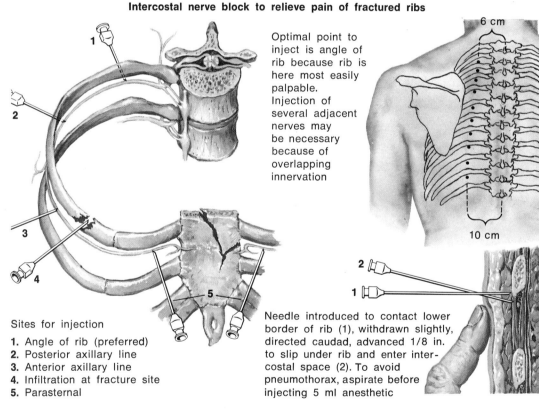

Intercostal nerve block to relieve pain of fractured ribs

Optimal point to inject is angle of rib because rib is here most easily palpable. Injection of several adjacent nerves may be necessary because of overlapping innervation

6 cm

10 cm

Sites for injection
1. Angle of rib (preferred)
2. Posterior axillary line
3. Anterior axillary line
4. Infiltration at fracture site
5. Parasternal

Needle introduced to contact lower border of rib (1), withdrawn slightly, directed caudad, advanced 1/8 in. to slip under rib and enter intercostal space (2). To avoid pneumothorax, aspirate before injecting 5 ml anesthetic

pneumonia, which is particularly dangerous in the elderly. If coughing is inadequate, tracheal aspiration by catheter or by bronchoscopy, and occasionally by endotracheal intubation or tracheostomy, may be necessary. The local anesthetic is injected into the fracture site, if possible, or as a nerve block. The needle is inserted under the rib to inject the anesthetic agent into the intercostal space, as the intercostal nerve runs along the lower border of the rib except posteriorly, where it lies midway between the ribs. Injection of one or two additional nerves above and below the fracture site may be required because of overlapping innervation. Complicating pneumothorax is always of concern.

Adhesive strapping of the chest wall should be avoided because it inhibits deep inspiration and may result in traumatic atelectasis. Medication for pain, however, is essential if the patient is to cough effectively. Drugs that depress the cough reflex must be used with great caution, and avoided altogether if possible. Patients should be encouraged to cough frequently and to breathe deeply, particularly if they receive sedation. The ribs usually become fairly stable within 10 days to two weeks, although some patients require ventilatory support longer, depending on the severity of the rib fractures. Firm healing with callus formation is seen after about six weeks.

Flail Chest

Flail chest is the result of a crushing injury in which the chest wall is "stove in," so that it loses its rigidity, causing severe respiratory distress. If the crushing force is from the lateral direction, the injury usually consists of fractures in at least two sites in multiple adjacent ribs on the involved side, resulting in a "floating" central portion of the chest wall, which goes in and out with respiration in a reverse or paradoxical manner to the rest of the chest wall. This type of respiration markedly decreases the efficiency of ventilation, and is usually accompanied by severe pain that renders the coughing mechanism ineffectual. If the crushing blow is directly over the sternum, as often happens in steering wheel injuries, fractures of the sternum may occur. Such an injury is most frequently associated with bilateral costochondral fractures, usually from the first rib down, resulting in extreme flailing of the anterior portion of the chest wall.

The physiologic effects of flail chest are a notable decrease in vital capacity, reduced functional residual capacity, ventilation-perfusion imbalance and resulting hypoxemia, decreased compliance, increased airway resistance, and increased breathing effort.

Clinically, the unsupported portion of the chest wall is seen to move paradoxically with respiration. On inspiration, the flail area moves in; on expiration or coughing, it moves outward. If the flail segment is large, the important effects are those of inadequate ventilation, inadequate perfusion resulting in progressive hypoxia and hypercapnia, and inefficient coughing with retained secretions.

Treatment of flail chest consists primarily in stabilization of the thorax and restoration of intrathoracic volume. The stabilization of the chest wall may be effected by either internal or external fixation.

Internal fixation is accomplished by use of an endotracheal tube or tracheostomy, with positive pressure respiration maintained by a ventilator. By this means, internal pneumatic stabilization of the chest wall may be achieved; however, two to three weeks are usually required for healing to occur. The ventilator assumes most of the work of breathing. If a pressure-limited ventilator is used, the increased airway pressure of the stiff lung syndrome will result in inadequate ventilation. To avoid this situa-

Flail Chest

Fracture of several adjacent ribs in two or more places. Flail may be complicated by lung contusion or laceration

Complete sternochondral separation with depression of sternum. Possibility of injury to heart and/or great vessels must also be considered

Pathologic physiology of lateral flail chest

Inspiration

As chest expands and diaphragm descends, flail section sinks in, impairing ability to produce negative intrapleural pressure. Mediastinum and trachea shift to uninjured side, decreasing expansion capability of lung on that side

Expiration

As chest contracts and diaphragm rises, flail segment bulges outward, impairing expiratory effect. Mediastinum and trachea shift to injured side. In severe flail chest air may shuttle uselessly from one lung to the other as indicated by broken lines (pendelluft)

tion, therefore, the patient should be placed on a volume-limited machine.

Pulmonary parenchymal complications are frequent after extensive chest trauma, and an adequate airway must be maintained. The airway is often plugged by secretions from bleeding or aspirated gastric contents, and repeated aspirations through an endotracheal or tracheostomy tube are necessary. The advantages of the endotracheal artificial airway are that it (1) reduces dead space, (2) decreases resistance during both inspiration and expiration, (3) permits stabilization of the chest wall and elimination of paradoxical respiration, (4) allows ready access to the trachea for aspiration, and (5)

consequently improves the relationship of alveolar ventilation to perfusion.

Surgical stabilization, or *external fixation,* of the chest wall is no longer widely done. It was effected by inserting steel pins through the pectoral muscles over the crushed area, or by passing towel clips or wires around the ribs or sternum.

The major ventilatory problem, however, may be not the paradoxical motion of the chest wall, but the severe pulmonary contusion which is often present. This must be treated with fluid restriction, diuretics, steroids, vigorous pulmonary toilet, supplemental oxygen and, frequently, mechanical ventilation.

Diaphragmatic Injuries

Once relatively uncommon, injuries of the diaphragm are occurring more frequently, paralleling the rise in frequency of automobile accidents. The diagnosis is often missed because of associated intraabdominal injuries as well as concomitant pelvic fractures. Diaphragmatic injuries may also be caused by penetrating (usually gunshot or stab injuries) or blunt trauma. The mechanism of diaphragmatic rupture varies greatly in these different types of trauma, and this significantly influences the size and side of the rupture. With gunshot wounds, as might be expected, the chances of involvement of the right or left side are approximately equal. In the majority of stab wounds, the left side of the diaphragm is involved; the assailant holds the stabbing instrument, usually a knife, in his right hand and faces his victim at close range, so that the victim's left side is in direct line with the blade. With blunt injuries, also, the left side is far more commonly involved than the right. The rent usually occurs through the dome of the diaphragm, and is much larger than is the case with penetrating wounds. As there is normally a pressure gradient across the diaphragm, with a higher pressure on the abdominal than on the thoracic side, the abdominal viscera herniate into the thorax. This gradient varies from 20 cm H_2O with quiet breathing to 100 cm H_2O with deep breathing. The possibility of intraabdominal injury, especially splenic rupture, in patients with left-sided thoracic injuries should also be remembered.

Isolated rupture of the diaphragm is rare. Far more common is life-threatening intraabdominal damage requiring immediate surgical correction. In 1679 Ambroise Paré described five diagnostic clinical signs that are still useful:

(1) prominence and immobility in the left chest,
(2) abnormal gurgling sounds in the left chest,
(3) displacement of the heart to the right,
(4) absent breath sounds in the left chest,
(5) tympany in the left lower chest on percussion.

In general, symptoms are related to the quantity of herniated viscera in the chest. The usual clinical manifestations are dyspnea, chest or shoulder pain and cyanosis. If the herniated organ is the stomach, the dyspnea can be relieved dramatically by insertion of a nasogastric tube for decompression. This may also help identify the location of the stomach on a plain chest x-ray film.

Suggestive or diagnostic roentgenographic signs of rupture of the diaphragm are acute diaphragmatic elevation, with or without pleural effusion; atelectasis with silhouetting of the ipsilateral diaphragm; evidence of an air-filled or solid viscus in the thorax. A stab wound to the anterior chest as high as the fourth intercostal space can perforate the diaphragm and enter the peritoneal cavity. Under conditions of stress and during forced expiration this is a possibility, particularly if the thrust of the knife is downward. Conversely, a stab wound high in the flank can also penetrate the diaphragm. The technique of artificial pneumoperitoneum can be useful for the diagnosis of a diaphragmatic lacer-

Thoracoabdominal penetrating wounds
Diaphragmatic injury is suspected in any penetrating thoracic wound (gunshot, stab, or accidental perforation) at or below 4th intercostal space anteriorly, 6th interspace laterally, or 8th interspace posteriorly, although sharply oblique wounds or missiles deflected by ribs may also penetrate diaphragm

Rupture of diaphragm
May result from blunt impact or compression or from penetrating wound. Stomach and other abdominal viscera herniated into left thorax; left lung collapsed, right lung compressed; mediastinum shifted and trachea deviated to right

ation. Several hundred milliliters of air are injected to produce a satisfactory roentgenogram. The pneumoperitoneum can be given along with either a diagnostic paracentesis or peritoneal lavage.

Management of rupture of the diaphragm depends largely on the associated injuries. For acute diaphragmatic injuries the abdominal approach may be preferable, since abdominal injuries requiring surgical repair are likely to be present. Most associated chest injuries can be managed by insertion of chest tubes and do not require surgery. The decision to repair an isolated diaphragmatic rupture in an acutely injured patient should depend on how the patient tolerates the loss of normal, nega-

tive intrathoracic pressure. Gross signs of cardiorespiratory embarrassment such as cyanosis, respiratory distress or shock are indications for repair.

Delay of surgery is a contributing factor to morbidity, particularly in patients with thoracic stab wounds. Guidelines to help reduce morbidity include: (1) increased awareness of the possibility of acute diaphragmatic injury, (2) careful evaluation of the plain chest roentgenogram and liberal use of appropriate contrast studies when indicated, (3) prompt repair of recognized diaphragmatic injuries, and (4) laparotomy as the operative approach of choice in an acute injury.

Rupture of Trachea or Major Bronchi

Rupture of the trachea or major bronchi is usually secondary to a nonpenetrating injury of the chest as a result of an automobile accident. It is a serious injury with an estimated overall mortality of 30%. More than 80% of the ruptures are within 2.5 cm of the carina. Injuries to the main bronchi and intrathoracic trachea are more prevalent than those to the cervical trachea because the latter is protected by the mandible and sternum anteriorly and by the vertebrae posteriorly.

Intrathoracic tracheal lacerations usually occur at the junction of the membranous and cartilaginous trachea within 2.5 cm of the carina. When lesions are vertical, they occur posteriorly, where the cartilage is deficient. The most common site of major bronchial rupture is also within 2.5 cm of the carina. Major bronchial rupture is usually unilateral, and more frequent on the right side. Accompanying important injuries have been reported in only 50% of cases of tracheobronchial rupture, despite the severity of these injuries.

The clinical picture appears in two patterns, depending on whether or not there is free communication between the rupture of the tracheobronchial tree and the pleural cavity. If there is free communication, a large pneumothorax results. Tube thoracostomy causes continuous bubbling of air in the water seal, and suction fails to reexpand the lung. The usual signs of tracheobronchial disruption are hemoptysis, dyspnea, subcutaneous and mediastinal emphysema, and occasionally cyanosis. Subcutaneous and mediastinal emphysema develops from the leakage of air into the cervical area. Hemoptysis is ordinarily mild and probably results from disruption of a bronchial artery. Dyspnea occurs from loss of functioning lung tissue. Tension pneumothorax is uncommon as the intrapleural air decompresses itself through the mediastinum. On auscultation, Hamman's sign is evident—a crunching sound synchronized with the heart beat; it is due to mediastinal emphysema. In the second pattern of injury, there is little or no communication between the torn bronchus and the pleural cavity, even though the transection may be complete. If pneumothorax does occur, it is relatively small. When an intercostal tube is inserted, the lung readily expands, and the pneumothorax does not recur after the tube is removed. The small rent in the pleura is quickly sealed off with fibrin and blood clot. The air generally escapes into the mediastinum and may produce surgical emphysema of varying severity.

If transection of the bronchus is complete and surgical repair is not performed promptly, the proximal and distal ends of the torn viscus are sealed by granulation tissue. As the granulation tissue obstructs the bronchus, the lung becomes atelectatic. If healing takes place without leaving any lumen in the bronchus, the collapsed lung does not become infected. However, if transection is incom-

plete and the granulation tissue forms a stricture, partial bronchial obstruction occurs and often results in pulmonary infection and eventually irreversible destruction of lung tissue.

A chest x-ray film does not demonstrate bronchial rupture. However, findings that indicate a need for other diagnostic procedures include deep cervical emphysema, pneumomediastinum, subcutaneous emphysema, pneumothorax, fractures of the upper five ribs, and air surrounding the bronchus. Air in the bronchus, visualized on a bronchogram, indicates a possible obstruction. Deep cervical emphysema is one of the earliest and most reliable of the indirect findings on the x-ray film.

Fractures of the first three ribs heighten suspicion of associated major airway damage.

Bronchoscopy should be carried out promptly when tracheobronchial rupture is suspected, since it is the most reliable means of establishing the diagnosis. If bronchoscopy indicates that the bronchial tear involves less than one-third of the lumen, and if the thoracostomy tube underwater-seal drainage results in complete expansion of the lung, treatment may be conservative. However, in all other types of tracheobronchial injury, thoracotomy should be performed as soon as the patient's condition permits. (See Plates 10, 11 and 12 for surgical management.)

Rupture of Trachea or Major Bronchi

Dyspnea
Cyanosis } may be present
Hemoptysis

Mediastinal and subcutaneous emphysema involving neck and anterior chest wall

Crepitus

Air escaping into mediastinum, thence to subcutaneous tissue and pleural cavity

Pneumothorax usually present

Tube to underwater-seal suction may or may not expand lung but prevents tension pneumothorax

Small tear of membranous portion of r. main bronchus (posterior view)

Almost complete rupture of thoracic trachea with continuity maintained by pretracheal fascia (anterior view)

Complete rupture of cervical trachea with recession of distal segment into thorax (anterior view)

Subcutaneous Emphysema

Laceration of both parietal and visceral pleura and of lung by fractured rib, torn adhesion, or puncture wound (may also be secondary to mediastinal emphysema resulting from rupture of trachea or bronchus, q.v.). "Frog-face" may occur in advanced cases

Crepitus

Air escaping to subcutaneous tissues

Subcutaneous Emphysema and Traumatic Asphyxia

Subcutaneous emphysema is a condition in which air is present in the tissues under the skin, particularly in the region of the head, neck and chest. It has several causes: (1) A fractured rib may damage the lung as well as the parietal pleura. (2) Tearing of pleural adhesions from a previous pleuritis may permit escaping air to enter the subcutaneous tissues. (3) It may result from positive pressure anesthesia or mechanical ventilation and is then known as "surgical emphysema." (4) It may occur before or after tracheostomy—airway obstruction prior to tracheostomy causes high alveolar pressures and may lead to alveolar rupture, with air traveling to the mediastinum by the interstitial route; following tracheostomy and neck surgery, air passes through the cervical incision along the outside of the trachea and into the mediastinum during inspiration; airway obstruction facilitates the passage of air by creating excessive negative intrathoracic pressure during inspiratory effort.

The diagnosis of subcutaneous emphysema is readily evident by the palpation of crepitus in the subcutaneous tissues and by the grotesque appearance of the face and head ("frog-faced man") which may develop. A chest x-ray film is mandatory to determine the presence or absence of a pneumothorax, which, if present, must be promptly treated.

If subcutaneous emphysema is well tolerated, there is minimal risk to the patient, and heroic methods of therapy are not needed. An additional chest tube is sometimes required for more efficient removal of air from a coexisting pneumothorax. If the condition is severe, a tracheostomy may be performed; this permits the escape of air by incision through the layers of cervical fascia and also allows adequate ventilation of the patient.

Traumatic asphyxia is a condition in which there is violaceous discoloration of the skin of the head, neck, shoulders and upper chest, together with bilateral subconjunctival hemorrhages and scattered petechiae over the upper part of the body. It results from a severe compressive force upon the thorax and upper abdomen. This clinical picture was first described by Ollivier in 1837, when he saw it in patients crushed to death by crowds in Paris. He coined the term *masque ecchymotique*. This form of crush injury may also occur from a heavy falling object, as in the case of an individual working under an automobile, which then slips and crushes the chest or upper abdomen. Deep-sea divers sustain similar injuries from underwater explosions. Depending on the cause, traumatic asphyxia may be critical, with death following immediately.

Traumatic Asphyxia

Ecchymotic mask. Conjunctival and pharyngeal hemorrhages and ocular proptosis may also occur

Theory of mechanism: Violent chest compression causes sudden, forceful expulsion of blood through superior vena cava into veins of head, neck, and upper chest, with rupture of venules

Of patients who survive the first few hours after injury, 90% will recover from traumatic asphyxia when it occurs as a single entity. Survival is directly related to the extent of associated injury.

Associated injuries are common and include injury to the chest wall, rib fractures, pulmonary contusion, pneumothorax and hemothorax. Damage to the heart and great vessels is rare. Sudden permanent loss of vision is attributed to retinal hemorrhage, and immediate transient loss of vision to retinal edema. The latter may be accompanied by papilledema, which is seen on funduscopic examination. There may be unilateral or bilateral subconjunctival hemorrhage, with or without conjunctival edema, and this is a fairly constant finding. Neurologic manifestations are frequent, as one-third of the patients become unconscious at the time of the injury. Intracranial or intracortical hemorrhages are rare even when injuries are fatal. Skeletal fractures are common.

No specific treatment is required for traumatic asphyxia, and all efforts are directed to management of associated injuries. However, the patient should be placed in an environment which will ensure a 40% oxygen concentration in the trachea. This concentration of oxygen not only provides safe oxygenation but also hastens absorption of any air within the mediastinum.

Open Pneumothorax

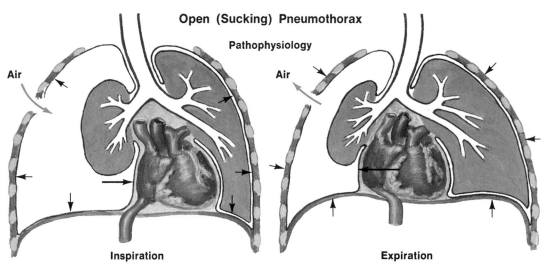

Open (Sucking) Pneumothorax

Pathophysiology

Inspiration

Air enters pleural cavity through open, sucking chest wound. Negative pleural pressure is lost, permitting collapse of ipsilateral lung and reducing venous return to heart. Mediastinum shifts, compressing opposite lung

Expiration

As chest wall contracts and diaphragm rises, air is expelled from pleural cavity via wound. Mediastinum shifts to affected side and mediastinal flutter further impairs venous return by distortion of venae cavae

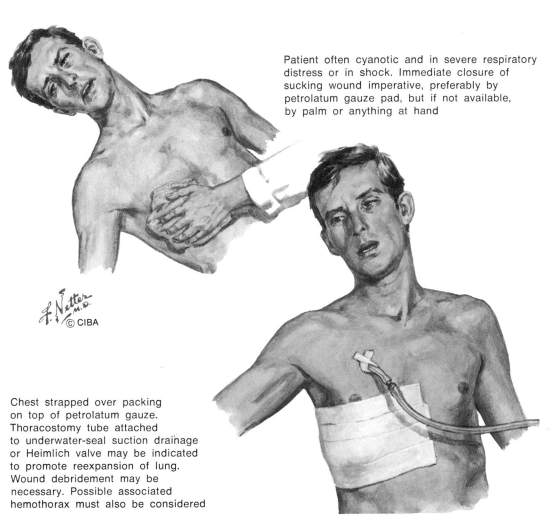

Patient often cyanotic and in severe respiratory distress or in shock. Immediate closure of sucking wound imperative, preferably by petrolatum gauze pad, but if not available, by palm or anything at hand

Chest strapped over packing on top of petrolatum gauze. Thoracostomy tube attached to underwater-seal suction drainage or Heimlich valve may be indicated to promote reexpansion of lung. Wound debridement may be necessary. Possible associated hemothorax must also be considered

Open pneumothorax usually results from a penetrating wound of the chest and is always a serious condition. Ancient warriors knew that if they could open an opponent's chest with a sword or lance the wound would always be fatal. In an open or "sucking" wound of the chest wall, the lung on the affected side is exposed to atmospheric pressure, which results in the lung's collapse and a shift of the mediastinum to the uninvolved side. Air passes into the chest more easily on inspiration than it can leave during expiration and this permits a progressive collapse of the lung. As the lung on the affected side is collapsed, the increased pleural pressure there pushes the mediastinum to the uninvolved side, thereby diminishing the contralateral lung volume. Because of the severe degree of venoarterial shunting that occurs in both lungs, resulting in profound ventilation-perfusion inequality, the patient becomes cyanotic and has serious respiratory distress.

The ability to tolerate the effects of a sucking wound of the chest depends on the patient's general condition and on whether previous fixation of the mediastinum has occurred. As the wound is sustained away from the hospital, the best first aid measure is the immediate restoration of the integrity of the chest wall by closure of the sucking wound with any material at hand such as a towel or other cloth, whether sterile or not; an occlusive dressing over the open wound is critically important to prevent death from anoxia.

Once the patient reaches the hospital emergency room, the sucking wound can be temporarily occluded with a massive dressing of petrolatum gauze, covered by dry gauze held in place by adhesive strips. A useful maneuver is to evacuate the pleural cavity by holding the wound open while the

patient coughs or exhales forcefully and then manually to reapproximate the wound when the patient inhales. A large amount of blood or air may be removed by this procedure. Once the open penetrating wound is converted to a closed wound, a thoracostomy tube must be placed in the chest for drainage of any associated hemothorax or pneumothorax. The tube is connected to an underwater seal for evacuation of air and measurement of the amount of blood loss. Examination of such a wound, which is usually the result of gunshot or stabbing, must be very thorough. A chest x-ray film is taken to disclose possible foreign bodies, fractured ribs or other intrathoracic damage.

The patient is next taken to the operating room, where sterile technique must be used to carry out careful cleansing, debridement, meticulous examination and repair. Clean wounds seen in the first 8 to 12 hours after injury may be sutured initially, but older or contaminated battlefield or disaster wounds are better handled by simple suture of the muscles of the chest wall. Closure of the skin is completed several days later if reexamination under sterile conditions shows that the wound is clean. Antitetanus therapy is carried out with toxoid and human tetanus immune globulin. All patients should also receive antibiotics, as these wounds must be considered contaminated.

Tension Pneumothorax

Tension pneumothorax may result from a variety of causes. In civilian life the most common cause is either a stab wound of the chest or a rib fracture, with the sharp end of the fractured rib lacerating the visceral pleura of the lung and permitting air to escape into the pleural space. In this cavity the rise above normal subatmospheric pressure, together with the lung elastic recoil, causes the lung to collapse partially or completely. Other traumatic causes of pneumothorax may be iatrogenic, such as the use of positive airway pressure during mechanical ventilation or anesthesia; cannulation of the subclavian or the internal jugular vein for hemodynamic monitoring; and performance of a tracheostomy, particularly in children. When respiratory distress or cyanosis is not relieved following establishment of a patent airway, pneumothorax should be suspected.

Thoracentesis is another relatively common cause of pneumothorax, usually by permitting air to enter through the needle. Laceration of the visceral pleura by the needle's point may also occur.

With any of these causes of pleural air leak the emergency situation of tension pneumothorax may arise. At each inspiration, intrapleural pressure increases because of a ball-valve mechanism that permits air to enter but not leave the pleural space. As the pressure constricts and distorts the venae cavae, the venous return to the heart is impaired, resulting in a decrease in stroke volume and cardiac output. Clinically, the patient experiences dyspnea, complains of chest pains, and becomes cyanotic because of shunting in the collapsed lung. The presence of hyperresonance and the absence of breath sounds, together with x-ray examination, should be useful in confirming the cause of the emergency.

On the electrocardiogram, four relatively consistent changes are observed: (1) a rightward shift in the mean frontal QRS axis, (2) a diminution in precordial voltage, (3) a diminution in QRS amplitude, and (4) an inversion of precordial T waves. A chest x-ray film indicates that the trachea and mediastinum are deviated to the side opposite the tension pneumothorax, while on the ipsilateral side the intercostal spaces are widened and the diaphragm is pushed downward. Since this critical emergency seldom permits time for x-ray confirmation, diagnostic needle insertion must be done. This distinct emergency requires immediate thoracostomy with underwater-seal drainage. Using local anesthesia a stab wound is made in the second anterior intercostal space on the affected side, two fingerbreadths lateral to the sternum to avoid the internal thoracic (internal mammary) vessels. A hemostat or scissors is used to separate the muscles, and the pleural space is entered just above the third rib to avoid bleeding from the intercostal vessels. A chest tube is then inserted into the pleural space and the incision closed with one or two sutures, which are additionally employed to

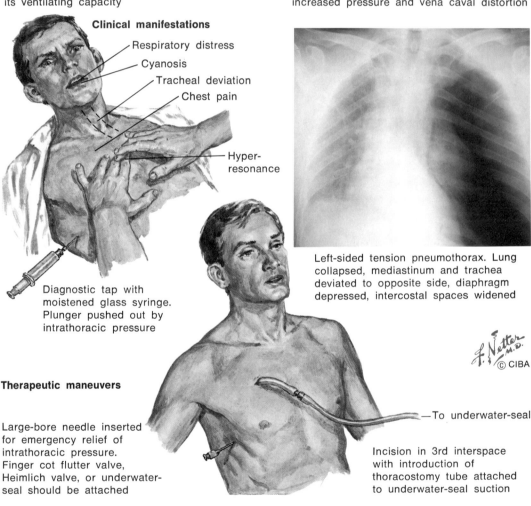

Tension Pneumothorax

Pathophysiology

Air
Air

Inspiration

Air enters pleural cavity through lung wound or ruptured bleb (or occasionally via penetrating chest wound) with valvelike opening. Ipsilateral lung collapses and mediastinum shifts to opposite side, compressing contralateral lung and impairing its ventilating capacity

Pressure

Expiration

Intrapleural pressure rises, closing valvelike opening, thus preventing escape of pleural air. Pressure is thus progressively increased with each breath. Mediastinal and tracheal shifts are augmented, diaphragm is depressed, and venous return is impaired by increased pressure and vena caval distortion

Clinical manifestations

Respiratory distress
Cyanosis
Tracheal deviation
Chest pain
Hyper-resonance

Diagnostic tap with moistened glass syringe. Plunger pushed out by intrathoracic pressure

Left-sided tension pneumothorax. Lung collapsed, mediastinum and trachea deviated to opposite side, diaphragm depressed, intercostal spaces widened

Therapeutic maneuvers

Large-bore needle inserted for emergency relief of intrathoracic pressure. Finger cot flutter valve, Heimlich valve, or underwater-seal should be attached

To underwater-seal

Incision in 3rd interspace with introduction of thoracostomy tube attached to underwater-seal suction

secure the chest tube. Trocars, once commonly used for this purpose, are less frequently used today as they may lacerate organs and vessels.

If the tube is to be placed in the lower lateral chest wall—a useful site if blood or fluid is also present—care must be taken to avoid placing it subdiaphragmatically or through the diaphragm, which could lead to penetration of the liver or spleen.

Any patient with trapped air in the pleural space who is to be given positive pressure anesthesia or supported by mechanical ventilation should have a thoracostomy tube inserted to prevent development of a tension pneumothorax. Positive pressure breathing can cause alveolar rupture due to pulmonary overinflation. This may produce surgical emphysema, with diffusion of air via the mediastinal pleura or pretracheal fascia into the subcutaneous tissues of the neck. Subsequent rupture of the mediastinal emphysema through the pleura will result in a pneumothorax. Bubbles in the pulmonary interstitium cause increased airway resistance and splinting of the lungs in the inspiratory position. As airway resistance increases, the patient exerts greater ventilatory effort, thus forcing more air into the pulmonary interstitium. However, high concentrations of inspired oxygen will reduce a pneumothorax by displacing nitrogen.

Hemothorax

Hemothorax

Hemothorax is common in both penetrating and nonpenetrating injuries to the chest. If the hemorrhage is large, it may not only cause hypovolemic shock but also dangerously reduce vital capacity by compressing the lung on the involved side. Persistent hemorrhage usually arises from an intercostal or internal thoracic (internal mammary) artery, and less frequently from the major hilar vessels. Bleeding from the lung generally stops within a few minutes, although initially it may be profuse. Depending on the direction of penetration, a hemothorax may come from a wound of the heart or from abdominal structures such as the liver or spleen if the diaphragm has been lacerated. Blood in the pleural cavity normally does not clot because of the smooth surfaces, the defibrinating action that occurs with the motions of respiration, and the presence of an anticoagulant enzyme.

The diagnosis of hemothorax is readily made from the clinical picture and x-ray evidence of fluid in the pleural space. Primary thoracentesis is carried out to confirm the diagnosis if the clinical picture indicates this is necessary. If the hemothorax is more than minimal or if hemopneumothorax is found, intercostal tube thoracostomy should be used. A large tube, preferably a silicone-coated No. 24 to 26 catheter, is inserted in either the fourth interspace laterally or the second intercostal space anteriorly. It is important not to use a lower point of insertion because there is a potential for penetration of the spleen or liver by perforation of the high-lying diaphragm, which is accentuated by expiration. Under local anesthesia a skin incision is made and blunt dissection carried out with a gloved finger to prevent inadvertent lung puncture by the tube should unsuspected pleural adhesions be present. When the tube is inserted, the skin should be sutured about the tube to secure an airtight seal. The tube is then connected to underwater-seal drainage. If the hemothorax is massive, two tubes are placed in the chest to evacuate the blood rapidly and permit the lung to expand.

Tube thoracostomy drainage allows constant monitoring of continuing blood loss and permits reexpansion of the lung. Patients with hemorrhage that initially measures more than 1500 ml or that bleeds faster than 100 ml per hour should be taken to the operating room for thoracotomy and control of the hemorrhage, as should patients with penetrating wounds of the heart causing hemothorax. If pericardial tamponade develops, a needle should be inserted into the pericardium and frequent measurements taken of venous as well as arterial blood pressure. If the pericardial tamponade recurs, a needle should be inserted again and left in place until the pericardium is opened during surgery. At that time any clots that may have formed are

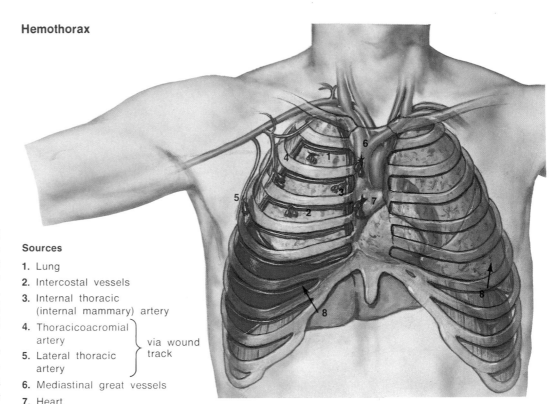

Sources

1. Lung
2. Intercostal vessels
3. Internal thoracic (internal mammary) artery
4. Thoracicoacromial artery
5. Lateral thoracic artery
6. Mediastinal great vessels
7. Heart
8. Abdominal structures (liver, spleen) via diaphragm

} via wound track

Degrees and management

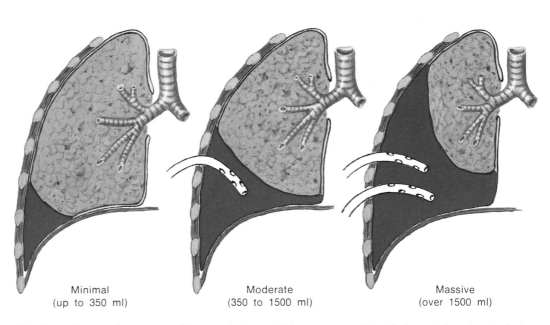

Minimal (up to 350 ml)

Blood usually resorbs spontaneously with conservative management. Thoracentesis rarely necessary

Moderate (350 to 1500 ml)

Thoracentesis and tube drainage with underwater-seal drainage usually suffices

Massive (over 1500 ml)

Two drainage tubes inserted since one may clog, but immediate or early thoracotomy may be necessary to arrest bleeding

rapidly removed from the pleural cavity, a search is made for all bleeding areas, and appropriate measures are taken to secure hemostasis. If blood is not readily available, the blood removed from the pleural cavity may be returned to the patient as an autotransfusion.

A small percentage of hemothoraces proceed to clot and cannot be evacuated by thoracentesis. Massive clots may lead to respiratory difficulty and infection, and should be evacuated surgically. Small clots will probably be resorbed and do not require operative removal. An infected hemothorax must be drained; in this case not only tube drainage but also operative intervention will be necessary.

If the hemothorax becomes organized, a peel of fibrous tissue or fibrothorax develops by the third or fourth week and completely encases the circumference of a lobe or the entire lung. At first this peel is only loosely adherent to the visceral and parietal pleurae but as time passes it increases in firmness and thickness and may become several millimeters thick. To restore the lung to normal function, decortication must be carried out. In this procedure, the peel or rind is removed from the visceral surface of the lung, leaving the pleural surface intact, with minimal air leakage. Decortication is easily accomplished in the first month after injury, but may be more difficult later.

Chylothorax

Chylothorax is ordinarily a complication of a thoracic surgical (usually mediastinal) procedure. It is remarkable that only rarely does penetrating or nonpenetrating trauma to the chest cause chylothorax, although the long-established triad of trauma, tuberculosis and tumor—especially lymphoma—is still valid as an etiologic concept. Cardiovascular surgery, particularly of the great vessels, is the most frequent cause of the condition. Other types of surgery resulting in chylothorax are esophageal, mediastinal and cervical. In general, chylothorax is most commonly a complication of mediastinal operations.

The development of chylothorax after such diverse procedures can probably be explained by the many anatomic variations of the thoracic duct (see CIBA COLLECTION, Volume 3/II, pages 39 and 74). In 50% of anatomic dissections there were such variations, including dual ducts and numerous lymphovenous anastomoses between the thoracic duct and the azygos and intercostal veins. Tributaries of the main thoracic duct are richly supplied from lymph nodes adjacent to the aortic isthmus and ligamentum arteriosum.

The diagnosis of chylothorax may be suspected from a roentgenogram of the chest showing widening of the mediastinum and the presence of pleural fluid. When aspirated, the pleural fluid is milky if the patient has been receiving fat in the diet. If the patient's diet has no fat, the fluid may be serous. Restoration of fat to the diet will quickly result in milky fluid in the pleura.

A remarkable clinical feature of chylothorax is the latent period between time of injury and onset of chylous effusion, which is usually 2 to 10 days, but sometimes extends to weeks or months. The reason, presumably, is that, following rupture of the duct, chyle accumulates in the mediastinum and only later extravasates into the pleural space. Enlargement of the cardiomediastinal shadow on a roentgenogram may represent this accumulation. Chyle is sufficiently radiopaque to be seen as a fluid collection in the posterior mediastinum on lateral roentgenograms of the chest.

Therapy for chylothorax remains controversial. Before the first successful ligation of the thoracic duct by Lampson in 1948, the overall mortality for traumatic chylothorax was 50%. In recent reports the mortality from either conservative or operative treatment is extremely low. However, considerable morbidity is still associated with this complication. Conservative therapy varies from multiple thoracenteses for three to four weeks, to continuous tube drainage with high negative pressure. The latter is used in the hope that a fully expanded lung will tampon the thoracic duct and promote early

Aspiration of milky (chylous) fluid from thoracic cavity (may be reintroduced into body by way of nasogastric tube or by well-monitored intravenous infusion)

Brachiocephalic (innominate) veins

Superior vena cava

Thoracic duct

Esophagus (cut away)

Azygos vein

Descending thoracic aorta

Diaphragm

Cisterna chyli

Normal course of thoracic duct

Ligation of thoracic duct after identification of rupture site by escape of intraabdominally injected dye

pleural symphysis by keeping the visceral and parietal pleura in constant opposition.

At present most surgeons advocate a maximum of seven days for nonoperative treatment, unless there is evidence that the volume of drainage is becoming progressively less. Early operation decreases morbidity, particularly in terms of hospitalization, while conservative treatment may require a hospital stay in excess of six weeks. If chylous drainage is copious, early surgery is indicated, as the extreme debility resulting from prolonged conservative treatment is best avoided. If the patient is seriously debilitated, surgery carries with it a formidable mortality.

On the evening before operative closure of the fistula, oral administration of olive oil (2 ml/kg of body weight), preferably with a dye added, facilitates identification of the leaking duct. When the defect is discovered, the duct should be mobilized only enough to permit its double transfixation ligation with nonabsorbable sutures. Reconstruction by end-to-end anastomosis or sidewall repair is not necessary, and is likely to fail. Search for the specific leaking point in an area of previous surgical dissection is difficult, protracted and unrewarding. The main thoracic duct may be ligated just above the aortic hiatus, where the channel is ordinarily single.

Pulmonary Contusion

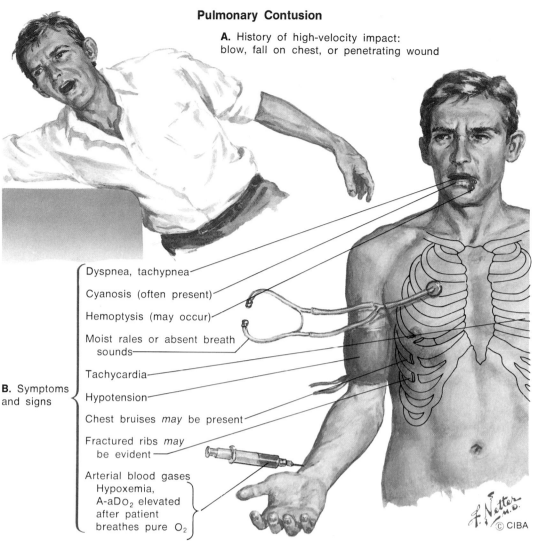

Pulmonary Contusion

A. History of high-velocity impact: blow, fall on chest, or penetrating wound

B. Symptoms and signs

Dyspnea, tachypnea

Cyanosis (often present)

Hemoptysis (may occur)

Moist rales or absent breath sounds

Tachycardia

Hypotension

Chest bruises *may* be present

Fractured ribs *may* be evident

Arterial blood gases Hypoxemia, A-aDo$_2$ elevated after patient breathes pure O$_2$

Pulmonary contusion is of primary importance in the field of major trauma to the chest. It is a life-threatening condition mainly because the onset of symptoms is insidious. Also, since the force required to produce a lung contusion must be great, the lesion is likely to occur principally in cases of high-speed accidents, falls from great heights and injuries by high-velocity bullets. Patients suffering such accidents often have so many other obvious injuries that a chest lesion may escape detection.

After seemingly negligible initial signs and symptoms, the outcome may be fatal. This type of reaction to trauma, which is peculiar to the lungs, is believed to be due to a number of factors, including lack of supporting cells in and around the alveoli, the low-pressure pulmonary perfusion system, sensitivity to reduction in cardiac output and the development of capillary wall damage. Hemorrhage, edema and atelectasis are the morphologic consequences of blunt injuries to the lung. While hemorrhage and microatelectasis are immediate results of the trauma, the most important factor in the often observed progressive deterioration of lung function in the 36 hours after injury seems to be interstitial and intraalveolar edema. Diffusion barriers, and especially shunts, result in potentially severe hypoxemia.

When symptoms of pulmonary contusion become obvious, the patient has dyspnea, tachypnea, cyanosis, tachycardia and hypotension. At that time a previously overlooked chest bruise may be noticed, and palpation may disclose fractures of the ribs or sternum. Moist rales are absent, but breath sounds are present at the site of the injury unless a complicating hemothorax or pneumothorax obscures them. Arterial blood gas analysis usually shows hypoxemia, often out of proportion to the extent of opacities on the chest x-ray film.

C. Pathology

Interstitial and intraalveolar edema the dominant factor; may cause impaired ventilation, shunts, and diffusion barrier, leading to hypoxemia

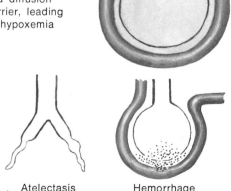

Atelectasis   Hemorrhage

Additional factors in hypoxemia

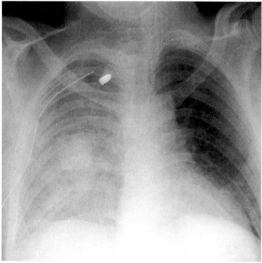

D. Ill-defined, patchy densities scattered throughout right lung (evidence of pulmonary edema) after bullet wound

A prompt diagnosis of pulmonary contusion is the main factor in initiating management and determining whether treatment will be effective. The diagnosis is first suspected from a history of major trauma. Young patients with elastic rib cages more often have pulmonary contusion without significant chest wall injuries, whereas in older patients an impact is more likely to cause serious injuries because the chest wall absorbs a great part of the applied force. The chest x-ray film is very important, and may show patchy, irregular, ill-defined densities or homogeneous consolidations. Frequently both appear simultaneously, and it is not unusual for contusions to be present in both lungs.

Lung scans may be helpful by demonstrating scattered areas of hypoperfusion. The most reliable and significant factors in confirming a diagnosis of pulmonary contusion are the *arterial blood gas analysis, chest roentgenogram* and *history.* As the symptoms immediately after the trauma may be obscure, serial blood gas analyses and chest roentgenograms are mandatory.

Mechanical ventilation and supplemental oxygen should be started immediately in cases of pulmonary contusion, even though symptoms are minimal. Later, if there is no hypoxemia and if the patient's pulmonary condition appears stable, ventilatory assistance can be withdrawn.

Posttraumatic Pulmonary Insufficiency (Adult Respiratory Distress Syndrome, Shock Lung)

Posttraumatic respiratory distress syndrome came into prominence in the management of combat casualties in the Vietnam War, when it was also known as "Da Nang lung." The syndrome is characterized by the development of acute respiratory failure (ARF) in the immediate postinjury period, usually in an individual with no preexisting pulmonary disease. It is associated with thoracic and nonthoracic trauma, including chest wall contusion, blast injury, multiple blood transfusions, fat embolism, aspiration, shock, cerebral hypoxia, and fluid and sodium overload. The common occurrence of shock during its course led to the term *shock lung*. It is recognized more accurately as one form of the adult respiratory distress syndrome (ARDS), which may complicate gram-negative sepsis, pancreatitis, congestive heart failure, pneumonia, intravascular coagulation, and prolonged exposure to high concentrations of inspired oxygen. Because loss of compliance, edema, intravascular cellular congestion, and alveolar collapse were frequently present, the terms *wet lung, stiff lung, congestive atelectasis* and others were used.

The condition is regarded as a form of noncardiogenic pulmonary edema, and the following etiologic factors play a role in its development:

1. *Vasoactive Substances.* Most pulmonary changes following shock, severe sepsis or trauma are probably related to vasoactive substances and lysosomal enzymes released from damaged, necrotic or infected cells or tissues. Permeability of the blood-air barrier and intravascular coagulation are believed to play a major role in the development of the syndrome. Some of the vasoactive substances thought to be implicated include catecholamines, kinins, serotonin, histamine and polypeptides.

2. *Fat Emboli.* Cerebral and respiratory dysfunction develops approximately 24 to 72 hours after severe injury, which usually includes long-bone fractures. The fat emboli act as a source of damaging vasoactive materials, such as fatty acids and serotonin.

3. *Fluid Overload and Congestive Heart Failure.* These problems increase the pulmonary interstitial edema and congestion that can develop in patients with shock, sepsis or trauma. Leakage of infused colloid into the interstitium establishes an adverse osmotic gradient which encourages the passage of additional fluid from the intravascular space. On the other hand, in the presence of an abnormally permeable blood-air barrier, the likelihood of further extravasation in the lungs is greatly increased.

4. *Massive Transfusions.* Banked blood, as it is stored, contains increasing quantities of aggregated WBC, RBC, platelets and fibrin which may occlude or damage small blood vessels in the lungs.

5. *Pulmonary Ischemia.* Severe prolonged pulmonary ischemia (due to shock and hypoperfusion) may eventually cause tissue necrosis and vascular damage, with development of the capillary leak syndrome characteristic of ARDS.

6. *Aspiration of Gastric Contents.* If aspirated vomitus is highly acid, pulmonary tissue damage can occur and may be severe or even fatal.

7. *Oxygen Toxicity.* Excessive concentrations of inspired oxygen are both wasteful and dangerous. A concentration of over 60% may damage the lung within three to four days, resulting in alveolar edema and collapse, with vascular congestion and hyaline membrane formation. It also decreases or stops ciliary action.

Pathology

Pulmonary capillary hypoxemia, microembolism and loss of surfactant have been regarded as possible precipitating mechanisms for ARDS, the bulk of the evidence incriminating the last two of these. In the first 18 hours after the onset of shock, petechial hemorrhages, scattered areas of congestion and atelectasis in dependent portions of lung are seen. These changes are associated with pulmonary venous and capillary engorgement, interstitial edema and thromboemboli. During the next 48 hours, the hemorrhagic consolidation progresses and intraalveolar hemorrhages appear. By the end of 72 hours, the changes are complete and the lungs resemble liver in color and consistency and are not inflatable. Hyaline membranes are formed, and bronchopneumonia is prominent. Throughout the process there is progressive reduction in numbers and size of alveoli due to interstitial edema and atelectasis. Fibroblasts and collagen appear when the condition has become irreversible.

Physiology

Acute respiratory failure (ARF) is present when there is impairment of blood-air gas exchange to the extent that the lungs can no longer support the metabolic needs of the body. In a healthy adult, breathing atmospheric air at sea level, a fall in the arterial oxygen tension (Pa_{O_2}) to less than 60 mm Hg or a rise in the arterial carbon dioxide tension (Pa_{CO_2}) to above 50 mm Hg is generally considered evidence of ARF. Since the presence and severity of blood gas changes cannot be assessed by clinical observation, serial determinations are indispensable in the management of ARDS. It should be borne in mind that if the patient's primary problem is relatively severe, with increased shunting in the lung due to ventilation-perfusion imbalance, the Pa_{O_2} will increase only slightly to moderately with a high inspired oxygen fraction. This is reflected in an increased alveolar-arterial oxygen tension difference ($A-aD_{O_2}$), and the shunt can be measured by using an appropriate equation.

Progressive stiffness of the lungs results in reduced tidal volumes and effective compliance, with a rise in respiratory frequency and peak airway pressures. Increasing disturbances in ventilation-perfusion relationships produce widening of the $A-aD_{O_2}$ and increasingly severe hypoxemia. Although there is an increase in total ventilation and pulmonary blood flow, it is made ineffective by an enlarged physiologic dead space and venoarterial shunting. In the terminal stages, hypercapnia is added to hypoxemia in spite of the use of mechanical ventilation and high inspired oxygen fractions.

Initially an alkalosis may be present and predispose to cardiac dysrhythmias. This is due to a combination of hyperventilation with resulting hypocapnia, along with excessive use of bicarbonate during resuscitation and stabilization. Later, acidosis supervenes from progressive hypercapnia and accumulation of lactic acid, and acts as a metabolic depressant.

Clinical Phases of ARDS

Phase I is characterized by altered tissue perfusion and metabolism. Unless there is a problem with CNS depression or damage to the airway, chest wall or lungs, a persistent moderate respiratory alkalosis is generally due to hyperventilation with a Pa_{CO_2} of 30 to 40 mm Hg. Arterial Po_2 may be slightly decreased or normal, and the $A-aD_{O_2}$ during breathing of room air is generally only slightly or moderately elevated to 20 to 40 mm Hg. The lungs are clear on physical examination except for a few basilar rales or rhonchi, and chest x-ray films as a rule appear to be normal.

In *phase II* hyperventilation continues and may be slightly increased, with a Pa_{CO_2} often in the range of 25 to 30 mm Hg. The $A-aD_{O_2}$ increases significantly, with hypoxemia unable to respond to simple oxygen therapy. Apart from the faster respiratory rate, there is no clinical evidence of severe respiratory distress, but some abnormalities are seen on x-ray examination of the chest. Mechanical ventilation now becomes necessary with the use of supplemental oxygen. The calculated shunt across the lungs may be 10 to 20% of cardiac output, but the patient can still recover.

In *phase III* (established respiratory distress) it is obvious that the patient has a serious respiratory problem. Hyperventilation may increase further, with a consequent drop in Pa_{CO_2}. Hypoxemia persists in spite of all attempts to correct it. The $A-aD_{O_2}$ is much bigger and the intrapulmonary shunt is generally 20% or greater. Increasing pulmonary edema with progressive confluence of the previously scattered diffuse infiltrates is noted on the chest x-ray film. Carbon dioxide retention subsequently develops, and the mortality is high.

Severe respiratory failure occurs in *phase IV,* with progressive hypoxemia, increasing lactic acidosis, carbon dioxide retention, and increased blood hydrogen ion concentration. Death results from cardiac arrhythmias or superimposed sepsis, which is frequently of gram-negative type. The mortality is usually in excess of 50%.

Treatment

The use of mechanical ventilation with positive end-expiratory pressure and supplemental oxygen has proved to be the most effective means of supporting life until the underlying problems can be corrected. Accurate assessment of the patient's hemodynamic status and fluid balance can be accomplished by means of a flotation catheter in the pulmonary artery. Corticosteroid drugs, anticoagulants, diuretics and appropriate antibiotics constitute the principal pharmacologic support. The recent use of extracorporeal membrane oxygenators has not proved any more successful than more conventional forms of treatment, but high frequency positive pressure ventilation may prove useful in the future.

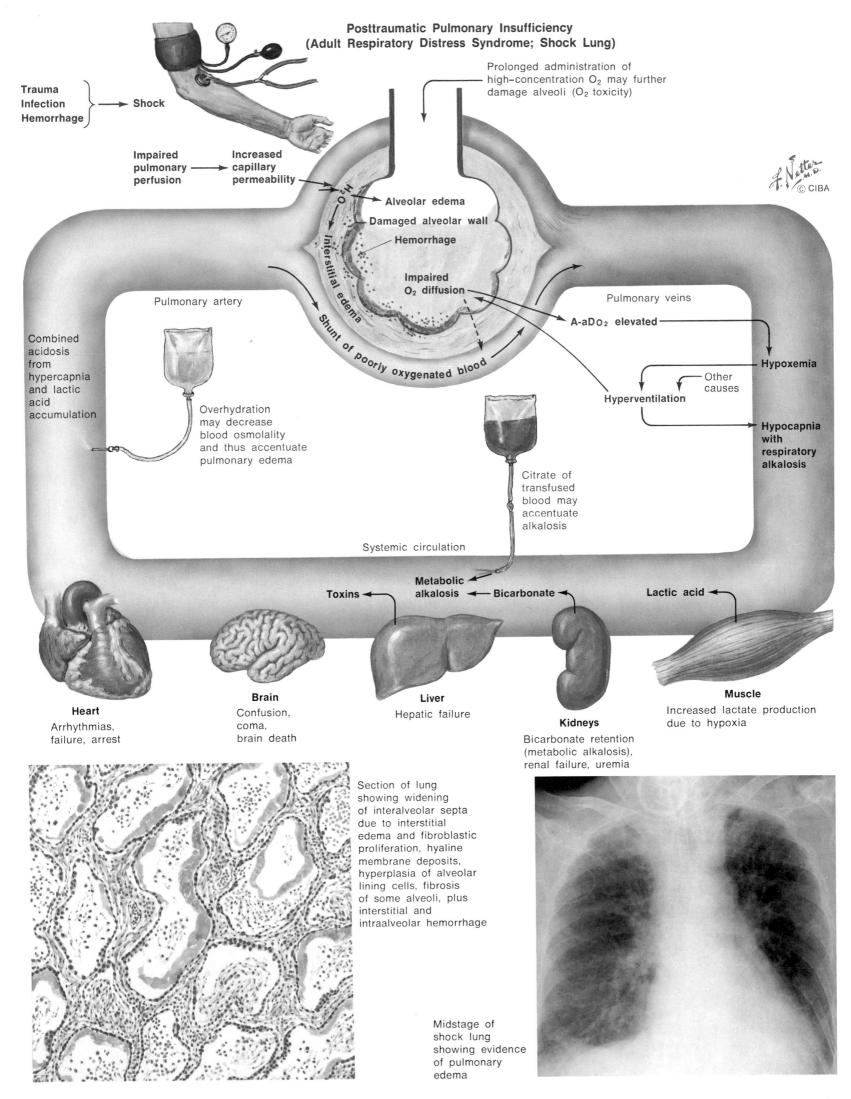

Posttraumatic Pulmonary Insufficiency
(Adult Respiratory Distress Syndrome; Shock Lung)

Trauma
Infection → Shock
Hemorrhage

Prolonged administration of
high–concentration O_2 may further
damage alveoli (O_2 toxicity)

Impaired → Increased
pulmonary   capillary
perfusion   permeability

H_2O

Alveolar edema

Damaged alveolar wall

Hemorrhage

Impaired
O_2 diffusion

Interstitial edema

Shunt of poorly oxygenated blood

Pulmonary artery

Pulmonary veins

A-aDO_2 elevated

Hypoxemia

Combined
acidosis
from
hypercapnia
and lactic
acid
accumulation

Overhydration
may decrease
blood osmolality
and thus accentuate
pulmonary edema

Hyperventilation

Other
causes

Hypocapnia
with
respiratory
alkalosis

Citrate of
transfused
blood may
accentuate
alkalosis

Systemic circulation

Metabolic
alkalosis ← Bicarbonate

Toxins

Lactic acid

Heart
Arrhythmias,
failure, arrest

Brain
Confusion,
coma,
brain death

Liver
Hepatic failure

Kidneys
Bicarbonate retention
(metabolic alkalosis),
renal failure, uremia

Muscle
Increased lactate production
due to hypoxia

Section of lung
showing widening
of interalveolar septa
due to interstitial
edema and fibroblastic
proliferation, hyaline
membrane deposits,
hyperplasia of alveolar
lining cells, fibrosis
of some alveoli, plus
interstitial and
intraalveolar hemorrhage

Midstage of
shock lung
showing evidence
of pulmonary
edema

Hyaline Membrane Disease

Hyaline membrane disease, sometimes referred to as respiratory distress syndrome (RDS), surfactant deficiency syndrome or neonatal atelectasis, is the result of lung ventilation in the presence of either inadequate stores of surfactant or insufficient capability for its continuous production. (See CIBA COLLECTION, Volume 3/II, page 114, and Volume 3/III, page 142.)

Epidemiology. Described in all populations of the world, hyaline membrane disease appears to be somewhat more common in prematurely born white infants than in black infants and nearly twice as common in males as females.

There is also the likelihood of familial recurrence in a subsequent prematurely born infant. The disorder accounts for about 10,000 deaths per year in the United States—a mortality of about 28% of those afflicted. Age at time of death is nearly always 72 hours or less, except for some infants who die of complications of the disease or its treatment later in the first few weeks of life.

Infants at special risk are those delivered prematurely, the incidence rising with greater prematurity. Delivery by cesarean section in the absence of previous labor also poses a risk if birth occurs before 37 weeks of gestation. Precipitous delivery after maternal hemorrhage, asphyxia or maternal diabetes is associated with a greater likelihood of hyaline membrane disease, and a second-born twin is at greater risk than the firstborn. Maternal conditions that are thought to have a sparing effect on the development of the disease are conditions associated with chronic intrauterine distress that lead to undersized infants, maternal steroid ingestion and, in some instances, prolonged labor following rupture of the membranes.

Pathology. On gross examination the lungs are found to be voluminous and liverlike, and they generally sink in water or formalin. Under the microscope much of the lung appears solid because of the tight apposition of most of the alveolar walls. Scattered throughout are dilated airspaces, respiratory bronchioles, alveolar ducts and a few alveoli, some of whose walls are lined with pink-staining "hyaline" material containing fibrin and cellular debris. The capillaries are strikingly congested, and there may be pulmonary edema and lymphatic distention.

Epithelial necrosis in the terminal bronchioles at sites underlying the hyaline membranes suggests that a reaction to injury has taken place. Hypersecretion of tracheobronchial mucus is evident, and reparative proliferation of type II cells is seen in infants who die on the second or third day of life.

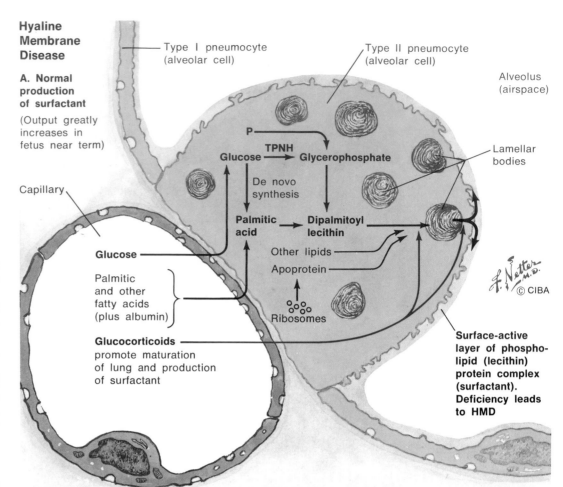

Hyaline Membrane Disease

A. Normal production of surfactant

(Output greatly increases in fetus near term)

- Type I pneumocyte (alveolar cell)
- Type II pneumocyte (alveolar cell)
- Alveolus (airspace)
- Lamellar bodies
- Capillary
- P
- TPNH
- Glucose → Glycerophosphate
- De novo synthesis
- Palmitic acid → Dipalmitoyl lecithin
- Glucose
- Other lipids
- Apoprotein
- Palmitic and other fatty acids (plus albumin)
- Ribosomes
- Glucocorticoids promote maturation of lung and production of surfactant
- Surface-active layer of phospholipid (lecithin) protein complex (surfactant). Deficiency leads to HMD

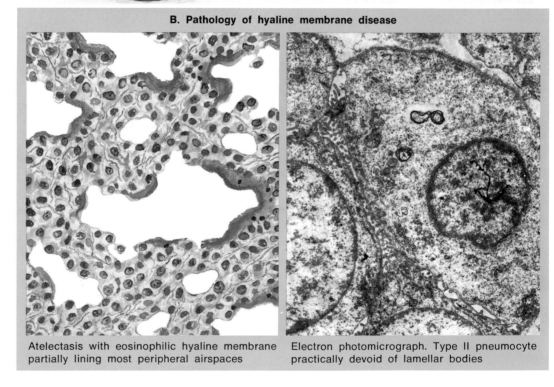

B. Pathology of hyaline membrane disease

Atelectasis with eosinophilic hyaline membrane partially lining most peripheral airspaces

Electron photomicrograph. Type II pneumocyte practically devoid of lamellar bodies

Pathogenesis. Although numerous theories of pathogenesis have been proposed since the first clinical description of hyaline membrane disease in 1949, the weight of evidence supports the central role of immaturity of the lung with respect to surfactant synthesis, or suppression of synthesis adequate to meet postnatal demands as, for example, by asphyxia. Surfactant deficiency results in failure of stabilization of small airways at end-expiration with consequent reduction of functional residual capacity. Each new inspiration requires the application of sufficient transpulmonary pressure to reinflate atelectatic airspaces. A high respiratory frequency and large applied pressures have to be employed to maintain effective ventilation. Uneven distribution of inspired air and perfusion of nonventilated alveoli result in poor gas exchange, characterized chiefly by hypoxemia. The infant grunts in an attempt to prolong end-inspiration, a pattern of breathing which can be shown experimentally to improve alveolar ventilation.

Pulmonary vascular resistance is increased by vasoconstriction due to hypoxia, with a resulting increase in right-to-left shunts through the persistent fetal vascular pathways, ductus arteriosus and foramen ovale. The hypoxemia is further

(Continued)

Clinical Manifestations of Hyaline Membrane Disease

Hyaline Membrane Disease
(Continued)

aggravated since as much as 80% of the cardiac output may be shunted past airless lungs.

Wasted ventilation and ineffective perfusion initiate a train of events that accounts for most of the findings in hyaline membrane disease. Reduced oxygenation of the myocardium impairs cardiac output and perfusion of the kidneys, whose ability to maintain acid-base homeostasis is compromised. Poor perfusion of peripheral tissues contributes to lactic acidemia and a profound metabolic acidosis. The association of intraventricular hemorrhage with hyaline membrane disease may be related to cerebral hypoxia and ischemia or to intravascular coagulation, which is seen in some seriously ill infants.

Diagnosis. The onset of symptoms is within minutes of birth, but often they are not recognized as significant for some hours. Duskiness, tachypnea, grunting and significant retraction of soft tissues are characteristic. Increasing cyanosis, often relatively unresponsive to greater inspired oxygen concentrations, is a notable feature of the disease. Air exchange may be present, and dullness to percussion may be detectable, particularly at the lung bases. Sometimes the upper sternum seems prominent as the lower sternum is sucked in with each inspiratory effort.

Radiologic Findings. The earliest roentgenographic finding is a fine miliary mottling of the lungs, with consolidation centrally. The air-filled tracheobronchial tree stands out in relief against the opacified lung roots, which often obscure the cardiothymic silhouette. The appearance may change from minute to minute, depending on the lung volume at which the x-ray film is taken. A good cry can aerate both lungs, and a deep inspiratory effort may produce an x-ray picture suggesting minimal disease. Expiration, particularly after oxygen-breathing, can lead to washing gas out of the lungs and a virtual "whiteout" of the thorax.

The miliary reticulogranularity of the lung parenchyma is usually present within minutes of birth. Occasionally the changes are more prominent on the right side than on the left, and sometimes more evident in lower lobes than in upper lobes.

During the course of the disease, chest roentgenograms may show a number of changes, including interstitial emphysema, pneumomediastinum and pneumothorax. In some infants recovery is slow, and complex radiologic changes occur over ensuing months.

Treatment. Of primary importance is the need to oxygenate the infant with whatever inspired mixture is required to keep arterial oxygen tensions at 50 to 70 mm Hg. This goal can be reached

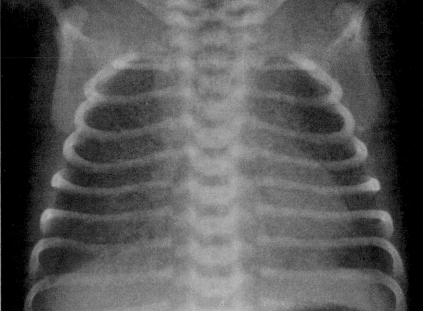

Expiratory grunt or whimper (may be clearly audible or heard only via stethoscope)

Respiratory rate accelerated (interposed apneic periods of over 10 sec indicate poor prognosis)

Retraction of soft tissues on inspiration (lower sternum may retract and abdomen distend "seesaw" fashion)

Umbilical artery sampling

O_2 desaturation
Acidosis (respiratory and metabolic)
Low serum protein (<4.6 g/100 ml) indicates likelihood of HMD

Flaring of nostrils

Cyanosis or ashen pallor (right-to-left shunts)

Breath sounds harsh; fine rales may be present

Pooling of circulation (darker discoloration of dependent areas)

Excessive peripheral edema

Radiologic findings

Granular pattern may be distributed throughout lung fields. Bronchial tree can often be visualized against opacified lung

Increasing confluence of density indicates poor prognosis

with inspired mixtures of modest concentration if continuous distending airway pressure is achieved by either positive pressure at the mouth or negative pressure around the thorax. Alternatively, prolonged inspiratory-expiratory ratios can do for the infant what he does with his own larynx in the act of grunting respiration.

Continuous distending airway pressure (not to be confused with intermittent positive pressure breathing) is obtained most commonly by imposing a resistance in the expiratory line if the infant is intubated or breathing through nasal cannulas. A head-hood under positive pressure achieves the same result.

Complications of Respiratory Therapy. Increasingly, infants are found to develop interstitial emphysema and pneumothorax during the course of ventilatory therapy. Alertness to the possibility of these complications, which are usually indicated by abrupt clinical deterioration, can lead to lifesaving intervention. Of prime importance is the awareness that the lungs themselves are changing during the course of the disease. Thus the 10 cm H_2O distending pressure found to be effective during early phases of treatment may cause tamponade of the pulmonary circulation during recovery. This leads to a worsening of hypoxemia
(Continued)

Risk Factors for Development of Hyaline Membrane Disease

Prematurity
Birth wt. > 2.5 kg; HMD not likely
Birth wt. < 2.5 kg; likelihood of HMD increases in relation to lower wt. (if viable)

Perinatal asphyxia
(2nd born of twins
∴ more susceptible)

Cesarean birth

Diabetes mellitus
(maternal)

Prenatal Predictability of Hyaline Membrane Disease

Amniocentesis

Lecithin-sphingomyelin ratio (L-S)

Mean L-S ratio

Respiratory distress (HMD) not likely

Some likelihood of mild respiratory distress

Likelihood of moderate to severe HMD increases with lower L-S ratio

Weeks of gestation

Shake test
1 ml amniotic fluid diluted in various ratios (1:1, 1:1.3, 1:2) with 1 ml 95% ethanol, shaken 15 sec and allowed to stand 15 sec. If stable foam forms, tube is called positive. Positive in all dilutions indicates little risk of HMD. Negative in all tubes indicates high risk

1:1 Positive   1:2 Positive   Little risk of HMD

1:1 Negative   1:2 Negative   High risk of HMD

1:1 Positive   1:2 Negative   Intermediate risk

Hyaline Membrane Disease
(Continued)

and so to stronger respiratory efforts, which may result in lung rupture and loculated air subcutaneously and in the pleural space.

Infants who survive the first week or so of illness may become respirator- and oxygen-dependent. Typically, their lungs undergo a series of changes that are characterized by air-trapping, atelectasis, fibrosis, cyst formation and basilar emphysema. Originally described by Northway and Rosan in 1967 as bronchopulmonary dysplasia, this condition is now well known to everyone caring for premature infants. The course is chronic, sometimes lasting months or years. Complete recovery is possible, but death from intercurrent illness is a continuing threat. At autopsy the lungs are found to be heavy, hypercellular and fibrotic, with squamous metaplasia of even the small airways. Since the cilia are gone, it is not surprising that secretions pool; either atelectasis or lobular emphysema is common.

Bronchopulmonary dysplasia is less often seen when the duration of exposure to high concentrations of inspired oxygen is reduced by the use of continuous distending airway pressure or prolonged inspiratory-expiratory ratios. The similarity of the lesion to that of chronic oxygen toxicity is striking, *and the lung changes may be related to oxygen alone.* That high applied airway pressures contribute to the pathogenesis of the lesion remains a possibility, and this is supported by the work of Reynolds, who reported a sharp diminution in the frequency of the lesion after airway pressures were limited to less than 25 cm H_2O.

Prognosis. Hyaline membrane disease is still a serious disorder. Approximately 20 to 30% of infants in whom the diagnosis is made succumb. Some of the deaths result from pulmonary failure; others are associated with, and perhaps caused by, intraventricular hemorrhage. The smallest infants usually die within 24 hours; larger ones may live longer, and some of these die from intercurrent infection. The majority of all deaths occur within 72 hours of birth; however, if mechanical ventilation is employed, death may occur much later. Survivors usually recover completely, but in rare instances recurrent pulmonary infection and fibrosis follow the illness.

Prenatal Diagnosis and Prevention. Lecithins synthesized by the fetal lung enter the amniotic fluid, and measurement of the lecithin-sphingomyelin (L-S) ratio in amniotic fluid has proved a useful index of lung maturity.

At about 34 to 35 weeks of normal gestation (but with considerable variability), lung lecithins increase in concentration and the L-S ratio rises. Values over 2 usually indicate lung maturity. The "shake test" offers the means to perform a quick

assessment of the presence of surface-active materials in amniotic fluid. The test depends on the ability of these materials to produce a stable foam on the surface of an aliquot of fluid shaken in air in a test tube. One milliliter of amniotic fluid undiluted, or diluted with 0.9% saline is shaken for 15 seconds with 1 ml of 95% ethanol. Bubbles at the air-liquid interface correlate with lung maturity.

The possibility of preventing hyaline membrane disease is at hand with the demonstration that glucocorticoids are the promoters of lung cell differentiation. Normally, the fetal adrenal gland produces these hormones toward the end of pregnancy, though they are produced earlier with

some kinds of intrauterine stress. Amniotic fluid levels reflect this activity by increasing after 35 weeks of gestation. Thus, premature birth deprives the infant of the physiologic surge in the glucocorticoid activity presumably necessary for alveolar cell differentiation and surfactant synthesis. Liggins and Howie first demonstrated that betamethasone given to a mother 24 hours before delivery could reduce deaths from hyaline membrane disease in infants less than 32 weeks old. It seems probable that this form of intervention, or prenatal treatment, will be indicated whenever delivery can be postponed 24 hours in the presence of a low L-S ratio.

Idiopathic Diffuse Interstitial Pulmonary Fibrosis (Hamman-Rich Disease)

Idiopathic Diffuse Interstitial Pulmonary Fibrosis (Hamman-Rich Syndrome, Cryptogenic Fibrosing Alveolitis)

Idiopathic diffuse interstitial pulmonary fibrosis (IDIPF) is a distinct clinical entity which probably represents a common "end stage" arrived at through different pathologic processes of varied causation. Known causes include viral pneumonias, drug reactions (nitrofurans, busulfan, bleomycin, methotrexate), chemical vapors, organic and inorganic dusts, radiation, connective tissue disorders, alveolar proteinosis and recovery from the adult respiratory distress syndrome (ARDS). When no cause is apparent, the disease is termed idiopathic, Hamman-Rich syndrome, or cryptogenic fibrosing alveolitis. The label *idiopathic* implies the exclusion of all other diseases known to cause diffuse pulmonary fibrosis; obviously, it must be applied with extreme caution. Rarely, the true systemic nature of a disease such as progressive systemic sclerosis does not become apparent until months or years after recognition of pulmonary changes.

Liebow and Carrington attempted to subdivide the pulmonary fibroses into UIP (usual interstitial pneumonia), which includes the idiopathic variety as well as the form that accompanies the connective tissue diseases; DIP (desquamative interstitial pneumonia), characterized by the desquamation of cells in alveolar spaces with varying degrees of interstitial reaction; LIP (lymphocytic interstitial pneumonia), manifested by a dense lymphocytic infiltration of the pulmonary interstitium often accompanied by a serologic monoclonal gammopathy; and GIP (giant cell interstitial pneumonia), seen almost exclusively in measles pneumonia. Scadding and others have objected to such fine subdivisions of IDIPF and maintain that these subclasses are merely different stages of the same idiopathic disease, which may eventually lead to profound fibrosis of the pulmonary interstitium.

IDIPF occurs slightly more often among women than men. It afflicts all ages, with predominance at 30 to 50 years of age. There are many reports of childhood disease as well as several instances of familial incidence.

The paramount pathologic feature of IDIPF is widespread distribution of patchy interstitial fibrosis. Grossly, the lungs are usually shrunken and stiff. Small (0.5 cm diameter) microcysts may be localized in the lung bases or scattered throughout the parenchyma, giving rise to the term *honeycomb lung*. The pleura is spared but may appear "cobblestoned" due to the underlying diseased lung. Early, there may be an alveolar exudate as well as interstitial edema and infiltration of the interstitium with lymphocytes, macrophages, eosinophils, neutrophils and fibroblasts. As the process continues, fibrotic thickening of the alveolar septa dominates. Relatively cellular areas may coexist with areas of dense fibrosis in the same lobe or lung. In the most fibrotic areas there is proliferation of cuboidal epithelium, derived from the type II alveolar cell, which results in "bronchiolization" of the alveolar lining. Marked

Diffuse bilateral fibrosis of lungs with multiple small cysts giving honeycomb appearance. Pleura thickened and adhesive in places with intervening nodularity

Advanced pulmonary fibrosis with almost complete loss of architecture. Small bronchus at left of picture

Clinical picture

Dyspnea
Cyanosis
Nonproductive hacking cough
Clubbing of fingers
Basilar inspiratory ("cellophane") rales
Diffuse pulmonary fibrosis on x-ray film; restrictive pulmonary function pattern
Loss of weight
Elevated diaphragm
Cor pulmonale (late)

peribronchiolar fibrosis may lead to airway narrowing. An increase in interstitial smooth muscle fibers and lymphoid aggregates takes place. Importantly, alveolar capillaries are obliterated by the interstitial process. In less involved portions the vessels leading to precapillary bronchopulmonary anastomoses may proliferate.

The small fibrotic lungs are mirrored physiologically by decreased lung volumes (TLC, VC, RV) and decreased pulmonary compliance. The loss of functioning alveolar-capillary units and ventilation-perfusion imbalance are marked by hypoxemia, which is accentuated by exercise. Relative sparing of the airways is noted in the

normal measurements of MVV, FEV_1, $FEF_{25-75\%}$, and pulmonary airway resistance. The flow-volume loop manifests a characteristic rapid rise to, and drop from, peak flow. Flow rates at low lung volumes may be decreased due to small airway disease or as a reflection of decreased lung volume.

The chest radiograph exhibits bilateral diffuse interstitial linear or nodular infiltrations with high diaphragm, giving the pattern of shrunken lungs. Radiologists frequently report "poor inspiratory effort." Occasionally the radiographic alterations may be confined to the lower lobes or

(Continued)

Idiopathic Diffuse Interstitial Pulmonary Fibrosis (Hamman-Rich Syndrome, Cryptogenic Fibrosing Alveolitis)
(Continued)

rarely to a single lung. Profusion of microcysts often allows the radiologist to make the diagnosis of honeycomb lung. The pleura and pericardium are normal. However, in the final stages of the disease, cardiomegaly and enlargement of the pulmonary arteries reflect pulmonary hypertension and cor pulmonale.

Interest continues to grow in the possibility that IDIPF is due to an immune reaction occurring in the alveolar walls and capillary endothelium. Several observers have demonstrated precipitation of immune complexes in these loci and lung biopsy specimens of patients with IDIPF. Moreover, serologic alterations suggesting altered immune responses have been reported: elevated erythrocyte sedimentation rate, the presence of antinuclear antibodies, rheumatoid factor and cryoglobulins, and elevated levels of serum IgG, IgA and IgM. Finally, Crystal has emphasized the finding of relatively large quantities of IgG as well as leukocytes and macrophages in the lavage field obtained from the bronchial washings.

All patients with IDIPF have dyspnea and a hacking nonproductive cough. Most are cyanotic, and clubbing of the fingers is common. Breathing is characteristically rapid and shallow. Subcrepitant rales (cellophane rales) are heard over all lobes. Wheezes and rhonchi are rare except with superimposed bronchitis. With the development of pulmonary hypertension the pulmonic valve sound becomes accentuated.

The diagnosis of IDIPF is established by the demonstration of interstitial pulmonary fibrosis by percutaneous needle, transbronchial or open lung biopsy in a patient with no other disease known to cause these changes. Since a large number of disorders may lead to pulmonary interstitial involvement, it is essential to prove the nature of the disease process histologically.

In patients with predominantly fibrotic lungs, oxygen is the mainstay of therapy. Most patients will show transient radiographic and functional improvement while receiving corticosteroid drugs. Improvement has also been reported with the addition of cyclophosphamide or azathioprine. However, the usual course in IDIPF is relentlessly downhill, with death occurring from a few months to as long as 20 years after onset. In the early stages response to steroids is often excellent, and several cures have been reported. With the demonstration of abnormal circulating proteins, elevated IgG in bronchial lavage fluid, increased pulmonary uptake of ^{67}Ga, and the presence of marked cellular infiltration rather than fibrosis on lung biopsy, Crystal has noted that a good response to corticosteroids can be expected. However, biopsy sampling may not be representative of all areas of the lungs, even when tissue is obtained by open lung biopsy. It is good practice, therefore, to administer a trial of steroid therapy to all patients with IDIPF.

Sarcoidosis

Sarcoidosis is a common disease of unknown origin characterized by the infiltration of many organs by noncaseating epithelioid granulomas. Although most accounts from the United States emphasize the predominance of the condition in blacks, it has been reported from five continents and among diverse ethnic groups, including Caucasians in Sweden, Orientals in Japan, and Puerto Ricans born in New York City. Women appear to contract the disease more often than men, and the majority of patients are less than 40 years of age at onset. There seems to be a familial incidence, several investigators encountering it among siblings and children. A childhood form is not uncommon, and an infant with "congenital" sarcoidosis has been reported. A constellation of fever, arthralgias and erythema nodosum is a traumatic mode of onset, occurring almost exclusively in young women.

In its usual benign form sarcoidosis runs its entire course without detection in an estimated 90% of patients. Its high prevalence is suggested by the large number of asymptomatic patients discovered by mass radiographic surveys.

Sarcoidosis presents as a variety of clinical syndromes, including erythema nodosum with radiographic evidence of hilar lymph node enlargement, cutaneous plaques and subcutaneous nodules, uveoparotid fever, isolated uveitis, salivary gland enlargement, central nervous system syndromes (usually seventh nerve palsy), cardiomyopathy and skeletal muscle myopathy, bone destruction, hepatosplenomegaly (with or without hypersplenism), arthritis, upper airway mucosal lesions, hypercalcemia, renal failure, generalized lymphadenopathy, and diffuse interstitial pulmonary disease. A single patient may demonstrate symptoms and signs referable to any one or a combination of features. It must be remembered that the most common initial presentation is an asymptomatic patient with an abnormal routine chest radiograph.

Because of the superficially similar pathologic and clinical pictures, early workers believed sarcoidosis was a manifestation of tuberculous infection. The absence of demonstrable tubercle bacilli, negative tuberculin skin test in the majority of patients, organ involvement not seen in infection by *Mycobacterium tuberculosis,* and salutary response to corticosteroid therapy have all marked sarcoidosis as an entity distinct from that disease. Similarly, claims for an etiologic role for the products of pine trees and atypical mycobacteria have been refuted.

Noncaseating epithelioid granulomas, often accompanied by giant cells and rarely by small calcified bodies (Schaumann's bodies), are the fundamental pathologic lesions in sarcoidosis, but are nonspecific. Since they often cannot be differentiated from the granulomas of fungal infections, berylliosis, leprosy, brucellosis, hypersensitivity lung diseases, the occasional instances of tuberculosis when caseation and acid-fast bacilli are not apparent, and from lymph nodes draining neoplastic tumors, the diagnosis requires a compatible clinical picture and negative smears and cultures for organisms causing the diseases. Granulomas may develop in almost every tissue, accounting for the multiple modes of clinical presentation when organ structure and function are impaired. In the majority of patients with disability, the organs primarily affected are the lungs, the eyes and the myocardium (see CIBA COLLECTION, Volume 5, page 205).

The intrathoracic presentations of sarcoidosis have been divided into three radiographic stages: (I) bilateral hilar and right paratracheal lymph node enlargement, (II) persistence of lymph nodes with concomitant pulmonary infiltrations, and (III) pulmonary infiltrations with no identifiable mediastinal adenopathy. A fourth stage has been proposed, manifested by fibrotic lungs often accompanied by bullae. Although the hilar lymphadenopathy seen in radiographic stages I and II is described as symmetric, the nodes at the right hilus are usually more prominent and are separated from the mediastinum by the air column formed by the intermediate and right lower lobe bronchi. Right paratracheal lymph node enlargement is common. This pattern of lymphadenopathy is typical for stage I sarcoidosis and is an aid in the radiographic differential diagnosis of mediastinal lymph node diseases. The parenchymal pulmonary infiltrations seen in stages II and III appear in a variety of patterns. The pulmonary densities are almost always bilateral and may be reticulonodular or confluent, or they may present as multiple large densities simulating metastatic carcinoma. Radiolucencies often appear scattered throughout the parenchymal shadows and range from small microcysts to large bullae. Occasionally, aspergillomas form in the bullae. With chronicity, fibrosis may be prominent, with retraction of the hilar areas upward and unilateral deviation of the trachea. This radiographic presentation (stage IV) can easily be confused with that seen in fibrocaseous pulmonary tuberculosis. There is a general parallel between the chronology of sarcoidosis and the radiographic stages, stage I usually occurring in early sarcoidosis and stage IV always indicating chronic disease. However, stages I, II and III have been noted within weeks of onset and may persist with little change for years.

Patients with radiographic stage I sarcoidosis are most often asymptomatic and ordinarily have normal pulmonary function tests despite the universal presence of granulomas on lung biopsy specimens at this stage of the disease. With radiographically discernible pulmonary lesions, a restrictive pattern of dysfunction is likely to emerge, with loss of lung volumes, decreased pulmonary compliance, hyperventilation, decreased diffusing capacity and, in the most severely afflicted patients, hypoxemia. In chronically scarred lungs, evidence of airway dysfunction usually appears, with decreased $FEF_{25-75\%}$ and diminished flow rates at low lung volumes.

Various alterations in cellular immunity occur in sarcoidosis. There is impaired delayed hypersensitivity to skin antigens, notably tuberculin, mumps, *Trichophyton* and oidiomycin. This relative anergy may persist for many years. Approximately

(Continued)

Sarcoidosis

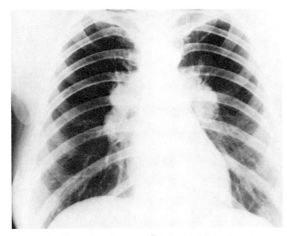

Radiologic stage I: Bilateral hilar lymph node enlargement

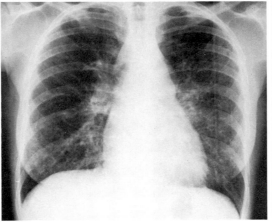

Stage II: Persistence of lymphadenopathy with reticular and nodular pulmonary infiltrations

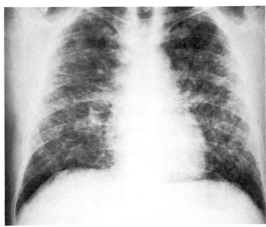

Stage III: Pulmonary infiltrations with no identifiable mediastinal lymphadenopathy

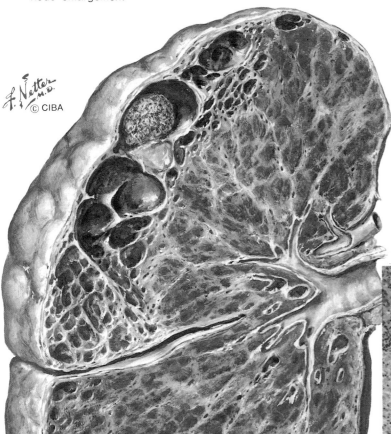

Stage IV: Fibrotic lungs with bullae

Sectioned lung in advanced sarcoidosis. Fibrosis in central zone with bullae near surface of upper lobe, one of which contains an aspergilloma

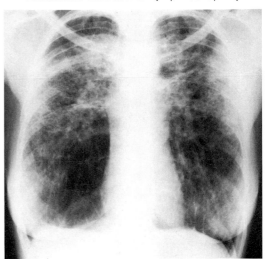

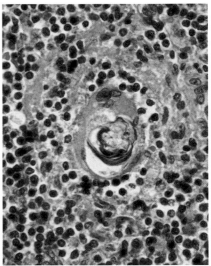

Typical epithelioid cell granulomas with occasional giant cells

Schaumann's body (concentrically laminated, calcified body) in a mediastinal lymph node giant cell

Sarcoidosis
(Continued)

two-thirds of all patients with active disease have a negative tuberculin skin test. When a patient with presumptive sarcoidosis and a negative tuberculin test subsequently manifests conversion to a positive tuberculin test, the onset of active *M. tuberculosis* infection obviously must be considered. Depressed

delayed hypersensitivity is probably related to abnormal T-lymphocyte function which can be shown by deficient response to phytohemagglutinin (PHA), an augmented rate of blast transformation, and increased release of migration inhibitory factor (MIF). Similarly, abnormal function of monocytes—probably the precursors of epithelioid cells—has been noted. On the other hand, there is an increase in circulating immunoglobulins, with frequent elevations of gamma globulin, IgA, IgM and IgG levels. Recently, elevated levels of serum angiotensin-converting enzyme (ACE) and serum lysozyme have been ob-

served in active sarcoidosis; a return toward normal values coincident with corticosteroid treatment or spontaneous improvement has been observed in some cases. Serum levels of ACE and lysozyme have been proposed as a good measure of disease activity.

The diagnosis of sarcoidosis rests on the demonstration of noncaseating epithelioid granulomas in tissues subjected to biopsy (skin, lymph nodes or lung) from a patient with a compatible clinical picture. During the past five years, lung biopsy via the fiberoptic bronchoscope has emerged as the premier diagnostic procedure in patients without
(Continued)

Sarcoidosis
(Continued)

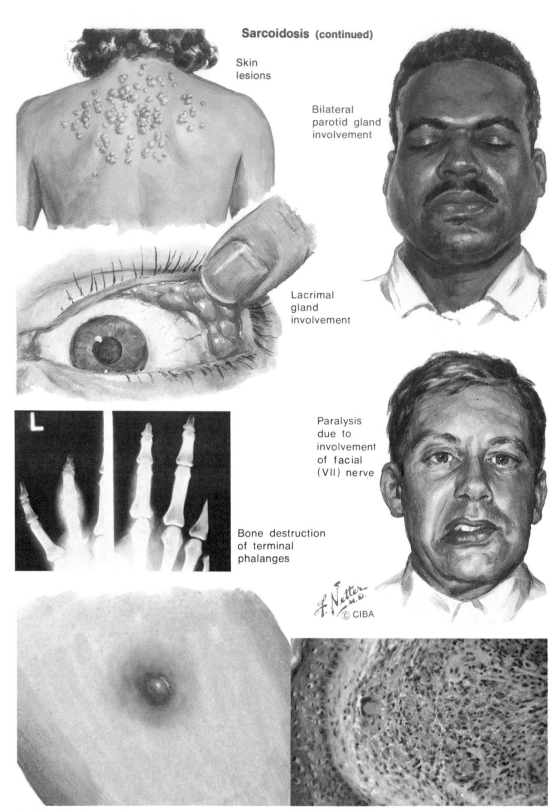

Sarcoidosis (continued)

Skin lesions

Bilateral parotid gland involvement

Lacrimal gland involvement

Paralysis due to involvement of facial (VII) nerve

Bone destruction of terminal phalanges

Positive Kveim test. Intracutaneous injection of saline suspension of human sarcoidal spleen or lymph nodes causes appearance of erythematous nodule in 2 to 6 weeks

Biopsy of nodule reveals typical sarcoidal granuloma (dense infiltration with macrophages, epithelioid cells, and occasional multinucleated giant cells)

easily accessible skin or peripheral lymph node lesions. Since the pathology is nonspecific, a properly standardized intracutaneous Kveim test is a valuable and reliable diagnostic tool. Siltzbach has shown that this test can be expected to be positive in 85% of patients with active, organ-biopsy-confirmed sarcoidosis. With reduced disease activity and the passage of time, its sensitivity decreases to 55% of positive reactors. The incidence of false positive Kveim tests is less than 0.2%. Reports of positive tests in other granulomatous diseases and nonsarcoid lymphadenopathies have proved to be due to faulty test antigen.

The vast majority of patients with sarcoidosis can expect a benign course, with complete clearing or nondisabling persistence of radiographic and other clinical abnormalities. However, a small but significant number of patients will be disabled, and approximately 4% will die of their sarcoidosis, usually from respiratory failure. Rarely, death oc-

curs from sarcoid cardiomyopathy or renal failure or from hemorrhage due to pulmonary aspergillomas that form in sarcoid bullae.

Active sarcoidosis responds well to corticosteroids. A relatively small dose of prednisone will shrink most granulomas. The usual course of therapy continues for six to nine months. Relapse is common after cessation of prednisone and may require reinstitution of treatment. This complication is particularly likely in cutaneous sarcoidosis. Since prolonged corticosteroid therapy is hazardous, chloroquine is preferred for skin involvement. Prompt treatment with corticosteroids is indicated for patients with uveitis, central nervous system

disease, hypercalcemia, cardiomyopathy, hypersplenism and progressive pulmonary dysfunction, but only 10% of patients with sarcoidosis require mandatory treatment of this kind. Approximately 20% more may be given this form of medication electively for persistent constitutional symptoms, disfiguring salivary gland and lymph node enlargement, upper airway mucosal lesions, and peripheral neuromuscular disease. Corticosteroid drugs are not indicated in patients with asymptomatic hilar lymphadenopathy or minor radiographic pulmonary shadows. Erythema nodosum can usually be controlled with aspirin, phenylbutazone or indomethacin.

Idiopathic Pulmonary Hemosiderosis

Idiopathic pulmonary hemosiderosis (IPH) is a disease of unknown origin, usually occurring in children but reported to begin as late as age 40 years. In children the disease occurs equally in both sexes, but in adults it is more common in the male. Repeated episodes of pulmonary hemorrhage with resultant blood-loss anemia and eventual respiratory failure characterize the illness. Multiple theories for the etiology of IPH have proved wanting. Because of the similarity between pulmonary manifestations of IPH and those of Goodpasture's syndrome, it has been proposed that IPH is also a disease of altered immunity. However, a search for an antilung antibody similar to the antiglomerular basement membrane antibody in Goodpasture's syndrome has been fruitless. Thus, the absence of a renal lesion and the usual childhood onset of IPH differentiates the two diseases.

During acute episodes of hemorrhage, the alveoli and smaller bronchi are filled with fresh blood in a patchy or lobar distribution. In addition to free red blood cells, numerous hemosiderin-laden pulmonary macrophages are present. The alveolar lining cells react with hyperplasia. Repeated hemorrhages bring proliferation of fibroblasts, resulting in the gradual development of severe interstitial pulmonary fibrosis. Alveolar capillaries become obliterated. With the eventual occurrence of pulmonary hypertension, the larger pulmonary arterial vessels exhibit intimal thickening and sclerosis. However, there is no evidence of true pulmonary vasculitis. Hemosiderin-impregnated nodules are scattered in the parenchyma, along the lymphatics, and in the draining hilar lymph nodes.

Physiologic abnormalities in IPH vary depending on the freshness of the hemorrhage, degree of fibrosis, and severity of vascular involvement. With the acute flooding of the lung with blood, the vital capacity, flow rates and arterial Po_2 may be diminished. As fibrosis ensues, a restrictive pattern of dysfunction emerges. Irreversible pulmonary hypertension and right ventricular failure are hallmarks of the end stage of the disease.

During acute hemorrhagic episodes the chest radiograph exhibits patchy or diffuse mottling as well as alveolus-filling shadows which may be a source of confusion with other diseases causing pulmonary consolidation. However, the shadows may clear rapidly in IPH, only to appear in the same or other locations with subsequent bouts of hemorrhage. Air bronchograms are frequently obtained. Where both lungs are diffusely involved, the pattern may resemble that of pulmonary edema. With repeated episodes a reticular interstitial pattern persists in the areas of prior hemorrhage. This parenchymal distribution gradually involves the majority of the lung fields and becomes indistinguishable from that found in other interstitial pulmonary diseases. The hilar lymph nodes may become enlarged. In the later stages right ventricular hypertrophy and enlarged pulmonary arteries are common.

IPH may begin with an explosive episode of hemoptysis, or it may be insidious at the onset. In some patients anemia, constitutional symptoms, cough and radiographic changes precede frank hemoptysis. During acute bleeding episodes, rales,

Idiopathic Pulmonary Hemosiderosis

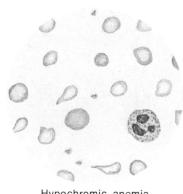

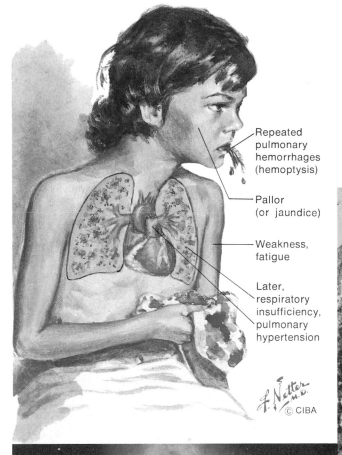

- Repeated pulmonary hemorrhages (hemoptysis)
- Pallor (or jaundice)
- Weakness, fatigue
- Later, respiratory insufficiency, pulmonary hypertension

Hypochromic anemia

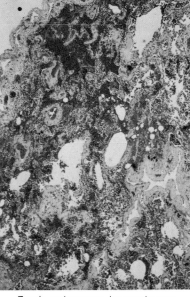

Fresh pulmonary hemorrhages

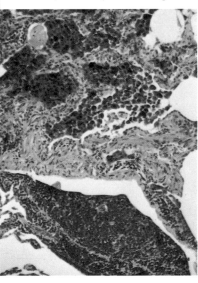

Fine reticular and mottled densities throughout both lungs. Diffuse fluffy shadows at both bases following acute hemorrhage

Intraalveolar macrophages full of hemosiderin plus septal fibrosis; lymphoid nodule at bottom

wheezes and rhonchi with dullness to percussion are noted over the involved lung areas. Later, dyspnea, tachypnea, hepatosplenomegaly and clubbing of the fingers may be observed.

Routine laboratory data are remarkable only in the presence of marked iron deficiency. In contrast to the situation in Goodpasture's syndrome, urinalysis and renal function studies are normal.

The diagnosis of IPH is strongly suggested by a history of recurrent episodes of hemoptysis, the demonstration of an iron deficiency anemia, and typical radiographic abnormalities in a child with normal renal function. Demonstration of sequestered blood in the pulmonary parenchyma by

radioactive isotope techniques and by the uptake and retention in the pulmonary parenchyma of an inhaled bolus of radiolabeled carbon dioxide ($^{15}CO_2$) is useful for making the diagnosis when these sophisticated techniques are available. Lung biopsy is the only unequivocal means of establishing the diagnosis, and may be accomplished by bronchoscopic percutaneous needle or open lung biopsy techniques. In patients who do not experience the typical episodes of hemoptysis, biopsy may be necessary for exact diagnosis.

The prognosis in IPH is poor. Death usually occurs within three years of diagnosis, although survivors have been reported for up to 20 years.

Pulmonary Alveolar Proteinosis

Pulmonary alveolar proteinosis (PAP) is an uncommon disease first described by Rosen, Castleman and Liebow in 1958. The hallmark of PAP is filling of alveoli with a grumous, white material which contains phospholipids, glycoproteins and cellular debris. This amorphous material stains with periodic acid–Schiff (PAS) reagent. The phospholipid is an important constituent of pulmonary surfactant which, like glycoproteins, is probably derived from type II alveolar cells. Thus, it has been proposed that the basic defect leading to PAP is increased destruction or decreased clearance of type II cells. There is little inflammatory reaction in the surrounding lung and almost a complete absence of alveolar macrophages.

PAP has recently been shown to represent a nonspecific pulmonary reaction to a number of different pulmonary insults. In addition to the generally reported idiopathic form, secondary PAP may develop in patients receiving alkylating agents and in those with fungal or *Pneumocystis carinii* infections, as well as in workers with silicosis.

Surprisingly, this alveolus-filling disease may cause little impairment of lung volumes. The vital capacity and FEV_1 have been slightly decreased in approximately one-half the reported patients. Similarly, lung mechanics are minimally impaired. The most marked abnormality is a reduced Pa_{O_2}, which may be profoundly lowered. Reduction in the diffusing capacity usually parallels the severity of the hypoxemia.

PAP represents a classic challenge to the radiologist—namely, the differentiation between an interstitial pulmonary disease and an alveolus-filling process. Both interstitial disease and PAP exhibit bilateral diffuse parenchymal densities. However, linear densities that are often punctuated by small radiolucencies (honeycombing) and are usually more prominent at the bases than in the upper lung zones indicate the presence of interstitial involvement. They stand in contrast to the "fluffy" rounded or rosette shadows and air bronchograms traversing areas of confluent consolidation seen in alveolus-filling diseases such as PAP. After the radiologist recognizes the presence of the densities, he still must choose among the similar roentgenographic patterns of several different conditions. These include pulmonary edema of cardiac and noncardiac origin, bacterial and mycoplasmal pneumonias, pulmonary hemorrhage, hypersensitivity pneumonitis, granulomatous lung disease and alveolar cell carcinoma.

There are no ancillary laboratory tests for PAP. Blood, urine and even sputum specimens fail to yield specific data, and the diagnosis can be unequivocally made only by lung biopsy.

While some patients are asymptomatic, with only an abnormal chest roentgenogram as the presenting complaint, most patients have a cough, which may produce unremarkable mucoid or whitish sputum. Dyspnea is frequent and may be disabling. Chest pain and hemoptysis are rare. In the more severely afflicted patients, constitutional symptoms of anorexia, weight loss and fatigue appear. Physical examination usually reveals a moderately to severely ill patient with a rapid respiratory

Alveolar Proteinosis

Alveoli and a small bronchus filled with eosinophilic fluid

Diffuse and nodular opacifications in both lungs

Large bottle of lavage fluid from lungs

Small bronchofiberscope can be used to identify correct positioning of Carlens tube and be advanced for sampling of alveolar fluid

Anesthesia and oxygen tube

Use of Carlens tube for lung lavage permits general anesthesia and ventilation to be supplied via opposite lung. Saline is instilled through tube by syringe or gravity flow

rate, cyanosis, rales over both lungs, tachycardia and occasionally clubbing.

There is a relatively high incidence of concomitant fungal infections. In such cases it is not clear whether PAP is a nonspecific pathologic reaction to the fungi or whether these organisms are opportunistic invaders. Biopsy tissue and secretions must be carefully examined and cultured for fungi, particularly *Nocardia* and *Cryptococcus*.

The course of PAP is variable. It is now apparent that many patients—perhaps the majority—may enjoy spontaneous remission. However, with persistence or worsening, treatment is required. Iodides and corticosteroid medications have failed

to clear the alveolar process consistently. To date, bronchial lavage with isotonic saline solution, alone or in combination with heparin and acetylcysteine, has been the most effective treatment. The procedure should be done under general anesthesia with the trachea intubated using a Carlens tube. Only one lung is washed out at each session while the contralateral lung receives oxygen as required. Often, a period of worsening is reflected in an aggravation of hypoxemia during and shortly after lavage. A few patients have improved after clearance of only one lung. Yet the efficacy of all lavage techniques is difficult to evaluate in a disease with such a high rate of natural remission.

Rheumatoid Arthritis

The exact incidence of pulmonary manifestations of the rheumatoid diathesis is unknown, but most authorities agree that there are three main intrathoracic complications of rheumatoid arthritis: (1) interstitial pulmonary infiltrations (rheumatoid lung), (2) pleuritis, with and without effusion, and (3) rheumatoid nodules.

Interstitial Pulmonary Infiltrations. Walker and Wright noted radiographic evidence of pulmonary fibrosis in approximately 1% of 516 patients with rheumatoid arthritis. Pulmonary function tests suggest the presence of interstitial involvement in a much larger number of patients with rheumatoid disease and normal chest radiographs. Frank has reported a restrictive type of dysfunction in 41% of these patients.

Rheumatoid arthritis is such a common disease that the appearance of nonspecific interstitial fibrosis may be coincidental. In approximately 25% of patients with idiopathic diffuse interstitial pulmonary fibrosis (cryptogenic fibrosing alveolitis), latex-fixing antibodies are present. Since some of these patients will manifest arthritis later in their course, several authors have suggested that the coincidental finding of pulmonary fibrosis and a positive latex fixation test is sufficient to establish the diagnosis of "rheumatoid lung," even in the absence of joint disease. However, both the pathologic and the serologic abnormalities are nonspecific, and the great majority of such patients never exhibit arthritis.

Roentgenographic manifestations of diffuse interstitial rheumatoid disease range from scattered nodules less than 5 mm in diameter to linear streaks densely infiltrating both lungs from base to apex. In its most chronic stage the lungs may assume a honeycombed pattern. This latter, far-advanced disease invariably leads to shrunken lungs which are reflected in physiologic studies showing small lung volumes, decreased pulmonary compliance ("stiff lungs"), and hypoxemia due to abnormalities in diffusion or in gas transfer. Patients with diffuse pulmonary fibrosis usually complain of cough and dyspnea. A shallow tachypnea and bilateral rales are observed. Subcutaneous rheumatoid nodules are frequent, and, rarely, clubbing of the digits is present.

Pleuritis. Pleuritis, with and without effusion, is the most common intrathoracic manifestation of rheumatoid arthritis. The effusion may precede, accompany or follow the onset of joint involvement. Despite the preponderance of females with this disease, rheumatoid pleural effusions are more prevalent in middle-aged males. The roentgenographic pattern does not differ from that of other pleural exudates except that the fluid tends to persist unchanged for months and even years. The effusion is usually unilateral, more common on the right than on the left, and often asymptomatic. The fluid is an exudate with high protein, elevated LDH (lactic dehydrogenase) and low complement levels, and mononuclear cells. As in the sera, an elevated latex fixation test in the pleural fluid is a nonspecific finding and is not diagnostic of rheumatoid arthritis. The occasional presence of "rheumatoid arthritis cells" or "ragocytes"

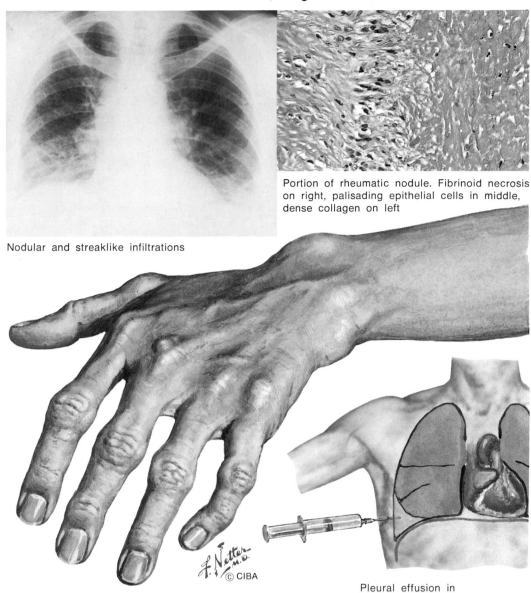

Nodular and streaklike infiltrations

Portion of rheumatic nodule. Fibrinoid necrosis on right, palisading epithelial cells in middle, dense collagen on left

Hand deformity in advanced rheumatoid arthritis

Pleural effusion in rheumatoid arthritis

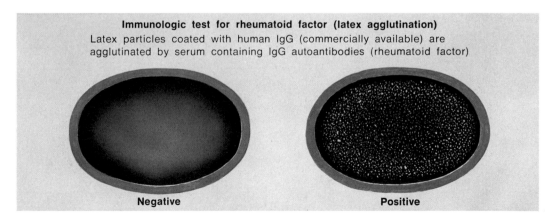

Immunologic test for rheumatoid factor (latex agglutination)
Latex particles coated with human IgG (commercially available) are agglutinated by serum containing IgG autoantibodies (rheumatoid factor)

Negative   **Positive**

(polymorphonuclear leukocytes with small black cytoplasmic inclusions) has been noted in the pleural exudate. Sometimes the fluid is pseudochylous—a milky effusion containing cholesterol but no true fat. In the presence of an effusion, pleural biopsy may reveal rheumatoid granulomas but usually shows only nonspecific inflammation. Fibrosing pleuritis may occur in the absence of free fluid. Rarely, this situation leads to a fibrothorax and a restrictive type of pulmonary dysfunction.

Rheumatoid Nodules. Well-circumscribed nodules, ranging in size from 0.5 to 5.0 cm and few in number, may be seen in the chest radiographs of

patients with chronic rheumatoid arthritis. On pathological examination they are identical to the nodules found in this disease in subcutaneous tissues and other viscera. Occasionally they cavitate, and spontaneous rupture leading to pneumothorax has been reported. Their size may wax and wane with the activity of the disease. Caplan has described a variant of this syndrome, occurring in coal miners with rheumatoid arthritis. Similar nodular shadows have been reported in workers exposed to talc, silica, asbestos, iron and brass who also have rheumatoid arthritis. Elevated serum rheumatoid factor and pulmonary nodules may precede joint symptoms.

Progressive Systemic Sclerosis (PSS; Scleroderma); Lung Involvement

Progressive Systemic Sclerosis (Diffuse Scleroderma)

Progressive systemic sclerosis (PSS) is a connective tissue disease that involves the skin (scleroderma), gastrointestinal tract, musculoskeletal system, kidneys, heart and lungs. Most patients are women in their middle years. Complaints include Raynaud's phenomenon; stiffness of the skin of the face, upper extremities and thorax; dysphagia; muscular pain and weakness; cough and dyspnea. Almost all patients manifest pulmonary involvement. Grossly, the lungs are scarred, with scattered small cystic areas present. With severe fibrosis the lungs are stiff and shrunken. Microscopic pulmonary changes, including those of arteritis, interstitial fibrosis and basilar bronchiolectasis, were found in all 28 patients studied at autopsy by Weaver.

As the name implies, PSS causes a sclerosis of involved organs. However, in most patients vasculitis, usually affecting arterioles and capillaries, precedes or coexists with fibrosis and is believed to be the initial pathologic lesion. As with other vascular or connective tissue diseases, this arteritis is probably due to an immunologic reaction of unknown causation. At autopsy and radiographically a nonspecific pleuritis may be evident, but, in contrast to rheumatoid arthritis and systemic lupus erythematosus, pleural effusion is unusual.

Wilson has reported physiologic dysfunction in as many as 90% of these patients. As with other pulmonary fibroses, a restrictive pattern of dysfunction predominates. Lung volumes are progressively diminished, flow rates remain normal and pulmonary compliance is reduced. Hypoxemia after exercise is the major arterial blood gas abnormality present, caused primarily by a reduced diffusing capacity for carbon monoxide. It has been reported that stiffness of the chest wall due to skin and muscle sclerosis may lead to alveolar hypoventilation, but this finding is exceedingly rare.

Up to 25% of patients will demonstrate radiographic reticular basilar infiltrations, progressive nodulations and/or linear streaks involving the major portions of both lungs. While most fibrotic and granulomatous lung diseases may show radiolucencies of varying size interspersed in fibrotic areas, PSS in particular demonstrates small (0.5 to 1.0 cm diameter) radiolucencies scattered throughout the *lower* lung fields. If the remainder of the lung fields are clear, this basilar infiltration and microcystic formation often suggest the diagnosis to the trained observer. Rarely, pneumothorax occurs when a cystic area ruptures. The sclerotic subcutaneous tissues of the thorax tend to become calcified, and these may be visible on the chest radiograph, as are the scattered calcifications throughout the pulmonary parenchyma.

The visceral organ most commonly affected is the esophagus. A sclerotic esophagus manifests

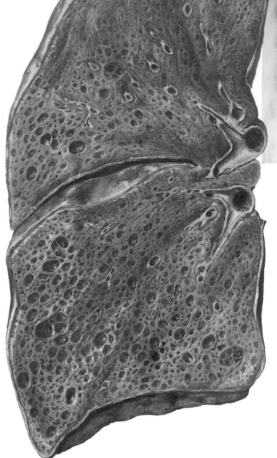

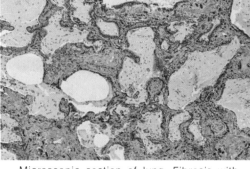

Reticular opacification in both lungs with small radiolucencies interspersed

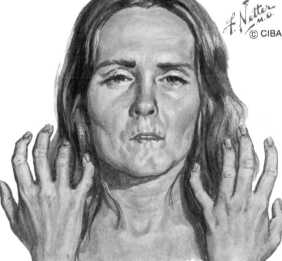

Microscopic section of lung. Fibrosis with formation of microcysts, many of which represent dilated bronchioles

Grossly-sectioned lung. Extensive fibrosis and multitudinous small cysts. Visceral pleura thickened but not adherent to chest wall

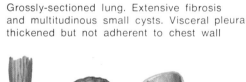

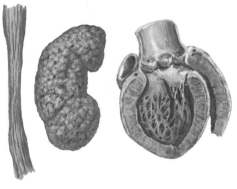

Esophagus, kidneys, heart, skin and other organs as well as joints may also be affected

Rigid, pinched facies and sclerodactyly

abnormal motility, leading to puddling of secretions, with resulting esophagitis and frequent regurgitation. Aspiration pneumonia is a common pulmonary complication in PSS patients with esophagitis independent of the degree of primary involvement of the lung.

Patients afflicted with pulmonary complications of PSS complain of shortness of breath—particularly with exercise—and a dry nonproductive cough. They may be cyanotic, but clubbing is not seen, perhaps because the terminal digits are often involved. The respiratory rate is rapid with a shallow tidal volume. Bilateral basilar rales reflect a tendency toward localization of bronchiolectasis in

the lower portions of the lung. However, such rales are often heard over all lobes.

There is no effective treatment. At some time in their course most patients are given corticosteroid medications. Recently, cyclophosphamide and azathioprine have been employed; neither has proved successful in the majority of patients. As the disease progresses, symptoms and signs of chronic pulmonary hypertension and cor pulmonale ensue. A salt-poor diet and diuretics offer some temporary relief of heart failure, but digitalis may be of little help if the myocardium is involved. Cardiorespiratory failure is second to renal failure as a leading cause of death in PSS.

Systemic Lupus Erythematosus

Systemic lupus erythematosus (SLE) is an immunologic disease characterized by multiple serologic alterations, including the lupus erythematosus (LE) cell, the presence of antinuclear and anticytoplasmic antibodies, and the hematoxylin-eosin body found scattered in the tissues of most organs. Serologic tests for syphilis often yield false positive results. Abnormal urinalysis, leukopenia, thrombocytopenia and anemia are common.

Fibrinoid necrosis in blood vessels, collagen and serosal surfaces leads to "onionskin" lesions in the spleen and "wire-loop" degeneration of kidney glomeruli. Renal involvement occurs in the majority of patients. Synovitis, serositis and skin and central nervous system lesions are also common. A minority of patients manifest endocarditis. Patients may present with fever, "butterfly" rash, arthritis, pleuritis, seizures and/or renal failure.

SLE occurs most frequently among women in the childbearing years. Although the course may be fulminant, it is usually marked by exacerbations and remissions, which may be stimulated by exposure to sunlight, drugs, infection or emotional disturbances.

Pleural and pulmonary complications are more frequent with SLE than in the other connective tissue disorders. At postmortem examination almost all patients manifest pleuritis with or without effusion, and clinically this may herald the onset of the disease and may continue as a marker of activity. Since pain usually accompanies lupus pleuritis, it is a particularly sensitive indicator of relapse. One may confuse the fever, chest pain and radiographic evidence of pleural disease with signs of idiopathic or viral pleurisy, recurrent pulmonary emboli or metastatic carcinoma. Pleural involvement, along with arthritis, appears to be an especially frequent manifestation of the lupus syndrome caused by reaction to medications—*e.g.,* procainamide and isoniazid. The fluid is a proteinaceous exudate with many polymorphonuclear cells and occasionally LE cells.

The altered immunologic status, often compounded by treatment with corticosteroid or immunosuppressive medications, leads to infections in patients with SLE more often than in those with other connective tissue diseases. Thus, pneumonia is the most common pulmonary abnormality. Bacterial, fungal, *Pneumocystis carinii* and tuberculous infections may develop. Acute pneumonic infiltrations sometimes occur in a febrile patient and are due to lupus "vasculitis" rather than infection. Such lesions may be demonstrated at autopsy. They may be clinically inferred by rapid clearing of the pulmonary densities with corticosteroid therapy, after failure to culture a bacterial pathogen or to attain improvement with antibiotic treatment.

Chronic diffuse interstitial pneumonitis is a rare clinical manifestation of pulmonary involvement in SLE. The interstitial inflammation and fibrosis differ from those seen in other connective tissue disorders: they are less apparent radiographically and clinically.

Pleuritic pain is the major symptom of intrathoracic involvement in SLE. Dyspnea and fever usually accompany both pleural and pulmonary involvement. In acute lupus pneumonitis or

Systemic Lupus Erythematosus (SLE); Lung Involvement

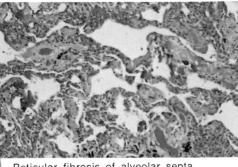

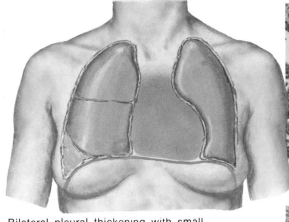

Bilateral pleural thickening with small effusion on right. Globular cardiac silhouette suggests pericardial or cardiac involvement

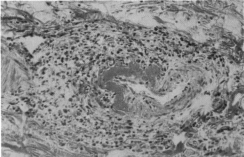

Reticular fibrosis of alveolar septa in SLE. Scattered anthracotic and iron deposits also present

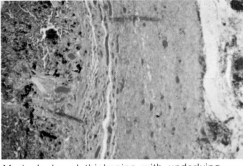

Marked pleural thickening with underlying pulmonary fibrosis

Arteritis involving small artery, showing segmental fibrinoid necrosis with layered concentric zone of inflammation

Pathogenesis of lupus (LE) cells and rosettes

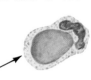

Polymorpho-nuclear leukocyte

Nucleus homogenized by LE factor (antinuclear antibody)

Homogenized nucleus extruded to form free nuclear (LE) body

Nuclear (LE) body phagocytized by granulocyte to form typical LE cell

Nuclear body encircled by granulocytes to form LE rosette

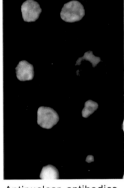

Antinuclear antibodies demonstrated by fluorescence

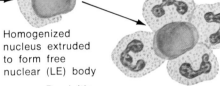

Normal serum
DNA
Precipitin line
Lupus serum

DNA antibodies demonstrated by precipitin test on agar plate

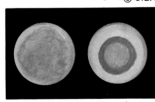

Positive   Negative

Hemagglutination of gamma globulin-coated red cells by SLE serum (tubes viewed from below). Latex agglutination test may also be done as for rheumatoid factor

interstitial inflammation and fibrosis, cyanosis reflects hypoxemia. Rales may be heard, but finger clubbing is not seen. With lupus pericarditis and endocarditis, cardiomegaly and pulmonary congestion may complicate the course. More often, however, pulmonary edema occurs secondary to renal failure in patients with chronic lupus nephritis. The classic butterfly rash, hepatosplenomegaly and arthritis are other common abnormalities detected on physical examination.

Despite the high frequency of pleural and pulmonary involvement, a chest radiograph often fails to reveal any abnormality. Effusions are seen in little more than one-half of the patients with

pleural disease and are usually small and bilateral, but occasionally become large. Bilateral pleural thickening without free fluid is common and persists throughout the patient's course. The cardiac silhouette may be globular or markedly widened when pericarditis is present. The typical pattern of pulmonary edema generally indicates renal or heart failure.

Both pleural and pulmonary manifestations of SLE may respond dramatically to corticosteroids. Recent reports of response to cyclophosphamide and azathioprine are encouraging. Unfortunately, with withdrawal or reduction in the dosage of medication, relapse is likely.

Dermatomyositis and Polymyositis

Dermatomyositis and polymyositis are diverse connective tissue disorders comprising (1) polymyositis without skin involvement or evidence of connective tissue disease, (2) polymyositis with mild skin and connective tissue changes, (3) polymyositis with florid dermatitis and connective tissue disease ("overlap" with systemic lupus erythematosus, progressive systemic sclerosis and/or rheumatoid arthritis), and (4) polymyositis and coexistent malignancy. The paramount finding is myositis manifested by weakness and often tenderness of the proximal muscles, usually those of the shoulder and pelvic girdles.

The etiology of dermatomyositis remains unknown, although the evidence suggests that it is a hypersensitivity disease occurring in an immunologically incompetent host in whom hyperreaction of cell-mediated immunity has been provoked.

In most cases onset is insidious, with the patient noting difficulty in performing routine acts such as climbing stairs or rising from bed or from an armless chair. In a minority of individuals the disease is relatively acute, causing disabling muscle pain and weakness, dysphagia and/or respiratory insufficiency in a few weeks. Symptoms often wax and wane without therapy, but the untreated course is usually progressive. When the disease is far advanced, the patient may be unable to hold his hands above his head to comb his hair or to lift his head from a pillow when reclining in bed. He may have a nasal voice, experience dysarthria and dysphagia, walk with a distinctive "waddle," fall frequently, and be unable to rise without assistance. Muscle atrophy ensues, and the patient may be confined to bed or a chair.

Dermatologic abnormalities occur in approximately one-third of patients. A unique periorbital, scaly, erythematous rash may be present. Hyperemia of the nail beds is also common, as are joint manifestations.

A final frequent visceral manifestation of this group of disorders also seen in dermatomyositis is diffuse interstitial pneumonitis. In all, the pulmonary manifestations of dermatomyositis may be broadly divided into three types: (1) aspiration pneumonia, (2) diffuse interstitial pneumonitis and (3) alveolar hypoventilation.

Aspiration pneumonia is directly related to weakness of the pharyngeal muscles and loss of the normal esophageal contraction waves leading to esophageal hypomotility. Patients usually present with consolidation and atelectasis of the basilar segments of the lower lobes, middle lobe and lingula. The involved areas may become necrotic, with abscess formation. Diffuse interstitial pneumonia is a rare manifestation occurring in less than 10% of patients with dermatomyositis. Pathologically, the alveolar septa are thickened and the interstitium is infiltrated with varying degrees of chronic inflammatory cells and fibroblasts. The pulmonary changes are the same as those described in rheumatoid arthritis, PSS, SLE, pulmonary reaction to drugs, and idiopathic pulmonary fibrosis (Hamman-Rich syndrome), all falling under the label of "usual interstitial pneumonia" (UIP) of Liebow and Carrington. As in other interstitial

Dermatomyositis and Polymyositis; Lung Involvement

Periorbital heliotrope discoloration and edema

Difficulty in swallowing due to pharyngeal muscle weakness may lead to aspiration pneumonia

Weakness of diaphragm and intercostal muscles causes respiratory insufficiency or failure

Weakness of central muscle groups evidenced by difficulty in climbing stairs, rising from chairs, combing hair, etc.

Erythematous or violaceous, scaly papules on dorsum of interphalangeal joints

Widely dispersed nodular and linear infiltrations. Abscess formation in areas of aspiration pneumonia

Longitudinal section of muscle showing intense inflammatory infiltration plus degeneration and disruption of muscle fibers

lung diseases, the lung volumes, diffusing capacity and pulmonary compliance are reduced. Hypoxemia is present, but flow rates, pulmonary airway resistance and maximum voluntary ventilation are well maintained. Rarely, a patient with dermatomyositis may have such severe weakness of the intercostal muscles and diaphragm that he suffers from "bellows failure." His inability to maintain a tidal volume adequate for alveolar ventilation leads to hypoxemia and eventually to hypercapnia. Although flow rates are normal when related to the reduced vital capacity, studies of the mechanics of breathing are abnormal.

Clinically, dermatomyositis may be differentiated from other proximal myopathies, myasthenia gravis and the myasthenia syndrome of malignancy. The diagnosis of dermatomyositis or polymyositis is established by muscle biopsy. However, serologic and electromyographic tests may aid in diagnosis and in assessing response to therapy.

Adrenocorticosteroid medications remain the standard treatment. The prognosis varies with the severity of the disease and the presence of associated malignancy. In patients without carcinoma, approximately 50% will benefit from therapy, and prolonged remission is common.

Polyarteritis Nodosa, Wegener's Granulomatosis and Allergic Granulomatosis

The pulmonary vasculitides include a number of multiple diseases of known and unknown origin that, for the present, defy classification. In view of this, the ensuing discussion will deal with conditions that have been accepted as recognizable entities because of more or less distinct clinical and pathologic presentations and characteristic responses to therapy.

Polyarteritis nodosa is characterized by necrotizing inflammation of medium-sized and small arteries. Patients usually present with multisystem involvement—kidneys, skin, muscles, central nervous system, gastrointestinal tract and pancreas. It is difficult to assess the prevalence of clinical pulmonary disease in polyarteritis nodosa. When present, the pulmonary manifestations vary from Löfflerlike pneumonia through diffuse interstitial reticulonodular infiltrations to larger patchy shadows probably representing areas of local infarction. Myocardial, pericardial and pleural involvement may be apparent on the chest x-ray film as cardiomegaly, pulmonary edema and pleural effusions.

Contrary to the relative paucity of clinical pulmonary manifestations in classic polyarteritis nodosa, lung involvement is frequently found in the two related conditions: Wegener's granulomatosis and allergic granulomatosis. By the criteria of Godman and Churg, *Wegener's granulomatosis* is characterized by necrotizing granulomatous lesions in the upper and lower respiratory tracts, widespread angiitis in arteries and veins, and focal necrotizing glomerulitis which often terminates in renal failure. The disease probably represents a hypersensitivity reaction that leads to necrosis and inflammation. In the "limited" form, the involvement is confined to the lungs.

Pulmonary manifestations of Wegener's granulomatosis are varied. Patients may complain of cough, hemoptysis, dyspnea, wheezing and pleuritic chest pain. However, an abnormal chest x-ray film may be the only clinical presentation of intrathoracic disease.

The most striking radiographic manifestation of Wegener's granulomatosis in the lungs is the appearance of parenchymal masses, 2 to 10 cm in size, which often show irregular cavitation. The lesions are often multiple and are easily mistaken for primary or metastatic carcinoma. Destruction of major bronchi may lead to atelectasis, further complicating the differentiation from carcinoma. Pleural effusions, diffuse linear or nodular densities, areas of consolidation, and infarction also may be seen.

There is no distinctive pattern of pulmonary dysfunction in Wegener's granulomatosis. When diffuse interstitial lesions predominate, a restrictive pattern of functional abnormality is present.

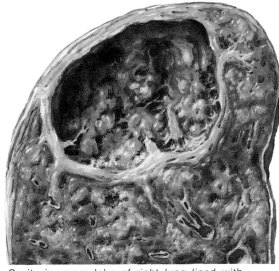

Cavity in upper lobe of right lung lined with necrotic material in Wegener's granulomatosis

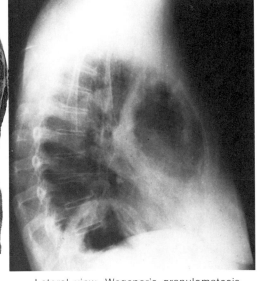

Lateral view. Wegener's granulomatosis of lungs with cavitation

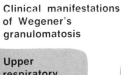

Wegener's granuloma with giant cells

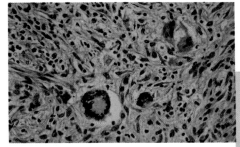

Severe arteritis with destruction of vessel wall in Wegener's granulomatosis

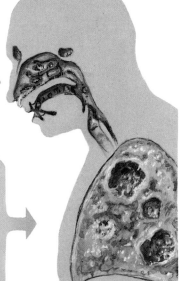

Clinical manifestations of Wegener's granulomatosis

Upper respiratory involvement
Ulcerative lesions of nose, sinuses, mouth, pharynx

Lower respiratory involvement
Necrotic areas and cavitation in lungs, cough, dyspnea, hemoptysis, chest pain

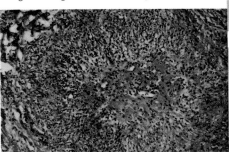

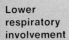

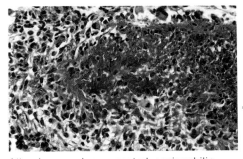

Allergic granuloma: central eosinophilic necrosis with palisading of epithelioid cells

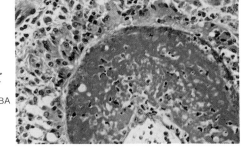

Allergic angiitis: fibrinoid necrosis of arterial wall with epithelioid reaction

With endobronchial involvement, airflow obstruction is seen.

Allergic granulomatosis differs from Wegener's granulomatosis in that it invariably begins with asthma and striking peripheral eosinophilia. Angiitis should be suspected in adult-onset asthma that is refractory to the usual therapies. Chest x-ray examination discloses a multiplicity of abnormalities, such as changing amorphous densities, areas of consolidation and reticular nodular infiltrations. In milder form these are similar to signs of Löffler's eosinophilic pneumonia. Rarely, pleural and pericardial effusions are detected by chest radiography. Renal failure is less common

than in Wegener's granulomatosis, but multisystem evidence of polyarteritis may be equally severe. As with all forms of polyarteritis, the diagnosis can be established by skin and muscle biopsy in approximately 50% of patients.

The prognosis for polyarteritis is generally poor, although some patients improve with steroid and/or immunosuppressive therapy. Spontaneous remissions have been reported. Corticosteroids have been effective in allergic granulomatosis but are less so in Wegener's granulomatosis. Remarkable remissions in Wegener's granulomatosis have been reported with cyclophosphamide.

Section V

Diagnostic and Therapeutic Procedures

Frank H. Netter, M.D.

in collaboration with

Murray D. Altose, M.D.   *Plates 1-2*

Hyun Taik Cho, M.D.   *Plates 13-16*

Albert Haas, M.D.   *Plates 19-21*

Jose F. Landa, M.D.   *Plates 8, 11*

Edward D. Michaelson, M.D.   *Plates 10, 23-26*

W. Spencer Payne, M.D.   *Plates 27-28*

Marvin A. Sackner, M.D.   *Plates 3-4, 12, 22*

William I. Wolff, M.D.   *Plates 7, 9, 17-18, 29-33*

Milton H. Uhley, M.D.   *Plates 5-6*

Tests of Pulmonary Function

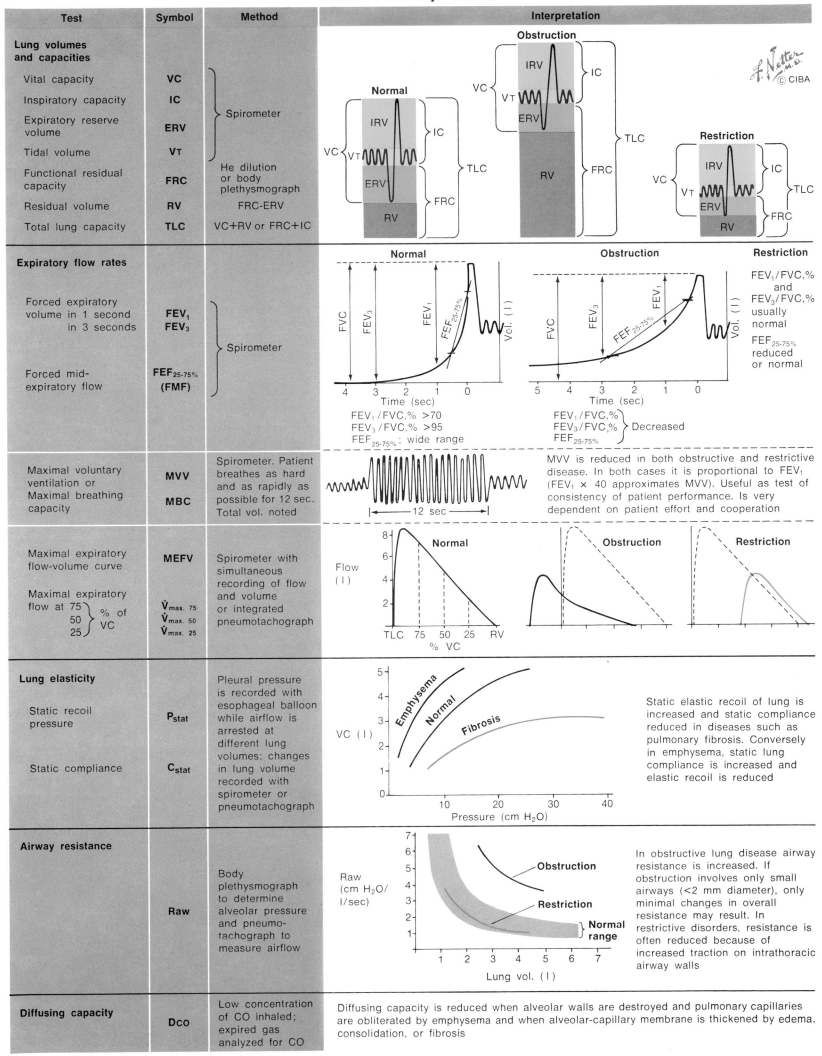

Test	Symbol	Method	Interpretation
Tests for small airway disease Closing volume Closing capacity	**CV** **CC**	Following a full inspiration of O_2, the expired lung volume from TLC to RV is plotted against the N_2 concentration	Airways in lower lung zones close at low lung volumes and only those alveoli at top of lungs continue to empty. Since concentration of N_2 in alveoli of upper zones is higher, slope of curve abruptly increases (phase IV). Phase IV begins at larger lung volumes in individuals with even minor degrees of airway obstruction increasing both CV and CC
Maximal expiratory flow-volume curve breathing 80% He and 20% O_2	$\Delta \dot{V}_{max.\ 50}$ **V iso $\dot{V}$**	Spirometer or pneumotachograph to record flow and volume	During a maximal expiratory maneuver, resistance to airflow is normally due to turbulence and convective acceleration. Breathing He, which is less dense than air, lowers resistance and increases flow at all but lowest volumes. In small airway disease, resistance to laminar flow makes up larger portion of total resistance and airflow is relatively independent of gas density. Increase in expiratory flow at 50% of VC while breathing $He-O_2$ ($\Delta \dot{V}_{max.\ 50}$) will be less, and volume at which flows while breathing $He-O_2$ and while breathing air are identical (V iso $\dot{V}$) will be higher in patients with small airway disease than in normal individuals
Frequency dependence of dynamic compliance	C_{dyn}	Esophageal balloon to measure pleural pressure and spirometer or pneumotachograph to record volume	Dynamic compliance is determined from changes in lung volume and difference in pleural pressure at end-inspiration and end-expiration. Normally C_{dyn} closely approximates C_{stat} and remains essentially unchanged as breathing frequency increases Small airway disease is characterized by patchy increases in airway resistance. During quiet breathing, ventilation may be evenly distributed throughout lung but as breathing frequency increases, alveoli will fill and empty unevenly and asynchronously as air tends to go to those areas which offer least resistance. Change in pleural pressure for a given change in lung volume increases and dynamic compliance falls

Test	Symbol	Method	Normal values	Abnormalities
Gas exchange Partial pressure of O_2 in arterial blood	Pa_{O_2}		60 to 100 mm Hg breathing room air at sea level. Falls slightly with age	Hypoxemia indicative of ventilation-perfusion abnormalities, shunts, diffusion defect, alveolar hypoventilation
Partial pressure of CO_2 in arterial blood	Pa_{CO_2}	Arterial blood is collected anaerobically in heparinized syringe	36 to 44 mm Hg	Pa_{CO_2} proportional to metabolic rate (CO_2 production) and inversely related to volume of alveolar ventilation

Arterial blood pH	**pH**		7.35 to 7.45 pH	Acidosis (pH < 7.35)
				  Respiratory (inadequate alveolar ventilation)
				  Metabolic (gain of acid and/or loss of base)
				Alkalosis (pH > 7.45)
				  Respiratory (excessive alveolar ventilation)
				  Metabolic (gain of base or loss of acid)

Alveolar-arterial O_2 difference	**A-aDO_2** **A-aPO_2**		<10 mm Hg breathing room air	Primarily reflects mismatching of ventilation and perfusion and/or shunts. May also be affected by diffusion defects
Dead space-tidal volume ratio	V_D/V_T	Determined from arterial and mixed expired P_{CO_2}	<0.3	Elevated ratio indicates wasted ventilation; i.e., that volume of gas which does not take part in gas exchange
Shunt fraction	$\dot{Q}_S/\dot{Q}_T$	Determined from Pa_{O_2} after a period of breathing 100% O_2	<5%	Elevation indicates increased amount of mixed venous blood entering systemic circulation without coming into contact with alveolar air, either because of shunting of blood past lungs to left side of heart or perfusion of regions of lung which are not ventilated

F. Netter
© CIBA

Psychotherapy

Patient reassurance and encouragement of slow, relaxed breathing often beneficial in milder degrees of bronchospasm

Psychotherapy and Administration of Bronchodilator Therapy

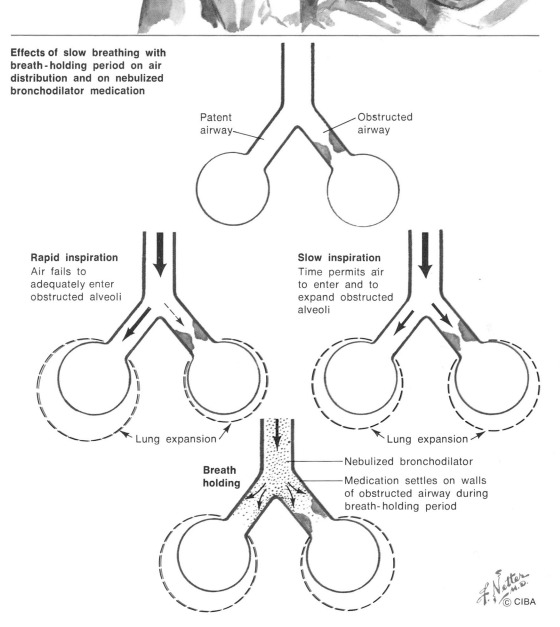

Effects of slow breathing with breath-holding period on air distribution and on nebulized bronchodilator medication

Patent airway — Obstructed airway

Rapid inspiration
Air fails to adequately enter obstructed alveoli

Slow inspiration
Time permits air to enter and to expand obstructed alveoli

←Lung expansion→

Breath holding

←Lung expansion→

Nebulized bronchodilator

Medication settles on walls of obstructed airway during breath-holding period

Psychotherapy

Minor degrees of bronchospasm often respond to psychotherapy. This may take the form of self-reassurance or of support from physicians and paramedical personnel. In a patient who is breathing rapidly during an acute episode of bronchospasm, the conscious voluntary change by the patient to a diaphragmatic breathing pattern often slows the frequency of respiration and promotes more even distribution of ventilation, not because of diaphragmatic breathing *per se* but because of the slowing of inspiratory flow. As the sensation of breathlessness subsides, the bronchospasm often disappears. The attending physician and paramedical personnel can also prevent the patient from panicking into the vicious circle of bronchospasm, feeling of suffocation, rapid breathing to "get more air," followed by further bronchospasm and dyspnea. There should be verbal encouragement to change breathing pattern from a rapid to a slow frequency—with a prolonged inspiratory phase—by coaxing, cajoling or ordering, using a tone of voice tailored to the patient's personality. It is important for the physician or paramedical attendant to "lay on the hands" while providing this verbal support. The frightened patient should be assured that he or she is not in a life-threatening situation and that the prompt treatment being given will relieve the breathlessness.

Bronchodilator Administration

The three modes of bronchodilator therapy depicted (Plate 4)—hand nebulizer, metered aerosol and intermittent positive pressure breathing—have the same basic physiologic principle for delivering bronchodilator agents. The agent is inhaled during a slow inspiratory maneuver in order to promote even distribution of ventilation and deposit the drug on the mucosa of obstructed airways. If the inspiration is performed with a rapid flow rate, lung units with high resistance will not be exposed to the drug. In hand nebulizer and metered aerosol systems, inhalation is voluntary,

whereas with intermittent positive pressure breathing, the ventilator mechanically forces the patient to inhale. Many investigators have shown that the degree of short-term bronchodilation achieved is similar with either hand-controlled systems or mechanical ventilators.

Hand-held delivery systems are widely used for the administration of inhalant bronchodilator therapy because they are cheaper and more convenient than, and as efficient as, intermittent positive pressure breathing. A metered aerosol dose of a bronchodilating agent is generated in a propellant by squeezing the container and the

(Continued)

Inhalant Bronchodilator Therapy

**Psychotherapy and
Administration of
Bronchodilator Therapy**
(Continued)

A. Hand nebulizer

Bulb squeezed
synchronously with
deep inhalation and
breath held briefly
to permit settling
of medication mist
on mucosa

B. Metered aerosol

**C. Intermittent positive
pressure breathing (IPPB)**

Nebulizer for
bronchodilator
medication

May be used with mask
or mouth tube as shown

nebulizer jet tube between the index finger and thumb. It is easier for an elderly patient with obstructive airway disease who lacks the manual dexterity to use a metered aerosol than to repeatedly squeeze and release the rubber bulb of a hand nebulizer while inhaling the medication. Perhaps only 70% of patients over 64 years of age can use a hand delivery unit properly; the other 30% may have to use an apparatus that delivers aerosol throughout a machine-generated slow inspiratory maneuver. Alternatively, the nebulizer may be driven by a compressed air pump while the medication is inhaled during tidal breathing. The administration of a drug by either intermittent positive pressure breathing or a powered nebulizer takes 10 to 15 minutes, whereas hand-held systems effect bronchodilation after a single inspiration.

Administration of medication by hand-held systems must be taught to the patient by a trained individual; it is not sufficient to prescribe a metered aerosol device and expect the patient to use it properly by reading the package insert. The patient should first exhale comfortably toward the residual volume position. The nozzle of the aerosol container is then placed loosely in the patient's mouth and squeezed two or three times while the patient inhales slowly toward total lung capacity. This action promotes a more even distribution of

inspired air, and the droplets are directed into both nonobstructed and obstructed airways. The breath is then held for about five seconds, allowing time for the droplets to settle on the mucosa. Then the patient exhales comfortably and resumes tidal breathing.

A variety of bronchodilator agents (isoproterenol, metaproterenol, isoetharine, epinephrine) is available in metered aerosol form and can be used safely as often as every three to six hours if required. Recent evidence indicates a wide margin of safety in the dosage forms currently being marketed in these units, as indicated by a lack of cardiovascular side effects—*e.g.,* tachycardia and increased cardiac

output—when these drugs are taken as recommended. In contrast, subcutaneous or oral administration of these drugs frequently causes cardiac irritability. Delivery of aerosolized bronchodilators by intermittent positive pressure breathing or powered nebulizer units is also done every three to six hours. The optimal volume put out by the first of these units has never been scientifically investigated. This may not be critically important, since the 15 minute period of breathing ensures that the drug reaches most airways, whether or not they are obstructed. In this respect both systems produce similar degrees of bronchodilation.

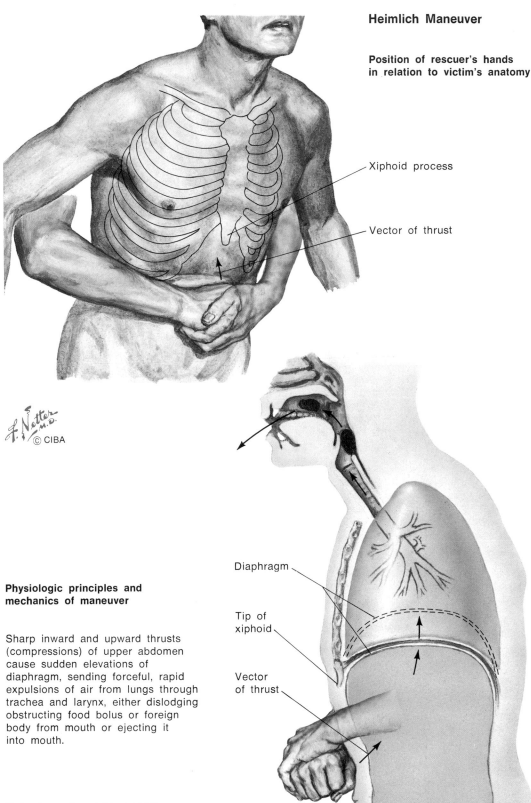

Heimlich Maneuver

Position of rescuer's hands in relation to victim's anatomy

Xiphoid process

Vector of thrust

f. Netter M.D.
© CIBA

Upper Airway Obstruction

Physiologic principles and mechanics of maneuver

Sharp inward and upward thrusts (compressions) of upper abdomen cause sudden elevations of diaphragm, sending forceful, rapid expulsions of air from lungs through trachea and larynx, either dislodging obstructing food bolus or foreign body from mouth or ejecting it into mouth.

Diaphragm

Tip of xiphoid

Vector of thrust

Navel

Note: lungs invariably contain appreciable amount of air consisting of both expiratory reserve volume and a portion of normal tidal volume

"How many persons have perished, perhaps in an instant, and in the midst of a hearty laugh, the recital of an amusing anecdote, or the utterance of a funny joke, from the interception at the glottis of a piece of meat, a crumb of bread, a morsel of cheese, or a bit of potato, without suspicion on the part of those around of the real nature of the case! Many a coroner's inquest has been held on the bodies of the victims of such accidents, and the verdict rendered that they died by the visitation of God, when the actual cause of death lay quietly and unobserved at the door of the windpipe of the deceased."

Although Gross wrote this comment in 1854, over a hundred years passed before Haugen, in 1963, used the term "café coronary" to describe sudden death—usually occurring in a restaurant—from food asphyxiation. Haugen and others advised that airway obstruction should immediately be suspected whenever an individual suddenly loses consciousness while dining and that, if death follows, one should question a diagnosis of "coronary" or "natural causes."

In 1974, after 20 years of development, a procedure for cardiopulmonary resuscitation (CPR) was described and widely adopted. The CPR procedure included the following steps as essential for basic life support: establishing and maintaining (1) an Airway, (2) Breathing, and (3) Circulation—the ABC's of CPR.

That same year, Heimlich first reported the results of animal studies on a new technique he proposed to relieve a completely obstructed airway. Over the next two years, Heimlich received reports of clinical experiences with the technique documenting approximately 500 instances of successful resuscitative efforts—including 11 cases of self-resuscitation. His technique is now known as the Heimlich maneuver.

Heimlich's work redirected attention to this important problem of food choking and foreign-body airway obstruction. His further contributions included (1) detailing the signs of choking for early recognition; (2) encouraging the use of a universal sign for food choking, the Heimlich "choke" sign, for which the victim brings his hand to his throat with the thumb and index

(Continued)

Upper Airway Obstruction
(Continued)

finger forming a V; (3) recommending immediate instead of delayed action; (4) demonstrating the specific manual maneuvers which could be life-saving; and (5) providing wide dissemination of explicit instructions for these simple maneuvers.

Heimlich Maneuver

The Heimlich maneuver is a technique whereby subdiaphragmatic compression, or abdominal "thrust," creates an expulsive force from the lungs to or through the upper airways. The consequent velocity of airflow is often sufficient to forcefully eject an obstructing object from the airway—to make it "pop" out.

Physiologic Principles and Mechanics. The anatomic basis for the Heimlich maneuver was established by observing that when a patient is in the lateral position during thoracotomy, pressure applied by the surgeon's fist upward into the abdomen below the rib cage causes the diaphragm to rise several inches into the pleural cavity. After studying airflow rates and pressures in conscious, healthy, adult volunteers, Heimlich concluded that the maneuver produced an average airflow of 205 liters/minute and pressure of 31 mm Hg, expelling an average of 945 ml of air in approximately 0.25 second. The projectile force thus generated propels any obstruction from the airway. It has been noted that, from an engineering standpoint, one could devise a mathematical formula to convert potential to kinetic energy. The momentum thereby generated is transmittable against a foreign body in the upper airway.

Recognizing the Obstructed Airway. The victim who has an obstructed airway cannot breathe, cough or speak. He may instinctively put his hand to his throat to indicate he is choking. He may stand immobilized in silent panic or, if embarrassed or shy, may try to walk away unobtrusively. If the victim is seated, he may try to stand but may not be able to do so. Within moments, all victims become ashen and progressively more cyanotic, lose consciousness and collapse over the table or onto the floor, at which time they are seconds away from dying.

Immediate action must be initiated upon *recognition of the obstructed airway crisis, or death will invariably ensue within four minutes.*

Specific Maneuvers

Adult Victim Standing. To perform the Heimlich maneuver on an adult who is standing, the rescuer stands directly behind the victim.

1. The rescuer puts one arm around the victim's waist and makes a closed fist, positioning the thumb side of his fist just above the victim's navel and *well below the tip of the xiphoid process.*

2. The rescuer encircles the victim's waist with his free arm and clasps his closed fist.

3. The rescuer gives a single, sharp, quick inward and upward compression or "thrust"; sometimes a series of two or more thrusts may be necessary.

The compressions almost invariably cause the food bolus or foreign body to be ejected completely, or to "pop" out, or else propel the object into the mouth where it is easily reached. A cleared airway is indicated by resumption of breathing, return of normal color, and restoration of consciousness.

The bolus of food or foreign body must be found and removed. If it is not, it may lodge in the oropharynx with danger of reaspiration.

Adult Victim Supine. A victim who collapses to the floor should immediately be turned to the supine position.

1. The rescuer kneels astride the victim so that his (the rescuer's) shoulders are over the victim's abdomen. The rescuer may straddle one or both thighs, depending on the victim's size.

2. The rescuer places the heel of one hand directly above the victim's navel—but well below the tip of the xiphoid—and the other hand on the dorsum of the first hand, both being in the midline.

3. The rescuer gives a single, sharp inward and upward thrust directed diagonally toward the victim's diaphragm; two or more thrusts may be required.

4. If regurgitation occurs, the victim should be turned completely to one side so that the vomitus may be wiped out of the mouth.

It is important that the rescuer's hands be in the midline position and not be shifted to one side or the other. In this way risk of injury to the victim's liver, spleen or visceral contents is minimized or avoided.

Adult Victim, Self-Save Technique. The instant an individual recognizes that his airway may be obstructed, he should do the following:

1. Make a fist and press it thumb side to the abdomen just above the navel and well below the xiphoid.

2. Grasp the fist with the other hand and make sharp, forceful, quick thrusts upward and inward toward the diaphragm.

If this is unsuccessful, the victim should immediately:

1. Position the body (at the level of the navel) across a structure with an edge such as a chair back, railing, table or sink, or any horizontal object that can sustain the body weight.

2. Lower the body sharply against the structure and repeat for two or more thrusts.

In effect, this action duplicates a rescuer's effort whereby subdiaphragmatic compression or thrust creates an expulsive force from the lungs toward the oropharynx.

Small Child or Infant Victim. The Heimlich maneuver for a small child or infant is essentially the same as for a supine adult.

1. The victim should be placed in a supine position if not already there.

2. The rescuer's extended index and middle fingers of one hand (or both, depending on the victim's size) are held closely together and positioned in the victim's midline, just above the navel. Abdominal thrust is applied, the thrust vector directed toward the diaphragm, with a "reasonable" amount of force. The maneuver may be repeated two or more times if necessary.

3. In case of regurgitation, the victim is turned to one side so that the vomitus may be cleared from the oropharynx.

As an alternative, children and infants may be held upright in the rescuer's lap, and the abdominal thrusts applied from behind (as with the standing adult victim) using the fingers. Criteria for success are the same as for adult resuscitation.

If a child or infant shows no response and death seems imminent, the victim may be draped over the rescuer's arm, knee or thigh and sharp but gentle blows struck against the spine. The rescuer must exercise judgment as to the force exerted. The back blow will impart a jarring force which will momentarily compress the subdiaphragmatic structures and create an abdominal thrust or vector force sufficient to eject the foreign body.

Only imminent death justifies using this technique. Otolaryngologists, surgeons and endoscopists have consistently cautioned about the possibility of converting a partial airway obstruction to a complete obstruction and consequent death. The danger of such an untoward event arises (1) when an infant or small child is held up by the heels and thumped or slapped on the back; (2) when finger probing is used, as it may result in laceration of an infant's tiny hypopharynx or impaction of a foreign body more deeply into the pharynx or tracheoesophageal tract; (3) when, as a result of inversion and percussion to the spine, a foreign body in the tracheobronchial tree is dislodged and becomes impacted in an upper bronchus or against the undersurface of the larynx.

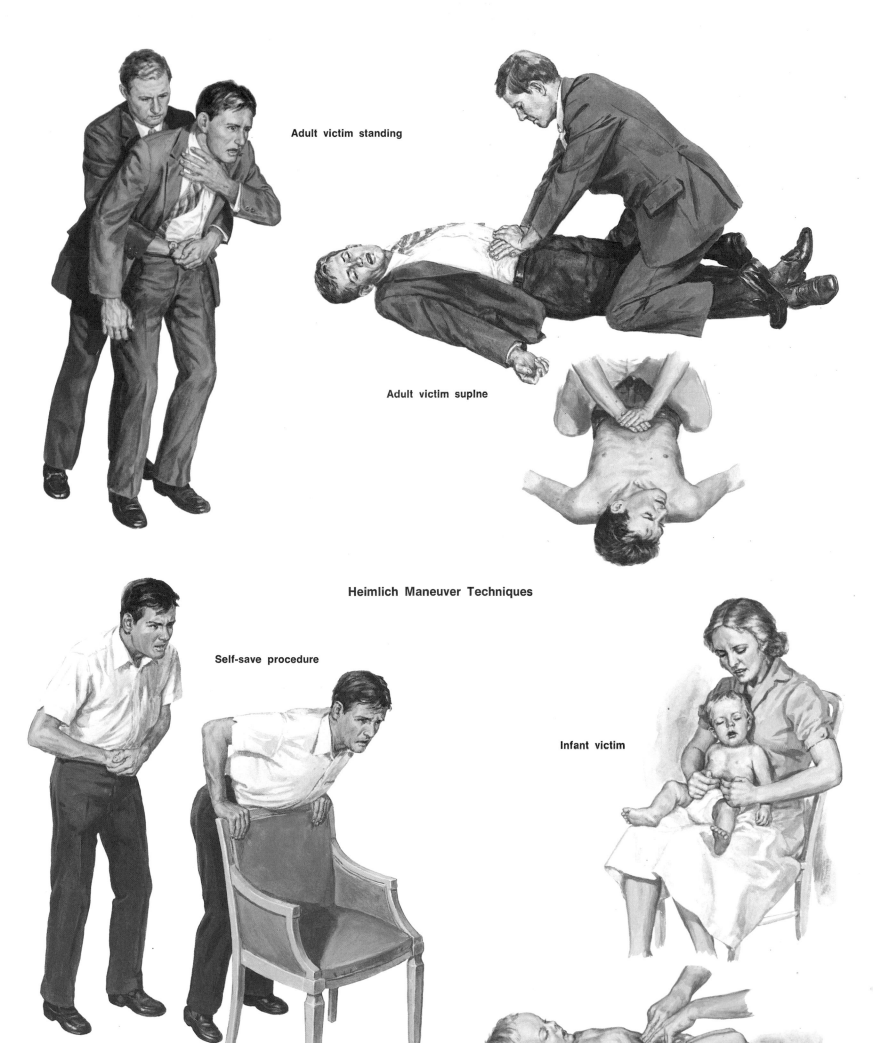

Adult victim standing

Adult victim supine

Heimlich Maneuver Techniques

Self-save procedure

Infant victim

Patent Airways

Maintenance of a patent airway is a primary supportive and resuscitative maneuver, and every physician should be able to insert an oropharyngeal airway, pass an orotracheal tube or perform a tracheostomy or cricothyrotomy. Loss of consciousness is associated with relaxation of the pharyngeal muscles when the tongue falls back to occlude the oropharynx. Asphyxiation will follow in a matter of minutes. Correction is accomplished by proper positioning of the head and jaw (neck extended, mandible supported) and displacement of the tongue to clear the air passages. The latter are maintained by passage of an oropharyngeal airway as illustrated.

For sustained ventilatory support, endotracheal intubation from above is the most rapid method of obtaining and maintaining an adequate airway. An endotracheal tube may be introduced by the oropharyngeal or by the nasopharyngeal route. Whenever possible, tracheal intubation is the procedure of choice, but outside a hospital setting this may not be feasible, and resort must be made to tracheostomy or cricothyrotomy.

Cricothyroid Stab

Cricothyrotomy requires only a sharp blade and is readily performed. The top of the thyroid cartilage or "Adam's apple" is usually easy to palpate. One carries the palpating finger inferiorly in the midline until an indentation is felt; this identifies the cricothyroid membrane, which extends from the thyroid cartilage above to the cricoid cartilage below. A transverse stab incision is made in the midline with the point of the blade directed inferiorly (to avoid laryngeal injury). Patency is

Oropharyngeal Airway

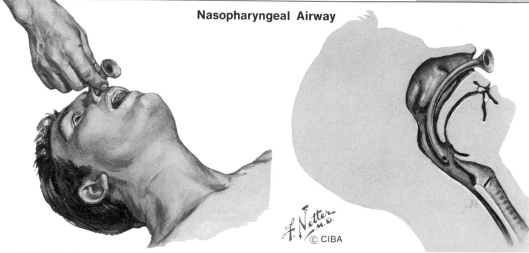

Nasopharyngeal Airway

Cricothyroid "Stab" or Cricothyrotomy

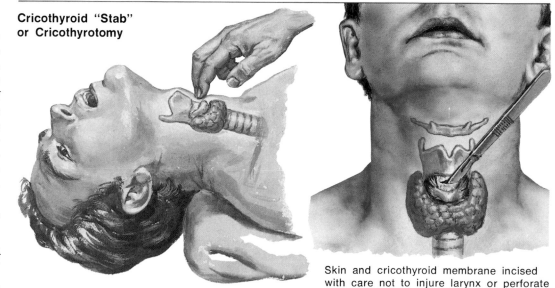

Cricothyroid membrane identified by palpating transverse indentation between thyroid and cricoid cartilages

Skin and cricothyroid membrane incised with care not to injure larynx or perforate esophagus. Patency is then maintained by inserting tube or, if not available, distending object

maintained by a tube or any blunt object (such as a ball-point pen).

The cricothyroid stab method of obtaining a patent airway carries the risk of permanent damage to the larynx and should be performed only by skilled personnel in an extreme emergency when all other methods of providing an artificial airway have been exhausted. Both spontaneous and artificial ventilation are possible by using a cannula of 6 mm maximum outside diameter and a standard 15 mm adapter.

In practice, a cricothyrotomy is seldom used because an endotracheal tube can usually be inserted to relieve airway obstruction. The cricoid

cartilage is the only complete tracheal ring in the airway and damage to it may produce significant obstruction. The problem of subglottic stenosis as an aftermath has been known for many years, and although recent observations indicate that it is not as frequent a complication as was once believed, the possibility of its occurrence has led to a conservative approach in the use of the procedure. Serious bleeding may occur into the tracheo-bronchial tree and life-threatening subcutaneous emphysema has been reported. However, success with its elective use has suggested that the procedure has value in selected circumstances and in competent hands.

Endotracheal Intubation

Endotracheal intubation is a lifesaving procedure that requires familiarity with the anatomy of the area as well as with the equipment to be used. However, knowing what to do is not enough; it is essential to be able to place an endotracheal tube rapidly and safely under the trying stress of an emergency. Only practice will provide the requisite skill before such a situation is encountered.

Choice of the correct size of endotracheal tube is fundamental. The average adult male will accept a cuffed tube, preferably of the low pressure type, with an inner diameter of 8.0 or 8.5 mm; for an adult female the tube diameter is 0.5 to 1.0 mm smaller. This will provide for adequate suctioning and for bronchofiberscopic examination during mechanical ventilation, if required. Some physicians prefer to use a nasal tube when it is evident that intubation will continue for a period of days. Nasal tubes can be "anchored" more securely, are better tolerated by patients, permit swallowing, and cannot be pinched or bitten off by the teeth.

Thorough familiarity with various laryngoscopes is necessary. The curved blade used in the McIntosh type is positioned in the vallecula, the space between the base of the tongue and the epiglottis; laryngoscopes with straight blades are designed to pick up the epiglottis. Patients with prominent incisor teeth may more readily admit a straight-bladed Miller laryngoscope, while the Bennett design is an ideal alternative.

Proper positioning with the patient's neck flexed and head tilted slightly backward is essential to provide a straight line from the oral cavity into the trachea.

To expose the larynx, the laryngoscope is held with the left hand, and the blade is first placed in the right side and then moved to the middle of the mouth, pushing the tongue to the left and out of the way. A straight blade is advanced as far as it will go along the posterior wall of the pharynx, then gently lifted and withdrawn against the anterior wall, elevating the epiglottis until the larynx is clearly seen. A curved blade is moved along the base of the tongue until the tip is in the vallecula, and the tongue is moved forward along with the epiglottis until the cords are in view. The laryngoscope should not be used to flex or extend the head by wrist movement, and introduction of an endotracheal tube should not be attempted unless the larynx is adequately exposed. The cuff should be pretested prior to intubation, and care must be exercised not to damage it against the patient's teeth. A soft-metal stylet facilitates orotracheal tube molding for introduction.

Nasotracheal intubation is performed in a similar fashion except that the tube is inserted through the larger nostril and a stylet cannot be used. The tip design of nasotracheal tubes differs from that of orotracheal tubes to facilitate blending of the tip during passage through the nasopharynx. Once the

Endotracheal Intubation

A. Endotracheal tube introduced into larynx under direct vision with laryngoscope to avoid false passage into esophagus

B. Oral view

To respirator

C. Scope withdrawn and cuff inflated with air by syringe with one-way valve adapter. Cuff tube may be clamped and then closed off or one-way valve left in line. Endotracheal tube connected to respirator

D. Transnasal introduction of endotracheal tube with aid of laryngoscope and Magill forceps

tube reaches the pharynx, it is grasped with a pair of curved forceps (Magill)—the balloon cuff being carefully avoided—and guided into the larynx and trachea.

If the patient is breathing during intubation, introduction should be attempted only during inspiration. Appropriate ventilation with supplemental oxygen should be instituted immediately before and between attempts. If the first attempt is unsuccessful, ventilation can be accomplished with a face mask and a ventilating or self-inflating bag.

Once the tube has passed the vocal cords, it is advanced to a point midway between the cords and the carina. The low pressure cuff is inflated with

sufficient air to overcome any leak during forced ventilation. It should be tested intermittently with a gauge to ensure that the cuff pressure does not exceed 20 mm Hg. Auscultation for breath sounds is then carried out over both lungs. A tube introduced too deeply into the airways will pass into the right main bronchus and occlude the left main bronchus, with resulting atelectasis and physiologic shunting of blood through a nonventilated area.

After the tube is correctly positioned, it should be adequately secured by tape. It is a sound practice to follow intubation with a chest x-ray examination to determine the tube's position.

Tracheostomy

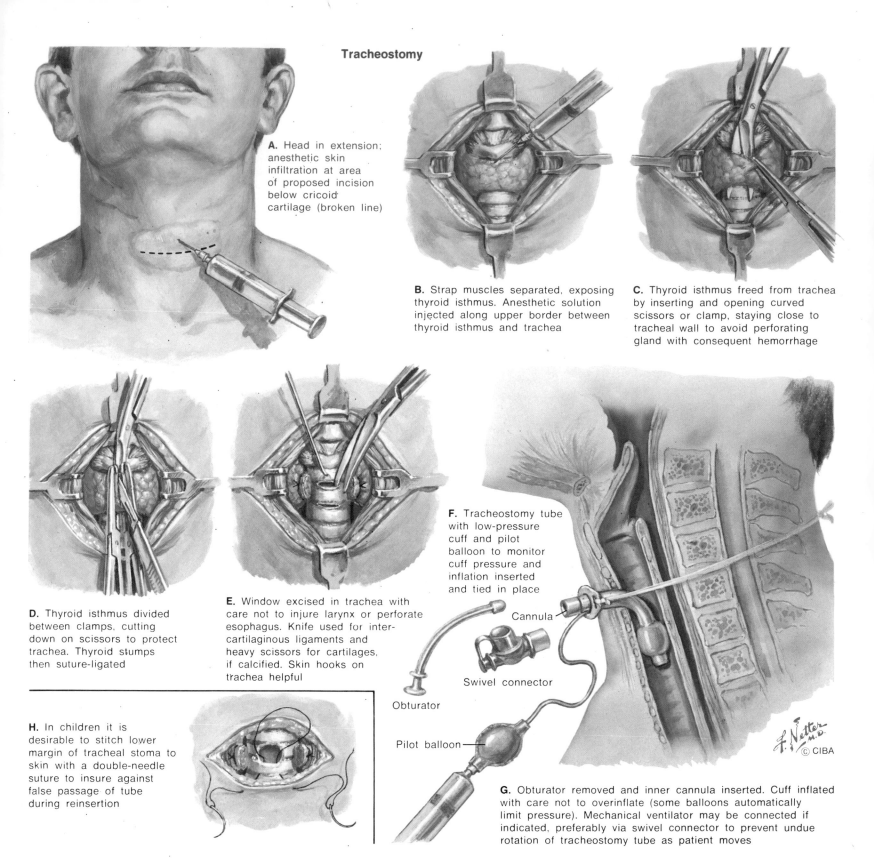

A. Head in extension; anesthetic skin infiltration at area of proposed incision below cricoid cartilage (broken line)

B. Strap muscles separated, exposing thyroid isthmus. Anesthetic solution injected along upper border between thyroid isthmus and trachea

C. Thyroid isthmus freed from trachea by inserting and opening curved scissors or clamp, staying close to tracheal wall to avoid perforating gland with consequent hemorrhage

D. Thyroid isthmus divided between clamps, cutting down on scissors to protect trachea. Thyroid stumps then suture-ligated

E. Window excised in trachea with care not to injure larynx or perforate esophagus. Knife used for intercartilaginous ligaments and heavy scissors for cartilages, if calcified. Skin hooks on trachea helpful

F. Tracheostomy tube with low-pressure cuff and pilot balloon to monitor cuff pressure and inflation inserted and tied in place

Cannula

Swivel connector

Obturator

Pilot balloon

H. In children it is desirable to stitch lower margin of tracheal stoma to skin with a double-needle suture to insure against false passage of tube during reinsertion

G. Obturator removed and inner cannula inserted. Cuff inflated with care not to overinflate (some balloons automatically limit pressure). Mechanical ventilator may be connected if indicated, preferably via swivel connector to prevent undue rotation of tracheostomy tube as patient moves

Tracheostomy

The tracheostomy incision is best made transversely (with the head extended) at a level midway between the notch at the superior border of the thyroid cartilage and the suprasternal notch. The strap muscles are separated in the midline, exposing the isthmus of the thyroid gland. This usually overlies the second and third tracheal cartilaginous rings, the optimal level at which to enter the trachea. If not retractable, the isthmus should be freed up, divided and ligated as illustrated. One should avoid entering the trachea at a level lower than the third tracheal ring since the trachea falls away from the surface to a deeper plane as it descends into the chest, making it less accessible. A window may be removed from the anterior tracheal wall with a scissors or knife, although in children and small adults a T or sideways H incision is preferred by many. Also useful is the inverted U opening, which provides a lower flap.

It is essential that the tracheal tube be of proper caliber and securely fixed. A traction suture through the lower edge of the tracheal incision and all other layers can be extremely useful.

The wound edges should be only loosely approximated, because a tight seal can drive air into the subcutaneous tissues or mediastinum during coughing or positive pressure ventilation.

The classic silver-plated Jackson tracheostomy tubes have been replaced over the past decade by a variety of nonirritating plastic tubes. These have balloon (or similar) cuffs providing a constant but low-pressure occlusion of the tracheal lumen, which is required for assisted or controlled ventilation. Thus chances of pressure necrosis on the tracheal wall are minimized.

Damage to the trachea from tracheostomy tubes can occur at the top of the tube, at the stoma, or at the level of the inflatable cuff. Erosion may occur into the esophagus, particularly if prolonged use of a nasogastric tube is also necessary, or into a major vessel with usually fatal results.

Morbidity of Endotracheal Intubation and Tracheostomy

Endotracheal Intubation. Nasotracheal tubes are more easily inserted, less easily dislodged and better tolerated than orotracheal tubes. However, they can cause nasal necrosis and maxillary sinusitis. "Blind insertion" may result in vocal cord trauma, which can be minimized by visualization—as with oral intubation. *Nasotracheal* tubes have small lumina, making suctioning and weaning from mechanical ventilation difficult. *Orotracheal tubes* are larger, and more readily permit suctioning or fiberoptic bronchoscopy than nasotracheal tubes. However, they are less comfortable, more easily dislodged, and can be kinked or damaged by the patient's teeth.

Complications of both types of endotracheal tubes include reaction to the local anesthetic, trauma, laryngospasm or laryngeal edema, aspiration of gastric contents, and intubation of the esophagus or right main bronchus. The oropharynx must be cleared of secretions or vomitus, as trauma and laryngospasm are minimized by full visualization of the vocal cords. Correct tube placement may be ascertained by auscultation over the chest and abdomen while an AMBU bag (Air-Mask-Bag-Unit) is squeezed. The cuff should be tested before intubation, and the tube secured to prevent slipping.

During mechanical ventilation several problems may occur. *Obstruction* of the tube can be secondary to kinking, mucus plugging, blood clots or slippage or overinflation of the cuff over the end of the tube. Obstruction causes respiratory distress and increased ventilator pressures, and may be recognized by inspection or by passing a suction catheter or fiberoptic bronchoscope. *Cuff leaks* due to rupture or uneven or improper cuff inflation will not allow a pressure-limited ventilator to cycle off, while the exhaled volume will be less than that set on a volume ventilator. *Aspiration* of secretions or gastric contents can occur with cuff leaks; the mouth and oropharynx should therefore be suctioned before cuff deflation.

A serious complication of both tracheostomy and endotracheal intubation is the development of a *tracheoesophageal fistula.* Fistulas usually occur when a nasogastric tube is in place. A fistula should be suspected when air leaks, aspiration of saliva or secretions, or any signs of respiratory distress are noted. The diagnosis may be confirmed by fiberoptic bronchoscopy.

Acute and chronic problems can follow *extubation.* An immediate complication is laryngospasm, which may require reintubation or tracheostomy. Minor problems such as sore throat and temporary hoarseness are frequent. Chronic problems include vocal cord incompetence, polyps or ulcerations; development of a subglottic membrane; and upper airway obstruction, which may be due to either tracheal stenosis or tracheomalacia. These can be diagnosed by indirect laryngoscopy or fiberoptic bronchoscopy. Pulmonary function studies, including evaluation of airway resistance and inspiratory and expiratory flow-volume loops, and studies of the distribution of ventilation can also help in the localization of the obstruction.

Tracheostomy. Bleeding and *tissue emphysema* are more or less unique to tracheostomy, and can be

Morbidity of Endotracheal Intubation and Tracheostomy

Tube in esophagus instead of in trachea

Tube in r. main bronchus

Kinking of tube either in pharynx or outside body

Overinflation with compression of tube or bulging of trachea

Rupture of cuff

Herniation of cuff over tube end

Blocking of tube by secretions

Tracheostomy tube misplaced in pretracheal tissues

Nasogastric tube

Ulceration into esophagus

Disconnection from respirator

Leakage of air and subcutaneous emphysema

Pressure necrosis with subsequent tracheal stenosis

minimized if the tracheostomy is performed electively, preferably under operating room conditions, and with an endotracheal tube already inserted. After tracheostomy, bleeding and subcutaneous and/or mediastinal emphysema can occur at any time. Bleeding at the incision site may be obvious, or it may occur internally, with aspiration of blood. If the tracheostomy tube becomes dislodged, reinsertion is sometimes difficult, especially with a fresh tracheostomy. If a dislodged tracheostomy tube cannot be quickly and easily reinserted, endotracheal intubation or ventilation by mask may be required until an experienced surgeon is available.

A common complication of tracheostomy is wound *infection,* which may remain localized or spread through the subcutaneous tissues or to the lung. It is usually not clear whether a pulmonary infection is caused by the same organism present in the tracheostomy wound, and transtracheal aspirates or selective cultures of the aspirate obtained by fiberoptic bronchoscopy may be helpful. The chance of infection is reduced if sterile technique is maintained during suctioning and manipulation of the tracheostomy. Cuffed tracheostomy tubes should be changed every five to seven days to prevent fixation by granulation tissue, and to help prevent infection.

Bronchofiberscopic Lavage

Tracheobronchial toilet is a very important aspect of bronchofiberscopy. Its role in the management of inflammatory pulmonary diseases was stressed by Jackson as long ago as 1928.

When compared with open-tube, rigid endoscopy, bronchofiberscopic lavage offers a safe, reasonably nontraumatic means of tracheobronchial toilet, even at the bedside. Passage through an endotracheal or tracheostomy tube adapter permits the removal of secretions even while the patient is on a mechanical ventilator.

Despite the small diameter of the instrument's inner channel, thick mucous plugs and inspissated secretions can be suctioned and removed. However, removal of these secretions and plugs is sometimes not done as readily as with the open tube, and the operator must exercise patience during the procedure. Irrigation with saline solution, 10 to 15 ml at a time, and hand suction with a large syringe (30 to 50 ml) will facilitate removal of tenacious plugs by allowing the application of higher pressures. Infrequently, the bronchofiberscope will have to be retrieved and reintroduced to get out very large, tenacious plugs. Adequate oxygenation should always be maintained with supplemental oxygen, which can be delivered through an appropriate adapter in intubated patients. A partial rebreathing mask or similar device may also be useful in achieving this in patients not supported by mechanical ventilation. Constant and careful monitoring of vital signs is necessary in these usually compromised situations. Where facilities are available, an ear oximeter will warn of sudden decreases in oxygen saturation. An ECG should always be used to detect life-threatening dysrhythmias due to hypoxemia.

True lavage of the lungs is not achieved with conventional bronchofiberscopic toilet unless a cuff is attached to the bronchoscope. Instead, aliquots of normal saline solution are instilled into the tracheobronchial tree, and as much as possible is recovered.

It is advisable to ask nonintubated patients to take frequent deep breaths to open dependent airways, which tend to close and promote hypoxemia because of increased shunting of blood through nonventilated areas. Mechanical sighs or high tidal volumes can be provided in mechanically ventilated patients.

Wanner and co-workers have reported radiographic evidence of reexpansion after flexible bronchoscopy in 85% of 27 patients with radiographic evidence of atelectasis.

Barrett and associates reported improvement in critically ill patients with unstable cardiopulmonary status. During spontaneous ventilation, transnasal examination for toilet purposes prevented subsequent endotracheal intubation and mechanical ventilation.

Indications for flexible fiberoptic bronchoscopy for toilet purposes include ineffective suctioning through an artificial airway, an abnormal chest x-ray film, persistent hypoxemia and ineffective nasotracheal suctioning.

An added advantage of flexible fiberoptic bronchoscopy is the ability to direct suctioning to areas of the lung—such as the left tracheobronchial

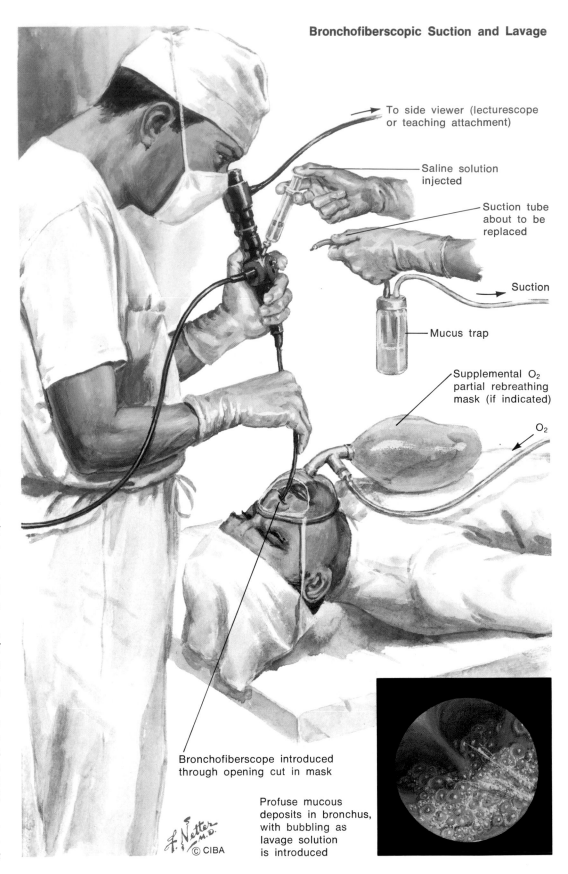

To side viewer (lecturescope or teaching attachment)

Saline solution injected

Suction tube about to be replaced

Suction

Mucus trap

Supplemental O$_2$ partial rebreathing mask (if indicated)

O$_2$

Bronchofiberscope introduced through opening cut in mask

Profuse mucous deposits in bronchus, with bubbling as lavage solution is introduced

tree—not readily reached by conventional suctioning means. Since bronchofiberscopy permits visual inspection of the tracheobronchial tree, the suctioning tip of the instrument can be directed to where secretions have accumulated.

In patients with the adult respiratory distress syndrome, Sackner and associates have used bronchofiberscopy combined with fluoroscopy for placement of a Metras suction balloon catheter, using a wire guide to facilitate introduction.

Cantrell and associates have obtained alveolar macrophages by the transnasal technique, introducing the 'scope into a dependent segmental bronchus and injecting saline in 50 ml aliquots. Also,

bronchofiberscopy is useful to establish drainage from lung abscesses. Penetration of the abscess cavity is not usual because of mucosal edema; nevertheless, probing the area with the tip of the instrument is frequently successful in initiating drainage in these situations.

In summary, bronchofiberscopy for toilet purposes is a valuable addition to the armamentarium of pulmonary medicine. Effective removal of secretions may be achieved through the suction channel of the instrument with minimal discomfort to the patient. Lavage solutions may be instilled into the tracheobroncheal tree to facilitate removal of secretions.

Nasotracheobronchial Suction

Nasotracheal Suction

Nasotracheal suction is rarely indicated today because of modern advances in respiratory care. The procedure aids the removal of retained bronchopulmonary secretions in patients who are unable to expectorate sputum voluntarily. However, chest physiotherapy including postural drainage, percussion or clapping, and aided coughing is more effective and acceptable to the oriented patient. Further, should such a patient require aspiration of secretions because cough is hindered by pain—as, for example, in trauma—fiberoptic bronchoscopy is preferred since all airways are directly visualized. The major indication for nasotracheal suction is the semicooperative patient who requires tracheobronchial toilet.

For nasotracheal suction a soft latex or polyvinyl No. 32 or 34 F. nasopharyngeal airway, lubricated with lidocaine jelly, is inserted into the nose and advanced so that its distal tip lies immediately above the vocal cords. A No. 14 F. suction catheter, held with a sterile-gloved hand, is then passed through the nasopharyngeal airway and advanced with each inspiratory phase of respiration. With passage through the vocal cords, the patient usually coughs. Introduction of the suction catheter in this way prevents trauma to the nasal mucosa, minimizes the deposition of upper airway secretions into the lung, and facilitates access to the major airways. Approximately 90% of attempts to reach the tracheobronchial tree by this method are successful, whereas the success rate for blind nasal passage ranges from 10 to 70% depending on the operator.

When it is beyond the vocal cords, the catheter is advanced farther until it reaches the main bronchi. It is then withdrawn while the operator intermittently makes and breaks the vacuum (set between 100 and 160 mm Hg) over a period of 15 to 25 seconds. The catheter is then removed and discarded after a single pass. Blind nasotracheal suctioning is generally effective in removing tracheal secretions. It also stimulates coughing, which facilitates clearance of secretions from the major bronchi. Because of the anatomic obliquity of the right compared with the left main bronchus, the suction catheter almost always passes down the right side. Blind nasotracheal suction of left-sided secretions usually fails, and fiberoptic bronchoscopic removal must be employed.

In the uncooperative, semiconscious or comatose patient, clearance of the tracheobronchial tree is best carried out after endotracheal intubation. This permits controlled access to the airways and connection to a mechanical ventilator for proper ventilation and oxygenation. In patients who are well oxygenated—*i.e.,* with an arterial oxygen saturation greater than 92% during spontaneous intermittent positive pressure breathing—it is quite safe to detach the endotracheal tube from the supplementary oxygen source. Suctioning can then be done using a sterile glove to pass the catheter through the endotracheal tube and thence into the main bronchi. Insignificant drops in arterial oxygen saturation occur for up to 25 seconds of interrupted suction. However, if positive end-expiratory pressure or continuous positive airway pressure is

Soft latex or polyvinyl nasopharyngeal airway

Vacuum tube

Intermittent closure of side vent on vacuum tube by operator's thumb causes suction to be discontinuous, permitting normal lung ventilation

To vacuum mucus trap

f. Netter © CIBA

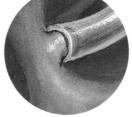

Bronchofiberscopic view showing how mucosa may invaginate into side or end hole of ordinary suction catheter

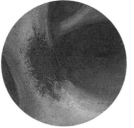

Hemorrhagic area at site of invagination after cessation of suction

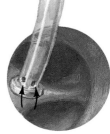

Special catheter tip with flange at end and 4 small vent holes proximal to it (magnified)

Flange prevents occlusion of small holes which serve as vents and no invagination occurs even if end hole directly abuts wall (at bifurcation). Air cushion on way to small holes enhances protection

required to maintain adequate oxygenation, marked hypoxemia may occur at these times, not primarily because of the suctioning procedure but because the end-expiratory lung volume has shifted closer to residual volume. Suctioning through a special connector will permit introduction of the catheter while still maintaining positive airway pressure. Hypoxemia may also be minimized by limiting the period of detachment from the positive pressure source to 15 seconds, including suctioning, and administering 100% oxygen for about one minute before the procedure.

It should be understoood that all suction catheters traumatize the tracheobronchial mucosa in two

ways: (1) by causing invagination of the mucosa into the end and/or side holes with consequent immediate ischemic necrosis of the area, and (2) by direct physical contact, which results in delayed sloughing of ciliated epithelium many hours later. Erosions caused by suctioning permit colonization and penetration of the mucosa by pathogens as well as cessation of the host mechanism of mucociliary transport. All commercially available catheters of end-hole and side-hole design produce this problem, as observed by fiberoptic bronchoscopy. Frequent interruption and use of a weaker vacuum tend to minimize the damage, but unfortunately efficiency of secretion aspiration also diminishes.

Bronchofiberscopy

Endoscopic examination of the tracheobronchial tree is an essential procedure in the diagnosis and treatment of diseases of the lungs and airways. The advantage of the recently introduced flexible bronchofiberscope is that it allows visualization and sampling of peripheral lesions which cannot be reached using a rigid instrument.

Equipment. Bronchofiberscopes are produced by several different manufacturers, making selection for specific needs possible. The main characteristics of the instrument are that: (1) it is slender enough to pass into an airway without significantly compromising it, (2) it is flexible and able to reach small airways, (3) it uses a cold light source (xenon or halogen) usually with a flash system to aid photography, (4) it has excellent optics and light transmission, with good resolution and field of vision, and (5) it has a channel for suction which also serves as a passageway for brush or forceps biopsy instruments.

Preparation of the Patient. Even with a small-diameter instrument, some degree of airway obstruction is unavoidable and a fall in arterial oxygen tension is frequently seen. Continuous suction may aggravate this problem, and preoperative arterial blood gas studies are essential for patients in whom there exists any suspicion of compromised lung function.

Premedication includes atropine sulfate to control secretions, minimize bronchospasm and block the vasovagal reflex. In addition, either morphine sulfate, meperidine hydrochloride or diazepam is given to allay anxiety. The premedication can be administered intravenously just before the procedure is begun. Good topical anesthesia is essential to reduce discomfort to the patient. Oxygen is supplied through a mask or nasal cannula or by the bronchoscopic channel. The fiberscope can be introduced transorally, in which case a bite block is usually necessary; transnasally; or through an endotracheal or tracheostomy tube which should have a minimum inside diameter of 8.5 mm. In patients with marginal pulmonary function, the procedure is best performed using endotracheal intubation and mechanical ventilation. A swivel adapter allows supplemental oxygen and inhalation anesthesia to be utilized.

Intubation Procedure. The position of the patient's head and neck is less important for flexible bronchoscopes than for rigid bronchoscopy. The instrument is treated with a suitable lubricant and antifogging agent, and its tip is introduced into whichever nostril is more patent. Under direct vision, it is advanced slowly and the nasopharynx carefully inspected. Familiarity with the controls of the instrument is important to enable its tip to be properly directed without damage to the instrument or the mucosal lining. After the uvula and base of the tongue have been seen and passed, the epiglottis is next identified and the flexible tip should be directed posteriorly. With slight advancement, both the arytenoids and the vocal cords come under direct vision, and further local anesthetic should be applied to this area. If the cords and larynx are normal, the fiberscope is introduced into the trachea. Inspection of the

Side viewer for observer

Fiberoptic tube from cold light source

Suction tube

Mucus trap

Flexible bronchoscopic tube inserted via nostril

Eye piece

Opening to channel for flexible biopsy forceps, cytology brush, suction, lavage, anesthesia, oxygen

Lever for angulation of tip

Fiberoptic tube from cold light supply box

Flexible tube for insertion into bronchi

Tip may be angulated up or down and scope rotated for entry into bronchial subdivisions

Biopsy forceps protruding from tip of tube (magnified)

Magnified section

Fiberoptic visualizing channel

Fiberoptic light guides

Open channel for anesthetic, oxygen, forceps, suction, lavage, cytology brush, etc.

lobar and segmental bronchi to the periphery is possible, and the upper lobes are more readily examined with this technique than is possible with a rigid bronchoscope.

Brush or forceps biopsy may be done by direct vision or, if this is impossible, under fluoroscopic control. Transbronchial lung biopsy is valuable in diffuse parenchymal lung diseases, particularly from the lower lobes. With proper experience, the incidence of a complicating hemorrhage or pneumothorax has been low. This procedure may also be done through a rigid bronchoscope, which allows better control of bleeding. Therapeutic bronchoscopy is most often carried out at the

bedside on mechanically ventilated patients. Saline lavage and suction through the fiberscope channel may be effective in removing retained secretions and clearing obstructed air passages.

Complications requiring immediate treatment include laryngospasm and bronchospasm, which usually respond to adequate topical anesthesia. Massive bleeding and discharge of abscess contents need prompt open-tube bronchoscopy. A pneumothorax, depending on its size, may call for placement of chest tubes. Severe hypoxemia and ventricular dysrhythmias usually require cessation of the procedure, oxygen and intravenous lidocaine.

Bronchofiberscopic Views

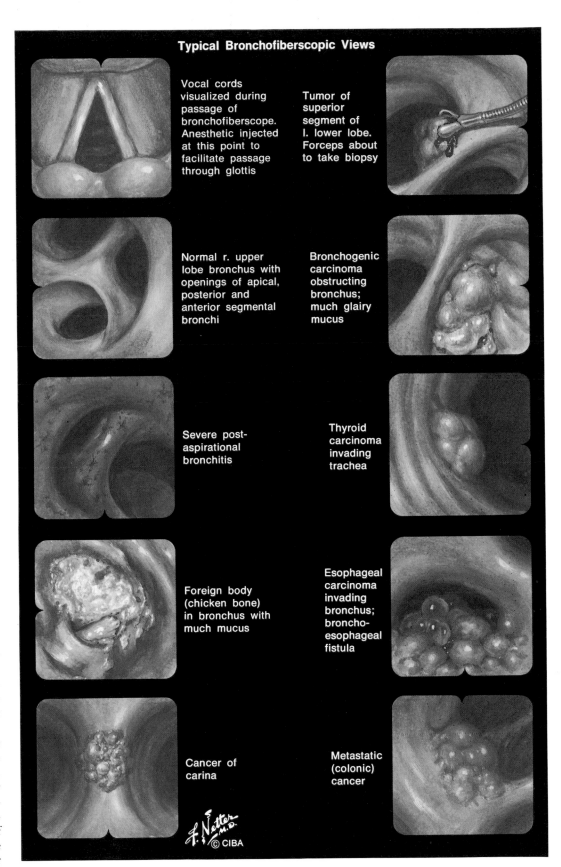

Typical Bronchofiberscopic Views

Vocal cords visualized during passage of bronchofiberscope. Anesthetic injected at this point to facilitate passage through glottis

Tumor of superior segment of l. lower lobe. Forceps about to take biopsy

Normal r. upper lobe bronchus with openings of apical, posterior and anterior segmental bronchi

Bronchogenic carcinoma obstructing bronchus; much glairy mucus

Severe post-aspirational bronchitis

Thyroid carcinoma invading trachea

Foreign body (chicken bone) in bronchus with much mucus

Esophageal carcinoma invading bronchus; broncho-esophageal fistula

Cancer of carina

Metastatic (colonic) cancer

While the bronchofiberscope is being passed down the tracheobronchial tree, careful attention is paid to the pattern of the mucosa, the size of the lumen and the elasticity of the walls. Normal bronchial mucosa is pale pink, but its color varies with the intensity of the light source. The surface follows the contours of tracheal and bronchial walls and becomes paler where it overlies cartilaginous rings. A small amount of mucus and a thin layer of surface lining fluid reflect the light from the bronchoscope. In the trachea and main bronchi, the shape of the lumen is an incomplete circle or arch with a membranous posterior portion; this portion disappears distally as the airways become surrounded first by irregular cartilaginous plates and eventually by concentric muscle and elastic tissue.

Inflammation may be diffuse or localized. The endobronchial changes seen are reddening, increased vascularity, edema, mucosal irregularity, augmented secretion production and occasionally ulceration. Swelling may lead to loss of the cartilaginous prominences and normal mucosal pattern and to blunting and associated narrowing of bronchial orifices. Excess secretions can be mucoid or purulent and either thin and watery or thick and viscid. Such changes are seen diffusely in chronic bronchitis and may be accompanied by collapse of major airways during expiration. Localized inflammation accompanies carcinomas, tuberculosis, foreign bodies, pneumonia, bronchiectasis and abscess formation. The most important lesion to be identified in these circumstances is a bronchogenic carcinoma. Healing of endobronchial inflammation may lead to permanent stenosis and obstruction. This occurs particularly following tuberculosis, and similar distortion is often seen after roentgen therapy for a carcinoma.

Extrabronchial compression is most commonly due to a mediastinal tumor or lymphadenopathy.

Widening of the carina with loss of its usual sharp edge because of enlarged subcarinal lymph nodes is confirmatory evidence of inoperability of a primary lung cancer. Extrinsic compression from any cause may reduce the bronchial lumen to a slitlike orifice, and displacement of bronchi often accompanies atelectasis of an adjacent lobe or follows resection. Occasionally a stitch granuloma is present in the bronchial stump and requires endoscopic removal of the retained suture.

Tissue involved by tumor growth is often fixed and rigid, and the mucosa may appear inflamed, or pale and yellow. There may be concentric narrowing of the lumen, or an irregular mass which at times is polypoid and occludes the bronchus entirely. Engorgement of superficial vessels is common and bleeding frequent. The great majority of tumors are primary bronchogenic carcinomas, but other less aggressive neoplasms are occasionally found. The possibility of multiple tumors should not be overlooked.

Material for bacteriologic and fungal culture and for microscopic examination can be obtained by suction through the operating channel of the fiberbronchoscope at the time of viewing. Biopsy by brushing or using suitable forceps introduced through the same channel produces tissue with a high diagnostic yield, especially for lung tumors.

Nomenclature for Peripheral Bronchi
(proposed by Ikeda)

For simplification, only a few bronchial subdivisions are labeled as far as 5th generation, but principle is demonstrated

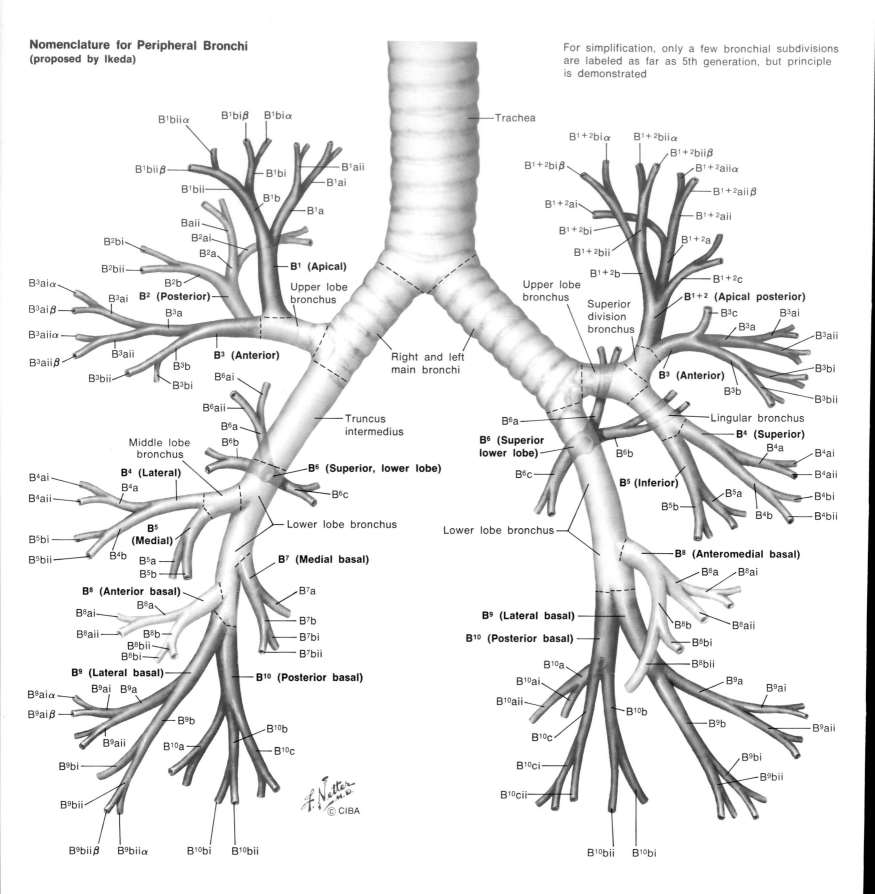

B^1biia $B^1bi\beta$ $B^1bi\alpha$

$B^1bii\beta$ B^1bi B^1aii

B^1bii B^1ai

Baii B^1b B^1a

B^2bi B^2ai

B^2bii B^2a

$B^3ai\alpha$ B^2b **B^1 (Apical)**

$B^3ai\beta$ B^3ai **B^2 (Posterior)**   Upper lobe bronchus

$B^3aii\alpha$ B^3a

$B^3aii\beta$ B^3aii **B^3 (Anterior)**

B^3bii B^3b

B^3bi

B^6ai

B^6aii

Middle lobe bronchus B^6a

B^6b

B^4 (Lateral)

B^4ai B^4a

B^4aii

B^5 (Medial)

B^5bi B^4b

B^5bii B^5a

B^5b

B^8 (Anterior basal)

B^8ai B^8a

B^8aii B^8b

B^8bii

B^8bi

B^9 (Lateral basal)

$B^9ai\alpha$ B^9ai B^9a

$B^9ai\beta$

B^9b

B^9aii

B^9bi

B^9bii

$B^9bii\beta$ $B^9bii\alpha$ $B^{10}bi$ $B^{10}bii$

Trachea

$B^{1+2}bi\alpha$ $B^{1+2}bii\alpha$

$B^{1+2}bi\beta$ $B^{1+2}bii\beta$

$B^{1+2}ai$ $B^{1+2}aii\alpha$

$B^{1+2}bi$ $B^{1+2}aii\beta$

$B^{1+2}bii$ $B^{1+2}aii$

$B^{1+2}b$ $B^{1+2}a$

Upper lobe bronchus $B^{1+2}c$

Superior division bronchus   **B^{1+2} (Apical posterior)**

B^3c B^3ai

B^3a

B^3aii

B^3 (Anterior) B^3bi

B^3b

B^3bii

Lingular bronchus

B^6a **B^4 (Superior)**

B^6 (Superior lower lobe) B^4a

B^6b B^4ai

B^6c **B^5 (Inferior)** B^4aii

B^5a B^4bi

B^5b B^4b B^4bii

Right and left main bronchi

Truncus intermedius

Lower lobe bronchus   Lower lobe bronchus

B^6 (Superior, lower lobe)

B^6c

B^8 (Anteromedial basal)

B^8a B^8ai

B^7 **(Medial basal)**

B^7a

B^7b

B^7bi

B^7bii

B^8b B^8aii

B^8bi

B^8bii

B^{10} (Posterior basal)

B^9 (Lateral basal)

B^{10} (Posterior basal)

$B^{10}a$

$B^{10}ai$ B^9a

$B^{10}aii$ $B^{10}b$ B^9ai

$B^{10}c$ B^9b

$B^{10}ci$ B^9aii

$B^{10}cii$ B^9bi

B^9bii

$B^{10}a$

$B^{10}b$ $B^{10}c$

f. Netter M.D.
© CIBA

$B^{10}bii$ $B^{10}bi$

SECTION V   PLATE 15

Nomenclature for Peripheral Bronchi

The nomenclature in common use for the segmental anatomy of the lungs is that of Jackson and Huber.

There are 10 segments in the right lung and eight in the left (see pages 16 and 17). Subdivisions of the bronchial tree correspond to the anatomic segments, and are named accordingly.

These tertiary bronchi were regarded by Jackson and Huber as the final branches, but the advent of the bronchofiberscope has led Ikeda to introduce additional nomenclature for the fourth, fifth and sixth divisions since these can now be visualized. A convenient numerical system is used in which segmental bronchi are numbered from 1 to 10 on each side and identified by the capital letter *B* for bronchus. This may be prefixed by a capital letter *R* for right and *L* for left, so that RB^3 identifies the bronchus to the anterior segment of the right upper lobe. The apical-posterior segment of the left upper lobe is LB^{1+2}, and the anteromedial basal segment of the same side becomes LB^8 since

each of these paired segments is supplied by a single tertiary bronchus. With rare exceptions, there is no LB designation.

Subsegmental or fourth-order bronchi are indicated by the lower case letter *a* for posterior and *b* for anterior. The letter *c* may also be used when necessary for additional bronchi.

Fifth-order bronchi are designated by the Roman numerals *i* (posterior) and *ii* (anterior). Finally, those at the level of the sixth order of division are characterized by α and β.

Endobronchial variations from the normal anatomy are not infrequent and are more common in peripheral airways.

Rigid Bronchoscopy

Attempts were made during the 1800s to visualize the tracheobronchial tree through an open tube, but it was not until the present century that Chevalier Jackson of Philadelphia perfected the technique of rigid bronchoscopy as we now know it. Much of today's expertise in endoscopy is based on his original methods or modifications of them.

As the use of the flexible instrument has increased, the open tube bronchoscope has had fewer routine functions, but it remains a very valuable diagnostic and therapeutic instrument. It is preferred in children because the hollow tube is much safer in ensuring an 'adequate airway through the small trachea and glottis. It is an essential piece of equipment for control of massive bleeding in the tracheobronchial tree since blood completely obscures the visual field of the bronchofiberscope. Similarly, thick secretions are better evacuated through it and a centrally located foreign body is more easily removed. On the other hand, it lacks the range and maneuverability of the flexible instrument and is more uncomfortable for the patient. The two methods of airway visualization should be regarded as complementary.

Instrument. The bronchoscope is an open tube with a proximal or distal lighting device and a side channel for oxygen or ventilation. The diameter of the bronchoscope used depends on the patient's size and age. A long suction tube for removing secretions or blood, biopsy or grasping forceps, and a sponge carrier are all necessary for adequate examination. Angled telescopes provide a better field of view in the bronchial tree, but upper lobe and peripheral lesions are more difficult to reach with this type of instrument.

Procedure. After explaining the procedure to the patient, the examination is begun. A premedication is given and should contain atropine sulfate to dry secretions and an agent to relieve anxiety. Local anesthesia is preferred by many since it is safe and allows a prolonged examination to be made, but general intravenous anesthesia is more comfortable for the patient. The risks of the latter have been greatly reduced by modern anesthetic technique.

Correct positioning of the head is important to bring the mouth, larynx and trachea in line with each other. A 3-inch thick foam rubber pillow allows flexion of the neck, and the head is then extended to accomplish this alignment. A rigid cervical spine may make this difficult. Dentures should have been removed previously, and the upper teeth are protected from injury, particularly by avoiding leverage against them. If general anesthesia and muscle relaxants have been used, the patient should be ventilated with high concentrations of oxygen and the constraints of time must be recognized.

The bronchoscope is lubricated at the distal end and introduced gently with one hand while the other hand keeps the mouth open and maintains head position. The bronchoscope is passed over the base of the tongue and its tip used to lift the epiglottis forward. Both arytenoepiglottic folds and the vocal cords are then visualized. At this point the bronchoscope is rotated through 90 degrees with its tip to the right. Thus the left

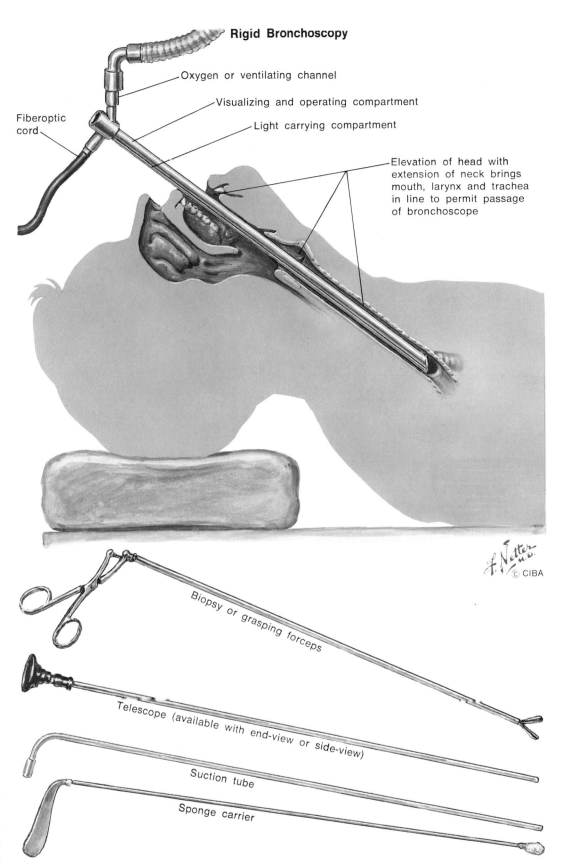

Rigid Bronchoscopy

Oxygen or ventilating channel

Visualizing and operating compartment

Fiberoptic cord

Light carrying compartment

Elevation of head with extension of neck brings mouth, larynx and trachea in line to permit passage of bronchoscope

Biopsy or grasping forceps

Telescope (available with end-view or side-view)

Suction tube

Sponge carrier

vocal cord becomes centered in the visual field, and the tip of the bronchoscope is brought between the two cords. With gentle progression, the instrument will pass into the trachea. At no time should its passage be forced; if there is difficulty, a smaller size of bronchoscope may be needed. As soon as the tracheal lumen is identified, ventilation is begun through the channel in the instrument provided for this purpose. Inspection and progression down the tracheobronchial tree is continued under direct vision.

It is easier to examine the right side where the main bronchus is more directly in line with the trachea. On either side, entrance is made simpler by rotation of the head in the opposite direction. The use of oblique, forward or lateral viewing telescopes is helpful for full visualization of the upper lobes and of smaller bronchi in all areas. Secretions and biopsy tissues are obtained from appropriate sites.

Withdrawal of the bronchoscope requires similar care to that used during insertion and should be carried out visually. If a general anesthetic has been given, its effects should have worn off before the instrument is removed. Finally, the vocal cords should be examined for evidence of trauma or for paralysis which might not have been apparent during anesthesia.

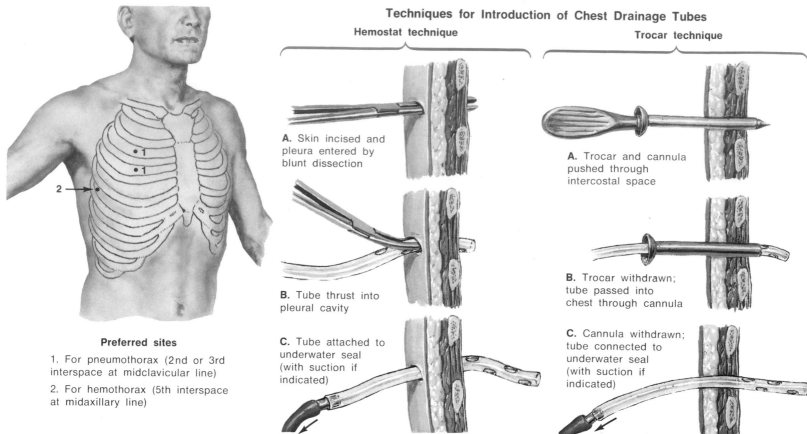

Techniques for Introduction of Chest Drainage Tubes

Hemostat technique

A. Skin incised and pleura entered by blunt dissection

B. Tube thrust into pleural cavity

C. Tube attached to underwater seal (with suction if indicated)

Trocar technique

A. Trocar and cannula pushed through intercostal space

B. Trocar withdrawn; tube passed into chest through cannula

C. Cannula withdrawn; tube connected to underwater seal (with suction if indicated)

Preferred sites

1. For pneumothorax (2nd or 3rd interspace at midclavicular line)
2. For hemothorax (5th interspace at midaxillary line)

Introduction of Chest Drainage Tubes

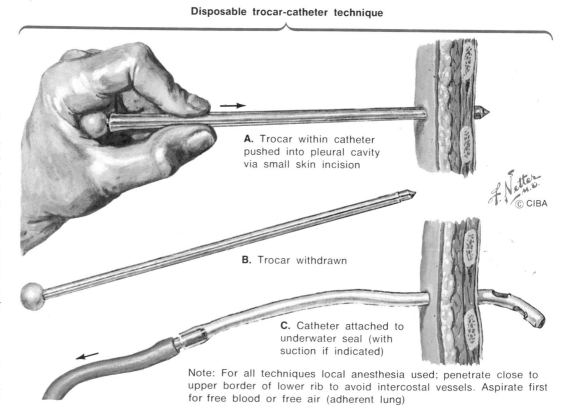

Disposable trocar-catheter technique

A. Trocar within catheter pushed into pleural cavity via small skin incision

B. Trocar withdrawn

C. Catheter attached to underwater seal (with suction if indicated)

Note: For all techniques local anesthesia used; penetrate close to upper border of lower rib to avoid intercostal vessels. Aspirate first for free blood or free air (adherent lung)

Pleural drainage tubes are inserted for evacuation of air or fluid from the pleural space in pneumothorax or hemothorax.

Placement of an intercostal tube or catheter for *pneumothorax* can be readily accomplished under local or intercostal nerve block anesthesia, or both. It may be done at the bedside, but strict aseptic precautions need be observed. The site for tube insertion should be one that is away from adherent lung. Generally preferred is the second or third anterior intercostal space in the midclavicular line or the fourth or fifth intercostal space in the midaxillary line. To help select the optimal point of entry, chest x-ray films should be reviewed unless the clinical situation is one of extreme urgency.

Under any circumstances, needle aspiration and ready withdrawal of air (or fluid) should precede any tube insertion. Such aspiration is simple and can be part of the process of local infiltration with an anesthetic agent. Failure to find a free pleural space necessitates choosing another site for tube insertion.

Anterior closed thoracotomies in the second and third intercostal space must be placed at least two fingerbreadths lateral to the sternal border in order to avoid injury to the internal mammary vessels. Lateral tube placements must not be made too low lest there be penetration of the sloping diaphragmatic attachment where it joins the chest wall. The act of tube insertion *should not be forceful* but done with delicacy and tactile control, to avoid stabbing of the diaphragm (or an enlarged heart on the left side).

Multifenestrated tubes should be checked carefully to be sure that all openings lie well within the pleural space. Thoracotomy tubes should be sutured to the skin, but such suture fixation cannot be depended upon to hold the tube securely in place; for this purpose, careful binding with adhesive tape is required. Also, protection against traction and tube angulation must be assured.

An underwater seal is attached to the tube and tube patency is present if there is bubbling under the water surface or if an oscillating column within the tube is observed. Having the patient cough or sniff is the best way to demonstrate small oscillations of tube fluid; barely detectable tube fluid oscillation signifies either full lung expansion or tube blockage.

Exacerbation of subcutaneous emphysema or an increasing pneumothorax with a tube in place signifies tube blockage or improper placement.

Once an intercostal tube is inserted, its position and effectiveness must be checked by AP and lateral x-ray studies as soon as possible.

Hemothoraces or large pleural effusions are best drained at a dependent site, usually in the seventh or eighth intercostal space in the posterior axillary line or the fourth or fifth intercostal space in the midaxillary line. Needle aspiration should always precede tube insertion, especially when infection is present, because evacuation is best assured by selecting a dependent site.

Underwater-Seal Drainage of Chest

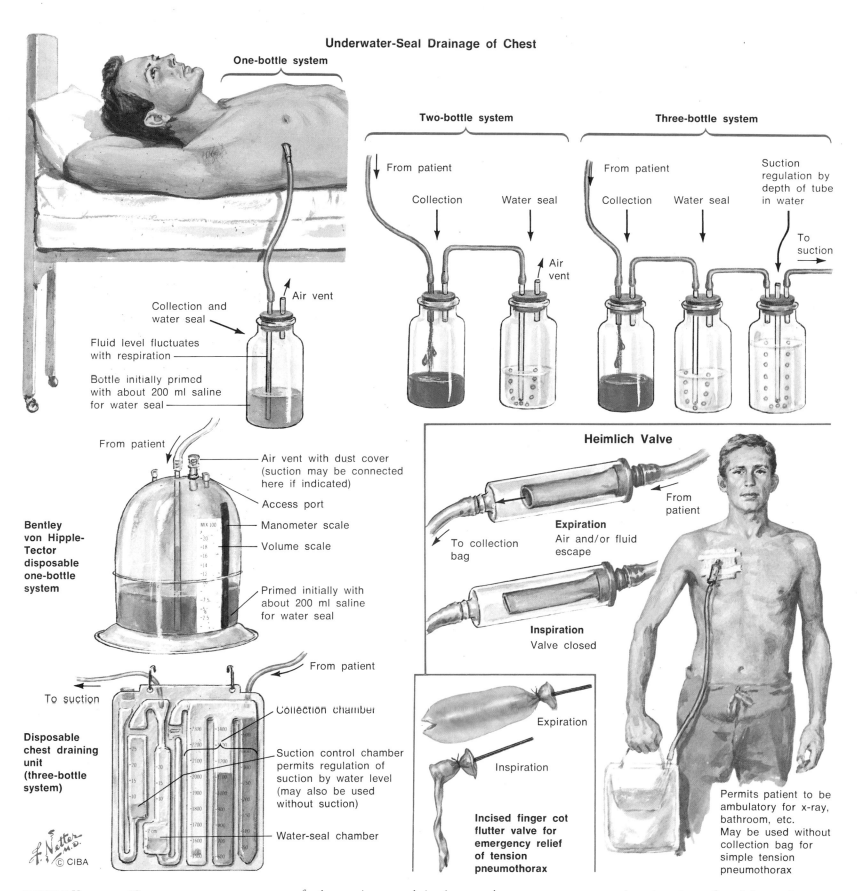

One-bottle system

Collection and water seal

Air vent

Fluid level fluctuates with respiration

Bottle initially primed with about 200 ml saline for water seal

From patient

Air vent with dust cover (suction may be connected here if indicated)

Access port

Manometer scale

Volume scale

Bentley von Hipple-Tector disposable one-bottle system

Primed initially with about 200 ml saline for water seal

To suction

From patient

Disposable chest draining unit (three-bottle system)

Collection chamber

Suction control chamber permits regulation of suction by water level (may also be used without suction)

Water-seal chamber

Two-bottle system

From patient

Collection

Water seal

Air vent

Three-bottle system

From patient

Collection

Water seal

Suction regulation by depth of tube in water

To suction

Heimlich Valve

To collection bag

Expiration
Air and/or fluid escape

From patient

Inspiration
Valve closed

Expiration

Inspiration

Incised finger cot flutter valve for emergency relief of tension pneumothorax

Permits patient to be ambulatory for x-ray, bathroom, etc.
May be used without collection bag for simple tension pneumothorax

Chest Draining Methods

Once an intercostal tube is inserted, the pleural contents are evacuated into an underwater trap or, in the case of a pneumothorax, through a one-way flutter valve of the Heimlich variety. The essential feature of the system is a means to permit escape of gas or fluid from the pleural space with no possibility of return, using gravity or suction.

If evacuation of fluid or air is impeded, there is a progressive increase in intrapleural pressure and further respiratory and circulatory embarassment. This may occur in a number of ways. A deeply submerged straw tip impedes air evacuation, and an air vent which is obstructed or too narrow has a similar effect. Soft chest drainage tubing may be occluded by kinking or outside pressure, or it may be of insufficient diameter to cope with the volume of a large air leak. Dependent loops of tubing containing fluid result in significant back pressure and accumulation of intrapleural fluid or air. More than one drainage tube is often needed, and although a one- or two-bottle system is effective, the use of suction pumps is common. In recent years, disposable suction systems of the under-water seal variety have found increasing acceptance, since both are practical.

A chest tube can usually be removed when there is less than 100-200 ml of serous fluid escaping daily. Occasionally, serosanguineous fluid may leak through the hole from which a tube has been removed, especially after coughing. This is not of concern since the leak almost always ceases spontaneously. If drainage occurs around a tube that is still in place, it indicates that the tip is no longer in communication with the intrapleural fluid and it needs to be repositioned or removed. Infection due to the presence of a drainage tube in the pleural space is unusual.

Postural Drainage and Breathing Exercises

The main symptoms of chronic obstructive pulmonary disease (COPD)—cough, easy fatigability, dyspnea—progressively worsen, especially following respiratory infections. Traditional treatment is primarily symptomatic. Antibiotics are administered to prevent or control infection, and various means are used to alleviate the discomfort caused by chronically impaired pulmonary ventilation (more severe in those with accumulated secretions); *i.e.,* expectorants, bronchodilators, intermittent positive pressure breathing (IPPB), and oxygen. Although these symptomatic depressants can be lifesavers and unquestionably provide temporary relief, at best their effect is of limited duration. Optimally, therapy should be oriented to the future as well as to the present, and one treatment procedure lies in the application of a relatively new specialty: rehabilitation medicine. The disabled person is taught to cope with his severely diminished cardiopulmonary reserves so as to regain performance capability in those activities still within his potential range. Physical therapy, the aspect of rehabilitation medicine discussed here, takes a three-pronged approach as it relates to the pulmonary cripple: (1) relaxation exercises, (2) postural drainage and (3) breathing exercises.

Relaxation Exercises

The COPD patient is a particularly tense and anxious individual because of dyspnea and fear of suffocation. The forward-bent body posture that facilitates his breathing leaves his trunk muscles taut and permanently contracted, so that he has the appearance of a quasi hunchback. To relieve the constant anxiety, decrease the compensatory muscular contraction, and significantly improve results in postural drainage and breathing, relaxation exercises are the essential first step in rehabilitation. The most effective techniques, described and used by Jacobson, place the patient in a supine or fetal position. (Orthopneic patients, who cannot easily tolerate the supine position, should have the upper trunk elevated 5 to 10 inches.)

Postural Drainage

The accumulation of excess bronchial secretions is a major complicating factor with COPD patients and is particularly critical when the disease has advanced so far that both the cough mechanism and bronchociliary action are greatly impaired. The accumulated mucoid and/or mucopurulent secretions constitute a permanent source for the reactivation of bacterial infection. In addition, they can interrupt airflow and cause temporary or permanent airway obstruction. The second step, therefore, in the rehabilitation of the pulmonary cripple involves the removal of these accumulated secretions from the bronchial tree by postural drainage.

(Continued)

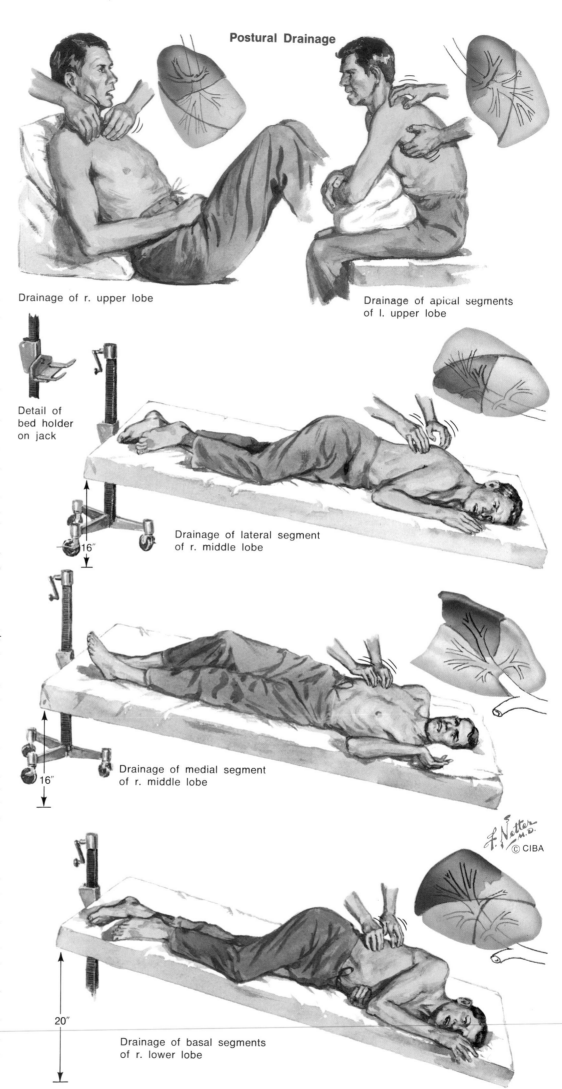

Postural Drainage

Drainage of r. upper lobe

Drainage of apical segments of l. upper lobe

Detail of bed holder on jack

Drainage of lateral segment of r. middle lobe

16″

Drainage of medial segment of r. middle lobe

16″

Drainage of basal segments of r. lower lobe

20″

Postural Drainage and Breathing Exercises
(Continued)

Postural drainage, also called gravitational drainage, is the preferred and best-tolerated means for clearing the bronchial tree. (Such techniques as suction or bronchial washing cause considerable discomfort, often requiring local anesthetic and specialized paramedical personnel.) It can be practiced effectively in the patient's home with the assistance of a family member. Indeed, the fact that the patient is able to participate actively in his own therapy, rather than being merely a passive recipient, is also of value. The bar graph (Plate 20), which reflects the significant increase in average sputum production following the use of postural drainage, quantitatively illustrates the procedure's therapeutic value.

Prior preparation of the patient is essential for reducing the viscosity of the tenacious secretions and obtaining spontaneous gravitational drainage of the bronchial tree. It involves inhalation of a heated aerosol, a bronchodilator and, if necessary, an appropriate mucolytic agent (the latter two being features of IPPB). Adequate hydration is also important in facilitating drainage. Drainage is then accomplished by means of the following manual and/or electrically operated maneuvers to dislodge and help propel the trapped secretions toward the trachea: (1) percussion with rapid vibration tap, (2) tapping with cupped hands, (3) high-frequency ultrasound. These techniques are applied where drainage is most necessary, over either the anterior or the posterior chest wall, and are repeated during the time each position or posture is held by the patient.

Proper positioning of the patient, which is paramount, is done according to the distribution and configuration of the bronchopulmonary segments. To achieve maximal drainage of the apical segments of the upper lobe, for example, a slightly reclining upright position is the most effective. For drainage of the trachea and major bronchi, the right-angled head-down position should be assumed. The head-down (Trendelenburg) position should be used in draining the middle and lower pulmonary lobes. This latter position, which is maintained (in hospital or at home) whenever the patient is prone or supine, requires a bed jack or a hospital bed for proper bed elevation.

Most patients tolerate these positions well, the exception being that the debilitated patient may initially experience difficulty in achieving the right-angled head-down position. In such cases this position should be attained very gradually, and only to the degree of the individual's tolerance.

Postural drainage should be practiced twice a day, preferably before both breakfast and dinner. Each position should be held for three to five minutes. If at all possible, a family member should

(Continued)

Postural Drainage
(continued)

Drainage of superior segment of l. lower lobe

16"

Drainage of inferior segment (lingula) of l. upper lobe

16"

Drainage of basal segments of l. lower lobe

20"

Drainage of major bronchi and of trachea

Sputum (ml/24 hr)

Postural drainage
No postural drainage

No sputum

Sputum production in 6 patients with and without postural drainage

Postural Drainage and Breathing Exercises
(Continued)

accompany the patient during his initial training for optimal preparation for assisting in home treatment.

Breathing Exercises

The breathing exercises for patients with COPD are designed to (1) increase alveolar ventilation to maintain adequate gas exchange, (2) restore the diaphragm to its normal and intended function as the main respiratory muscle, and (3) reestablish a well-coordinated and efficient breathing pattern to decrease the effort of breathing.

During normal quiet breathing, the diaphragm actively contracts and descends during inhalation. It passively ascends against gravity during exhalation, assisted synergistically by the recoiling properties of the lung and the expiratory muscles of the chest. Diaphragmatic mobility in quiet breathing is about 1 to 3 cm and is responsible for 65 to 70% of pulmonary ventilation, with the respiratory muscles carrying the remaining 30 to 35%. Because of the structural changes characterizing COPD, the lung loses its elastic and recoiling properties and becomes pathologically distended, and the diaphragm is weakened and depressed. The debilitated diaphragm, unable to ascend against both gravity and the distended lung, loses its normal capacity for excursion and consequently its role as the primary respiratory muscle. The respiratory and accessory muscles of the chest, normally fully utilized only during periods of extra effort, are increasingly called into action in a compensatory attempt to maintain adequate pulmonary ventilation. This gradual change continues until the chest respiratory and accessory muscles carry 70% of the respiratory effort and the diaphragm only 30%. Such role reversal both increases the overall cost of breathing and decreases the respiratory volume available for proper pulmonary ventilation. The diminished respiratory volume, in turn, generates a compensatory increase in respiratory rate. The result is a rapid, shallow breathing pattern that fails to make up for the decreased volume and generates air hunger. Air hunger disrupts the respiratory cycle and further diminishes adequate ventilation, because inhalation continually recommences before exhalation is complete. Breathing becomes panicky and uncoordinated, and the stricken individual constantly gasps for air. In order to approach adequate alveolar ventilation and improved gas exchange, as well as to decrease the cost of breathing, (1) the diaphragm must be assisted in its ascent so that it can resume its former work load and increase the available respiratory volume, and (2) the respiratory rate must be decreased to permit a coordinated and efficient breathing pattern.

The first step in the basic breathing exercises is to thoroughly master abdominal breathing,

Breathing Exercises

A. Basic abdominal breathing

Lie on back, legs drawn up, one hand on chest, other on abdomen, with thumb at or just below navel. Breathe in deeply through nose, letting abdomen protrude fully as felt by hand. Chest remains stationary. Breathe out slowly through pursed lips, abdomen drawing inward, assisted by hand pressure. Do for 3 min morning and evening, and after mastery without aid of hands. Also do exercise lying on each side with legs drawn up for 3 min

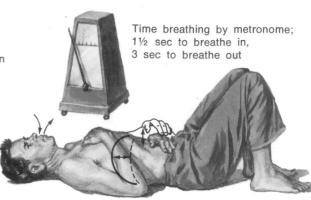

Time breathing by metronome; 1½ sec to breathe in, 3 sec to breathe out

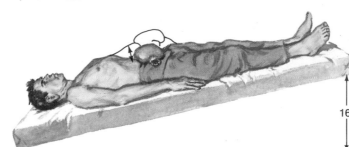

B. Abdominal weight exercise

Foot of bed raised about 16 in. About 1 lb weight (sandbag, hot water bottle, or book) on abdomen. Do basic breathing as in "A," pushing abdomen against weight when exhaling. Do for 5 to 10 min b.i.d. and every 3rd day add ½ lb to weight up to 5 lb. When it becomes easy, prolong exercise period gradually up to 10 min

16″

C. Candle blowing

Lighted candle on table, flame level with and about 5 in. from mouth. Blow gently through pursed lips using abdominal breathing as in "A," not extinguishing flame but bending it away. Do for 3 min at bedtime, increasing distance 3 to 4 in. nightly up to 3 ft. Then do standing up with flame raised to mouth level

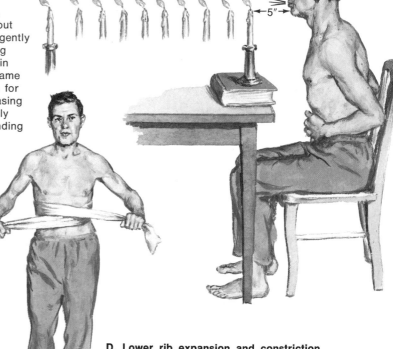

36″   5″

D. Lower rib expansion and constriction

Strip of cloth, 5 ft. long around lower ribs, ends crossed. Do basic breathing, letting belt out with inspiration and tightening it firmly on expiration. Do this sitting, then standing, and then walking around room. Take one step with inspiration and two with expiration. Practice until chest movement can be done without belt and without thinking about it

including pursed-lip exhalation. The latter trick both slows the respiratory rate and, by significantly prolonging the expiratory cycle, allows exhalation to continue to completion. The result is a relaxed and coordinated breathing pattern that makes optimal use of the available respiratory volume. Abdominal breathing with pursed-lip exhalation is then used during the abdominal weight and candle-blowing exercises. Abdominal breathing is initially taught for the head-down supine position, and mastery must occur first at that level and then progressively during sitting, standing and walking. Once this has been achieved, mastery of exercises involving lower costal breathing can proceed

in the same order of progress. It is advisable that a family member attend the initial training sessions so that the patient can be supervised in the exercises once he returns home.

It must be emphasized as strongly as possible to the patient that the practice of these exercises is not limited to the official training period. Since their purpose is to effect and then maintain significant changes in diaphragmatic function and in breathing pattern, they must be practiced conscientiously. Participation of a family member can aid in achieving this goal. Basic exercises and postural drainage are the mainstays of a home care physical therapy program.

Arterial Puncture for Blood Gas Analysis

Arterial Blood Gas Analysis

Analysis of arterial blood gases and determination of pH and base excess constitute the most important information to assist the clinical management of patients with respiratory and metabolic problems. The radial artery is preferred for obtaining blood; alternatively, the brachial and femoral arteries can be used.

Techniques of Arterial Puncture

For single-stick arterial blood punctures, the technique to be described can be employed by physicians, nurses, respiratory therapists and technicians. The material used includes a 5 ml glass syringe wetted with heparin solution (1000 units/ml) and attached to a 22 gauge 1 inch needle; a 2 ml plastic disposable syringe filled with a 2% lidocaine solution and fitted with a 25 gauge 9.5 inch needle; alcohol sponges; and a round toothpick.

The patient is preferably supine or semirecumbent, and the wrist is extended to about 45 degrees. The area over the radial artery 0.5 to 1 inch above the wrist crease is cleansed with alcohol and infiltrated with 1 to 2 ml of 2% lidocaine solution to make a skin wheal. The artery is palpated with the fingers of one hand and the 5 ml syringe and needle advanced gently with the other hand, so that it enters the artery at a 45 degree angle. Generally there is a paucity of veins and large nerve trunks in the vicinity. Occasionally penetration into the artery can be sensed by the operator, but puncture of the blood vessel is usually detected by slow entrance of blood into the syringe as a result of arterial pressure. Because of the small size of the needle, pulsations are generally damped. However, the syringe barrel will be forced backward by arterial but not by venous pressures. Plastic syringes should therefore not be used since their greater friction may hinder this movement. After 3 to 5 ml of blood is withdrawn, firm pressure is applied for about two minutes at the puncture site. If air bubbles are seen in the syringe, they are flushed out, with the syringe held vertically, since the entrapped air will alter the analysis. The needle is removed from the syringe and a round toothpick inserted in its place so that the blood is not exposed to the atmosphere. The specimen is immediately transported to the laboratory, preferably in ice, for analysis.

Gas Analysis

The pH is the negative logarithm of the hydrogen ion concentration and is normally fixed between 7.38 and 7.42. It is affected by a change in P_{CO_2} and accumulation of nonvolatile acids or bases.

Arterial oxygen tension (Pa_{O_2}) is measured by a polarographic apparatus which consists of a cell

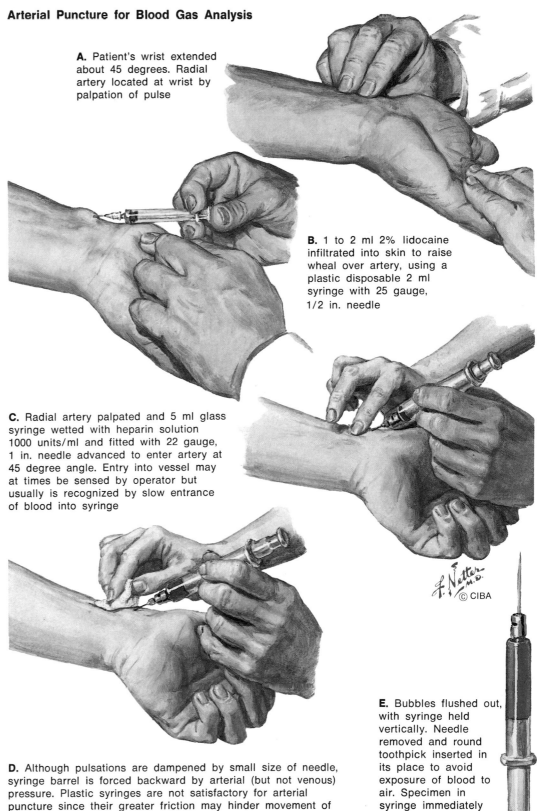

A. Patient's wrist extended about 45 degrees. Radial artery located at wrist by palpation of pulse

B. 1 to 2 ml 2% lidocaine infiltrated into skin to raise wheal over artery, using a plastic disposable 2 ml syringe with 25 gauge, 1/2 in. needle

C. Radial artery palpated and 5 ml glass syringe wetted with heparin solution 1000 units/ml and fitted with 22 gauge, 1 in. needle advanced to enter artery at 45 degree angle. Entry into vessel may at times be sensed by operator but usually is recognized by slow entrance of blood into syringe

D. Although pulsations are dampened by small size of needle, syringe barrel is forced backward by arterial (but not venous) pressure. Plastic syringes are not satisfactory for arterial puncture since their greater friction may hinder movement of syringe barrel. When 3 to 5 ml blood has been collected, syringe is withdrawn and immediate pressure with gauze applied and maintained for about 2 minutes to prevent hematoma formation

E. Bubbles flushed out, with syringe held vertically. Needle removed and round toothpick inserted in its place to avoid exposure of blood to air. Specimen in syringe immediately placed in ice and transported to laboratory

formed by a silver anode and a platinum cathode, both in contact with an electrolyte in dilute solution. If about 700 mv is applied to the cell, a current develops that is directly proportional to the oxygen tension of the electrolyte in the region of the cathode. The electrolyte is separated from the blood sample by a thin membrane permeable to oxygen and thus attains the same tension; the current passed is proportional to the blood oxygen tension. In young normal adults Pa_{O_2} is greater than 90 mm Hg, but in the elderly it may be as low as 70 mm Hg in the absence of disease. The reason is that basal airway closure occurs in the aged in the presence of adequate perfusion and results in

right-to-left intrapulmonary shunt. Arterial oxygen tension may be reduced by ventilation-perfusion defects, right-to-left shunts, alveolar hypoventilation, and limitations to the diffusion of oxygen. The breathing of 100% oxygen usually raises the Pa_{O_2} to over 550 mm Hg. Lesser values of Pa_{O_2} during this procedure indicate a right-to-left shunt, but it should be appreciated that quantitation is extremely dependent on cardiac output, particularly at low levels of arterial oxygen tension. For example, a Pa_{O_2} of 100 mm Hg attained while breathing 100% oxygen and with a normal oxygen capacity of hemoglobin would be associated with a

(Continued)

Arterial Blood Gas Analysis
(Continued)

right-to-left shunt of 14% in the presence of a low cardiac output (pulmonary arteriovenous oxygen difference of 10 volumes/100 ml), while with a high cardiac output (pulmonary arteriovenous oxygen difference of 2.5 volumes/100 ml) the shunt would have to be 38%. Thus a high cardiac output can minimize the effect of a large right-to-left shunt.

The oxygen saturation is the percentage of the content of oxygen in the arterial blood relative to the oxygen capacity of hemoglobin and is normally greater than 96%. Although it was measured by manometric techniques in the past, it is usually either calculated from the Pa_{O_2}, pH and a standard oxyhemoglobin dissociation curve or measured directly by spectrophotometric methods. In the presence of an abnormal hemoglobin such as carboxyhemoglobin, the oxygen saturation calculated from the Pa_{O_2} will be spuriously high since oxygen tension is unaltered. However, a spectrophotometric determination will be accurate and indicate the discrepancy between a normal Pa_{O_2} and a reduced saturation. Because of the sigmoid nature of the oxyhemoglobin dissociation curve, there may be a considerable fall in Pa_{O_2} with minimal change in oxygen saturation. For example, with a normal pH, Pa_{O_2} must fall to 60 mm Hg before the saturation drops from 96 to 89%. In addition, for a given Pa_{O_2}, oxygen saturation is higher for an alkaline than an acid pH.

Arterial carbon dioxide tension (Pa_{CO_2}) is determined with a P_{CO_2}-sensitive electrode. The P_{CO_2} of a film of bicarbonate solution is allowed to equilibrate with that of blood across a membrane permeable to carbon dioxide. The pH of the bicarbonate solution is constantly monitored with a glass electrode, and the log of the P_{CO_2} is inversely proportional to the recorded pH. The partial pressure of carbon dioxide in the arterial blood ranges from 38 to 42 mm Hg and is inversely related to alveolar ventilation. Hypercapnia ($Pa_{CO_2} > 42$ mm Hg) is due to hypoventilation; hypocapnia ($Pa_{CO_2} < 38$ mm Hg), to hyperventilation.

Base excess is defined as zero for a blood pH of 7.40 and a Pa_{CO_2} of 40 mm Hg. Theoretically it can be determined by titration of the blood to a pH of 7.40 at a Pa_{CO_2} of 40 mm Hg and a temperature of 38°C, but in practice it is calculated from a nomogram relating values for pH, Pa_{CO_2} and hemoglobin concentration. Positive base excess values (> 2.5 mEq/liter) are present in a metabolic alkalosis, whereas negative base excess or base deficit values (< -2.5 mEq/liter) indicate a metabolic acidosis. *In vivo* carbon dioxide–buffering studies indicate that the base excess is lower than that calculated *in vitro* because of the presence of buffers in the extracellular fluid. However, from a clinical standpoint this discrepancy does not seem great enough to mitigate against the value of applying base excess as the indicator of metabolic and Pa_{CO_2} of respiratory acid-base disturbances.

Interpretation of Arterial Blood Gas Analysis

To describe the acid-base disturbance, one notes the value for blood pH first. An elevated value of pH—*i.e.,* greater than 7.42—indicates alkalosis; a value less than 7.38 indicates acidosis. A low value of Pa_{CO_2}—*i.e.,* less than 38 mm Hg—indicates hyperventilation while a value greater than 42 mm Hg denotes hypoventilation. A high pH and low Pa_{CO_2} signify respiratory alkalosis; a low pH and high Pa_{CO_2}, respiratory acidosis. Positive base excess, which usually implies bicarbonate accumulation, together with a high pH indicates metabolic alkalosis, while a negative base excess with a low pH shows metabolic acidosis. Respiratory and metabolic disturbances may occur simultaneously, or one disturbance may be primary and the other compensatory. Under such circumstances a clinical history leading up to the arterial blood gas determination must be taken into account.

Compensation by the body is an attempt to adjust the arterial pH to 7.40. Respiratory compensation to metabolic disturbances may occur within minutes whereas renal adjustments to hypoventilation and hyperventilation take at least 8 to 24 hours to develop. The respiratory response to metabolic acidosis—*i.e.,* a low pH and a base deficit—is hyperventilation, and the adjustment to a pH of 7.40 may be complete or partial. Metabolic alkalosis is characterized by an elevation in pH and a base excess, but respiratory compensation is usually only partial to a Pa_{CO_2} of about 47 mm Hg in individuals with normal lungs, because hypoventilation leads to hypoxemia. In patients with chronic hypoxemia, Pa_{CO_2} may reach 55 mm Hg. Acute respiratory acidosis is typified by a low pH and elevated Pa_{CO_2}; base excess may initially be negative because coexistent hypoxemia leads to accumulation of lactic acid. The kidney compensates for the respiratory acidosis over an 8 to 24 hour period by retention of bicarbonate as manifested by a positive base excess. Respiratory alkalosis—*i.e.,* high pH and low Pa_{CO_2}—is slowly compensated by the kidneys through excretion of base.

Respiratory Alkalosis. The most common cause of acute respiratory alkalosis is anxiety reaction with hyperventilation. The diagnosis is established by the findings of a high pH, low Pa_{CO_2} and normal base excess in the presence of a normal Pa_{O_2}. Although the normal arterial oxygen tension helps to establish the diagnosis of this acid-base disorder, many patients with chronic pulmonary diseases also overbreathe as a result of anxiety, and clinical examination is necessary to substantiate the diagnosis. In status asthmaticus the most frequent acid-base disturbance is acute respiratory alkalosis with hypoxemia due to ventilation-perfusion upset. Cerebrovascular accidents may be associated with either hyperventilation or hypoventilation. In postoperative atelectasis, hypoxemia is usually combined with respiratory alkalosis. Also, such drugs as progesterone, salicylates and prochlorperazine may cause stimulation of the respiratory center with marked hyperventilation and the same acid-base abnormality. Restrictive lung diseases—pulmonary fibrosis, for example—are characterized by hypoxemia and a partially compensated fall in hydrogen ion concentration from the high minute

ventilation present. In congestive heart failure, there is often combined respiratory and metabolic alkalosis. The latter is due to salt restriction and diuretic therapy. With multiple pulmonary emboli or primary pulmonary hypertension, chronic respiratory alkalosis and a negative base excess are found, along with minimal resting hypoxemia. Gram-negative bacteremia is likely to be associated with a rapid respiratory rate even without fever. Systemic hypotension may cause hyperventilation, usually in association with metabolic acidosis. Acute respiratory alkalosis may be produced iatrogenically through the use of mechanical ventilators.

Respiratory Acidosis. Acute respiratory acidosis is characterized by a low pH and an elevated Pa_{CO_2} and is due to alveolar hypoventilation. Arterial oxygen tension is low if the patient is breathing room air but may be normal or elevated if supplementary oxygen is used. It commonly occurs after an overdose of sedatives and frequently can be rapidly reversed by mechanical ventilators without resort to intravenous administration of sodium bicarbonate if metabolic acidosis is not also present. Respiratory acidosis may worsen with oxygen-breathing because a Pa_{O_2} above 50 mm Hg depresses the neuronal activities of the carotid body chemoreceptors, an important secondary source of respiratory stimulation when the respiratory center is depressed by elevation of Pa_{CO_2}. The acute form may be superimposed on a chronic respiratory acidosis (elevation of Pa_{CO_2} and base excess and acid pH) as a result of infection, sedation or congestive heart failure. Under such circumstances the goal of therapy is slow correction to a normal pH over several hours. Combined respiratory and metabolic acidosis occurs in about 25% of patients with pulmonary edema associated with arteriosclerotic heart disease, and when the pH is less than 7.25, both mechanical ventilation and administration of intravenous sodium bicarbonate are indicated.

Metabolic Alkalosis. This condition is frequently the result of diuretic therapy, corticosteroid administration, and large losses of gastrointestinal fluids. It is often seen in association with hypokalemia. The primary compensation for it is hypoventilation in order to effect an elevation in Pa_{CO_2}. However, increasing degrees of hypoventilation diminish Pa_{O_2}, and therefore complete respiratory compensation for a severe metabolic alkalosis rarely takes place. This form of alkalosis can also be produced by excessive sodium bicarbonate administration, particularly in the treatment of cardiac arrest, in which it is often necessary to begin emergency resuscitation prior to knowledge of the arterial blood gas analysis.

Metabolic Acidosis. The chief cause of metabolic acidosis is renal insufficiency. With mild degrees, the lungs can completely compensate to a pH of 7.40 by lowering the Pa_{CO_2}. It occurs in diabetic coma and occasionally in association with phenformin ingestion as a result of lactic acid accumulation. Necrosis of abdominal viscera due to acute pancreatitis, mesenteric embolus and shock, for example, is accompanied by marked metabolic acidosis generally refractory to sodium bicarbonate administration. Cardiac arrest is almost always accompanied by acidosis of this type. Near-drowning in either salt or fresh water is frequently associated with severe metabolic acidosis and hypoxemia and occasionally with coexisting respiratory acidosis.

Oxygen Therapy in Acute Respiratory Failure

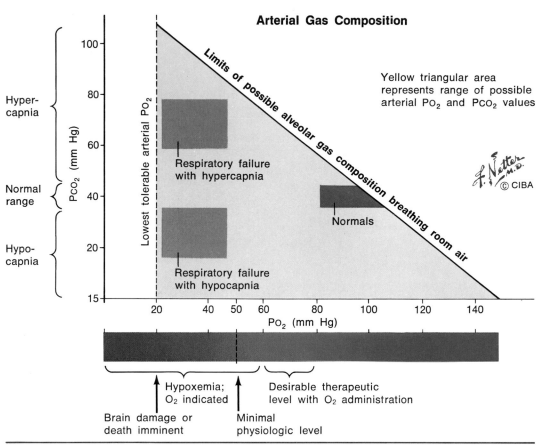

Arterial Gas Composition

Yellow triangular area represents range of possible arterial PO_2 and PCO_2 values

Arterial Blood Gas Composition. In patients with chronic bronchitis and emphysema, acute respiratory failure is usually due to infection, retained secretions, heart failure or some combination thereof. These patients are usually severely hypoxemic (with an arterial oxygen tension [Pa_{O_2}] of 20 to 40 mm Hg), have only moderate hypercapnia (with an arterial carbon dioxide tension [Pa_{CO_2}] of 60 to 80 mm Hg), and have mild respiratory acidosis. Most patients are alert or arousable, have a preserved cough reflex and may not need mechanical ventilation.

The blood gas findings can be explained by the carbon dioxide:oxygen diagram shown at the top of the illustration. Since there is no uptake or excretion of nitrogen during respiration and the alveolar partial pressure of water vapor is a function of body temperature only, there is a reciprocal relationship between the alveolar PCO_2 and PO_2, as indicated by the alveolar gas composition line. As prolonged survival is not possible when the Pa_{O_2} is less than 20 mm Hg, the range of arterial gas tensions compatible with life is confined to the yellow triangle. Initial arterial blood gas values of air-breathing patients with decompensated chronic obstructive pulmonary disease (COPD) will fall in the upper shaded area. With higher oxygen concentrations the alveolar gas composition line is shifted to the right, and much higher Pa_{CO_2} values are possible.

Fortunately, due to the shape of the hemoglobin dissociation curve, only a small rise in oxygen tension is necessary to produce a marked increase in arterial oxygen content. In most patients a 15 mm Hg increase in arterial oxygen tension can be produced by raising the inspired oxygen fraction by only 4 to 7%. This increase in Pa_{O_2} is associated with minimal carbon dioxide retention but the use of higher oxygen concentrations can cause severe hypercapnia. Administration of low oxygen concentrations (24 to 35%) can be achieved by use of a Venturi mask or nasal cannula (Plate 24). Hypoxemic patients with mild COPD, asthma and pulmonary fibrosis may have a low Pa_{CO_2}, and higher concentrations of oxygen may be safely administered in such cases.

Until the patient's clinical and arterial blood gas response to oxygen therapy has been evaluated, oxygen should not be interrupted because the body's unequal storage capacity for oxygen and carbon dioxide can result in a rapid fall in alveolar oxygen tension. Intermittent positive pressure breathing (IPPB) should be given with compressed air rather than oxygen in patients who retain carbon dioxide. Rapid lowering of the Pa_{CO_2} should be avoided, since this can produce alkalosis and a reduction of cerebral blood flow.

Care and Monitoring During Oxygen Therapy. While measurement of arterial blood gases is of prime importance in patients receiving

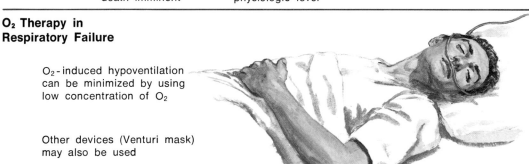

O₂ Therapy in Respiratory Failure

O₂-induced hypoventilation can be minimized by using low concentration of O₂

Other devices (Venturi mask) may also be used

Ear Oximetry

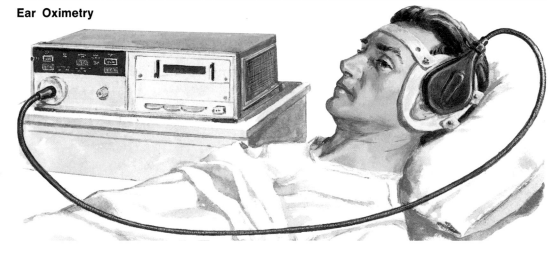

oxygen for respiratory failure, a reduction in cardiac output, hemoglobin concentration or local blood flow, a shift in position of the oxygen dissociation curve, or an increase in tissue requirements can result in inadequate oxygen delivery to the tissues even if the Pa_{O_2} is normal. Although there is no specific way to assess the level of tissue oxygenation, tissue hypoxia probably exists if the mixed venous PO_2 is less than 35 mm Hg. Monitoring and correcting abnormalities of cardiovascular function and hemoglobin concentration will minimize tissue hypoxia.

Oxygen requirements may change during therapy, and a patient's respiratory, cardiovascular

and mental status should be evaluated often. Patients should be observed during sleep, when their breathing patterns may be different. Sedation is to be avoided.

Recently, ear oximetry has become popular for indirect assessment of arterial oxygen saturation. Modern ear oximeters are reliable and do not require a blood sample for calibration. Although ear oximetry gives no indication of Pa_{O_2}, hemoglobin concentration or local blood flow, it is sometimes useful to continuously monitor relative changes in oxygen saturation. Ear oximetry may also be used to assess exercise hypoxia and the effects of supplementary oxygen administration.

Methods of Oxygen Administration

Various types of oxygen masks, cannulas and tents are available. With a flow rate of 6 to 10 liters/minute of 100% oxygen, it is possible to achieve inspired oxygen concentrations (F_{IO_2}) of 25 to 95%. The actual F_{IO_2} depends on the system used and the oxygen flow rate relative to the patient's demand and rate of ventilation.

The *simple mask* fits over the mouth and nose, and exhaled gas escapes via side ports. Carbon dioxide may accumulate if the oxygen flow rate is too low. Simple masks deliver an F_{IO_2} of 35 to 50% with a flow rate of 6 to 10 liters/minute. The *partial rebreathing mask* is similar to the simple mask, but has a reservoir bag. On inspiration, oxygen from the bag is mixed with air entering via the exhalation ports. The oxygen flow rate is adjusted so that the bag does not collapse with inspiration; most of the exhaled gas escapes via exhalation ports. Partial rebreathing masks deliver an F_{IO_2} of 50 to 70% with an oxygen flow rate of 6 to 10 liters/minute. The *nonrebreathing mask* is a modification of the partial rebreathing mask and incorporates one-way valves between the mask and the reservoir bag and at the exhalation ports. Thus, oxygen is inspired only from the bag, while exhaled gas may escape only via the ports. The oxygen flow rate is adjusted so that the bag does not collapse. The nonrebreathing mask can deliver an F_{IO_2} of up to 95%. The *rebreathing mask* is a closed-circuit system incorporating a carbon dioxide absorber and is used only for anesthesia administration. The *face tent* or shield is equipped with large-bore tubing, and is used to administer supplemental oxygen (40 to 70%) together with high humidity, and for aerosol therapy. The *Venturi mask* (see below) is used to deliver a *fixed* low concentration (24 to 40%) of oxygen.

The *nasal catheter* or oropharyngeal catheter, so called because its tip lies in the oropharynx, is not in common use. The nasal catheter delivers about 30 to 50% oxygen at 6 to 8 liters/minute. The *nasal cannula* (nasal prongs) is perhaps the most common mode of oxygen delivery, and can provide 30 to 50% oxygen with flow rates of 6 to 8 liters/minute; higher flow rates may cause nasal irritation. The nasal cannula and Venturi mask are best suited for administering the low concentrations of oxygen necessary to minimize carbon dioxide retention in patients with COPD.

The *Venturi mask* works on the principle of air entrainment; 100% oxygen is directed through a tube in a center jet stream which pulls in room air through side ports. The relative amounts of air and oxygen are determined by the size of the jet and side ports. Venturi masks deliver oxygen concentrations of 24, 28, 35 or 40%. The amount of air entrained by the Venturi mask is high, and this flushes the environment around the patient's face—preventing rebreathing—and maintains a fixed oxygen concentration over a wide range of oxygen flow rates and independent of the patient's rate of ventilation, thus minimizing the danger of inadvertently supplying too much oxygen. Disadvantages of the Venturi and other masks include difficulty with talking, eating, washing, expectoration and administration of aerosol medications.

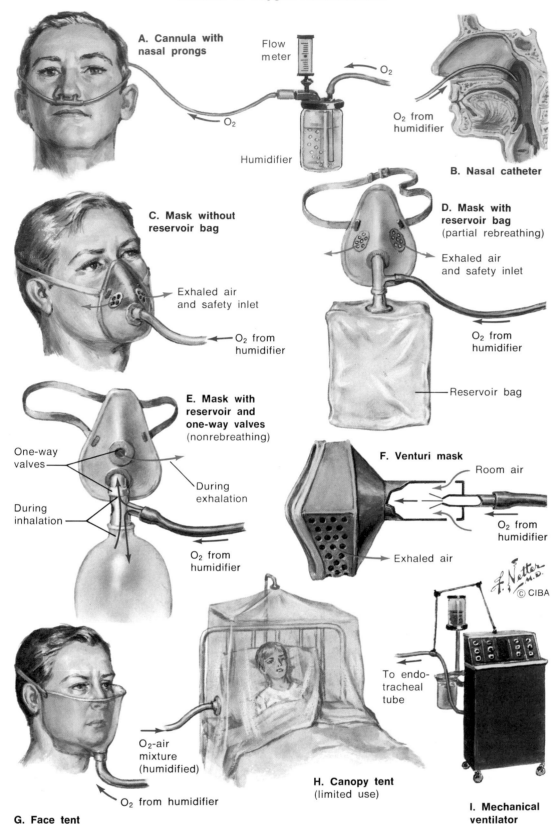

A. Cannula with nasal prongs

Flow meter

O_2

O_2

Humidifier

B. Nasal catheter

O_2 from humidifier

C. Mask without reservoir bag

Exhaled air and safety inlet

O_2 from humidifier

D. Mask with reservoir bag (partial rebreathing)

Exhaled air and safety inlet

O_2 from humidifier

Reservoir bag

E. Mask with reservoir and one-way valves (nonrebreathing)

One-way valves

During exhalation

During inhalation

O_2 from humidifier

F. Venturi mask

Room air

O_2 from humidifier

Exhaled air

G. Face tent

O_2-air mixture (humidified)

O_2 from humidifier

H. Canopy tent (limited use)

To endotracheal tube

I. Mechanical ventilator

Since the Venturi mask delivers a fixed low oxygen concentration, it is ideal for the *initial* treatment of almost all spontaneously breathing patients who require supplementary oxygen. The Venturi mask should be used by paramedical personnel as the first approach to oxygen therapy in emergency rooms and by rescue squads. After the arterial blood gas analysis is available, another form of oxygen therapy may be substituted.

Use of a nasal cannula to administer 100% oxygen at flow rates of 1 to 3 liters/minute is a reasonable alternative to the Venturi mask for administering low concentrations of oxygen. The nasal cannula is more comfortable and does not interfere with eating, washing or expectorating. However, the actual F_{IO_2} depends on the amount of flow relative to the patient's demand and the amount of air taken in through the mouth or nose.

Other less common types of oxygen delivery available include *tents,* which are most frequently used to provide children with oxygen concentrations of up to 50% and to allow for control of temperature and humidity, and the *hood,* which fits over the head and neck and is useful for achieving higher oxygen concentrations. The *T tube* and *tracheostomy collar* (also available in a Venturi mode) are used to deliver supplementary oxygen to patients with tracheostomies (Plate 26).

Ambulatory and Home Use of Oxygen

Short-Term Oxygen Therapy. Patients with stable chronic obstructive pulmonary disease (COPD) have increased requirements for oxygen during sleep, exercise and air travel, or at high altitude. Insomnia, headaches or irritability may indicate nocturnal hypoxemia. During exercise, oxygen improves tolerance in patients with COPD and may reduce exercise-induced pulmonary hypertension. Patients with a resting Pa_{O_2} of 55 mm Hg or less may benefit from supplementary oxygen, but hypoxemia and relief by oxygen should be demonstrated first.

Continuous Oxygen Therapy. Administration of oxygen for 15 to 24 hours each day, in low concentrations via a nasal cannula (1 to 3 liters/minute) or Venturi mask (24 to 28% oxygen), for periods longer than four weeks is generally regarded as continuous "low flow" oxygen therapy. Complications are minimal, and many patients with COPD derive beneficial effects, including improved pulmonary hemodynamics, exercise tolerance and neuropsychiatric status, as well as reduced hemoglobin concentration, better control of congestive heart failure, and fewer hospital admissions despite no change in pulmonary function. It is not known whether mortality is reduced.

Long-term oxygen therapy is controversial and expensive, and careful selection of patients is important. Patients with severe exertional dyspnea, recurrent congestive heart failure, marked polycythemia, impaired mental function, and restlessness or insomnia are likely to benefit, while patients with a Pa_{O_2} greater than 55 mm Hg at rest and during exercise probably will not. The following criteria should be met before a patient is committed to continuous oxygen therapy: (1) demonstration of severe airway obstruction by pulmonary function tests; (2) in-hospital trial of all types of respiratory care, including stopping of smoking, control of secretions, infection and congestive heart failure, and maximum bronchodilator therapy; (3) signs and symptoms of hypoxemia, including polycythemia, pulmonary hypertension and exercise intolerance relieved by oxygen; (4) resting hypoxemia less than 55 mm Hg.

Patients living at high altitude should consider moving to sea level; patients with hypoxemia at rest with an FEV_1 of less than 1 liter after treatment with bronchodilators will probably benefit.

Sources of Ambulatory and Home Oxygen. Compressed gas cylinders and liquid oxygen are most widely used for home therapy. The liquid oxygen reservoir contains approximately 14,000 liters of oxygen, which supplies about 110 hours of 100% oxygen at a flow rate of 2 liters/minute. Two standard-sized H cylinders, at 2200 psi, contain a similar amount. Because of evaporation, the liquid oxygen reservoir loses about 5% or 700 liters of oxygen in 24 hours. Thus, if it is used intermittently, less oxygen will be available.

Recently, several oxygen concentrator systems have become available that separate oxygen from room air with a molecular sieve bed. The units are designed like furniture, do not require refilling, but need a continuous source of electricity. Maintenance requirements are uncertain at this time but

Ambulatory and Home Use Oxygen Equipment

Walker system employing liquid O_2

Walker system employing O_2 gas

Mask or nasal prongs may be used with any apparatus depicted here

Home refill reservoir of liquid O_2 for walker. May also be used for O_2 supply at home in place of tank (as below)

Duo-pak with extra O_2 gas cylinder for longer use or when one cylinder is being refilled

Flow meter (l O_2/min)

Tank pressure

O_2 tank equipment

Long tube permits mobility around home

Apparatus concentrates O_2 from atmosphere

appear to be minimal. The units are somewhat noisy and intermittently make a peculiar "sighing" noise. Most units have power-failure alarms; some have oxygen concentration monitors; most do not have emergency power sources, and a reserve oxygen tank is recommended. The oxygen concentration delivered by the units varies with the flow rate, ranging from 80 to 90% at 2 liters/minute to 40 to 50% at 10 liters/minute.

Portable oxygen delivery systems improve patient mobility and are useful in emergencies. The two basic portable systems use liquid oxygen or small compressed gas cylinders. Most units weigh between 7 and 10 pounds, may be carried by the

patient with a shoulder strap, and deliver between 50 and 200 minutes of oxygen at a flow rate of 2 liters/minute. The main advantage of the liquid oxygen walker is a relatively large amount of oxygen for its weight. The walker unit may be refilled from a large reservoir, which also may be used at home. The walker loses about 150 liters of oxygen from evaporation over 24 hours, impairing range and storage capability.

Portable compressed gas tanks contain less oxygen for a given weight, are somewhat less expensive, easier to use and relatively maintenance-free, and may be stored indefinitely. Some models can be refilled from universally available large cylinders.

Mechanical Ventilation

Indications. Although various physiologic criteria for tracheal intubation and mechanical ventilation have been proposed, the decision to institute this form of support must include *clinical* assessment of the patient and his *sensorium.* Regardless of the physiologic abnormalities, few alert patients require mechanical ventilation. If there is *progression* of hypoxemia and acidosis or if the patient becomes unresponsive or somnolent, it is indicated.

Goals. The main goal of mechanical ventilation is to maintain the patient's oxygenation and acid-base balance in a physiologic range. The $F_{I_{O_2}}$ should be kept as low as possible to maintain Pa_{O_2} in the range of 60 to 80 mm Hg. The Pa_{CO_2} should not be lowered too rapidly since alkalosis, tetany, seizures, cardiac arrhythmias, reduced cerebral blood flow and a shift of the hemoglobin dissociation curve to the left may result.

Ventilators and Delivery of Ventilation. Most ventilators deliver intermittent positive pressure (IPPB) to the airway during inspiration. The *pressure-limited* ventilator delivers positive pressure until a preset airway pressure is reached, and the amount of ventilation delivered will vary if the mechanical properties of the lung change. The *constant volume* ventilator, which delivers a preset volume up to a preset pressure limit, is more flexible, allows better control of $F_{I_{O_2}}$, and delivers the same volume if the mechanical properties of the lung change. The inspired gas should be warmed, humidified and sterile.

Positive end-expiratory pressure (PEEP) is a variation of IPPB, wherein at the end of exhalation a positive pressure (usually 5 to 20 cm H_2O) is maintained in the airways. This results in a higher lung volume, minimizes airway closure and atelectasis, and improves gas exchange. PEEP is most useful in patients with the adult respiratory distress syndrome (ARDS, shock lung).

Care and Monitoring of Patients. The patient's general medical and respiratory status must be continuously assessed.

There should be repeated physical examinations, monitoring of vital signs, and measurement of fluid intake and output. Ventilator settings, clinical observations and appropriate laboratory values should be recorded on a *flow sheet* along with spontaneous breathing rate, volume and vital capacity. $F_{I_{O_2}}$ must be monitored continuously. The most useful studies are arterial blood gas-pH analyses and the chest x-ray examination. The hoses and humidifier should be changed daily. Every one to two hours tracheal cuff deflation, suctioning and draining of condensation in the ventilator tubing should be done and the patient's position changed. Aseptic techniques in airway care must be observed and an extra sterile endotracheal or tracheostomy tube kept at the bedside.

Tracheostomy should be considered if mechanical ventilation is needed for more than three days.

If mechanical ventilation is prolonged, adequate nutrition must be provided and may be given through a nasogastric tube or feeding gastrostomy, or by intravenous hyperalimentation. Skin care is

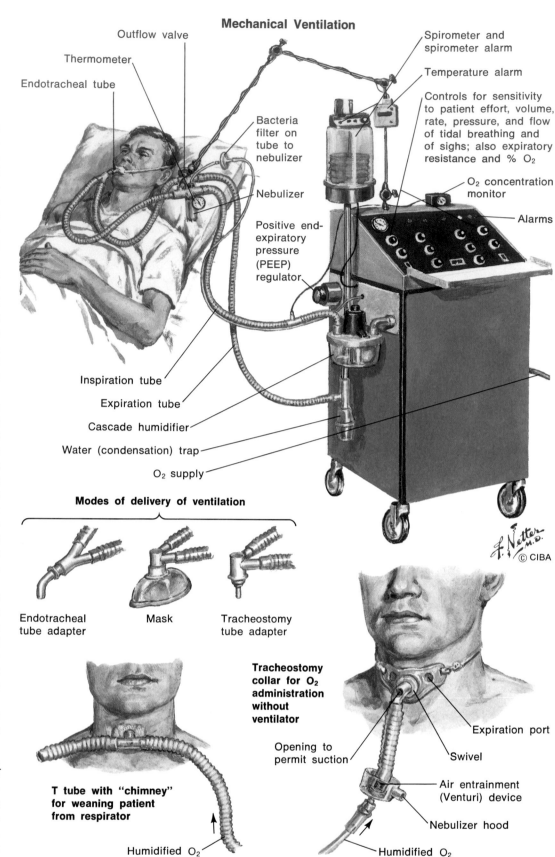

Mechanical Ventilation

Outflow valve
Thermometer
Endotracheal tube
Bacteria filter on tube to nebulizer
Nebulizer
Positive end-expiratory pressure (PEEP) regulator
Inspiration tube
Expiration tube
Cascade humidifier
Water (condensation) trap
O_2 supply

Spirometer and spirometer alarm
Temperature alarm
Controls for sensitivity to patient effort, volume, rate, pressure, and flow of tidal breathing and of sighs; also expiratory resistance and % O_2
O_2 concentration monitor
Alarms

F. Netter M.D. © CIBA

Modes of delivery of ventilation

Endotracheal tube adapter
Mask
Tracheostomy tube adapter

T tube with "chimney" for weaning patient from respirator

Humidified O_2

Tracheostomy collar for O_2 administration without ventilator

Opening to permit suction
Expiration port
Swivel
Air entrainment (Venturi) device
Nebulizer hood
Humidified O_2

important, and padding should be applied to the elbows, heels and knees. Paralyzed or comatose patients on long-term mechanical ventilation should have passive-range motion exercises.

Psychological aspects of caring for patients on mechanical ventilation cannot be overemphasized. Patients are under extreme physical and emotional stress and are unable to communicate effectively. Although many may seem unconscious or poorly responsive, they may be quite aware of their surroundings and able to hear conversation. It is important to treat them kindly, offer repeated assurance, and periodically attempt to communicate with them.

Sudden deterioration of a patient on mechanical ventilation may be manifested by tachypnea, agitation, cyanosis, hypotension or a cardiac arrhythmia. Causes include electric or mechanical failure of or disconnection from the ventilator, air leaks, obstruction of an endotracheal or tracheostomy tube, bronchospasm, retained secretions, pneumothorax and pulmonary embolism.

Complications. Other common complications include infection, hypotension, fluid overload, ARDS, oxygen toxicity, cardiac arrhythmias, gastrointestinal bleeding, acute gastric or cecal dilatation, ileus, acid-base/fluid-electrolyte imbalance, and emotional problems.

Mediastinotomy and Mediastinoscopy

Surgical ablation is the only known cure for bronchogenic carcinoma. To be effective, resection must be performed under appropriate circumstances: not only must the patient be able to tolerate the required operation but the cancer must be sufficiently well localized for complete surgical removal. For this reason staging or definition of the extent of the tumor is essential.·

Staging in Managment of Carcinoma of Lung. For the modern thoracic specialist, the selection of patients for lung cancer operations involves a definition and an assessment of certain discriminating factors related to the primary tumor and its lymphatic and hematogenous metastases. In recent years an effective and meaningful system for staging lung cancer has evolved, largely through the efforts of the American Joint Committee for Cancer Staging and End Results Reporting.

Essentially, the system is based on the summation of statistically significant risk factors expressed in terms of a code designation: T-N-M. T refers to risk factors related to the primary lung tumor itself. N refers to the status of the regional lymphatic drainage system of the primary lung cancer. M refers to the tumor status in terms of definable distant (hematogenous) metastasis. Thus, by summation of T-N-M risk factors, various stages of lung cancer can be defined.

Surgical Evaluation of Regional Lymphatic System. Of particular interest is the surgical investigation of the lymphatic drainage of the lung (see pages 32 and 33) as it relates to data collection for clinical staging prior to thoracotomy and resection. The lymphatic drainage system provides distinct predictable routes or pathways for the spread of malignancies from each lobe of the lung to the hilus and up the mediastinum to the base of the neck. Daniels is credited with early surgical attempts to assess this lymphatic system, which were restricted to the exploration of the supraclavicular prescalene space to define the terminal few centimeters of the system. Harken attempted to investigate the system retrograde through the lateral supraclavicular incision at the time of scalene node biopsy, but it was Carlens who devised the more direct approach to mediastinal lymphatics used today. Usually performed under general anesthesia, Carlens' *mediastinoscopy* involves a horizontal suprasternal low cervical skin incision to expose the lower cervical part of the trachea. Through this, either a cervical or a thoracic duct lymph node can be visualized, and biopsies can be performed by simple retraction of the incision to the right or left as specific conditions dictate. More often, however, the strap muscles are retracted from the midline, exposing the anterior aspect of the trachea in the neck. In the absence of thyroid enlargement, nothing need be done to the thyroid, although significant thyroid ima veins may require individual ligation and division in the midline to gain access to the trachea. Rare anomalies in brachiocephalic vessels should be kept in mind lest their presence confound or frustrate surgical dissection and

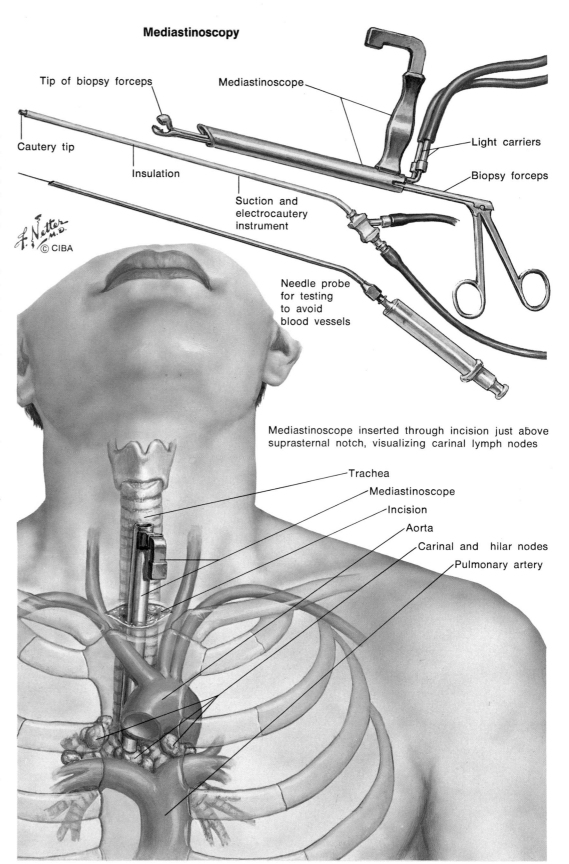

Mediastinoscopy

Tip of biopsy forceps
Mediastinoscope
Cautery tip
Light carriers
Insulation
Biopsy forceps
Suction and electrocautery instrument
Needle probe for testing to avoid blood vessels

Mediastinoscope inserted through incision just above suprasternal notch, visualizing carinal lymph nodes

Trachea
Mediastinoscope
Incision
Aorta
Carinal and hilar nodes
Pulmonary artery

exposure. With care, the pretracheal space is explored and dissected, the index finger being used to develop a midline pretracheal dissection plane from neck to tracheal bifurcation. Much information is to be gleaned through initial palpation of this developed tract. Usually, the presence and location of enlarged lymph nodes can best be identified by this means, as can their size, fixation and relation to neighboring structures. Indeed, one can detect the presence of significant abnormalities by palpation long before they are visualized by introduction of a lighted speculum or mediastinoscope. Futhermore, their localization by preliminary palpation will greatly facilitate

subsequent endoscopic dissection, visualization and biopsy.

Following digital development of a pretracheal tract and its careful digital exploration, the lighted speculum is introduced. If preliminary digital exploration is complete, the 'scope should advance without resistance or need for force. As with other endoscopic maneuvers, the lumen of the tract to be explored must be under direct vision as the instrument is advanced. To assure orientation, the anterior aspect of the trachea should be continually under direct vision. If further dissection is required to advance the 'scope *(Continued)*

Mediastinotomy and Mediastinoscopy
(Continued)

caudad, this is best accomplished by blunt dissection with either the rounded tip of a long rigid suction instrument or the closed jaw end of a pair of biopsy forceps. The latter has the added advantage of permitting the spread of soft tissues because its jaws can be opened during withdrawal. Bleeding can develop from minor injury to minute tracheal and bronchial vessels and requires suction clearing of blood from the operative field with electrocautery of bleeding sites. Massive bleeding can occur as a consequence of injury to major arteries or veins, but it can generally be controlled by packing the mediastinal space tightly with a long gauze pack and closing the cervical wound, thus leading to hemostasis or—if necessary—allowing enough time to perform the thoracotomy needed for repair of the blood vessels. Often the use of a long needle probe to detect major vessels prior to biopsy of a mass is extremely helpful. Although mediastinoscopy involves risk, information obtained may obviate the need for thoracotomy when resection for potential cure is clearly not feasible.

Debate continues regarding the indications for mediastinoscopy and how to interpret and utilize the information gained. Most physicians would agree that patients with clearly resectable clinical stage I cancers are unlikely to benefit from the examination. Almost all would concur in the view that a contralateral mediastinal lymph node metastasis or any metastasis fixed to adjacent structures is nonresectable. Less certain is the interpretation of ipsilateral, freely movable, intracapsular nodal metastases that might be included in a radical mediastinal lymph node dissection at the time of thoracotomy and lung resection. In these circumstances, more enthusiasm for resection might be evoked if the tumor is squamous cell in type, rather than large cell undifferentiated or adenocarcinoma. Still, current knowledge clearly defines mediastinal lymph nodal metastasis as stage III disease, and despite radical resection less than 10% of patients will experience long-term survival—a fact that certainly must be considered in selecting patients.

Mediastinoscopy should not be resorted to in the presence of clinically palpable cervical or scalene lymphadenopathy. Direct surgical biopsy of these nodes can be accomplished at minimal risk, and if malignancy is present, the assumption of inoperability is conclusive. Biopsy of the scalene nodes should not be carried out on patients with bronchogenic carcinoma when the nodes are not palpable. Furthermore, for a left upper lobe neoplasm, mediastinoscopy is less often definitive in establishing operability than is the case for left lower and right lung tumors.

For left upper lobe lesions the left anterior extrapleural *mediastinotomy* developed by Chamberlain has proved most helpful. This procedure, too, is usually performed under general anesthesia, often at the same time as mediastinoscopy, since it can be done without repositioning the patient. By wide preparation and draping of the

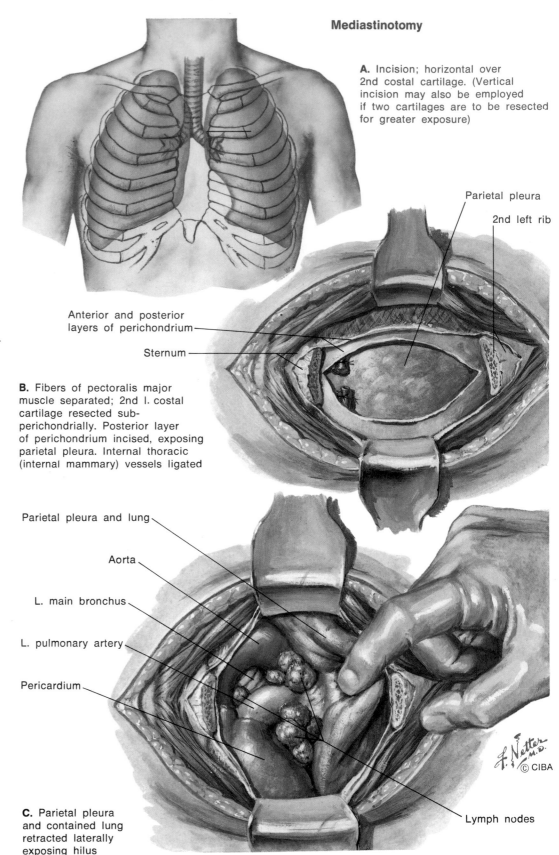

Mediastinotomy

A. Incision; horizontal over 2nd costal cartilage. (Vertical incision may also be employed if two cartilages are to be resected for greater exposure)

Parietal pleura

2nd left rib

Anterior and posterior layers of perichondrium

Sternum

B. Fibers of pectoralis major muscle separated; 2nd l. costal cartilage resected subperichondrially. Posterior layer of perichondrium incised, exposing parietal pleura. Internal thoracic (internal mammary) vessels ligated

Parietal pleura and lung

Aorta

L. main bronchus

L. pulmonary artery

Pericardium

Lymph nodes

C. Parietal pleura and contained lung retracted laterally exposing hilus

neck and anterior thorax, either one or both procedures can be done, depending on the particular circumstances.

Ordinarily, mediastinotomy is accomplished through a horizontal incision over the second anterior costal cartilage. Pectoralis muscle is separated in the direction of its fibers and retracted. The underlying costal cartilage is resected subperichondrially. The posterior perichondrium is incised horizontally in the axis of the major incision. Medially, this exposes the internal thoracic (internal mammary) artery and vein, which should be individually ligated and divided. The parietal pleura and contained lung can now be

dissected free of mediastinal connective tissue so that it may be retracted laterally to expose the root of the lung. Mediastinal lymph nodes overlying the left pulmonary artery, phrenic nerve and subaortic and low paratracheal areas are exposed, and a biopsy can readily be performed. Findings on mediastinotomy are interpreted in the same way as those detected by mediastinoscopy. Single-layer closure of the wound is effected at the end of the procedure.

It should be apparent that either of the foregoing methods can be selectively employed in the diagnosis of hilar or mediastinal adenopathy due to causes other than lung malignancy.

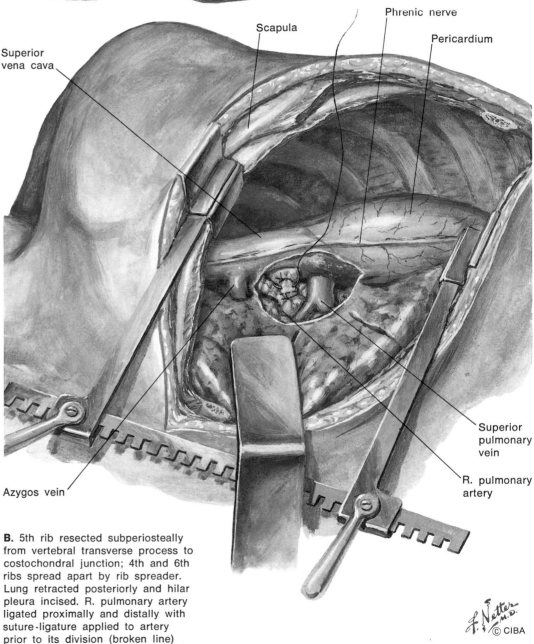

Pneumonectomy (Right Lung)

A. Patient in lateral recumbent position, inflatable bag or bolster under chest. Curved posterolateral ("hockey-stick") incision. Trapezius, latissimus dorsi, and rhomboid muscles will be divided and fibers of serratus anterior separated (postero-lateral thoracotomy)

Pneumonectomy

Superior vena cava

Scapula

Phrenic nerve

Pericardium

Superior pulmonary vein

R. pulmonary artery

Azygos vein

B. 5th rib resected subperiosteally from vertebral transverse process to costochondral junction; 4th and 6th ribs spread apart by rib spreader. Lung retracted posteriorly and hilar pleura incised. R. pulmonary artery ligated proximally and distally with suture-ligature applied to artery prior to its division (broken line)

Pneumonectomy was first successfully performed in 1933 by Evarts Graham. The procedure was carried out for bronchogenic carcinoma in a fellow physician who eventually outlived his surgeon. The event is a milestone in surgical history. The technique of pneumonectomy has been improved and standardized in the intervening years and the results are quite gratifying when the operation is carefully performed in appropriately selected cases. Current indications are chiefly as an operation for cure for lung cancer or for a destroyed lung derived from a variety of causes. Palliative pneumonectomy is generally not warranted unless it is directed at alleviation of sepsis or control of recurrent hemorrhage. Before embarking upon resection of an entire lung the surgeon must have a reasonably reliable assessment of the patient's cardiopulmonary reserve; little is gained if the pneumonectomized patient survives but only as a respiratory cripple.

While operability, in terms of ability to carry out a definitive surgical resection, may ultimately have to be determined by the results of a exploratory thoracotomy, the nonresectability rate has been reduced to an acceptably low level by currently available diagnostic techniques. Thus, the modern surgeon embarks upon thoracotomy more frequently than not with a known histologic diagnosis and a sophisticated understanding of cardiopulmonary function and extent of tumor involvement.

Pneumonectomy, as now practiced, is routinely performed via a standard posterolateral thoracotomy incision. The anterior approach has long

been abandoned because of inadequate access to critical hilar structures; the posterior approach, with the patient in a face-down or prone position—once favored because it afforded better control of secretions from the operative side—is no longer required, as a result of improvements in anesthesiologic control.

Posterolateral thoracotomy is performed with the patient securely fixed in a lateral recumbent position. An inflatable bag or bolster under the chest greatly improves access and exposure and is removed when it is time to close the incision. A curved "hockey stick" incision is made, starting midway between the vertebral border of the

scapula and the vertebral spines, clearing the angle of the scapula by at least two fingerbreadths and continuing forward in a transverse direction to a submammary position. The lower fibers of the trapezius and rhomboid muscles and the latissimus dorsi are divided, in the performance of which the use of electrocautery can be a timesaving maneuver. The serratus anterior fibers are divided and separated.

With exposure of the subscapular space the ribs are counted from above downward, using the origin of the serratus posterior superior muscle from the second rib as a starting point of reference.

(Continued)

Pneumonectomy, Right Lung (continued)

Superior vena cava

Phrenic nerve

C. R. pulmonary artery and superior pulmonary vein divided after ligature and suture - ligature, exposing r. main bronchus

Superior pulmonary vein

R. pulmonary artery

Pneumonectomy
(Continued)

D. Lung retracted superiorly, pulmonary ligament incised, exposing inferior pulmonary vein, which has been ligated and suture - ligated preparatory to division

E. R. main bronchus clamped distally and stapling device placed across it, close to carina (or is closed by over-end, nonabsorbable sutures). After driving staples home, bronchus is divided and lung removed

Resection of a rib, customarily the fifth, generally provides favorable exposure in older patients (who have a less resilient chest wall) and allows for a good airtight closure of the chest wall. The rib is subperiosteally resected from the transverse process (deep to the erector spinal muscles) posteriorly to the costal cartilage anteriorly. Insertion of a rib spreader provides the exposure illustrated, once any pleural adhesions present are divided.

At this point a biopsy and frozen section of the lesion may be in order, if a positive histologic diagnosis is not already available. The hilus is carefully studied by both visual examination and palpation for extension of tumor into the mediastinum—a sign of nonresectability. Infrequently, the pericardium has to be opened to complete this assessment. The superior mediastinum is similarly explored by entering via an incision through the parietal pleura dorsad to the superior vena cava. Suspicious lymph nodes may be removed and submitted for frozen section and, while nodes in this area may be removed with the lung, the presence of extensive mediastinal lymphatic spread bodes for a poor prognosis and may influence the surgeon's decision whether or not to remove the lung.

Once the lesion is evaluated as being resectable for cure, the lung is retracted posteriorly and inferiorly and the right main pulmonary artery exposed behind the lower superior vena cava. Division between ligatures, of the uppermost tributary of the right superior pulmonary vein, may facilitate exposure. The perivascular sheath is entered—a most important maneuver—and the artery is freed up by sharp and blunt dissection using a right-angle clamp. The artery is then divided between ligatures, leaving a long proximal stump.

The superior pulmonary vein is similarly freed up and divided, exposing the anterior aspect of the right main bronchus.

The lung is then retracted superiorly and anteriorly to expose the inferior pulmonary vein in its anatomic position along the superior margin of the inferior pulmonary ligament. This vessel too is exposed within its vascular sheath for a suitable extent and divided, leaving a long proximal stump after suitable proximal and distal ligation.

The right main bronchus is cleared and clamped after lymph nodes and areolar tissue have been swept distally. The bronchus is exposed to the level of the carina and a stapling device placed across it immediately below its origin. After the staples are driven home, the bronchus is amputated distal to the line of staple closure and the lung removed from the chest. The bronchial stump is then tested under saline for air leakage by having the anesthesiologist increase the intrabronchial pressure via his endotracheal tube. No attempt is made to cover or reinforce the bronchial stump closure, and with this technique stump leaks are uncommon.

Lobectomy

Lobectomy is a more difficult procedure to perform than pneumonectomy, particularly in the presence of chronic inflammatory changes or where tumor (or involved lymph nodes) occupies the lobar hilus. Not only must the critical lobar structures be identified and controlled by the operator but the remaining structures must be painstakingly protected and preserved. Incomplete fissures may add to the problem, and the surgeon must possess a precise knowledge of hilar anatomy and common anomalies.

The standard posterolateral thoracotomy approach is favored by most. Of historical interest is an early report on technique alleging that a proper dissection lobectomy could not be carried out for the left upper lobe, because an anterior thoracotomy incision was then being used.

Resection of the left upper lobe can be more difficult than a similar procedure on the right side. The main pulmonary artery is exposed as it emerges from beneath the arch of the aorta and care is exercised to avoid the recurrent nerve as it arises from the vagal trunk and passes beneath the aortic arch. In contrast to the right side, the artery passes behind the bronchus. The arterial branches of the main pulmonary artery may number five or more and there are considerable variations in their location. (Should a problem situation be anticipated, the main pulmonary artery should be freed up and an umbilical tape passed around it. Thus, should there be an arterial tear or hemorrhage later on, it becomes a simple matter to place a vascular clamp across the main vessel.)

The perivascular sheath surrounding the pulmonary artery is entered and, with the lobe drawn downward and backward, each arterial branch is dissected free with a right-angle clamp as it is encountered. The segmental artery is then ligated close to its point of origin. Once proximal ligation is accomplished, it is usually possible to dissect distally along the branch so that placement of the distal tie will permit leaving a long proximal stump when the branch artery is divided.

The first branch found is usually the apical posterior artery. Often segmental branch arteries have a common trunk.

The main artery is followed down the oblique fissure exposing its anterior and posterior aspects. The lowermost branches to the upper lobe supply the lingular and come off anteriorly. Directly opposite, on the posterior aspect of the continuing main pulmonary artery, the artery to the superior segment of the lower lobe takes origin, and this should be carefully preserved.

The lung is then retracted posteriorly for dissection of the superior pulmonary vein, which drains only the upper lobe on the left side. This vein is proximally and distally ligated and divided. A useful practice is to place a Cooley ductus clamp across the vein deep to the proximal liga-

Lobectomy (Left Upper Lobe)

Pericardium
Phrenic nerve
Superior pulmonary vein
L. main pulmonary artery
Aortic arch
Ligamentum arteriosum
Recurrent laryngeal nerve
Vagus nerve
Apical-posterior segmental artery

A. L. upper lobe retracted downward and backward; hilar pleura incised. Anterior and apical-posterior segmental arteries ligated, suture ligated and divided

B. Upper lobe retracted anteriorly and downward, opening fissure. Segmental arteries successively ligated and divided from above downward with care to preserve superior segmental artery of lower lobe

Lingular artery
Anterior segmental artery
Apical posterior segmental artery
Basal arteries
Superior segmental artery of lower lobe

C. Lung again drawn downward and superior pulmonary vein doubly ligated and divided

D. Upper lobe bronchus clamped preparatory to division and stapling close to its origin (as indicated by broken line), thus freeing upper lobe for removal

ture before dividing the vein, and then ligating the vein again beneath this clamp after division.

Once dissection of the fissures is completed, the lung is left attached only by the bronchus, which is cleared by sweeping lymph nodes and connective tissue distally. An atraumatic bronchial clamp is then placed across the bronchus, and the anesthesiologist is asked to inflate the lung. Correct identification of the bronchus clamped is assured when the lower lobe inflates and the upper remains collapsed. Release of the clamp is followed by inflation of the upper lobe. Despite the confidence of the surgeon in his dissection and perception of the anatomy, this simple maneuver,

requiring only a few moments, may avoid considerable trouble later on.

The stapling device is then placed across the bronchus close to its origin and the bronchus is amputated after stapling.

When an upper lobe lobectomy is performed for cancer, the mediastinum should be opened and all lymph nodes cleared to the carina (or beyond) if suspicion of lymphatic metastasis exists. When an upper lobectomy is a feasible resection for cancer, no added advantage is gained by performing a pneumonectomy since dissection of the area of lymphatic drainage is as adequate with one procedure as with the other.

Resection and Biopsy

Segmental Resection

Resection of lung tissue anatomically less than a lobe is carried out for localized lesions such as benign tumors, granulomas, tuberculous foci, bronchiectasis, metastatic cancers and others, and to obtain tissue specimens required for the diagnosis of diffuse pulmonary disease processes.

Segmentectomy requires a detailed anatomic knowledge of secondary and tertiary hilar structures. Intersegmental cleavage planes are best defined at operation when, by selective bronchial occlusion, adjacent portions of lung tissue are maintained, one inflated and the other atelectatic. Resection of only one or more segments has the advantage of removing only diseased structures and leaving healthy, functioning lung tissue which ordinarily would be removed if the excision involved the whole lobe.

Segmental resection is best performed through the standard posterolateral thoracotomy incision. Depending upon individual circumstances, the segmental bronchus is identified and approached first, by palpation; or the segmental artery first, by dissection. To assure correct identification of the proper bronchus once it is dissected free, one carries out temporary atraumatic occlusion of this structure while the remainder of the lobe is being inflated by the anesthesiologist. After division and closure by stapling or by suture, a clamp is left on the distal portion of the severed bronchus, subsequently to be used for traction. The segmental artery lies close to the bronchus; it is identified, dissected free and divided between ligatures.

Whenever feasible it is preferable to locate and divide the arterial supply to the segment first as this minimizes chances of major bleeding during the procedure. The main pulmonary artery, or the continuing pulmonary artery, is identified in its proper anatomic location and the perivascular sheath entered. The segmental artery or arteries are located, carefully dissected free and divided after appropriate proximal and distal ligation. The segmental bronchus is closely adjacent and then may be palpated and dissected free. If the draining vein or veins are seen, these are divided between ligatures. However, the veins are frequently identified only as branches in the intersegmental plane.

Separation of the intersegmental plane is performed largely by blunt dissection with the fingers, working toward the pleural surface while exercising traction on the clamp attached to the distal divided bronchus. Venous branches on the segmental surface are grasped by small hemostats before cutting and subsequently ligated with fine suture material. These veins can serve as a helpful guide to the intersegmental plane as dissection proceeds.

Often it is possible to close the defect created by removal of the segment and to reconstruct the lobe once the segment is taken out.

Wedge Resection

Wedge resections are useful when one is dealing with small peripheral lesions or for diagnosis of a diffuse disease process. Less lung tissue is re-

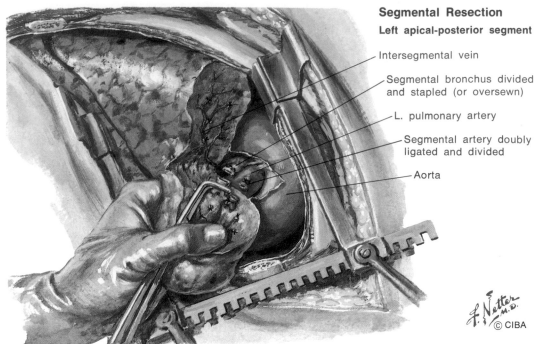

Segmental Resection
Left apical-posterior segment

- Intersegmental vein
- Segmental bronchus divided and stapled (or oversewn)
- L. pulmonary artery
- Segmental artery doubly ligated and divided
- Aorta

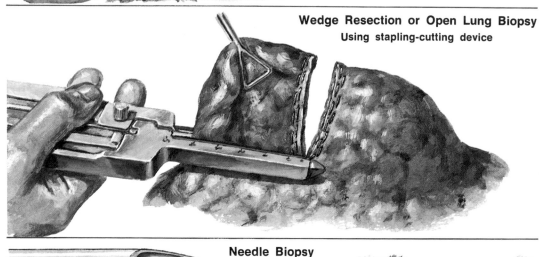

Wedge Resection or Open Lung Biopsy
Using stapling-cutting device

Needle Biopsy

Needle tip (greatly magnified)

Mandrin withdrawn

Biopsy needle 0.9 to 1.1 mm in diameter, 9 to 16 cm long, with long, bevelled, sharp-edged tip which causes little trauma but cuts tissue when rotated. A mandrin within needle during insertion under fluoroscopic television control prevents picking up tissue until needle tip reaches target. Mandrin then withdrawn, needle rotated, and suction applied. A 3-way stopcock may facilitate this. Insertion close to top of rib avoids intercostal vessels

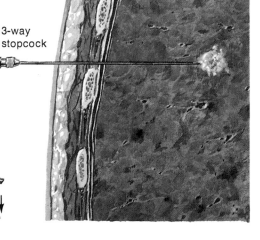

3-way stopcock

moved, as a rule, than with segmental resection, and the procedure is simpler, safer and quicker.

Wedge resection has been made easier by the availability of stapling-cutting instruments which lay down a double row of staples on either side and divide lung tissue in between these rows. Bleeding is rarely a problem—requiring only one or two suture ligatures should it be present—and air leaks are negligible.

Needle Biopsy

Generally, needle aspiration has not been reliably diagnostic, except in the hands of a few groups, and is not widely used. However, needle biopsy of localized dense infiltrates is an extremely useful procedure, especially when reading of the aspirate is done by an experienced cytopathologist. The question most commonly posed is: Is it a lung cancer and, if it is not, what is it? Results obtained by needle biopsy can prove diagnostic in as many as 80% of patients.

The technique, as shown in the illustration, is carried out under fluoroscopic control using an image intensifier screen. It is quite safe. Complications are few: pneumothorax is an occasional sequel, which generally responds to conservative management. Bleeding occurs rarely, and it, too, is best managed by conservative measures.

Removal of Mediastinal Tumors

Tumors of the mediastinum are a challenging group both diagnostically and in terms of treatment. A host of pathologic entities is involved, and for many of these, surgical excision is the treatment of choice. Recognition and identification of mediastinal abnormalities are almost always based on the chest roentgenogram. While the radiologic appearance is sometimes characteristic or (rarely) pathognomonic, most often it is the location within the mediastinum that is most influential in correct diagnostic interpretation.

Radiologic evaluation depends on the lateral film of the chest, and no assessment should be made without this view. If the chest, on lateral view, is divided into three roughly equal compartments in an anteroposterior plane, the most common tumors are as follows: (1) anterior mediastinum—thymoma, teratoid tumor (dermoid, teratoma), intrathoracic thyroid (including substernal thyroid) and pericardiocoelomic cyst; (2) midmediastinum—bronchogenic cyst (respiratory reduplication cyst), and tumors of lymphoid involvement (lymphomas, benign and malignant, primary and metastatic); (3) posterior mediastinum—tumors of neurogenic origin (neurofibroma) and esophageal lesions. Vascular tumors (aneurysms, anomalies, angiomas) may occur anywhere in the mediastinum.

Most mediastinal tumors are best approached surgically by the standard posterolateral incision with the hemithorax entered at an appropriate level on the side of maximal projection of the lesion.

The illustration shows removal of a neurofibroma, the most common mediastinal tumor,

Removal of Mediastinal Tumors

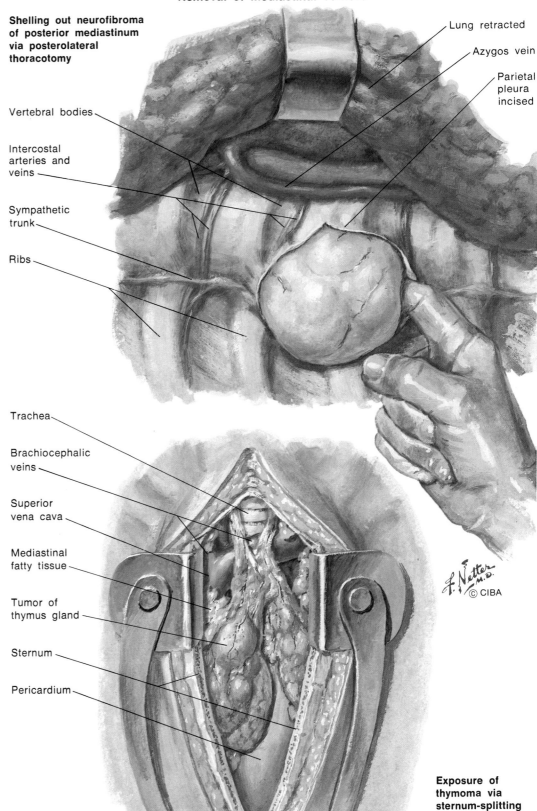

Shelling out neurofibroma of posterior mediastinum via posterolateral thoracotomy

Lung retracted

Azygos vein

Parietal pleura incised

Vertebral bodies

Intercostal arteries and veins

Sympathetic trunk

Ribs

Trachea

Brachiocephalic veins

Superior vena cava

Mediastinal fatty tissue

Tumor of thymus gland

Sternum

Pericardium

Exposure of thymoma via sternum-splitting incision

which, characteristically, hugs the posterior costovertebral angle. Most such tumors are readily shelled out, and their blood supply is easily identified. The presence of an intraspinal component ("dumbbell" tumor) should be ruled out preoperatively by means of lateral views of the spine showing the intervertebral foramina.

Most anterior mediastinal lesions can be handled by the lateral approach, particularly if they are large, for this affords access to the plane between the tumor and the heart and great vessels, to which it may be attached.

An anterior, sternal splitting approach, as shown, is preferred by some thoracic surgeons for

thymic tumors, particularly in the presence of myasthenia gravis where complete extirpation of all components of thymic origin is desired. When the tumor is large or densely adherent, this approach may present difficulties since the tumor lies between the operator and the vital structures from which it must be freed. Sternal splitting thoracotomy, on the other hand, is now quite commonly employed (for open-heart surgery), is reasonably rapid and affords access to both pleural cavities. Therefore, the operating surgeon must base his preference for one approach or the other on the facilities available and the particular tumor presentation involved.

Selected References

General References

BATES DV, MACKLEM PT, CHRISTIE RV: *Respiratory Function in Disease*, 2nd ed. Philadelphia, WB Saunders, 1971

BAUM GL (Ed): *Textbook of Pulmonary Diseases*, 2nd ed. Boston, Little, Brown, 1974

CHERNIACK RM, CHERNIACK L, NAIMARK A: *Respiration in Health and Disease*, 2nd ed. Philadelphia, WB Saunders, 1972

COMROE JH JR: *Physiology of Respiration*, 2nd ed. Chicago, Yearbook Medical Publishers, 1974

COMROE JH JR, FORSTER RE, DUBOIS AB, et al (Eds): *The Lung*, 2nd ed. Chicago, Yearbook Medical Publishers, 1972

GORDON BL, CARLETON RA, FABER LP (Eds): *Clinical Cardiopulmonary Physiology*, 3rd ed. New York, Grune & Stratton, 1969

MURRAY JF: *The Normal Lung: the Basis for Diagnosis and Treatment of Pulmonary Disease*. Philadelphia, WB Saunders, 1976

PAPPENHEIMER JR, et al: *Standardization of definitions and symbols in respiratory physiology*. Fed Proc 9:602-605, 1950

SHIELDS TW (Ed): *General Thoracic Surgery*. Philadelphia, Lea & Febiger, 1972

WEST JB: *Respiratory Physiology: the Essentials*. Baltimore, Williams & Wilkins, 1974

Section I

	Plate Number

AREY LB: *Developmental Anatomy*, 7th ed. Philadelphia, WB Saunders, 1965 — 32-41

AVERY ME, FLETCHER BD: *The Lung and its Disorders in the Newborn Infant*, 3rd ed. Philadelphia, WB Saunders, 1974 — 32-41

BOYDEN EA: *The developing bronchial arteries in a fetus of the twelfth week*. Am J Anat 129:357-368, 1970 — 26

BOYDEN EA: *The intrahilar and related segmental anatomy of the lung*. Surgery 18:706-731, 1945 — 14, 15

BOYDEN EA: *Segmental Anatomy of the Lungs*. New York, McGraw-Hill, 1955 — 21, 26

BRASH JC, JAMIESON EB (Eds): *Cunningham's Text-Book of Anatomy*, 9th ed. New York, Oxford University Press, 1951 — 1-19

BROCK RC: *The nomenclature of broncho-pulmonary anatomy*. Thorax 5:222-228, 1950 — 21

CRELIN ES: *Anatomy of the Newborn: an Atlas*. Philadelphia, Lea & Febiger, 1969 — 32-41

CRELIN ES: *Functional Anatomy of the Newborn*. New Haven, Yale University Press, 1973 — 32-41

ELLIOTT FM, REID LM: *Some new facts about the pulmonary artery and its branching pattern*. Clin Radiol 16:193-198, 1965 — 26

FOSTER CARTER AF: *Broncho-pulmonary anatomy*. In HOLMES SELLERS T, PERRY KM (Eds): *Chest Diseases*. London, 1963 — 21

GARDNER E, GRAY DJ, O'RAHILLY R: *Anatomy: A Regional Study of Human Structure*, 4th ed. Philadelphia, WB Saunders, 1975 — 1-19

GODFREY S: *Growth and development of the respiratory system. Functional development*. In DAVIS A, DOBBING J (Eds): *Scientific Foundations of Paediatrics*. Philadelphia, WB Saunders, 1974 — 32-41

GRAY HG: *Anatomy of the Human Body*, 26th ed,

Section I (continued)

	Plate Number

GOSS CM (Ed). Philadelphia, Lea & Febiger, 1954 — 1-19

GUYTON AC: *Textbook of Medical Physiology*, 4th ed. Philadelphia, WB Saunders, 1971 — 32-41

HAMILTON WJ, BOYD JD, MOSSMAN HW: *Human Embryology*, 3rd ed. Baltimore, Williams & Wilkins, 1964 — 32-41

HAYWARD J, REID LM: *Cartilage of the intrapulmonary bronchi in normal lungs, in bronchiectasis, and in massive collapse*. Thorax 7:98-110, 1952 — 21

HISLOP A, MUIR DC, JACOBSON M, et al: *Postnatal growth and function of the pre-acinar airways*. Thorax 27:265-274, 1972 — 22

HISLOP A, REID LM: *Formation of the pulmonary vasculature*. In LENFANT C (Exec ed): *Lung Biology in Health and Disease*. Vol 6: *Development of the Lung*, HODSON WA (Section ed). New York, Marcel Dekker, 1977, pp 37-86 — 26

HISLOP A, REID LM: *Growth and development of the respiratory system. Anatomical development*. In DAVIS JA, DOBBING J (Eds): *Scientific Foundations of Paediatrics*. Philadelphia, WB Saunders, 1974 — 32-41

HUBER CG (Ed): *Piersol's Human Anatomy*, 9th ed. Philadelphia, JB Lippincott, 1930 — 1-19

HUBER JF: *Practical correlative anatomy of the bronchial tree and lungs*. J Natl Med Assoc 41, 1949 — 14, 15

HYMAN LH: *Comparative Vertebrate Anatomy*, 2nd ed. Chicago, University of Chicago Press, 1946 — 32-41

JACKSON CL, HUBER JF: *Correlated applied anatomy of the bronchial tree and lungs with a system of nomenclature*. Dis Chest 9:319-326, 1943 — 14, 15

JEFFERY PK, REID LM: *New observations of rat airway epithelium: a quantitative and electron microscopic study*. J Anat 120:295-320, 1975 — 24

JONES R, REID LM: *The effect of pH on Alcian Blue staining of epithelial acid glycoproteins. II. Human bronchial submucosal gland*. Histochem J 5:19-27, 1973 — 25

LAMBERT MW: *Accessory bronchiole-alveolar communications*. J Path & Bact 70:311-314, 1955 — 22

MEYRICK B, REID LM: *Ultrastructure of cells in the human bronchial submucosal glands*. J Anat 107:281-299, 1970 — 25

MEYRICK B, STURGESS JM, REID LM: *A reconstruction of the duct system and secretory tubules of the human bronchial submucosal gland*. Thorax 24:729-736, 1969 — 25

MILLER WS: *Distribution of lymphoid tissue in the lung*. Anat Rec 5:99-119, 1911 — 30, 31

MILLER WS: *The Lung*, 2nd ed. Springfield Ill, CC Thomas, 1947 — 22

NAGAISHI C: *Functional Anatomy and Histology of the Lung*. Baltimore, University Park Press, 1972 — 23, 30, 31

PATTEN BM: *Human Embryology*, 3rd ed. New York, McGraw-Hill, 1968 — 32-41

ROUVIÉRE H: *Anatomy of the Human Lymphatic System*. Translated by TOBIAS MJ. Ann Arbor, Edwards Brother, 1938 — 30, 31

RYAN JW, DAY AR, SCHULTZ DR: *Localization of angiotensin converting enzyme (kininase II). I. Preparation of antibody-hemeoctapeptide conjugates*. Tissue Cell 8:111-124, 1976 — 27-29

Section I (continued)

	Plate Number

RYAN JW, RYAN US: *Metabolic activities of plasma membrane and caveolae of pulmonary endothelial cells with a note on pulmonary prostaglandin synthetase*. In JUNOD AF, DE HALLER R (Eds): *Lung Metabolism*. New York, Academic Press, 1976, pp 399-424 — 27-29

RYAN US, RYAN JW: *Pulmonary macrophage and epithelial cells*. In SANDERS CL, et al (Eds): *16th Annual Hanford Biological Symposium*. Springfield Va, US Dept Commerce, 1977, pp 115-140 — 27-29

RYAN US, RYAN JW, CHIU A: *Localization of angiotensin converting enzyme (kininase II). II Immunocytochemistry and immunofluorescence*. Tissue Cell 8:125-146, 1976 — 27-29

SLEIGH MA: *The nature and action of respiratory tract cilia*. In LENFANT C (Exec ed): *Lung Biology in Health and Disease*, Vol 5: *Respiratory Defense Mechanisms*, BRAIN JD, PROCTOR DF, REID LM (Section eds). New York, Marcel Dekker, 1977, pp 247-288 — 24

SMITH DS, SMITH U, RYAN JW: *Freeze-fractured lamellar body membranes of the rat lung great alveolar cell*. Tissue Cell 4:457-468, 1972 — 27-29

SMITH U, RYAN JW: *Electron microscopy of endothelial and epithelial components of the lungs: correlations of structure and function*. Fed Proc 32:1957-1966, 1973 — 27-29

SMITH U, RYAN JW, MICHIE DD, et al: *Endothelial projections: as revealed by scanning electron microscopy*. Science 173:925-927, 1971 — 27-29

SMITH U, RYAN JW, SMITH DS: *Freeze-etch studies of the plasma membrane of pulmonary endothelial cells*. J Cell Biol 56:492-499, 1973 — 27-29

SOROKIN S: *A morphologic and cytochemical study on the great alveolar cell*. J Histochem Cytochem 14:884-897, 1966 — 27-29

STURGESS JM, REID LM: *An organ culture study of the effect of drugs on the secretory activity of the human bronchial submucosal gland*. Clin Sci 43:533-543, 1972 — 25

TOBIN CE: *Human pulmonic lymphatics: an anatomic study*. Anat Rec 127:611-633, 1957 — 30, 31

TOBIN CE, ZARIGUIEY MO: *Bronchopulmonary segments and blood supply of the human lung*. Med Radiogr Photogr 26:38-45, 1950 — 14, 15

TRAPNELL DH: *Peripheral lymphatics of the lung*. Br J Radiol 36:660-672, 1963 — 30, 31

VON HAYEK H: *The Human Lung*. New York, Hafner, 1960 — 23

WARWICK R, WILLIAMS P (Eds): *Gray's Anatomy*, 35th ed. Philadelphia, WB Saunders, 1973 — 32-41

WEISS EB: *Bronchial Asthma*. Clinical Symposia 27(1,2): 1-72, 1975 — 20

Section II

AGOSTONI E, SANT'AMBROGIO G: *The diaphragm*. In CAMPBELL EJ, et al (Eds): *The Respiratory Muscles: Mechanics and Neural Control*, 2nd ed. Philadelphia, WB Saunders, 1970 — 1

AMERICAN COLLEGE OF CHEST PHYSICIANS (Committee on Pulmonary Physiology):

Section II (continued)

Plate Number

Clinical Spirometry. Dis Chest 43:214-219, 1963 — 11, 12

ANTHONISEN NR, DANSON J, ROBERTSON PC, et al: *Airway closure as a function of age.* Respir Physiol 8:58-65, 1969 — 13, 17

ANTHONISEN NR, MILIC-EMILI J: *Distribution of pulmonary perfusion in erect man.* J Appl Physiol 21:760-766, 1966 — 14, 15

ASMUSSEN E: *Muscular exercise.* In *Handbook of Physiology: Respiration.* Washington DC, Am Physiol Soc, 1965, Sec 3, Vol 2, pp 939-978 — 27

BISCOE TJ: *Carotid body: structure and function.* Physiol Rev 51:437-495, 1971 — 25

BLACK LF, HYATT RE: *Maximal respiratory pressures: normal values and relationship to age and sex.* Am Rev Respir Dis 99:696-702, 1969 — 1

BRODOVSKY D, MACDONELL JA, CHERNIACK RM: *The respiratory response to carbon dioxide in health and in emphysema.* J Clin Invest 39:724-729, 1960 — 31

BROWN HW, PLUM F: *The neurologic basis of Cheyne-Stokes respiration.* Am J Med 30:849-860, 1961 — 29, 30

BURNS BD: *The central control of respiratory movements.* Br Med Bull 19:7-9, 1963 — 26

CALDWELL PR, SEEGAL BC, Hsu KC, et al: *Angiotensin-converting enzyme: vascular endothelial localization.* Sci 191:1050-1051, 1976 — 24

CAMPBELL EJ, DAVIS JN: *The intercostal muscles and other muscles of the rib cage.* In CAMPBELL EJ, et al (Eds): *The Respiratory Muscles: Mechanics and Neural Control,* 2nd ed. Philadelphia, WB Saunders, 1970 — 1

CAMPBELL EJ, WESTLAKE EK, CHERNIACK RM: *Simple methods of estimating oxygen consumption and efficiency of the muscles of breathing.* J Appl Physiol 11:303-308, 1957 — 12

CHERNIACK NS, FISHMAN AP: *Abnormal breathing patterns.* Med Clin North Am 59:1-45, 1975 — 31

CHERNIACK NS, LONGOBARDO GS: *Cheyne-Stokes breathing: an instability in physiologic control.* N Engl J Med 288:952-957, 1973 — 29, 30

CHOW CK, TAPPEL AL: *Activities of pentose shunt and glycolytic enzymes in lungs of ozone-exposed rats.* Arch Environ Health 26:205-208, 1973 — 22

CLEMENTS JA: *Surface phenomena in relation to pulmonary function.* Physiologist 5:11-28, 1962 — 6

COURNAND A, RICHARDS DW, BADER RA, et al: *Oxygen cost of breathing.* Trans Assoc Am Physicians 67:162-173, 1954 — 12

CROSS CE: *The granular type II pneumocyte and lung antioxidant defense.* Ann Intern Med 80:409-411, 1974 — 22

CUNNINGHAM DJ: *The control system regulating breathing in man.* Q Rev Biophys 6:433-483, 1974 — 22

DAVENPORT HW: *The ABC of Acid-Base Chemistry: the Elements of Physiological Blood-Gas Chemistry for Medical Students and Physicians,* 5th ed. Chicago, University of Chicago Press, 1969 — 21

DEJOURS P: *Control of respiration in muscular exercise.* In *Handbook of Physiology: Respiration.* Washington DC, Am Physiol Soc, 1964, Sec 3, Vol 1, pp 631-648 — 27

DESPAS PJ, LEROUX M, MACKLEM J: *Site of airway obstruction in asthma.* Chest 63 (Suppl):28, 1973 — 11, 12

DUBOIS AB, BOTELHO SY, BEDELL GN, et al: *A rapid plethysmographic method for measuring thoracic gas volume: a comparison with a nitrogen washout method for measuring functional residual capacity in normal subjects.* J Clin Invest 35:322-326, 1956 — 2, 3

DUBOIS AB, BOTELHO SY, COMROE JH JR: *A new method for measuring airway resistance in man using a body plethysmograph: values in normal subjects in patients with respiratory disease.* J Clin Invest 35:327-355, 1956 — 3, 8, 9

EDELMAN NH, LAHIRI S, BRAUDO L, et al: *The blunted ventilatory response to hypoxia in cyanotic congenital heart disease.* N Engl J Med 282:405-411, 1970 — 28

ERDÖS EG: *Angiotensin I converting enzyme.* Circ Res 36:247-255, 1975 — 24

FERRIS BG JR, MEAD J, OPIE LH: *Partitioning of respiratory flow resistance in man.* J Appl Physiol 19:653-658, 1964 — 3, 8, 9

FILLEY GF: *Acid-base and blood gas regulation.* Philadelphia, Lea & Febiger, 1971 — 21

FILLEY GF, MACINTOSH DJ, WRIGHT GW: *Carbon monoxide uptake and pulmonary diffusing capacity in normal subjects at rest and during exercise.* J Clin Invest 33:530-539, 1954 — 16

FINCH CA, LENFANT C: *Oxygen transport in man.* N Engl J Med 286:407-415, 1972 — 20

FISHMAN AP: *Dynamics of the pulmonary circulation.* In *Handbook of Physiology: Circulation.* Washington DC, Am Physiol Soc, 1963, Sec 2, Vol 2, pp 1667-1743 — 14, 15

FISHMAN AP: *Respiratory gases in the regulation of the pulmonary circulation.* Physiol Rev 41:214-280, 1961 — 14, 15

FISHMAN AP, PIETRA GG: *Handling of bioactive materials by the lung.* N Engl J Med 291:884-889, 953-959, 1974 — 23

FORSTER RE: *Exchange of gases between alveolar air and pulmonary capillary blood.* Physiol Rev 37:391-405, 1957 — 16

GAENSLER EA, WRIGHT GW: *Evaluation of respiratory impairment.* Arch Environ Health 12:146-189, 1966 — 11, 12

GIBSON GJ, PRIDE NB: *Lung distensibility. The static pressure-volume curve of the lungs and its use in clinical assessment.* Br J Dis Chest 70:143-184, 1976 — 4, 5

GLAZIER JB, HUGHES JM, MALONEY JE, et al: *Vertical gradient of alveolar size in the lungs of dogs frozen intact.* J Appl Physiol 23:694-705, 1967 — 13, 17

HEAF PJ, PRIME FJ: *Compliance of thorax in normal human subjects.* Clin Sci Mol Med 15:319-327, 1956 — 7

HURTADO A: *Animals in high altitudes: Resident man.* In *Handbook of Physiology: Adaptation to Environment.* Washington DC, Am Physiol Soc, 1964, Sec 4, p 843 — 28

HUTCHEON M, GRIFFIN P, LEVISON H, et al: *Volume of isoflow. A new test in detection of mild abnormalities of lung mechanics.* Am Rev Respir Dis 110:458-465, 1974 — 11, 12

HYATT RE, BLACK LF: *The flow-volume curve: a current perspective.* Am Rev Respir Dis 107:191-199, 1973 — 10, 11

HYATT RE, FLATH RE: *Relationship of air flow to pressure during maximal respiratory effort in man.* J Appl Physiol 21:477-482, 1966 — 10, 11

JUNOD AF: *Metabolism, production, and release of hormones and mediators in the lung.* Am Rev Respir Dis 112:93-108, 1975 — 24

KAPANCI Y, WEIBEL ER, KAPLAN HP: *Pathogenesis and reversibility of the pulmonary lesions of oxygen toxicity in monkeys. II. Ultrastructural and morphometric studies.* Lab Invest 20:101-118, 1969 — 22

KORY RC, CALLAHAN R, BOREN HG, et al: *The veterans administration-army cooperative study of pulmonary function: I. Clinical spirometry in normal men.* Am J Med 30:243-258, 1961 — 11, 12

KROGH M: *The diffusion of gases through the lungs.* J Physiol (Lond) 49:271-300, 1915 — 16

LAHIRI S: *Physiological responses and adaptations to high altitude.* In ROBERTSHAW D (Ed): *Environmental Physiology.* Baltimore, University Park Press, 1974, pp 271-312 — 28

LAHIRI S, DELANEY RG, BRODY JS: *Relative role of environmental and genetic factors in respiratory adaptation to high altitude.* Nature 261:133-135, 1976 — 28

LANGE RL, HECHT HH: *The mechanism of Cheyne-Stokes respiration.* J Clin Invest 41:42-52, 1962 — 29-30

LENFANT C: *Measurement of ventilation/perfusion with alveolar-arterial differences.* J Appl Physiol 18:1090-1094, 1963 — 18

LEUSEN I: *Regulation of cerebrospinal fluid composition with reference to breathing.* Physiol Rev 52:1-56, 1972 — 25

LOURENÇO RV, TURINO GM, DAVIDSON LA, et al: *The regulation of ventilation of diffuse pulmonary fibrosis.* Am J Med 38:199-216, 1965 — 31

MACKLEM PT, MEAD J: *Resistance of central and peripheral airways measured by a retrograde catheter.* J Appl Physiol 22:395-401, 1967 — 3, 8, 9

MCCARTHY DS, SPENCER R, GREENE R, et al: *Measurement of closing volume as a simple and sensitive test for early detection of small airway disease.* Am J Med 52:747-753, 1972 — 13, 17

MCILROY MB, MARSHALL R, CHRISTIE RV: *The work of breathing in normal subjects.* Clin Sci Mol Med 13:127-136, 1954 — 12

MARGARIA R, CERRETELLI P: *The respiratory system and exercise.* In FALLS HB (Ed): *Exercise Physiology.* New York, Academic Press, 1968, pp 43-54 — 27

MARSHALL R: *A comparison of methods of measuring the diffusing capacity of the lungs for carbon monoxide: investigation by fractional analysis of the alveolar air.* J Clin Invest 37:394-408, 1958 — 16

MARSHALL R: *Effect of lung inflation on bronchial dimensions in the dog.* J Appl Physiol 17:596-600, 1962 — 3, 8, 9

MASSON RG, LAHIRI S: *Chemical control of ventilation during hypoxic exercise.* Respir Physiol 22:241-262, 1974 — 27

MEAD J, TURNER JM, MACKLEM PT, et al: *Significance of the relationship between lung recoil and maximum expiratory flow.* J Appl Physiol 22:95-108, 1967 — 10, 11

MENEELY GR, BALL CO, KORY RC, et al: *A simplified closed circuit helium dilution method for the determination of the residual volume of the lungs.* Am J Med 28:824-831, 1960 — 2, 3

MERRIL EG: *Finding a respiratory function for the medullary respiratory neurons.* In BELLAIRS R, GREY EG (Eds): *Essays on the Nervous System.* Oxford, Clarendon Press, 1974, pp 451-486 — 26

MILIC-EMILI J, HENDERSON JA, DOLOVICH MB, et al: *Regional distribution of inspired gas in the lung.* J Appl Physiol 21:749-759, 1966 — 13, 17

MILIC-EMILI J, MEAD J, TURNER JM, et al: *Improved technique for estimating pleural pressure from esophageal balloons.* J Appl Physiol 19:207-211, 1964 — 4, 5

MITCHELL RA, BERGER AJ: *Neural regulation of*

Section II (continued)

	Plate Number

respiration. Am Rev Respir Dis 111:206-224, 1975 26

NG KK, VANE JR: *Conversion of angiotensin I to angiotensin II.* Nature 216:762-766, 1967 24

OGILVIE CM, FORSTER RE, BLAKEMORE WS, et al: *A standardized breath holding technique for the clinical measurement of the diffusing capacity of the lung for carbon monoxide.* J Clin Invest 36:1-17, 1957 16

OTIS AB: *Work of breathing.* Physiol Rev 34:449-458, 1954 12

PATTLE RE: *The lining layer of the lung alveoli.* Br Med Bull 19:41-44, 1963 6

PERMUTT S, RILEY RL: *Hemodynamics of collapsible vessels with tone: the vascular waterfall.* J Appl Physiol 18:924-932, 1963 14, 15

PITTS RF: *Physiology of the Kidney and Body Fluids,* 3rd ed. Chicago, Yearbook Medical Publishers, 1974 21

PRIDE NB: *The assessment of airflow obstruction. Role of measurements of airways resistance and of tests of forced expiration.* Br J Dis Chest 65:135-169, 1971 11, 12

PRIDE NB, PERMUTT S, RILEY RL, et al: *Determinants of maximum expiratory flow from the lungs.* J Appl Physiol 23:646-662, 1967 10, 11

PUGH LG: *Animals in high altitudes: Man above 5000 meters—mountain exploration.* In *Handbook of Physiology: Adaptation to Environment.* Washington DC, Am Physiol Soc, 1964 28

RADFORD EP: *Recent studies of mechanical properties of mammalian lungs.* In REMINGTON JW (Ed): *Tissue Elasticity.* Washington DC, Am Physiol Soc, 1957 6

RAHN H, FENN WO: *Graphical analysis of the respiratory gas exchange: The O_2-CO_2 diagram.* Washington DC, Am Physiol Soc, 1955 18

RAHN H, OTIS AB, CHADWICK LE, et al: *The pressure-volume diagram of the thorax and lung.* Am J Physiol 146:161-178, 1946 7

READ DJ: *A clinical method for assessing the ventilatory response to carbon dioxide.* Aust Ann Med 16:20-32, 1967 25

REBUCK AS, CAMPBELL EJ: *A clinical method for assessing the ventilatory response to hypoxia.* Am Rev Respir Dis 109:345-350, 1974 25

RILEY RL, COURNAND A: *"Ideal" alveolar air and the analysis of ventilation—perfusion relationships in the lung.* J Appl Physiol 1:825-847, 1949 18

ROUGHTON FJ: *Transport of oxygen and carbon dioxide.* In *Handbook of Physiology: Respiration.* Washington DC, Am Physiol Soc, 1964, Sec 3, Vol 1, pp 767-825 20

ROUGHTON FJ, FORSTER RE: *Relative importance of diffusion and chemical reaction rates in determining rate of exchange of gases in the human lung with special reference to true diffusing capacity of pulmonary membrane and volume of blood in the lung capillaries.* J Appl Physiol 11:290-302, 1957 16

RYAN JW, SMITH U, NIEMEYER RS: *Angiotensin I: metabolism by plasma membrane of lung.* Science 76:64-66, 1972 24

SAID SI: *The lung in relation to vasoactive hormones.* Fed Proc 32:1972-1976, 1973 23

SENIOR RM, FISHMAN AP: *Disturbances of alveolar ventilation.* Med Clin North Am 51:403-425, 1967 31

SMITH G, WINTER PM, WHEELS RF: *Increased normobaric oxygen tolerance of rabbits following oleic acid-induced lung damage.* J Appl Physiol 35:395-400, 1973 22

STARLING EH, VERNEY EB: *The excretion of urine as studied on the isolated kidney.* Proc R Soc Lond (Biol) 97:321, 1924/1925 23

STRUM JM, JUNOD AF: *Radioautographic demonstration of 5-hydroxytryptamine–^3H uptake by pulmonary endothelial cells.* J Cell Biol 54:456-467, 1972 23

STUBBS SE, HYATT RE: *Effect of increased lung recoil pressure on maximal expiratory flow in normal subjects.* J Appl Physiol 32:325-331, 1972 10, 11

TURNER JM, MEAD J, WOHL ME: *Elasticity of human lungs in relation to age.* J Appl Physiol 25:664-671, 1968 4, 5

VANE JR: *The release and fate of vaso-active hormones in the circulation.* Br J Pharmacol 35:209-242, 1969 23

VON EULER C, HAYWARD JN, MARTTILA I, et al: *Respiratory neurones of the ventrolateral nucleus and of the solitary tract of cat: vagal input, spinal connections and morphological identification.* Brain Res 61:1-22, 1973 26

WEST JB, DOLLERY CT, NAIMARK A: *Distribution of blood flow in isolated lung: relation to vascular and alveolar pressures.* J Appl Physiol 19:713-724, 1964 14, 15

WITSCHI H, CÔTÉ MG: *Biochemical pathology of lung damage produced by chemicals.* Fed Proc 35:89-94, 1976 22

WOOLCOCK AJ, VINCENT NJ, MACKLEM PT: *Frequency dependence of compliance as a test for obstruction in the small airways.* J Clin Invest 48:1097-1106, 1969 12

Section III

DENARDO GL, GOODWIN DA, RAVASINI R, et al: *The ventilatory lung scan in the diagnosis of pulmonary embolism.* N Engl J Med 282:1334-1336, 1970 1-17

FAVIS EA: *Planigraphy (body section radiography) in detecting tuberculosis pulmonary cavitation.* Dis Chest 27:668-673, 1955 1-17

FELSON B: *Principles of Chest Roentgenology: A Programmed Text.* Philadelphia, WB Saunders, 1965 1-17

FELSON B: *The roentgen diagnosis of disseminated pulmonary alveolar disease.* Seminars Roentgen 2:3, 1967 1-17

GREENSPAN RH, CAPPS JH: *Pulmonary angiography: its use in diagnosis and as a guide to therapy in lesions of the chest.* Radiol Clin North Am 1:315, 1963 1-17

KREEL L: *Selective thymic venography: new method for visualization of the thymus.* Br Med J 1:406-407, 1967 1-17

LUBERT M, KRAUSE GR: *Patterns of lobar collapse as observed radiographically.* Radiology 56:165-181, 1951 1-17

LYNCH PA: *A different approach to chest roentgenography: triad technique (high kilovoltage, grid, wedge filter).* J Amer J Roentgen 93:965-971, 1965 1-17

MILNE EN: *Correlations of physiologic findings with chest roentgenology.* Radiol Clin North Am 11:17-47, 1973 1-17

NADEL JA, WOLFF WG, GRAF PD: *Powdered tantalum as a medium for bronchography in canine and human lungs.* Invest Radiol 3:229-238, 1968 1-17

RHODES BA, ZOLLE I, BUCHANAN JW, et al: *Radioactive albumin microspheres for studies of the pulmonary circulation.* Radiology 92:1453-1460, 1969 1-17

RIGLER LG: *Roentgen diagnosis of small pleural effusions; new roentgenographic position.* JAMA 96:104-108, 1931 1-17

STEELE JD: *The solitary pulmonary nodule. Report of a cooperative study of resected asymptomatic solitary pulmonary nodules in males.* J Thorac Cardiov Surg 46:21-39, 1963 1-17

STORCH CB: *Fundamental aids in roentgen diagnosis: emphasizing spot filming and fluoroscopy.* New York, Grune & Stratton, 1964 1-17

WESTERMARK N: *On roentgen diagnosis of lung embolism.* Acta radiol 19:357-372, 1938 1-17

ZISKIND MM, WEILL H, PAYZANT AR: *The recognition and significance of acinus-filling processes of the lungs.* Am Rev Respir Dis 87:551-559, 1963 1-17

Section IV

ADAMS JT, DEWEESE JA: *Experimental and clinical evaluation of partial vein interruption in the prevention of pulmonary emboli.* Surgery 57:82-102, 1965 122

ADAMS JT, FEINGOLD BE, DEWEESE JA, et al: *Comparative evaluation of ligation and partial interruption of inferior vena cava.* Arch Surg 103:272-276, 1971 122

ADHIKARI PK, BIANCHI FA, BOURSHY SF, et al: *Pulmonary function in scleroderma. Its relations to changes in the chest roentgenogram and in the skin of the thorax.* Am Rev Respir Dis 86:823-831, 1962 146

AMERICAN THORACIC SOCIETY: *Statement on guidelines for long term institutional care of tuberculosis patients.* Am Rev Respir Dis 113:253-254, 1976 88-96

AMERICAN THORACIC SOCIETY: *Statement on BCG vaccination for tuberculosis.* Am Rev Respir Dis 112:478-480, 1975 88-96

AMERICAN THORACIC SOCIETY: *Statement on tuberculosis control programs for low incidence areas.* Am Rev Respir Dis 112:480-481, 1975 88-96

AMERICAN THORACIC SOCIETY: *Statement on preventive therapy of tuberculous infection.* Am Rev Respir Dis 110:371-374, 1974 88-96

AMERICAN THORACIC SOCIETY: *Statement on intermittent chemotherapy for adults with tuberculosis.* Am Rev Respir Dis 110:374-376, 1974 88-96

AMERICAN THORACIC SOCIETY: *Statement on quality of laboratory services for mycobacterial diseases.* Am Rev Respir Dis 110:376-377, 1974 88-96

ANDERSON AE JR, FORAKER AG: *Centrilobular emphysema and panlobular emphysema: two different diseases.* Thorax 28:547-550, 1973 29, 33, 35, 45

ANDRUS CH, MORTON JH: *Rupture of the diaphragm after blunt trauma.* Amer J Surg 119:686-693, 1970 128

ATKINS P, HAWKINS LA: *Detection of venous thrombosis in the legs.* Lancet 2:1217, 1965 111

AUSTEN KF, ORANGE RP: *Bronchial asthma: the possible role of the chemical mediators of immediate hypersensitivty in pathogenesis of subacute chronic disease.* Am Rev Respir Dis 112:423-436, 1975 13-27

AUSTRIAN R, DOUGLAS RM, SCHIFFMAN G, et

Section IV (continued)

Plate Number

al: *Prevention of pneumococcal pneumonia by vaccination.* Trans Assoc Am Physicians 89:184-194, 1976 — 66-76

AUSTRIAN R, GOLD J: *Pneumococcal bacteremia with special reference to bacteremic pneumococcal pneumonia.* Ann Intern Med 60:759-776, 1964 — 66-76

AVERY ME, FLETCHER BD: *The Lung and its Disorders in the Newborn Infant,* 3rd ed. Philadelphia, WB Saunders, 1974 — 1, 7, 137, 139

BARTLETT JG, GORBACH SL, TALLY FP, et al: *Bacteriology and treatment of primary lung abscess.* Am Rev Respir Dis 109:510-518, 1974 — 77, 78

BARNES RW, COLLICOTT PE, MOZERSKY DJ, et al: *Noninvasive quantitation of maximum venous outflow in acute thrombophlebitis.* Surgery 72:971-979, 1972 — 112, 113

BATES DV: *Chronic bronchitis and emphysema.* N Engl J Med 278:546-555, 1968 — 43, 44

BATES DV, et al: *Respiratory Function in Disease,* 2nd ed. Philadelphia, WB Saunders, 1971 — 97-104

BEAMIS JF JR, STEIN A, ANDREWS JL JR: *Changing epidemiology of lung cancer. Increasing incidence in women.* Med Clin North Am 59:315-325, 1975 — 50

BECKLAKE MR: *Asbestos-related disease of the lungs and other organs: their epidemiology and implications for clinical practice.* Am Rev Respir Dis 114:187-227, 1976 — 97-104

BENNETT DE, SASSER WF, FERGUSON TB: *Adenocarcinoma of the lung in men. A clinicopathologic study of 100 cases.* Cancer 23:431-439, 1969 — 54

BERGOFSKY EH, TURINO GM, FISHMAN AP: *Cardiorespiratory failure in kyphoscoliosis.* Medicine 38:263-317, 1959 — 2, 3

BETTMANN MA, PAULIN S: *Leg phlebography: the incidence, nature and modification of undesirable side effects.* Radiology 122:101-104, 1977 — 110

BISNO AL: *Hyposplenism and overwhelming pneumococcal infection: a reappraisal.* Am J Med Sci 262:101-107, 1971 — 66-76

BLADES B: *Surgical Diseases of the Chest,* 3rd ed. St. Louis, CV Mosby, 1974 — 4, 7

BLOCK AJ, CASTLE JR, KEITT AS: *Chronic oxygen therapy. Treatment of chronic obstructive pulmonary disease at sea level.* Chest 65:279-288, 1974 — 36, 43, 44

BODE FR, PARÉ JA, FRASER RG: *Pulmonary diseases in the compromised host. A review of clinical and roentgenographic manifestations in patients w/impaired host defense mechanisms.* Medicine (Baltimore) 53:255-293, 1974 — 66-76

BOUCOT KR, WEISS W, SEIDMAN W, et al: *The Philadelphia pulmonary neoplasm research project: basic risk factors of lung cancer in older men.* Am J Epidemiol 95:4-16, 1972 — 50

BOWMAN BH, MANGOS JA: *Current concepts in genetics. Cystic fibrosis.* N Engl J Med 294:937-938, 1976 — 48, 49

BOYD PH: *Idiopathic pulmonary hemosiderosis in adults and adolescents.* Br J Dis Chest 53:41-51, 1959 — 143

BRUNTON FJ, MOORE ME: *A survey of pulmonary calcification following adult chickenpox.* Br J Radiol 42:256-259, 1969 — 66-76

BUECHNER HA: *Treating systemic fungus diseases.* Compr Ther 2:22-28, 1976 — 79-84, 86

BUECHNER HA: *Management of Fungus Diseases of the Lungs.* Springfield Ill, Charles C Thomas, 1971 — 79-86, 105-106

BUECHNER HA: *Clinical aspects of fungus diseases of the lungs including laboratory diagnosis and*

Section IV (continued)

Plate Number

treatment. In *Advances in Cardiopulmonary Diseases.* Chicago, Yearbook Medical Publishers, 1966, Vol 3, pp 123-157 — 79-86

BUECHNER HA, FURCOLOW ML, FARNESS OJ, et al: *Epidemiology of the pulmonary mycoses.* Chest 58:68-70, 1970 — 81-84, 86

BUECHNER HA, SEABURY JH, CAMPBELL CC, et al: *The current status of serologic, immunologic and skin tests in the diagnosis of pulmonary mycoses.* Chest 63:259-271, 1973 — 81-85

BYRD RB, MILLER WE, CARR DT, et al: *The roentgenographic appearance of squamous cell carcinoma of the bronchus.* Mayo Clin Proc 43:327-332, 1968 — 53

BYRD RB, MILLER WE, CARR DT, et al: *The roentgenographic appearance of large cell carcinoma of the bronchus.* Mayo Clin Proc 43:333-336, 1968 — 52

BYRD RB, MILLER WE, CARR DT, et al: *The roentgenographic appearance of small cell carcinoma of the bronchus.* Mayo Clin Proc 43:337-341, 1968 — 51

CAMPBELL GD, FERRINGTON E: *Rheumatoid pleuritis with effusion.* Dis Chest 53:521-527, 1968 — 145

CAPLIN M: *Ammonia gas poisoning; 47 cases in a London shelter.* Lancet 2:95-96, 1941 — 97-104

CARR DT, MAYNES JG: *Pleurisy with effusion in rheumatoid arthritis, with reference to the low concentration of glucose in pleural fluid.* Am Rev Respir Dis 85:345-350, 1962 — 145

CARRINGTON CB, LIEBOW AS: *Limited forms of angiitis and granulomatosis of Wegener's type.* Am J Med 41:497-527, 1966 — 149

CATTERALL M, ROWELL NR: *Respiratory function in progressive systemic sclerosis.* Thorax 18:10-15, 1963 — 146

CEVESE PG, VECCHIONI R, D'AMICO DF, et al: *Postoperative chylothorax. Six cases in 2,500 operations, with a survey of the world literature.* J Thorac Cardiovasc Surg 69:966-972, 1975 — 134

CHANDLER FW, HICKLIN MD, BLACKMON JA: *Demonstration of the agent of legionnaires' disease in tissue.* N Engl J Med 297:1218-1220, 1977 — 66-76

CHANOCK RM: *Mycoplasma infections of man.* N Engl J Med 273:1257-1264, 1965 — 66-76

CHOPRA D, CLERKIN EP: *Hypercalcemia and malignant disease.* Med Clin North Am 59:441-447, 1975 — 58, 59

CHURG J, STRAUSS L: *Allergic granulomatosis, allergic angiitis and periarteritis nodosa.* Am J Path 27:277-302, 1951 — 149

CLARK TJ, GODFREY S (Eds): *Asthma.* Philadelphia, WB Saunders, 1977 — 13-27

CLOWES GH JR, HIRSCH E, WILLIAMS L, et al: *Septic lung and shock lung in man.* Ann Surg 181:681-692, 1975 — 136

COATES EO JR, WATSON JH: *Diffuse interstitial lung disease in tungsten carbide workers.* Ann Intern Med 75:709-716, 1971 — 97-104

COLMAN RW, OXLEY L, GIANNUSA P: *Statistical comparison of the automated activated partial thromboplastin time and the clotting time in the regulation of heparin therapy.* Am J Clin Pathol 53:904-907, 1970 — 121

COLMAN RW, WILLIAMS G, WYLLIE J: *Statistical comparison of the fibrometer and the Electra 600 for prothrombin time determination.* Am J Clin Pathol 64:108-112, 1975 — 121

COOPER WC, et al: *Pneumoconiosis in diatomite mining and processing.* (DHEW Publication No. 601), Washington DC, Government Printing Office, 1958 — 97-104

COURTNEY LD: *Amniotic fluid embolism.* Obstet

Section IV (continued)

Plate Number

Gynecol Surv 29:169-177, 1974 — 123

COTTOM DG, MYERS NA: *Congenital lobar emphysema.* Br Med J 5032:1394-1396, 1957 — 9

CROFTON J: *Respiratory tract disease. Bronchiectasis. I. Diagnosis.* Br Med J 5489:721-723, 1966 — 46, 47

CROFTON J: *Respiratory tract disease. Bronchiectasis. II. Treatment and prevention.* Br Med J 5490:783-785, 1966 — 46, 47

DANIEL RA, DIVELEY WL, EDWARDS WH, et al: *Mediastinal tumors.* Ann Surg 151:783-795, 1960 — 64

DEREMEE RA, HARRISON EG JR, ANDERSON HA: *The concept of classical interstitial pneumonitis-fibrositis (CIP-F) as a clinicopathologic syndrome.* Chest 61:213-220, 1972 — 140

DINES DE, BURGHER LW, OKAZAKI H: *The clinical and pathologic correlation of fat embolism syndrome.* Mayo Clin Proc 50:407-411, 1975 — 123

DIVERTIE MB: *Lung involvement in the connective tissue disorders.* Med Clin North Am 48:1015-1030, 1964 — 140-149

DONTAS NS: *The Pancoast syndrome.* Br J Tuberc 51:246-250, 1957 — 55

DREWS JA, BENFIELD JR, MERCER EC: *Acute diaphragmatic injuries.* Ann Thorac Surg 16:67-78, 1973 — 128

DUFFELL GM, MARCUS JH, INGRAM RH JR: *Limitation of expiratory flow in chronic obstructive pulmonary disease. Relation of clinical characteristics, pathophysiological type, and mechanisms.* Ann Intern Med 72:365-374, 1970 — 33-35, 40, 41

DUNHILL MS: *The pathology of asthma, with special reference to changes in the bronchial mucosa.* J Clin Pathol 13:27-33, 1960 — 13-27

EAGAN RT, MAURER LH, FORCIER RJ, et al: *Proceedings: small cell carcinoma of the lung: staging, paraneoplastic syndromes, treatment, and survival.* Cancer 33:527-532, 1974 — 53

EDMONDSON EB, SANFORD JP: *The Klebsiella-Enterobacter (Aerobacter)-Serratia group. A clinical and bacteriological evaluation.* Medicine (Baltimore) 46:323-340, 1967 — 66-76

EINHORN LH, FEE WH, FARBER MO, et al: *Improved chemotherapy for small-cell undifferentiated lung cancer.* JAMA 235:1225-1229, 1976 — 53

EISENBERG H, DUBOIS EL, SHERWIN RP, et al: *Diffuse interstitial lung disease in systemic lupus erythematosus.* Ann Int Med 79:37-45, 1973 — 147

ELLIS K, RENTHAL G: *Pulmonary sarcoidosis. Roentgenographic observations on the course of the disease.* Am J Roentgenol 88:1070-1083, 1962 — 141

ELMES PC, SIMPSON MJ: *The clinical aspects of mesothelioma.* Q J Med 69:427-449, 1976 — 65

ESTERLY JR, OPPENHEIMER EH: *Cystic fibrosis of the pancreas: structural changes in peripheral airways.* Thorax 23:670-675, 1968 — 48, 49

EWAN PW, JONES HA, RHODES CG: *Detection of intrapulmonary hemorrhage with carbon monoxide uptake.* N Engl J Med 295:1391-1396, 1976 — 143

FARRELL PM, AVERY ME: *Hyaline membrane disease.* Am Rev Respir Dis 111:657-688, 1975 — 137-139

FAUCI AS, WOLFF SM: *Wegener's granulomatosis. Studies in eighteen patients and a review of the literature.* Medicine (Baltimore) 52:35-61, 1973 — 149

FINLAND M: *The significance of specific pneumococ-*

Section IV (continued)

Plate Number

cus types in disease, including types IV to XXXII.
Ann Intern Med 10:1531-1543, 1937 — 66-76

FINLAND M, PETERSON OL, STRAUSS E: *Staphylococcic pneumonia occurring during epidemic of influenza.* Arch Int Med 70:183-205, 1942 — 66-76

FISHER AM, TREVER RW, CURTIN JA, et al: *Straphylococcal pneumonia; a review of 21 cases in adults.* N Engl J Med 258:919-928, 1958 — 66-76

FISHMAN AP: *Chronic cor pulmonale.* Am Rev Respir Dis 114:775-794, 1976 — 36

FISHMAN AP: *Pulmonary edema: the water-exchanging function of the lung.* Circulation 46:390-408, 1972 — 124, 125

FISHMAN AP: *Shock lung: a distinctive nonentity.* Circulation 47:921-923, 1973 — 124, 125

FLANC C, KAKKAR VV, CLARKE MB: *The detection of venous thrombosis of legs using ^{125}I-labelled fibrinogen.* Br J Surg 55:742-747, 1968 — 111

FLETCHER DE, EDGE JR: *The early radiological changes in pulmonary and pleural asbestosis.* Clin Radiol 21:355-365, 1970 — 97-104

FORSYTH BR, BLOOM HH, JOHNSON KM, et al: *Etiology of primary atypical pneumonia in a military population.* JAMA 191:364, 1965 — 66-76

FOX W: *Changing concepts in the chemotherapy of tuberculosis.* Am Rev Respir Dis 97:767-790, 1968 — 86-96

FOY HM, KENNEY GE, MCMAHON R, et al: *Mycoplasma pneumoniae pneumonia in an urban area. Five years of surveillance.* JAMA 214:1666-1672, 1970 — 66-76

FRASER RG: *The radiologist and obstructive airway disease.* Am J Roentgenol 120:737-775, 1974 — 40, 41

FRASER RG, PARÉ JA: *Diagnosis of Diseases of the Chest.* Philadelphia, WB Saunders, 1970 — 4, 58, 59

FRAZIER AR, MILLER RD: *Interstitial pneumonitis in association with polymyositis and dermatomyositis.* Chest 65:403-407, 1974 — 148

FRIDY WW JR, INGRAM RH JR, HIERHOLZER JC, et al: *Airways function during mild viral respiratory illnesses. The effect of rhinovirus infection in cigarette smokers.* Ann Intern Med 80:150-155, 1974 — 37

GAENSLER EA, CADIGAN JB, SASAHARA AA, et al: *Graphite pneumoconiosis of electrotypers.* Am J Med 41:864-882, 1966 — 97-104

GAMSU G, NADEL JA: *The roentgenologic manifestations of emphysema and chronic bronchitis.* Med Clin North Am 57:719-733, 1973 — 40, 41

GALLUS AS, HIRSH J: *Treatment of venous thromboembolic disease.* Seminar Thromb Hemostas 2:291-331, 1976 — 107

GEOGHEGAN T, LAM CR: *Mechanism of death from intracardiac air and its reversibility.* Ann Surg 138:351-359, 1953 — 123

GIBSON LE, DI SANT'AGNESE PA, SHWACHMAN H: *Procedure for the quantitative iontophoretic sweat test for cystic fibrosis.* Atlanta, Cystic Fibrosis Foundation, 1975 — 48, 49

GILSON JC: *Occupational bronchitis.* Proc R Soc Med 63:857-864, 1970 — 97-104

GOLD WM, JENNINGS DB: *Pulmonary function in patients with systemic lupus erythematosus.* Am Rev Respir Dis 93:556-567, 1966 — 147

GOLD WM, KESSLER GF, YU DY: *Role of vagus nerves in experimental asthma in allergic dogs.* J Appl Physiol 33:719-725, 1972 — 13-27

GOMEZ-URIA A, PAZIANOS AG: *Syndromes resulting from ectopic hormone-producing tumors.* Med Clin North Am 59:431-440, 1975 — 58, 59

GOOD CA, HOLMAN CB: *Cavitary carcinoma of*

Section IV (continued)

Plate Number

the lung: roentgenologic features in 19 cases. Dis Chest 37:289-293, 1960 — 57

GREENBERG SD, SMITH MN, SPJUT HJ: *Bronchiolo-alveolar carcinoma–cell of origin.* Am J Clin Pathol 63:153-167, 1975 — 61

GRILLO HC: *Management of tracheal stenosis following assisted respiration.* J Thorac Cardiovasc Surg 57:52-71, 1969 — 10-12

GRILLO HC: *Surgical approaches to the trachea.* Surg Gynecol Obstet 129:347-352, 1969 — 10-12

GRIMBY G, OXHOJ H, BAKE B: *Effects of abdominal breathing on distribution of ventilation in obstructive lung disease.* Clin Sci Mol Med 48:193-199, 1975 — 36, 43, 44

GUENTER CA, WELCH MH, HAMMARSTEN JF: *Alpha$_1$-antitrypsin deficiency and pulmonary emphysema.* Annu Rev Med 22:283-292, 1971 — 39

GUYTON AC, GRANGER HJ, TAYLOR AE: *Interstitial fluid pressure.* Physiol Rev 51:527-563, 1971 — 124, 125

HAEGER K: *Problems of acute deep venous thrombosis. I. The interpretation of signs and symptoms.* Angiology 20:280-286, 1969 — 112, 113

HALE LW, GOUGH J, KING EJ, et al: *Pneumoconiosis of kaolin workers.* Br J Ind Med 13:251-259, 1956 — 97-104

HALL WJ, HYDE RW, SCHWARTZ RH, et al: *Pulmonary abnormalities in intermediate alpha$_1$-antitrypsin deficiency.* J Clin Invest 58:1069-1072, 1976 — 39

HALLBOOK T, GOTHLIN J: *Strain gauge plethysmography and phlebography in diagnosis of deep venous thrombosis.* Acta Chir Scand 137:37-52, 1971 — 112, 113

HALLER JA JR, DONAHOO JS: *Traumatic asphyxia in children: pathophysiology and management.* J Trauma 11:453-457, 1971 — 130

HALLSTRAND HO: *Crushing chest injuries.* Int Surg 58:316-321, 1973 — 132

HAMMAN L, RICH AR: *Acute diffuse interstitial fibrosis of the lungs.* Bull Johns Hopkins Hosp 74:177-212, 1944 — 140

HARRIS WH, SALZMAN EW, ATHANASOULIS C, et al: *Comparison of ^{125}I fibrinogen count scanning with phlebography for detection of venous thrombi after elective hip surgery.* N Engl J Med 292:665-667, 1975 — 111

HARVEY AM, et al: *Systemic lupus erythematosus: review of the literature and clinical analysis of 138 cases.* Medicine (Baltimore) 33:291-437, 1954 — 147

HATCH TF, GROSS P: *Pulmonary Deposition and Retention of Inhaled Aerosols.* New York, Academic Press, 1964 — 97-104

HEPPER NG, FERGUSON RH, HOWARD FM JR: *Three types of pulmonary involvement in polymyositis.* Med Clin North Am 48:1031-1042, 1964 — 148

HIGGINS CB, MULDER MD: *Chylothorax after surgery for congenital heart disease.* J Thorac Cardiovasc Surg 61:411-418, 1971 — 134

HILARIS BS, MARTINI N, LUOMANEN RK, et al: *The value of preoperative radiation therapy in apical cancer of the lung.* Surg Clin North Am 54:831-840, 1974 — 55

HO M, DOWLING JN, ARMSTRONG JA, et al: *Factors contributing to the risk of cytomegalovirus infection in patients receiving renal transplants.* Yale J Biol Med 49:17-26, 1976 — 66-76

HOCHBERG LA, SCHACTER B: *Benign tumors of bronchus and lung.* Am J Surg 89:425-438, 1955 — 63

HOLLINGER P: *Congenital anomalies of the*

Section IV (continued)

Plate Number

tracheobronchial tree. Post Grad Med 362:454-462, 1964 — 5

HORN BR, ROBIN DR, THEODORE J, et al: *Total eosinophil counts in the management of bronchial asthma.* N Engl J Med 292:1152-1155, 1975 — 13-27

HOURIHANE DO: *The pathology of mesotheliomata and an analysis of their association with asbestos exposure.* Thorax 19:268-278, 1964 — 65

HOWELL JF, CRAWFORD ES, JORDAN GL JR: *The flail chest: an analysis of 100 patients.* J Surg 106:628-635, 1963 — 127

HUANG CT, LYONS HA: *Comparison of pulmonary function in patients with systemic lupus erythematosus, scleroderma and rheumatoid arthritis.* Am Rev Respir Dis 93:865-875, 1966 — 140-149

HUANG CT, HENNIGAR GR, LYONS HA: *Pulmonary dysfunction in systemic lupus erythematosus.* N Engl J Med 272:288-293, 1965 — 147

HUDSON LD, SBARBARO JA: *Twice weekly tuberculosis chemotherapy.* JAMA 223:139-143, 1973 — 88-96

HUSSEY HH: *Pulmonary confusion.* JAMA 230:264, 1974 — 137

INGRAM RH JR: *Chronic bronchitis, emphysema and chronic airways obstruction.* In *Harrison's Principles of Internal Medicine,* 8th ed. Philadelphia, McGraw-Hill, 1977 — 36, 43, 44

INGRAM RH JR, GROSSMAN GD: *Chronic cor pulmonale.* In *The Heart,* 3rd ed. New York, McGraw-Hill, 1974 — 36

INGRAM RH JR, O'CAIN CF: *Frequency dependence of compliance in apparently healthy smokers versus non-smokers.* Bull Physiopathol Resp 7:195-212, 1971 — 37

INGRAM RH JR, O'CAIN CF, FRIDY WW JR: *Simultaneous quasi-static lung pressure-volume curves and "closing volume" measurements.* J Appl Physiol 36:135-141, 1974 — 37

INGRAM RH JR, SCHILDER DP: *Effect of pursed lips expiration on the pulmonary pressure-flow relationship in obstructive lung disease.* Am Rev Respir Dis 96:381-388, 1967 — 34, 43

ISRAEL HL, PATCHEFSKY AS, SALDANA MJ: *Wegener's granulomatosis, lymphomatoid granulomatosis and benign lymphocytic angiitis and granulomatosis of lung.* Ann Int Med 87:691-699, 1977 — 149

JACOBSON G, LAINHART WS: *ILO U/C 1971 international classification of radiographs of the pneumoconioses.* Med Radiogr Photogr 48:67-76, 1972 — 97-104

JAFFE HJ, KATZ S: *Current ideas about bronchiectasis.* Am Fam Physician 7:69-76, 1973 — 46, 47

JANOWER ML, BLENNERHASSETT JB: *Lymphangitic spread of metastatic cancer to the lung. A radiologic-pathologic classification.* Radiology 101:267-273, 1971 — 57

JAY SJ, JOHANSON WG JR, PIERCE AK: *The radiographic resolution of Streptococcus pneumoniae pneumonia.* N Engl J Med 293:798-801, 1975 — 66-76

JOHNSON RM, LINDSKOG GE: *100 cases of tumor metastatic to lung mediastimum. Treatment and results.* JAMA 202:94-98, 1967 — 60

JONES JC, ALMOND CH, SNYDER HM, et al: *Lobar emphysema and congenital heart disease in infancy.* J Thorac Cardiovasc Surg 49:1-10, 1965 — 9

JONES MJ, JAMES EC: *The management of traumatic asphyxia: case report and literature review.* J Trauma 16:235-238, 1976 — 130

Section IV (continued)

JONES RJ, SAMPSON PC, DUGAN DJ: *Current management of civilian thoracic trauma.* Am J Surg 114:289-296, 1967 — 131

JOSEPH WL, MURRAY JF, MULDER DG: *Mediastinal tumors–problems in diagnosis and treatment.* Dis Chest 50:150-160, 1966 — 64

KAKKAR VV: *The diagnosis of deep vein thrombosis, using the ^{125}I fibrinogen test.* Arch Surg 104:152-159, 1972 — 110

KAKKAR VV, CORRIGAN TP: *Detection of deep vein thrombosis: survey and current status.* Prog Cardiovasc Dis 17:207-217, 1974 — 111

KAKKAR VV, NICOLAIDES AN, RENNEY JT, et al: *^{125}I-labelled fibrinogen test adapted for routine screening for deep-vein thrombosis.* Lancet 1:540, 1970 — 111

KILBOURNE ED: *The molecular epidemiology of influenza.* J Infect Dis 127:478-487, 1973 — 66-76

KIRSH MM, ORRINGER MB, BEHRENDT PM, et al: *Management of tracheobronchial disruption secondary to nonpenetrating trauma.* Ann Thorac Surg 22:93-101, 1976 — 129

KOUTRAS P, URSCHEL HC JR, PAULSON DL: *Hamartoma of the lung.* J Thorac Cardiovasc Surg 61:768-776, 1971 — 63

KOVATS F, BUGYI B: *Occupational Mycotic Diseases of the Lungs.* Budapest, Akademiai Kiado, 1968 — 105, 106

KURITZKY P, GOLDFARB AL: *Unusual electrocardiographic changes in spontaneous pneumothorax.* Chest 70:535-537, 1976 — 132

LAMBIE JM, MAHAFFEY RG, BARBER DC: *Diagnostic accuracy in venous thrombosis.* Br Med J 2:142-143, 1970 — 110

LAMPSON RS: *Traumatic chylothorax.* J Thorac Cardiovasc Surg 17:778, 1948 — 134

LAU WK, YOUNG LS: *Trimethoprim-sulfamethoxazole treatment of Pneumocystis carinii pneumonia in adults.* N Engl J Med 295:716-718, 1976 — 66-76

LEHAR TJ, CARR DT, MILLER WE, et al: *Roentgenographic appearance of bronchogenic adenocarcinoma.* Am Rev Respir Dis 96:245-248, 1967 — 54

LEIGH TF, WEENS HS: *Roentgen aspects of mediastinal lesions.* Semin Roentgenol 4:59-73, 1969 — 64

LEMAY M, PIRO AJ: *Cavitary pulmonary metastases.* Ann Intern Med 62:59-66, 1965 — 60

LERTZMAN MM, CHERNIACK RM: *Rehabilitation of patients with chronic obstructive pulmonary disease.* Am Rev Respir Dis 114:1145-1165, 1976 — 36, 43, 44

LESTER W: *Treatment of drug-resistant tuberculosis.* DM:1-43, 1971 — 88-96

LEVITT SH, JONES TK, KILPATRICK SJ JR, et al: *Treatment of malignant superior vena caval obstruction. A randomized study.* Cancer 24:447-457, 1969 — 56

LICHTENSTEIN L, AUSTEN KF (Eds): *Asthma: Physiology, Immunopharmacology, and Treatment.* New York, Academic Press, 1977 — 13-27

LIE JT: *Nosology of pulmonary vasculitides,* Mayo Clin Proc 52:520-522, 1977 — 149

LIEBOW AA: *Bronchiolo-alveolar carcinoma.* Adv Intern Med 10:329-358, 1960 — 61

LIEBOW AA, CARRINGTON CB: *Alveolar diseases. The interstitial pneumonias.* In SIMON M (Ed): *Frontiers of Pulmonary Radiology.* New York, Grune & Stratton, 1967, pp 102-141 — 140

LIEBOW AA, HALES MR, LINDSKOG GE: *Enlargement of the bronchial arteries and their anastomoses with pulmonary arteries in bronchiectasis.*

Section IV (continued)

Am J Pathol 25:211-231, 1949 — 46, 47

LIGGINS GC, HOWIE RN: *A controlled trial of antipartum glucocorticoid treatment for prevention of the respiratory distress syndrome in premature infants.* Pediatrics 50:515-525, 1972 — 137-139

LOFGREN S: *Erythema nodosum. Studies on etiology and pathogenesis in 185 adult cases.* Acta Med Scand (Suppl) 174:1-197, 1946 — 141

LOKICH JJ, GOODMAN R: *Superior vena cava syndrome. Clinical management.* JAMA 231:58-61, 1975 — 56

LOURIA DB, BLUMENFELD HL, ELLIS JT, et al: *Studies on influenza in the pandemic of 1957-1958. II. Pulmonary complications of influenza.* J Clin Invest 38:213-265, 1959 — 66-76

MCBURNEY RP, MCDONALD JR, CLAGETT OT: *Bronchogenic small-cell carcinoma.* J Thorac Cardiovasc Surg 22:63-73, 1951 — 53

MCFADDEN ER JR, LYONS HA: *Arterial blood gas tensions in asthma.* N Engl J Med 278:1027-1032, 1968 — 13-27

MCFADDEN ER JR, INGRAM RH JR: *Peripheral airway obstruction.* JAMA 235:259-260, 1976 — 37

MCFARLANE RG: *An enzyme cascade in the blood clotting mechanism and its function as a biochemical amplifier.* Nature (London) 202:498-499, 1964 — 107

MCGREGOR MB, SANDLER G: *Wegener's granulomatosis. A clinical and radiological survey.* Br J Radiol 37:430-439, 1964 — 149

MACKLEM PT: *The pathophysiology of chronic bronchitis and emphysema.* Med Clin North Am 57:669-670, 1973 — 33-35, 40, 41

MAHRER PR, EVANS JA, STEINBERG I: *Scleroderma: relation of pulmonary changes to esophageal disease.* Ann Intern Med 40:92-110, 1954 — 146

MANFREDI F, DALY WJ, BEHNKE RH: *Clinical observations of acute Friedländer pneumonia.* Ann Intern Med 58:642-653, 1963 — 66-76

MARCUS JH, MCLEAN RL, DUFFELL GM, et al: *Exercise performance in relation to pathophysiologic type of chronic obstructive pulmonary disease.* Am J Med 49:14-22, 1970 — 33-35, 40, 41

MARDER VJ, SHULMAN NR: *High molecular weight derivatives of human fibrinogen produced by plasmin.* J Biol Chem 244:2120-2124, 1969 — 109

MARKEL SF, ABELL MR, HAIGHT C, et al: *Neoplasms of bronchus commonly designated as adenomas.* Cancer 17:590-608, 1964 — 62

MARTEL W, ABELL MR, MIKKELSEN WM, et al: *Pulmonary and pleural lesions in rheumatoid disease.* Radiology 90:641-653, 1968 — 145

MELLINS RB, LEVIN OR, INGRAM RH JR, et al: *Obstructive disease of the airways in cystic fibrosis.* Pediatrics 41:560-573, 1968 — 48, 49

MEYERS JD, SPENCER HC JR, WATTS JC, et al: *Cytomegalovirus pneumonia after human marrow transplantation.* Ann Intern Med 82:181-188, 1975 — 66-76

MILES RM, RICHARDSON RR, WAYNE L, et al: *Long-term results with the serrated Teflon vena caval clip in the prevention of pulmonary embolism.* Ann Surg 169:881-891, 1969 — 122

MILNE JE: *Nitrogen dioxide inhalation and bronchiolitis obliterans. A review of the literature and report of a case.* J Occup Med 114:538-547, 1969 — 97-104

MITCHELL DN, SCADDING JG: *Sarcoidosis.* Am Rev Respir Dis 110:774-802, 1974 — 141

MITCHELL RS: *Control of tuberculosis.* N Engl J

Section IV (continued)

Med 276:842-848 & 905-11, 1973 — 88-96

MITCHELL RS, STANFORD RE, JOHNSON JM, et al: *The morphologic features of the bronchi, bronchioles, and alveoli in chronic airway obstruction: a clinicopathologic study.* Am Rev Respir Dis 114:137-145, 1976 — 29-33, 35, 45

MITENKO PA, OGILVIE RI: *Rational intravenous doses of theophylline.* N Engl J Med 289:600-603, 1973 — 13-27

MOBIN-UDDIN K: *Present status of the inferior vena cava umbrella filter.* Surgery 70:914-919, 1971 — 122

MOORE JD, MAYER JH, GAGO O: *Traumatic asphyxia.* Chest 62:634-635, 1972 — 130

MOORE FJ, et al: *Posttraumatic Pulmonary Insufficiency.* Philadelphia, WB Saunders, 1969 — 136

MORETZ WH, RHODE CM, SHEPHERD MH: *Prevention of pulmonary emboli by partial occlusion of the inferior vena cava.* Am Surg 25:617-626, 1959 — 122

MORGAN WK, LAPP NL: *Respiratory disease in coal miners.* Am Rev Respir Dis 113:531-559, 1976 — 97-104

MORGAN WK, SEATON A: *Occupational Lung Diseases.* Philadelphia, WB Saunders, 1975 — 105, 106

MOSER KM, STEIN M (Eds): *Advances in Cardiopulmonary Diseases, Pulmonary Thromboembolism.* Chicago, Yearbook Medical Publishers, 1973 — 114-120

MUELLER RE, PETTY TL, FILLEY GF: *Ventilation and arterial blood gas changes induced by pursed lips breathing.* J Appl Physiol 28:784-789, 1970 — 34, 43

MULDER J, HERS JF: *Influenza.* Groningen, Walters-Noordhoff, 1972 — 66-76

MUSTARD WT, et al: *Pediatric Surgery,* 2nd ed. Chicago, Year Book Medical Publishers, 1963 — 1, 4

NAGAYA H, ELMORE M, FORD CD: *Idiopathic interstitial pulmonary fibrosis. An immune complex disease?* Am Rev Respir Dis 107:826-830, 1973 — 140

NASH ES, BRISCOE WA, COURNAND A: *The relationship between clinical and physiological findings in chronic obstructive disease of the lungs.* Med Thorac 22:305-327, 1965. — 33-35, 40, 41

NASH G, LANGLINAIS PC, GREENAWALD KA: *Alveolar cell carcinoma: does it exist?* Cancer 29:322-326, 1972 — 61

NICE CM JR, MENON AN, RIGLER LG: *Pulmonary manifestations in collagen diseases.* Am J Roentgenol 81:264-279, 1959 — 140-149

NORTHWAY WH, ROSAN RC, PORTER DY: *Pulmonary disease following respiratory therapy of hyaline membrane disease. Bronchopulmonary dysplasia.* N Engl J Med 276:357-368, 1967 — 137-139

OCHSNER A: *Bronchiectasis. Disappearing pulmonary lesion.* NY State J Med 75:1683-1689, 1975 — 46, 47

OGNIBENE AJ, JOHNSON DE: *Idiopathic pulmonary hemosiderosis in adults. Report of case and review of literature.* Arch Intern Med 111:503-510, 1963 — 143

OLLIVIER: *Relation medicale des évènements survenus au Champs-de-Mars le 14 juin, 1837.* Ann Hyg 18:485-489, 1837 — 130

ORANGE RP, AUSTEN WG, AUSTEN KF: *The immunologic release of histamine and slow reacting substance of anaphylaxis from human lung. I. Modulation by agents influencing cyclic 3', 5'-adenosine monophosphate.* J Exp Med 134 (Suppl):136, 1971 — 13-27

OSEASOHN R, ADELSON L, KAJI M:

Section IV (continued)

Plate Number

Clinicopathologic study of thirty-three fatal cases of Asian influenza. N Engl J Med 260:509-518, 1959   66-76

OSTROW D, CHERNIACK RM: *Resistance to airflow in patients with diffuse interstitial lung disease.* Am Rev Respir Dis 108:205-210, 1973   140

PADOVAN IF, DAWSON CA, HENSCHEL EO, et al: *Pathogenesis of mediastinal emphysema and pneumothorax following tracheotomy.* Chest 66:553-556, 1974   130, 132

PAMRA SP, PRASAD G, MATHUR GP: *Relapse in pulmonary tuberculosis.* Am Rev Respir Dis 113:67-72, 1976   88-96

PANCOAST HK: *Superior pulmonary sulcus tumor; tumor characterized by pain, Horner's syndrome, destruction of bone and atrophy of hand muscles.* JAMA 99:1391-1396, 1932   55

PARASKOS JS, ADELSTEIN SJ, SMITH RE, et al: *Late prognosis of acute pulmonary embolism.* N Engl J Med 289:55-58, 1973   114-120

PATTON MM, McDONALD JR, MOERSCH HJ: *Bronchogenic adenocarcinoma.* J Thorac Cardiovasc Surg 22:83-87, 1951   54

PATTON MM, McDONALD JR, MOERSCH HJ: *Bronchogenic large cell carcinoma.* J Thorac Cardiovasc Surg 22:88-93, 1951   52

PELEG H, PAUZNER Y: *Benign tumors of the lung.* Dis Chest 47:179-186, 1965   63

PERLMAN LV, LERNER E, D'ESOPO N: *Clinical classification and analysis of 97 cases of lung abscess.* Am Rev Respir Dis 99:390-398, 1969   77, 78

PETTY TL, ASHBAUGH DG: *Adult respiratory distress syndrome. Clinical features, factors influencing prognosis and principles of management.* Chest 60:233-239, 1971   136

PETTY TL, WILKINS M: *The five manifestations of rheumatoid lung.* Dis Chest 49:75-82, 1966   145

PHIBBS BP, SUNDIN RE, MITCHELL RS: *Silicosis in Wyoming bentonite workers.* Am Rev Respir Dis 103:1-17, 1971   97-104

PIERCE JA, EISEN AZ, DHINGRA HK: *Relationship of antitrypsin deficiency to the pathogenesis of emphysema.* Trans Assoc Am Physicians 82:87-97, 1969   9

PIERCE AK, SANFORD JP: *Aerobic gram-negative bacillary pneumonias.* Am Rev Respir Dis 110:647-658, 1974   66-76

RABINOV K, PAULIN S: *Roentgen diagnosis of venous thrombosis in the leg.* Arch Surg 104:134-144, 1972   110

RAWLINGS W JR, KREISS P, LEVY D, et al: *Clinical, epidemiologic, and pulmonary function studies in alpha$_1$-antitrypsin–deficient subjects of Pi Z type.* Am Rev Respir Dis 114:945-953, 1976   35

REBUCK AS, READ J: *Assessment and management of severe asthma.* Am J Med 51:788-798, 1971   13-27

REES HA, MILLAR JS, DONALD KW: *A study of the clinical course and arterial blood gas tensions of patients in status asthmaticus.* Q J Med 37:541-561, 1968   13-27

REYNOLDS EO: *Management of hyaline membrane disease.* Br Med Bull 31:18-24, 1975   137-139

RICKMAN FD, HARDIN R, HOWE JP, et al: *Fibrin split products in acute pulmonary embolism.* Ann Intern Med 79:664-668, 1973   109

RITCHIE B: *Pulmonary function in scleroderma.* Thorax 19:28-36, 1964   146

ROBIN ED, CROSS CE, ZELIS R: *Pulmonary edema.* N Engl J Med 288:239-246 & 292-304, 1973   124, 125

ROGERS DE: *The current problems of staphylococcal*

Section IV (continued)

Plate Number

infections. Ann Intern Med 45:748-781, 1956   66-76

ROGOFF SM, DEWEESE JA: *Phlebography of the lower extremity.* JAMA 172:1599-1606, 1960   110

ROSCHER R, BITTNER R, STOCKMAN U: *Pulmonary confusion. Clinical experience.* Arch Surg 109:508-510, 1974   135, 136

ROSE AL, WALTON JN: *Polymyositis: A survey of 89 cases with particular reference to treatment and prognosis.* Brain 89:747-768, 1966   148

ROSE GA: *Clinical features of polyarteritis nodosa with lung involvement.* Br J Tuberc 51:113-122, 1957   149

ROSE GA, SPENCER H: *Polyarteritis nodosa.* Q J Med 26:43-81, 1957   149

ROSEN P, ARMSTRONG D, RAMOS C: *Pneumocystis carinii pneumonia. A clinicopathologic study of twenty patients with neoplastic diseases.* Am J Med 53:428-436, 1972   66-76

ROSEN SH, CASTLEMAN B, LIEBOW AA: *Pulmonary alveolar proteinosis.* N Engl J Med 258:1123-1142, 1958   144

RUBIN EH, LUBLINER R: *The Hamman-Rich syndrome: review of the literature and analysis of 15 cases.* Medicine 36:397-463, 1957   140

RUBIN P: *Lung cancer: histopathologic analysis as related to treatment policy and radiation response.* Front Rad Ther Onc 9:151, 1974   52

RUBIN P, GREEN J, HOLZWASSER G, et al: *Superior vena caval syndrome. Slow low-dose versus rapid high-dose schedules.* Radiology 81:388-401, 1963   56

RUBIN PE, BLOCK AJ: *Nonspecific lung abscess. A perspective.* Geriatrics 27:125-136, 1972   77, 78

RUCKLEY CV, DAS PC, LEITCH AG, et al: *Serum fibrin-fibrinogen degradation products associated with postoperative pulmonary embolus and venous thrombosis.* Br Med J 4:395-398, 1970   109

RYLAND D, REID LM: *The pulmonary circulation in cystic fibrosis.* Thorax 30:285-292, 1975   48, 49

SAGEL SS, ABLOW RC: *Hamartoma: on occasion a rapidly growing tumor of the lung.* Radiology 91:971-972, 1968   63

SALSALI M, CLIFFTON EE: *Superior vena caval obstruction with carcinoma of the lung.* Surg Gynecol Obstet 121:783-788, 1965   56

SALYER DC, SALYER WR, EGGLESTON JC: *Bronchial carcinoid tumors.* Cancer 36:1522-1537, 1975   62

SASAHARA AA: *Current problems in pulmonary embolism: introduction.* Prog Cardiovasc Dis 17:161-165, 1974.   114-120

SCADDING JG: *Diffuse pulmonary alveolar fibrosis.* Thorax 29:271-281, 1974   140

SCHWARTZ HJ, LOWELL FC, MELBY JC: *Steroid resistance in bronchial asthma.* Ann Intern Med 69:493-499, 1968   13-27

SEIDMAN H, SILVERBERG E, HOLLEB AI: *Cancer Statistics, 1976. A comparison of white and black populations.* CA 26:2-30, 1976   50

SEVITT S, GALLAGHER N: *Venous thrombosis and pulmonary embolism. A clinicopathologic study in injured and burned patients.* Br J Surg 48:475-489, 1961   111

SHAPIRO R, WILSON GL, YESNER R, et al: *A useful roentgen sign in the diagnosis of localized bronchioloalveolar carcinoma.* Am J Roentgenol 114:516-524, 1972   61

SHARNOFF JG, SCHNEIDER L: *Wegener's granulomatosis.* Am Rev Respir Dis 86:553-556, 1962   149

SHULMAN JA, PHILLIPS LA, PETERSDORF RG: *Errors and hazards in the diagnosis and treatment*

Section IV (continued)

Plate Number

of bacterial pneumonias. Ann Intern Med 62:41-58, 1965   66-76

SILTZBACH LE: *Sarcoidosis: clinical features and management.* Med Clin North Am 51:483-502, 1967   141

SILTZBACH LE: *The Kveim test in sarcoidosis. A study of 750 patients.* JAMA 178:476-482, 1961   141

SOERGEL KH, SOMMERS SC: *Idiopathic pulmonary hemosiderosis and related syndromes.* Am J Med 32:499-511, 1962   143

SOM ML, KLEIN SH: *Primary anastomosis of the trachea after resection of a wide segment; an experimental study.* J Mt Sinai Hosp NY 25:211-220, 1958   10-12

SOM ML, NUSSBAUM M: *Tracheal resection and reanastomosis. Cervical approach.* Arch Otolaryngol 99:19-22, 1974   10-12

SPENCER FC, JUDE J, RIENHOFF WF III, et al: *Plication of the inferior vena cava for pulmonary embolism: long-term results in 39 cases.* Ann Surg 161:788-801, 1965   122

SPENCER H: *Pulmonary lesions in polyarteritis nodosa.* Br J Tuberc 51:123-130, 1957   149

SPENCER H: *Pathology of the Lung,* 2nd ed. Oxford, Pergamon Press, 1968   7, 6, 51

STAUB NC: *Pulmonary edema.* Physiol Rev 54:678-811, 1974   124, 125

STEIN M (Ed): *New Directions in Asthma.* Park Ridge Ill, American College of Chest Physicians, 1975   13-27

STRANDNESS DE JR, SUMNER DS: *Acute venous thrombosis.* JAMA 233:46-48, 1975   112, 113

STRANDNESS DE JR, SUMNER DS: *Ultrasonic velocity detector in the diagnosis of thrombophlebitis.* Arch Surg 104:180-183, 1972   112, 113

SZENTIVANYI A: *The adrenergic theory of the atopic abnormality in bronchial asthma.* J Allergy 42:203-232, 1968   13-27

TEIRSTEIN AS, SILTZBACH LE: *Sarcoidosis of the upper lung fields simulating pulmonary tuberculosis.* Chest 64:303-308, 1973   141

THURLBECK WM: *Chronic bronchitis and emphysema.* Med Clin North Am 57:651-668, 1973   29-33, 36, 39

TIMMES JJ, GRAY JA: *Developmental anatomy and diseases caused by maldevelopment of the tracheobronchial tree.* In BAUM GL (Ed): *Textbook of Pulmonary Diseases,* 2nd ed. Boston, Little, Brown, 1974, pp 885-892   1, 6, 9

TIMMES JJ, GRAY JA: *Congenital diseases caused by anomalies of the pulmonary vasculature, the pleural fissures, and the thoracic cage.* In BAUM GL (Ed): *Textbook of Pulmonary Diseases,* 2nd ed. Boston, Little, Brown, 1974, pp 893-899   6

TRAPNELL DH: *Radiological appearances of lymphangitic carcinomatosa of the lung.* Thorax 19:251-260, 1964   57

TRIEBWASSER JH, HARRIS RE, BRYANT R, et al: *Varicella pneumonia in adults. Report of seven cases and a review of literature.* Medicine 46:409-423, 1967   66-76

TRINKLE JK, FURMAN RW, HINSHAW MA, et al: *Pulmonary contusion. Pathogenesis and effect of various resuscitative measures.* Ann Thorac Surg 16:568-575, 1973   136

TRINKLE JK, RICHARDSON JD, FRANZ JL, et al: *Management of flail chest without mechanical ventilation.* Ann Thorac Surg 19:355-363, 1975   126, 127

TURNBULL AD, HUVOS AG, GOODNER JT, et al: *The malignant potential of bronchial*

Section IV (continued)

adenoma. Ann Thorac Surg 14:453-464, 1972 — 62

VISWANATHAN R, JAIN SK, SUBRAMANIAN S: *Pulmonary edema of high altitude. 3. Pathogenesis.* Am Rev Respir Dis 100:342-349, 1969 — 124, 125

WALKER WC, WRIGHT V: *Rheumatoid pleuritis.* Ann Rheum Dis 26:467-474, 1967 — 145

WALZER PD, PERL DP, KROGSTAD DJ, et al: *Pneumocystis carinii pneumonia in the United States. Epidemiologic, diagnostic, and clinical features.* Ann Intern Med 80:83-93, 1974 — 66-76

WASSERMAN K, BLANK N, FLETCHER G: *Lung lavage (alveolar washing) in alveolar proteinosis.* Am J Med 44:611-617, 1968 — 144

WEAVER AL, DIVERTIE MB, TITUS JL: *Pulmonary scleroderma.* Dis Chest 54:490-498, 1968 — 146

WEBB WR: *Thoracic trauma.* Surg Clin North Am 54:1179-1192, 1974 — 126, 127, 131-133

WEBB-JOHNSON DC, ANDREWS JL JR: *Drug therapy–bronchodilator therapy.* N Engl J Med 297:476-482 & 758-764, 1977 — 13-27

WEILL H, GEORGE R, SCHWARZ M, et al: *Late evaluation of pulmonary function after acute exposure to chlorine gas.* Am Rev Respir Dis 99:374-379, 1969 — 97-104

WEISS EB (Ed): *Status Asthmaticus.* Baltimore, University Park Press, 1978 — 13-27

WEISS EB, SEGAL MS (Eds): *Bronchial Asthma: Mechanisms and Therapeutics.* Boston, Little, Brown, 1976 — 13-27

WEISS W: *Oral antibiotic therapy for acute aspiration lung abscess.* Tex Med 74:110-114, 1978 — 77, 78

WEISS W: *Cavity behavior in acute, primary, nonspecific lung abscess.* Am Rev Respir Dis 108:1273-1275, 1973 — 77, 78

WEISS W, BOUCOT KR, COOPER DA: *The histopathology of bronchogenic carcinoma and its relation to growth rate, metastasis and prognosis.* Cancer 26:965-970, 1970 — 51

WEISS W, CHERNIACK NS: *Acute nonspecific lung abscess: a controlled study comparing orally and parenterally administered penicillin G.* Chest 66:348-351, 1974 — 77, 78

WEISZ GM: *Fat embolism.* Curr Probl Surg: 1-54, 1974 — 123

WESSLER S, YIN ET: *Theory and practice of minidose heparin in surgical patients. A status report.* Circulation 47:671-676, 1973 — 107

WHEELER HB, PEARSON D, O'CONNELL D, et al: *Impedance phlebography: technique, interpretation and results.* Arch Surg 104:164-169, 1972 — 110, 112, 113

WHITWELL F, RAWCLIFFE RM: *Diffuse malignant pleural mesothelioma and asbestos exposure.* Thorax 26:6-22, 1971 — 65

WIENER ES, OWENS L, SALZBERG AM: *Chylothorax after Bochdalek herniorrhaphy in a neonate. Treatment with intravenous hyperalimentation* J Thorac Cardiovasc Surg 65:200-206, 1973 — 134

WILLIAMS DM, KRICK JA, REMINGTON JS: *Pulmonary infection in the compromised host. Part II.* Am Rev Respir Dis 114:593-627, 1976 — 66-76

WILLIAMS JS, MINKEN SL, ADAMS JT: *Traumatic asphyxia, reappraised.* Ann Surg 167:384-392, 1968 — 130

WILLIAMS WJ: *Venography.* Circulation 47:220-221, 1973 — 110

WILLIS RA: *Secondary Tumours of the Lungs.* London, Butterworth, 1952 — 60

WILSON RJ, RODMAN GP, ROBIN ED: *An early pulmonary physiologic abnormality in progressive*

Section IV (continued)

systemic sclerosis (diffuse scleroderma). Am J Med 36:361-369, 1964 — 146

WISE L, CONNORS J, HWANG YH, et al: *Traumatic injuries to the diaphragm.* J Trauma 13:946-950, 1973 — 128

WITZLEBEN CL: *Aplasia of the trachea.* Pediatrics 32:31-35, 1963 — 5

WOOD RE, BOAT TF, DOERSHUK CF: *Cystic fibrosis.* Am Rev Respir Dis 113:833-878, 1976 — 48, 49

WOOLCOCK AJ, VINCENT NJ, MACKLEM PT: *Frequency dependence of compliance as a test for obstruction in small airways.* J Clin Invest 48:1097, 1969 — 37

ZISKIND MM: *Occupational pulmonary disease.* Clinical Symposia 30(4):1-32, 1978 — 97-104

ZISKIND MM, JONES RN, WEILL H: *Silicosis.* Am Rev Respir Dis 113:643-665, 1976 — 97-104

ZUCKERMAN HS, WURTZEBACK LR: *Kartagener's triad: review of literature and report of a case.* Dis Chest 19:92-97, 1951 — 46, 47

Section V

ALDRETE JA: *Nasotracheal intubation.* Surg Clin North Am 49:1209-1215, 1969 — 8

ALLEY RD: *Thoracic surgical incisions and postoperative drainage.* In Cooper P (Ed): *The Craft of Surgery,* 2nd ed. Boston, Little, Brown, 1971 — 17, 18

AROM KV, FRANZ JL, GROVER FL, et al: *Subxiphoid anterior mediastinal exploration.* Ann Thorac Surg 24:289-290, 1977 — 27, 28

ATTIA RR, RATTIT GE, MURPHY JD: *Transtrachial ventilation.* JAMA 234:1152-1153, 1975 — 7

AVERY WG, SAMET P, SACKNER MA: *The acidosis of pulmonary edema.* Am J Med 48:320-324, 1970 — 22

BAIER H, BEGIN R, SACKNER MA: *Effect of airway diameter, suction catheters, and the bronchofiberscope on airflow in endotracheal and tracheostomy tubes.* Heart Lung 5:235-238, 1976 — 8

BARRETT CR JR, VECCHIONE JJ, BELL AL JR: *Flexible fiberoptic bronchoscopy for airway management during acute respiratory failure.* Am Rev Respir Dis 109:429-434, 1974 — 11

BLOCK AJ: *Low flow oxygen therapy. Treatment of the ambulant patient.* Am Rev Respir Dis 110:71-84, 1974 — 25

BLOCK AJ, BURROWS B, KANNER RE, et al: *Oxygen administration in the home.* Am Rev Respir Dis 115:897-899, 1977 — 25

BRANTIGAN CO, GROW JB: *Cricothyroidotomy: elective use in respiratory problems requiring tracheostomy.* J Thorac Cardiovasc Surg 71:72-81, 1976 — 7, 9

BRYANT LR, SPENCER FC, BOYD AB, et al: *Tracheostomy and assisted ventilation.* In SABISTON DC JR, SPENCER FC (Eds): *Gibbon's Surgery of the Chest,* 3rd ed. Philadelphia, WB Saunders, 1976 — 7, 9

BURROWS B: *Arterial oxygenation and pulmonary hemodynamics in patients with chronic airways obstruction.* Am Rev Respir Dis 110:64-70, 1974 — 23

CAMPBELL EJ: *The mangement of acute respiratory failure in chronic bronchitis and emphysema.* Am Rev Respir Dis 96:626-639, 1967 — 23

CANTRELL ET, WARR GA, BUSBEE DL, et al: *Induction of aryl hydrocarbon hydroxylase in*

Section V (continued)

human pulmonary alveolar macrophages by cigarette smoking. J Clin Invest 52:1881-1884, 1973 — 8

CARLENS E: *Mediastinoscopy: a method for inspection and tissue biopsy in the superior mediastinum.* Dis Chest 36:343-352, 1959 — 27, 28

CHAMBERLAIN JM: *Pulmonary resection.* In COOPER P (Ed): *The Craft of Surgery,* 2nd ed. Boston, Little, Brown, 1971 — 29-31

CHAMBERLAIN JM, STOREY CF, KLOPSTOCK R, et al: *Segmental resection for pulmonary tuberculosis.* J Thorac Surg 26:471-485, 1953 — 32

CRAWLEY BE, CROSS DE: *Tracheal cuffs. A review and dynamic pressure study.* Anaesthesia 30:4-11, 1975 — 8

CUTCHAVAREE A, SACKNER MA: *Adult respiratory distress syndrome: report of 18 cases.* J Fla Med Assoc 61:429-436, 1974 — 22

D'ABREU AL, COLLIS JL, CLARKE DB: *A Practice of Thoracic Surgery,* 3rd ed. London, Edward Arnold, 1971 — 32

DANIELS AC: *A method of biopsy useful in diagnosing certain intrathoracic diseases.* Dis Chest 16:360-366, 1949 — 27, 28

DESLAURIERS J, BEAULIEU M, DUFOUR C, et al: *Mediastinopleuroscopy: a new approach to the diagnosis of intrathoracic diseases.* Ann Thorac Surg 22:265-269, 1976 — 27, 28

EGAN DF: *Fundamentals of Respiratory Therapy,* 3rd ed. St. Louis, CV Mosby, 1977 — 10, 24, 26

GRAHAM EA, SINGER JJ: *Successful removal of the entire lung for carcinoma of the bronchus.* JAMA 101:1371, 1933 — 30, 31

GROSS S: *A Practical Treatise on Foreign Bodies in the Air-passages.* Philadelphia, Blanchard & Lea, 1854 — 5, 6

HARKEN DE, BLACK H, CLAUSS R, et al: *Simple cervicomediastinal exploration for tissue diagnosis of intrathoracic disease with comments on recognition of inoperable carcinoma of the lung.* N Engl J Med 251:1041-1044, 1954 — 27, 28

HASAN S, AVERY WA, SACKNER MA: *Near drowning in humans: report of 36 patients.* Chest 59:191-197, 1971 — 22

HAUGEN RK: *The café coronary. Sudden deaths in restaurants.* JAMA 186:142-143, 1963 — 5, 6

HAYATA Y, OHO K, ICHIBA M, et al: *Percutaneous pulmonary puncture for cytologic diagnosis: its diagnostic value for small peripheral pulmonary carcinoma.* Acta Cytol (Baltimore) 17:469-475, 1973 — 32

HEIMLICH HJ: *Heimlich maneuver: lecture at conference on emergency airway management.* Washington DC, National Academy of Sciences, 1976 — 5, 6

HEIMLICH HJ: *A life-saving maneuver to prevent food-choking.* JAMA 234:398-401, 1975 — 5, 6

HEIMLICH HJ: *"Pop goes the café coronary."* Emergency Medicine 6:154-155, 1974 — 5, 6

IKEDA S, ONO Y, MIYAZAWA S, et al: *Flexible bronchofiberscope.* Otolaryngology (Tokyo) 42:855-861, 1970 — 13-16

JACKSON C: *Bronchoscopy; past, present and future.* N Engl J Med 199:759-763, 1928 — 11

JACKSON C, JACKSON CL: *Bronchoesophagology.* Philadelphia, WB Saunders, 1950 — 11

JACKSON CL: *Foreign bodies in the air and food passages.* In MALONEY WH (Ed): *Otolaryngology.* New York, Harper & Row, 1973 — 5, 6

JACKSON CL, HUBER J: *Correlated applied anatomy of the bronchial tree and lungs with a system of nomenclature.* Dis Chest 9:319-326, 1943 — 13-16

JACOBSON E: *Anxiety and Tension Control: A*

Section V (continued)

Plate Number

Physiologic Approach. Philadelphia, JB Lippincott, 1964 — 20, 21

JENSEN V, ENGE I, LEXOW P: *The value of percutaneous lung puncture cytology in clinical work: an analysis of 120 cases.* Scand J Respir Dis 51:233-241, 1970 — 32

JOHNSON J, KIRBY CK: *Surgery of the Chest,* 3rd ed. Chicago, Yearbook Medical Publishers, 1964 — 29-31

MCNEILL TM, CHAMBERLAIN JM: *Diagnostic anterior mediastinotomy.* Ann Thorac Surg 2:532-539, 1966 — 27, 28

MCPHERSON SP: *Respiratory Therapy Equipment.* St. Louis, CV Mosby, 1977 — 24

MALONEY JV JR, FRANKS R, MAKOFF D: *Biopsy of the scalene lymph nodes and the right thoracic duct lymph node for the diagnosis of pulmonary disease.* J Thorac Cardiovasc Surg 47:438-445, 1964 — 27, 28

MARSH BR, FROST JK, EROZAN YS, et al: *Flexible fiberoptic bronchoscopy—its place in the search for lung cancer.* Ann Otol Rhinol Laryngol 82:757-764, 1973 — 13-16

MAYER JH JR: *"Artery First" pulmonary resection.* In Cooper P (Ed): *The Craft of Surgery,* 2nd ed. Boston, Little, Brown, 1971 — 29-31

MITHOEFER JC: *Indications for oxygen therapy in chronic obstructive pulmonary disease.* Am Rev Respir Dis 110:35-39, 1974 — 23, 25

NGAI SH: *Down the hatch in a hurry.* Emergency Medicine 23, 1971 — 8

OLDHAM HN JR, SABISTON DC JR: *Primary tumors and cysts of the mediastinum.* Monogr Surg Sci 4:243-279, 1967 — 33

PADULA RT: *Postoperative management.* In SABIS-

Section V (continued)

Plate Number

TON DC JR, SPENCER FC (Eds): *Gibbon's Surgery of the Chest,* 3rd ed. Philadelphia, WB Saunders, 1976 — 17, 18

PEMBERTON LB: *A comprehensive view of tracheostomy.* Am Surg 38:251-256, 1972 — 7, 9

PINCUS S: *Respiratory Therapist Manual.* New York, Bobbs-Merrill, 1975 — 24

PONTOPPIDAN H, WILSON RS, RIE MA, et al: *Respiratory intensive care.* Anaesthesiology 47:96-116, 1977 — 26

RUSK HA (Ed): *Rehabilitation Medicine,* 3rd ed. St. Louis, CV Mosby, 1971 — 19

SACKNER MA: *Bronchodilator agents.* Clin Notes Respir Dis 15:3-14, 1976 — 3, 4

SACKNER MA: *Bronchofiberscopy.* Am Rev Respir Dis 111:62-88, 1975 — 11, 12

SACKNER MA: *Management of pulmonary insufficiency.* J Iowa Med Soc 54:352-354, 1969 — 22

SACKNER MA: *Arterial blood gas analysis.* Med Times 95:79-87, 1967 — 22

SACKNER MA, LANDA JF, GREENELTCH N, et al: *Pathogenesis and prevention of tracheobronchial damage with suction procedures.* Chest 64:284-290, 1973 — 12

SACKNER MA, WANNER A, LANDA JF: *Applications of bronchofiberscopy.* Chest 62(Suppl):70-78, 1972 — 8, 13-16

SAHN SA, LAKSHMINARAYAN S, PETTY TL: *Weaning from mechanical ventilation.* JAMA 235:2208-2212, 1976 — 26

SANDERS DE, THOMPSON DW, PRUDDEN BJ: *Percutaneous aspiration lung biopsy.* Can Med Assn J 104:139-142, 1971 — 32

SANDERSON DR, FONTANA RS, WOOLNER LB, et al: *Bronchoscopic localization of radio-*

Section V (continued)

Plate Number

graphically occult lung cancer. Chest 65:608-612, 1974 — 27, 28

SHENFIELD GM, EVANS ME, WALKER SR, et al: *The fate of nebulized salbutamol (albuterol) administered by intermittent positive pressure respiration to asthmatic patients.* Am Rev Respir Dis 108:501-505, 1973 — 3, 4

SMELZER TH, BARNETT TB: *Bronchodilator aerosol: comparison of administration methods.* JAMA 223:884-889, 1973 — 3, 4

STRADLING P: *Diagnostic Bronchoscopy,* 3rd ed. New York, Churchill Livingstone, 1976 — 13-16

TIMMIS HH: *Tracheostomy: an overview of implications, management and morbidity.* In *Advances in Surgery, VII.* Chicago, Yearbook Medical Publishers, 1973 — 7, 9

TUCKER GF, TURTZ MG. *Foreign bodies in the air and food passages.* In *Pediatric Otolaryngology, II.* Philadelphia, WB Saunders, 1976, pp 1242-1246 — 5, 6

WANNER A, LANDA JF, NEIMAN RE JR, et al: *Bedside bronchofiberscopy for atelectasis and lung abscess.* JAMA 224:1281-1283, 1973 — 11

WANNER A, ZIGHELBOIM A, SACKNER MA: *Nasopharyngeal airway: a facilitated access to the trachea.* Ann Intern Med 75:593-595, 1971 — 12

WYCHULIS AR, PAYNE WS, CLAGETT OT, et al: *Surgical treatment of mediastinal tumors: a 40 year experience.* J Thorac Cardiovasc Surg 62:379-392, 1971 — 33

ZAVALA DC: *Flexible Fiberoptic Bronchoscopy.* Cedar Rapids Ia, Pepco Litho Press, 1978 — 13-16

ZELCH JV, LALLI AF, MCCORMACK LJ, et al: *Aspiration biopsy in diagnosis of pulmonary nodules.* Chest 63:149-152, 1973 — 32

Subject Index

(Numerals refer to pages, not plates)

aorta—*continued*
  dorsal, 34, 39, 114
  thoracic, 12, 114, 246
  ventral, 34
aortography, 94
aplasia, tracheal and pulmonary, 111,
  112
apnea, 81, 82, 113, 133
  see also asphyxia; breathlessness
apneustic center, 76, 77
apoproteins, 250
appendectomy, 190
arachidonic acid, 124
arch
  aortic, 15, 18, 19, 20, 21, 22, 32,
    34, 75, 299
  of cricoid cartilage, 37
  lumbocostal, 12
  mandibular, 34, 35, 37, 38
argon, 65
arsenic, 158, 212
arteries
  agenesis of, 91
  angiotensin in, 74
  arterial puncture, 289
  axillary, 7
  basal, 299
  brachiocephalic (innominate), 8, 18,
    20, 114
  bronchial, 15, 19, 20, 21, 25, 28,
    69
  carotid, 7, 18, 20, 21, 22, 34, 75
  coronary, 94
  dorsalis pedis, 220
  emboli in, 63, 226, 227
  enlarged, 172, 257
  epigastric, 7, 8
  esophageal, 12, 19
  and gas analysis, 268, 289-290
  gas composition in, 291
  hypoplasia of, 91
  intercostal, 5, 6, 7, 8, 10, 11, 19,
    20, 21, 114, 301
  internal thoracic (internal
    mammary), 6, 7, 8, 11, 12, 18,
    20, 21, 245, 296
  laryngeal, 117
  musculophrenic, 7, 8, 11
  necrotizing inflammation of, 263
  obstructed, 100, 220, 237, 257
  pericardiacophrenic, 8, 12, 18, 20,
    21
  pressure in, 61, 62, 75, 80, 81, 123,
    131-132, 231, 232
  pulmonary, 3, 15, 16, 18, 19, 20,
    21, 28, 31, 32, 33, 34, 35, 37,
    43, 69, 94, 114, 226, 227, 296,
    298
  segmental, 299, 300
  and shunting, 68-69
  subclavian, 3, 5, 7, 8, 10, 15, 18,
    19, 20, 21, 163
  supernumerary, 19
  thoracoacromial, 6, 7
  thyroid, 116
  umbilical, 251
  see also aorta
arteriography, 94, 102
arterioles, 62, 63, 74, 123, 237
arteriosclerosis, 114
arteriosclerotic heart disease, 290
arteriovenous malformation, 99
arteritis, 260
arthralgias, 254

arthritis, 254, 261
  costovertebral, 82
  pneumococcal, 176
  rheumatoid, 101, 208, 209, 210,
    259, 262
arthrospores, 194
arytenoids, 38, 116, 280, 283
asbestos; asbestosis, 100, 101, 103,
  158, 173, 211, 259
aspergillomas, 198, 254, 255, 256
aspergillosis, 157
  allergic, 98, 121, 130, 198
  invasive, 198
Aspergillus, 174, 183
  fumigatus and other species, 120,
    198, 218
asphyxia, 274
  food, 272
  perinatal, 250, 252
  traumatic, 242
aspiration
  abscess due to, 188, 189
  needle, 284, 300
  of secretions or gastric contents,
    248, 277
aspirin, 256
  sensitivity to, 119, 126
asterixis, 129
asthma, 26, 47, 59, 82, 115, 263,
  291
  allergic (extrinsic), 119, 120-121,
    125-126, 130, 133, 134, 198
  baker's, 129
  bronchial, 36, 98, 119-135, 198
  clinical forms of, 119-120
  clinical and laboratory
    considerations in, 128-129
  differential diagnosis in, 128,
    129-130
  exercise-induced, 120, 134
  general causes of, 125-126
  infective (idiopathic; intrinsic), 119,
    120, 125
  long-term management of, 133, 135
  mixed, 119
  pathogenesis of, 120-125
  pathologic changes in, 126, 127
  pathophysiologic effects of, 126-128
  spirometry in, 127-128
  treatment of, 130-135
  ventilatory function in, 127-128
  see also status asthmaticus
ataxia, 167
atelectasis, 52, 68, 180, 275
  in ARDS, 248
  with aspergillosis, 198
  in asthma, 126, 127, 129, 130
  basilar, 262
  congestive, 248
  in emphysema, 115
  focal, 130
  in hyaline membrane disease, 250,
    252
  in kyphoscoliosis, 108
  with lung tumors, 159, 160, 170,
    171
  with metal sensitivities, 213
  neonatal, 43, 110, 250-252
  postoperative, 290
  with pulmonary edema, 237
  and pulmonary embolism, 227, 228
  roentgenologic signs of, 97, 98, 99
  with scleroderma, 263
  with trauma, 238, 240, 241, 247

atherosclerosis, 231
atopy, 119, 120, 122, 198
atresia
  esophageal, 111
  of vas deferens, 156
atropine, 123, 280, 283
ATS medium, 205
auramine O staining, 204-205, 206
Aureobasidium pullulans, 218
autoimmunity, 208, 209
autolysis, 174
autonomic nervous system, 22, 36,
  63, 123
autotransfusion, 244
axonemes, 26
azathioprine, 254, 260, 261
azotemia, 184

B

Bacillus subtilis, 218
bacteremia, 174, 176, 178, 290
bacteria, 125, 126, 134, 152,
  190-191, 203, 205, 206, 207,
  209, 261
  pneumonias caused by, 174-178,
    179, 180, 182, 184, 186, 258
  thermophilic, 216, 217, 218
Bacteroides, 174
bagasse; bagassosis, 198, 216,
  217-218
barium enema, 110
barium swallow, 86, 89, 90-91, 102,
  111
baroreflex, 77
basement membrane, 29, 42, 219,
  236
  airway, 25, 26, 27, 65
  bronchial, 25, 26, 27
  capillary, 30, 31
  in chronic bronchitis, 137
  hyaline thickening of, 127
basophils, 121, 122, 123, 124
Battey bacillus, 209
BCG vaccination, 207
"bellows failure," 262
Bennett laryngoscope, 275
Bentley von Hipple-Tector system,
  285
bentonite, 214
Bernheim phenomenon, reverse, 144
beryllium; berylliosis, 72, 174, 213
betamethasone, 252
Bible printer's disease, 218
bicarbonate
  intravenous administration of, 131
  levels of, 70, 71, 75, 79, 82, 290
  retention of, 248, 249
bilirubin, 228
biopsy
  bronchoscopic, 158, 162, 257
  brush, 162, 280, 281
  forceps, 280, 281, 295, 296
  in legionnaires' disease, 184
  lung, 159, 160, 185, 254, 255-256,
    258, 280
  lymph node, 255-256, 296
  with mediastinoscopy, 295, 296
  needle, 173, 185, 300
  open lung, 185, 254, 257, 300
  pleural, 95, 101, 259
  in sarcoidosis, 255-256
  scalene node, 295
  skin and muscle, 255-256, 262, 263

biopsy—*continued*
  transbronchial, 185, 254
bladder
  carcinoma of, 168
  tuberculous spread to, 199
blast injury, 248
Blastomyces dermatitidis, 174, 195
blastomycosis
  North American, 195
  South American, 196
blast transformation, 255
bleomycin, 161, 253
block
  alveolar-capillary, 165
  bundle-branch, 130, 227, 231
  intercostal or paravertebral, 238
  spinal, 220
blockade
  beta adrenergic, 121, 122-123, 124,
    125-126, 130
  thyroid, 223
blood
  antinuclear factor in, 208, 209
  circulation of, 28, 60-64, 80-81,
    251
  coagulation system, 219
  histamine in, 124
  in pleural cavity, 244 (*see also*
    hemothorax)
  serotonin in, 73
  shunting of, 18, 68-69 (*see also*
    shunts)
  supplied to airways, 25, 35
  supplied to submucosal glands, 27
  transfused, 183, 235, 237, 244,
    248 (*see also* hemorrhage)
blood-air barrier, 29, 30, 40-41, 42,
  64, 248
blood flow
  and acid-base regulation, 70-71
  distribution of, 62-63, 68, 100
  exercise and, 77
  fetal and neonatal, 43
  in hypercapnia and hypocapnia, 80,
    82
  measured by radioisotopes, 95
  and oxygen transport, 69-70
  and oxyhemoglobin dissociation
    curve, 68, 69-70, 290, 291
  systemic and pulmonary, 61-62
  and ventilation-perfusion
    relationships, 67, 68
blood gas analysis, 247, 268,
  289-290, 291, 294
  arterial oxygen and carbon dioxide
    tensions, 80, 81, 123, 131-132,
    289-290
  arterial puncture, 289
blood gas levels, 75, 79, 80, 81, 109,
  123
  disturbances of, 131-132, 148-149,
    260
Bochdalek hernia, 112
bodies
  aortic, 22, 75, 80
  asbestos, 211
  carotid, 22, 78, 80
  Creola, 126, 127
  hematoxylin-eosin, 261
  inclusion, 29-30, 41, 182, 183, 259
  lamellar, 29-30, 41, 250
  multivesicular, 30, 31
  postbranchial, 36
  Schaumann's, 213, 254, 255

bodies—*continued*
Weibel-Palade, 30
body plethysmography, 49-50, 53, 61, 134
body temperature, pressure and saturation (BTPS), 49
bones
beryllium deposits in, 213
destruction of, 101, 102, 254, 256
hyoid, 117
metastatic disease to, 166, 199
new, subperiosteal, 167
occipital, 10
sarcomas of, 168
bone marrow embolism, 235
bony thorax, 4, 14, 43
see also thorax
bowel, malrotation of, 110
see also colon
Boyle's law, 50, 65, 141
bradykinin, 63, 74, 124
brain lesions, 71, 134, 155, 183, 188, 191, 237, 249, 251, 291
brass, 259
breast
carcinomas of, 168
enlargement of, 164
breathing
abdominal, 269, 288
Cheyne-Stokes, 79-81, 82
cost of, 59, 108, 109, 288
exercises, 286, 288
in hyaline membrane disease, 250, 251
positive pressure, 62, 152, 244, 286, 287
pursed-lip, 142, 148, 151, 288
quiet, 50, 58, 59, 67, 268, 288
tidal, 140, 141, 145, 270
work of, 58-59, 60, 108, 109, 128, 132, 141, 239
see also respiration; ventilation
breathlessness, 48, 173, 211, 212, 227, 230, 260, 269
breath sounds
amphoric, 189
in asthma, 119, 120, 129
in COPD, 148, 149
in hyaline membrane disease, 251
in pneumonia, 175, 177, 180
with pulmonary contusion, 247
with pulmonary embolism, 228
suppressed, 188
brewer's lung, 218
bronchi, 3, 15, 16, 24
accessory, 114
airway resistance in, 52
in aplastic or hypoplastic lungs, 112
arteries of, 15, 19, 20, 21, 25, 28, 69
benign tumors of, 170, 171
destruction of, 263
development of, 34, 35, 36, 37
eparterial, 23
epithelium of, 26
generations of, 24, 35, 52, 282
irritant receptors in, 22
lobar, 16-17, 18
in lobectomy, 299
lymph channels in, 32, 33
main, 3, 16, 17, 18, 19, 20, 21, 23, 27, 32, 35, 37
malignant tumors of, 97, 98, 99, 158-168, 170, 188, 189, 211, 212, 281, 295, 296, 297

bronchi—*continued*
peripheral, nomenclature for, 282
in pneumonectomy, 298
relations of trachea and, 18
rupture of, 241, 242
segmental, 35, 36, 37, 39, 112, 300
in status asthmaticus, 126
structure of, 23, 25
submucosal glands of, 25, 27
tuberculous spread to, 199
visualization of, 278, 280, 281, 283
bronchial provocation tests (BPT), 134
bronchiectasis, 91, 157, 215, 300
acquired and congenital, 154-155
with aspergillosis, 198
with asthma, 128, 130
with COPD, 136
inflammation with, 281
with lung abscess or cyst, 113, 188, 189
nontuberculous, 155
with pectus excavatum, 107
with tuberculosis, 207
bronchiolectasis, 260
bronchioles, 22, 24, 25, 53
carcinoma of, 169
in COPD, 136, 137
dilated, 260
epithelium of, 26
in hyaline membrane disease, 250
respiratory, 24, 25, 28, 32, 33, 39, 40, 41, 137, 138
in status asthmaticus, 126
terminal, 24, 25, 28, 32, 33, 36, 39, 41, 137, 138
bronchiolitis, 115, 126, 128, 186, 215
bronchitis, 59, 82, 108, 109, 126, 128, 213
the "blue bloater," 149, 150
chronic, 60, 100, 107, 115, 119, 136-137, 138-139, 141, 142, 143, 144, 148, 149-151, 157, 215, 281, 291
destructive, 154
industrial, 210
postaspirational, 281
transitory, 147
bronchoarterial bundle, 28
bronchoconstriction, 22, 73, 121, 122, 123, 124, 125, 130
bronchodilatation, 22, 122
bronchodilators, 119, 120, 124, 125, 127, 130-131, 132, 134, 152, 269-270, 286, 287, 293
sympathomimetic, 134
bronchography, 91, 92, 97, 112, 139, 154, 155, 188, 189, 241
air, 257, 258
bronchopneumonia, 174-176, 180, 186, 215, 248
bronchorrhea, 144
bronchoscopy, 111, 112, 132, 155, 170, 189, 204, 238, 241
biopsy by, 158, 162, 257
excision through, 171
fiberoptic, 91, 158, 159, 160, 161, 162, 255, 258, 275, 277, 278, 279, 280, 281, 282, 283
lavage by, 278
open tube, 278, 280, 283
rigid, 158, 159, 160, 161, 278, 280, 283

bronchoscopy—*continued*
therapeutic, 280
bronchospasm, 119, 121, 124, 125, 126, 127, 134, 269, 280, 294
brushing, bronchial, 185
budgerigar fancier's disease, 216, 218
busulfan, 72, 174, 253

C

cachexia, 166, 203
cadmium, 213
caisson disease, 235
calcification, 89, 90, 101, 168, 171, 260
in asbestosis, 211
central or concentric, 99
cerebral, 183
in cryptococcosis, 197
eccentric, 99
in histoplasmosis, 192, 193
multiple punctate, 99
in silicosis, 208
in tuberculosis, 200
calcitonin, 167
calcium, 121, 124, 171, 219, 233
calcium montmorillonite, 214
Candida, 198
candle-blowing exercise, 288
capillaries, 25, 39-40, 41, 75
alveolar-capillary membrane, 40-41, 42, 47, 49, 64, 72, 143, 165, 218, 236-237, 267
and angiotensin conversion, 74
bleeding from, 181
and diffusion, 65
and gas exchange, 65-66
in hyaline membrane disease, 250
increased permeability of, 124, 248, 249
leaks from, 248
obliterated, 143, 253, 257, 267
pressure in, 61, 62
and shunting, 69
structure of, 29-31
thromboses of, 180
transcapillary exchange, 236, 237
and vascular resistance, 63
Caplan's syndrome, 209
capreomycin, 206
carbamino-hemoglobin, 70
carbolfuchsin, 204, 206
carbon, 212, 214
carbon dioxide
carried in blood, 70, 71
control of, in ventilation, 75, 80, 81
and diffusing capacity, 64, 65, 260, 267
dissociation curve, 68
and growth of actinomycetes, 190
and oxygen, exchange between, 19, 31, 34, 41, 42, 47, 65-69, 228, 248, 268, 289-290, 291
prolonged exposure to, 78, 82
radiolabeled, 257
retention of, 71, 76, 79, 127, 128, 132, 150, 291, 292
in spirometry, 49
carbonic acid, 70
carbon monoxide, diffusing capacity for, 64-65, 143
carboxyhemoglobin, 290
carcinoid syndrome, 167

carcinomas, 94, 97, 198
adenocarcinoma, 158, 160, 162, 165, 166, 167, 169
adenocystic, 170
alveolar cell (bronchiolar), 97, 99, 102, 169, 258
bronchial adenoma, 170
bronchogenic, 97, 99, 158-168, 188, 189, 211, 212, 281, 295, 296, 297
endobronchial, 98, 99
epidermoid (squamous cell), 158, 159, 164, 165, 166, 167, 211, 212, 296
esophageal, 281
inflammation with, 281
large cell anaplastic, 158, 160
lymphangitic spread and cavitation of, 159, 161, 165
malignant mesothelioma, 173
mediastinal, 172
metastatic, 99, 168, 261, 281, 295, 296, 300
neuromuscular syndromes, 167
nonmetastatic extrapulmonary manifestations of, 166-167
Pancoast's syndrome, 159, 163
pancreatic, 166, 220
small cell anaplastic (oat cell), 158, 161, 162, 164, 166, 167
staging in management of, 295
superior vena cava syndrome, 164
surgical removal of, 295, 296
thyroid, 166, 281
visualization of, 295-296
cardiac notch, 13, 15, 39
cardiomegaly, 129; see also heart, enlarged
cardiomyopathy, 130, 254, 256
cardiopulmonary resuscitation (CPR), 272
cardiorespiratory failure, 108, 109, 231, 240, 260
see also heart failure
carina, cancer of, 281
Carlens tube, 258
carotid body; carotid sinus, 22, 290
cartilages
arytenoid, 116
bronchial, 25, 115
costal, 3, 4, 5, 6, 7, 12, 13, 16, 107, 296
cricoid, 13, 18, 23, 37, 274, 276
development of, 35-36
distribution of, and airways, 24, 25, 27
ensiform (xiphoid), 13
fragmentation of, 116
hyoid, 37
to support tracheal and bronchial walls, 23, 53
thyroid, 13, 18, 23, 37, 117, 274, 276
tracheal, 23, 34, 37, 53, 111
caseation, 200, 202, 203
cataracts, 134
catecholamines, 22, 77, 82, 122, 123, 124, 125, 128, 133, 248
catheterization
arterial, 91, 94
flotation, 248
heart, 91, 94, 232
in hernia surgery, 110
intercostal, 284

cough—*continued*
  in PSS, 260
  in pulmonary fibrosis, 212
  in rheumatoid arthritis, 259
  and rib fractures, 238
  in silicosis, 208
  stimulation of, 279
  in tuberculosis, 203
  in Wegener's granulomatosis, 263
Coxiella burnetii, 174
coxsackie virus, 179
Creola bodies, 126, 127, 130
crepitus, 238, 241, 242
cricoid lamina, 37
cricothyrotomy, 274
cristobalite, 214
cromolyn sodium, 120, 134
croup, 128
crushing injuries, 238, 239, 242
cryoglobulins, 254
cryptococcosis, 197
Cryptococcus, 258
  neoformans, 197
Cryptostroma corticale, 218
culturing of sputum, 205-206, 207
Curschmann's spirals, 126, 127, 129, 130
Cushing's syndrome, 166
cyanosis
  with airflow obstruction, 284
  with amniotic fluid embolism, 235
  in asthma, 119, 120, 128
  in bronchitis, 149
  in cor pulmonale, 231
  with diaphragmatic hernia, 110
  with diaphragmatic injury, 240
  in emphysema, 115, 143
  in hyaline membrane disease, 251
  in IDIPF, 253, 254
  with lymphangiectasis, 113
  with mechanical ventilation, 294
  with metal sensitivity, 213
  in PAP, 258
  in pneumonia, 177, 178, 180, 182, 185
  in pneumothorax, 243, 244
  in PSS, 260
  in pulmonary contusion, 247
  in SLE, 261
  with tracheal strictures, 111
  with tracheobronchial disruption, 241
cyclophosphamide, 161, 254, 260, 261, 263
cycloserine, 206
cylindroma, 170
cystic adenomatous malformation, 113
cystic disease of lungs, 110
cystic fibrosis, 129, 130, 154, 156-157
cysts
  Baker's, 223
  bronchogenic, 99, 112, 113, 172, 301
  dermoid, 172
  duplication, 102, 301
  emphysematous, 153, 198
  enterogenous, 172
  in hyaline membrane disease, 252
  laryngeal, 128
  microcysts, 253, 254, 260
  pericardial, 102, 110, 172
  pericardiocoelomic, 301

cysts—*continued*
  pneumatoceles, 113, 178
  in pulmonary sequestration, 114
  tension, 115
cytolysis, 123
cytomegalovirus, 179, 183, 186
cytoplasm, 26, 30, 42, 159, 161
  vacuolated, 217, 218
cytotropism, 121, 122

D

damping, 80
Da Nang lung, 248-249
dead space, 61, 66-67, 268
  anatomic, 66
  physiologic, 66, 67, 68, 71, 76, 128, 248
deafness, 183
death, due to
  amniotic fluid embolism, 235
  ARDS, 248
  asthma, 134, 135
  chylothorax, 246
  hyaline membrane disease, 42, 250, 252
  IDIPF, 254
  IPH, 257
  lung carcinoma, 158, 159, 161, 162, 163, 173
  nocardiosis, 191
  pneumonia, 176, 177, 185
  respiratory failure, perinatal, 34
  sarcoidosis, 256
  silicosis, 208, 209
  stage III cancer, 296
  tracheal or bronchial rupture, 241
  tuberculosis, 199
  upper airway obstruction, 272
decompression sickness, 235
decongestants, 134
dehydration, 126, 128, 130, 132
delirium, 184
dementia, 167
deoxyribonucleic acid (DNA), 130, 261
depressants, 82, 109
dermatomyositis, 262
detergent disease, 218
dexamethasone, 166
dextrocardia, 154
diabetes, 71, 201, 207
  mellitus, 134, 177, 250, 252
diaphragm, 3, 8, 12, 13, 14, 15, 20, 21, 75, 246
  in asthma, 36
  depressed, 115, 129, 130, 150, 153, 244, 288
  development of, 37-38, 40
  dome of, 12, 13, 14, 38, 47, 89, 110
  electric activity of, 79, 80
  elevated, 110, 227, 228, 240, 253
  esophageal hiatus of, 18
  herniated, 110, 112
  injuries to, 240
  innervation of, 40
  lesions of, 95, 101
  paralysis of, 89
  as principal respiratory muscle, 37, 38, 42, 47, 153, 288
  transverse septum and, 36
diarrhea, 71, 130, 170, 184
diazepam, 280

Dieterle silver impregnation method, 184
diethylnitrosamine, 72
diffuse alveolar consolidation, 52
diffuse pulmonary disease, 212, 254
diffusion, 64-65
  barriers to, 64, 247
  blood phase and gas phase, 64
  capacity for, 64-65, 79, 80, 143, 155, 254, 260, 267
  problems of, 76, 268, 289
digitalis, 260
dilution (helium) technique, 141, 267
dinitrophenol, 77
dipalmitoyl lecithin, 41, 52, 250
2, 3-diphosphoglycerate (DPG), 70, 78, 79
discs
  intervertebral, 4, 5, 12
  optic, 109
dislocations, bone, 238
diuretics, 239, 248, 260, 290
diverticula, esophageal, 102
doghouse disease, 218
dopamine, 122
Doppler method of diagnosis, 222, 224
dorsal respiratory group (DRG) of neurons, 76
double diffusion tests, 216
doxorubicin, 161
drainage
  chest, 284, 285
  postural, 135, 152, 155, 157, 189, 286-288
  underwater-seal, 241, 243, 244, 245, 285
  see also intubation
drugs
  antihistamine, 124, 134
  beta adrenergic, 130-131, 134
  narcotic, 235, 237
  reactions to, 119, 121, 126, 174, 253, 262
  resistance to, 206-207
  sympathomimetic, 36, 125, 130, 131, 134
  toxicity of, 206
drug susceptibility tests, 205, 206, 207
ducts
  alveolar, 33, 39, 41
  arterial (ductus arteriosus), 18, 21, 43, 112, 115
  ciliated; collecting, 27
  lymphatic, 32
  thoracic, 12, 32, 246
dura mater, 3
dusts, 119, 120, 125, 126, 133, 134, 135, 198, 208, 209, 210, 212, 214, 216, 253
dwarfing, 108
dynein, 26
dysarthria, 167, 262
dysautonomia, familial, 82
dysphagia, 114, 260, 262
dysplasia
  bronchopulmonary, 252
  chondroectodermal (Ellis–Van Creveld syndrome), 115
dyspnea
  in asthma, 119, 120, 127, 128
  in bronchiectasis, 155

dyspnea—*continued*
  in COPD, 148, 149
  with diaphragmatic hernia, 110
  with diaphragmatic injury, 240
  with embolism, 227, 228, 232, 235
  exertional, 293
  in IDIPF, 253, 254
  in IPH, 257
  in kyphoscoliosis, 108, 109
  in lobar emphysema, 115
  with lung abscess, 189
  with lung cancer, 159, 161, 164, 165, 173
  in PAP, 258
  in pneumonia, 177, 178, 180, 182, 183, 185
  in pneumoconiosis, 208, 210, 211, 213, 215, 218
  with pneumothorax, 244
  in PSS, 260
  in pulmonary contusion, 247
  in rheumatoid arthritis, 259
  in SLE, 261
  with tracheal disorders, 111, 241
  in Wegener's granulomatosis, 263
dysrhythmias, 130, 131, 231, 248, 278, 280
dystrophy, thoracic-pelvic-phalangeal, 107

E

ear, tuberculous spread to, 199
ear oximetry, 278, 291
Eaton agent, 186
ecchymosis, 238
echovirus, 179
ectopia cordis, 107
eczema, 119, 121
edema, 52, 82, 181
  in asthma, 124, 126, 127, 128, 129, 134
  in bagassosis, 217, 218
  bronchial wall, 119
  cerebral, 109
  conjunctival, 242
  in COPD, 149
  facial, 166
  hemodynamic, 237
  hemorrhagic, 180
  high altitude, 237
  hyperventilation and, 79, 80
  interstitial, 100, 248, 249, 253
  laryngeal, 128, 277
  mucosal, 53, 136, 137, 278
  overtransfusion, 237
  periorbital, 262
  peripheral, 129, 143, 144, 167, 251
  in pneumonia, 174, 177
  pulmonary, 64, 97, 99, 100, 102, 213, 215, 236-237, 247, 248, 249, 250, 258, 261, 263
  in pulmonary contusion, 247
  retinal, 242
  in SLE, 261
  in superior vena cava syndrome, 164
  in thrombophlebitis, 220
effusions
  chylous, 246
  pericardial, 263
  pleural, 173, 176, 184, 193, 194, 197, 227, 230, 238, 259, 261, 263, 284
  synovial, 167

elastase, 147
elasticity, of lung and respiratory system, 40, 41, 51-53, 54, 127, 140, 141, 142, 143, 145, 146, 149, 267
elastin, 52, 148
electrocardiography, 130, 144, 227, 229, 231, 232, 244, 278
electrolytes, 134, 166, 294
electromyography, 79
Ellis-Van Creveld syndrome, 115
embolectomy, 231
embolism, pulmonary, 63, 91, 97, 100, 220, 226-232, 290
  in asthma, 123, 128, 129, 130
  clinical manifestations of, 227-228
  and cor pulmonale, 227, 230-232
  fibrin degradation products and, 221
  laboratory tests for, 228-229
  with lung abscess, 188, 189
  and mechanical ventilation, 294
  phlebothrombosis and, 222
  and pneumonia, 178
  prophylaxis and treatment for, 229-230, 233, 234
  and SLE, 261
  sources of, 226-227, 235
  transfusion, 235
embolus, 82
  air; amniotic fluid; bone marrow, 235
  eye, 235
  fat, 235, 248
  foreign body, 235
  mesenteric, 290
  saddle, 229
embryology, 34-43
emphysema, 59, 60, 64, 82, 97, 267, 291
  antitrypsin deficiency, 147-148
  basilar, 252
  bullous, 153, 213, 217, 218
  centriacinar (centrilobular), 137-138, 139, 151, 153
  cervical, 241
  congenital lobar, 115
  in COPD, 136, 137-138, 139, 141, 142, 143, 148-149, 152
  interstitial, 251
  with kyphoscoliosis, 108
  lobular, 252
  mediastinal, 241, 242, 244, 277
  panacinar (panlobular), 138, 139, 140, 147, 149
  paraseptal, 138, 153
  the "pink puffer," 148, 150
  in pneumoconiosis, 210, 214, 215
  pulmonary, 52, 53, 100, 130, 181
  smoking and, 145, 146
  subcutaneous, 238, 241, 242, 274, 277, 284
  surgical, 241, 242, 244, 277
empyema, 101, 176, 177, 178, 188, 190, 191
encephalitis, 82, 182, 183
encephalopathy, 167, 180
endocarditis, 176, 178, 261
endocrine disorders, 166-167
endothelial fuzz, 29
endotheliomas, 171
endothelium
  capillary, 30-31, 40, 41, 65, 74, 236

endothelium—*continued*
  pulmonary, and serotonin exposure, 73
enophthalmos, 163
environmental factors, 126, 133, 135, 151
  see also allergens
enzymes
  angiotensin-converting, 31, 255
  lysosomal, 248
  proteolytic, 147
  thyroid, 82
eosinophil chemotactic factor (ECF), 121, 122, 124
eosinophilia, 99, 100, 119, 120, 198, 263
eosinophils, 121, 124, 126, 127, 129, 130, 170, 185, 253, 258
  total eosinophil counts, 130
ephedrine, 131
epiglottis, 3, 35, 38
  visualization of, 280
epinephrine, 22, 63, 122, 123, 124, 130, 131, 132, 134, 135, 270
epithelioma, transitional cell, 165, 168
epithelium, 23, 25, 26, 27, 33, 34
  alveolar, 29, 65, 74, 236
  capillary, 40
  ciliated, 25, 35, 113, 130
  columnar, 25, 39, 114, 130, 169
  cuboidal, 25, 39, 41, 113, 114, 171, 253
  desquamated, 127, 137, 183
  goblet cells in, 156, 157
  hyperplastic, 155
  metaplasia of, 212, 213
  and squamous cell carcinoma, 158, 159
  tumors of, 165, 168, 173
  ultrastructure of, 26
equal pressure point, 56, 57
equilibration technique, 141
erythema nodosum, 194, 254, 256
erythroblastosis fetalis, 183
erythrocytes, 42, 65, 72, 78, 174, 179-180, 186, 248
erythrocyte sedimentation rate, 254
erythrocytosis, 144, 149
erythromycin, 134, 184, 186, 190
erythropoiesis, 149
Escherichia coli, 174, 178
esophagitis, 260
esophagus, 3, 12, 15, 18, 19, 20, 21, 114, 116, 117, 246
  development of, 34, 35, 38, 39, 40
  hiatus of, 12, 18, 101, 110
  hypomotility of, 262
  lesions of, 102, 111, 172, 260, 301
  roentgenologic examination of, 85, 89, 90, 102
ethambutol, 206, 207
ethionamide, 206
exercise(s)
  asthma and, 120, 133, 134
  blood flow and, 63, 64
  breathing, 135, 153, 286, 288
  COPD and, 151
  diffusing capacity during, 65
  intolerance for, 293
  and kyphoscoliosis, 108, 109
  leg, for thromboembolic disease, 232
  passive-range motion, 294

exercise(s)—*continued*
  relaxation, 286
  respiratory response to, 77-78
expectorants, 131, 132, 134, 152, 286
expiration
  in asthma, 36, 126, 127, 129
  flow-volume curves, 55, 57, 58, 59, 116, 127, 139-141
  forced, 55, 56, 58, 59, 120, 127, 128, 129, 131, 134, 139-142, 215, 253, 254, 258, 267, 293
  laminar flow during, 55
  muscles of, 47-48, 57, 59
  passive nature of, 38
  positive end-expiratory pressure (PEEP), 294
  pursed-lip, 142, 148, 151, 288
  in quiet breathing, 50, 58, 60
  see also breathing; respiration; ventilation
expiratory reserve volume (ERV), 48-49, 141, 267, 271
"extrapleural sign," 102
eyes
  lesions of, 196, 199, 213, 235, 242, 262
  optic discs, 109

F

face tent, 292
falx cerebri, 3
farmer's lung, 128, 198, 216, 217
fascia
  cervical; clavipectoral, 6
  infraspinatus, 9
  lumbodorsal, 9, 10
  Sibson's, 20, 21
fat embolism, 235, 248
fatigue, 127, 129, 203, 232, 257, 258
fat pad, 21, 102
fat stains, 235
fatty acids, 72, 248, 250
fatty tissue, 15, 301
feather plucker's disease, 218
feedback control system, 79-80
fever
  in asthma, 132
  in bagassosis, 218
  in coccidioidomycosis, 194
  with lung abscess, 188
  with mediastinal masses, 172
  in nocardiosis, 191
  in North American blastomycosis, 195
  in pneumonia, 175, 178, 180, 183, 184, 185, 186
  in sarcoidosis, 254
  in SLE, 261
  in thrombophlebitis, 220
  with toxic gas inhalation, 215
  in tuberculosis, 203
fever blisters, 175
fiberoptics, 280, 281, 283
  see also bronchoscopy, fiberoptic
fibrin, 184, 221
fibrin degradation products, 221, 228
fibrinogen, 219
fibrinogen scan, 220, 221, 222, 223, 225, 229
fibrinolysis, 221, 231

fibrinopeptides, 219, 221
fibroblasts, 30, 40, 41, 171, 208, 209, 248, 249, 253, 257, 262
fibroemphysema, residual, 196
fibromas, 171
fibrometer, 233
fibrosarcomas, 173
fibrosis
  cystic, 129, 130, 154, 156-157
  in hyaline membrane disease, 252
  idiopathic diffuse, 100, 253-254, 262
  interstitial, 213, 218, 253-254, 257, 260, 261
  peribronchiolar, 136, 137, 253
  in pneumoconiosis, 208, 209, 210, 211, 212, 214, 216, 217, 218
  pulmonary, 52, 58, 59, 60, 63, 64, 79, 82, 267, 290, 291
  and pulmonary edema, 237
  and rheumatoid arthritis, 259
  in sarcoidosis, 254
  septal, 253, 257, 261
  with tracheostomy, 276
  and tuberculosis, 203
fibrothorax, 244, 259
Fick method, 61
finger cot flutter valve, 244, 285
fissures
  dissection of, 299
  extra, 13, 17
  horizontal, 13, 14, 15, 16
  interlobar, 97, 98, 99
  oblique, 13, 14, 15, 16, 17, 23
fistulas
  arteriovenous, 68, 69, 89, 171
  bronchoesophageal, 281
  bronchopleural, 188
  tracheoesophageal, 111, 277
flail chest, 238, 239
flow-volume curves, 55, 57, 58, 59, 116, 127, 139-141, 253, 267, 268
flucytosine, 197, 198
fluid-electrolyte imbalance, 294
fluids
  amniotic, 42, 235, 252
  edema, 174, 177, 181, 236, 237 (*see also* edema)
  eosinophilic, 258
  interstitial, 75, 82, 165, 236, 237
  overload of, 248, 294
  pleural, 42, 43, 100-101, 246
  protein-rich, 183
  replacement, 132
  restricted, 239
  spinal, 75, 78, 79, 109, 197
  surface tension of, 41, 43
  see also effusions
fluorescent-antibody test, 184, 186
5-fluorocytosine, 197
fluorography, 111
fluoroscopy, 89-90, 100, 101, 162, 222, 278, 280, 300
flushing, facial, 119, 120, 163, 164, 170
fog fever, 216, 218
foods
  allergenic, 119, 121, 125, 126, 134, 135
  aspiration of, 128
  see also nutrition
foramina
  of Bochdalek, 101, 110
  cecum (of tongue), 35, 36, 38

hyaline membrane disease, 42, 43, 250-252
hyalinization, 208
hyaluronic acid, 173
hydration, 132, 151, 152, 155, 287
hydrocephalus, 194
hydrocortisone, 193
hydrogen ions, 70-71, 75, 82, 248, 290
hydrogen sulfide, 215
hydropneumothorax, loculated, 110
5-hydroxyindoleacetic acid, 73
17-hydroxysteroids, 166
hydroxystilbamidine isethionate, 195
5-hydroxytryptamine, 73, 170
   see also serotonin
5-hydroxytryptophan, 170
hyperalimentation, intravenous, 294
hypercalcemia, 166, 254, 256
hypercapnia, 63, 75, 76, 77, 80, 81, 82, 290, 291
   in ARDS, 248, 249
   in asthma, 129, 131-132
   in COPD, 143
   in dermatomyositis, 262
   with flail chest, 239
   in kyphoscoliosis, 108-109
   with pulmonary edema, 237
   and respiratory failure, 291
hyperchromatism, 161
hyperemia, 137, 180, 181, 262
hyperglycemia, 166
hyperinflation, 119, 126, 127, 128, 129, 136, 139, 150, 156, 157, 244
   compensatory, 35
hyperparathyroidism, 172, 238
hyperplasia
   adrenal gland, 166
   alveolar, 249, 257
   basal cell, 159
   fibrous tissue, 165
   mucous gland, 53, 136, 137, 139, 145, 156
   smooth muscle, 53, 126
hyperpnea, 81, 146
hyperresonance, 115, 119, 120, 129, 148, 244
hypersensitivity
   to coccidioidin, 194
   diseases of, 262, 263
   in Mantoux test, 203
   in pneumonitis, 198, 216-218
   in sarcoidosis, 254-255
   tungsten, 212
   type I, type III, 120-122
   see also reactions
hypersplenism, 256
hypertension, 64, 79, 100, 290, 293
   with asthma, 128, 129, 130, 134
   with bronchogenic carcinoma, 166
   in COPD, 144, 153
   in hemosiderosis, 257
   in IDIPF, 254
   in kyphoscoliosis, 108, 109
   in pneumoconiosis, 208, 209, 212, 213
   with pulmonary edema, 235, 236
   with pulmonary embolism, 230, 232
   pulmonary venous, 237
   with scleroderma, 260
   systemic, 237

hypertrophic pulmonary osteoarthropathy, 167, 171
hypertrophy
   glandular, 27, 53, 136, 137, 139, 145, 156
   muscular, 53, 126, 127, 136, 232
   see also heart, enlarged
hyperventilation, 71, 76, 79, 81, 82, 290
   in ARDS, 248, 249
   in asthma, 132
   in bagassosis, 218
   in kyphoscoliosis, 108
   in lobar emphysema, 115
   in pulmonary edema, 79, 80
   in pulmonary embolism, 228
   in sarcoidosis, 254
   voluntary, 59
hypervolemia, 109
hyphae
   filamentous, 196
   fungal, 198
hypnotics, 129
hypocapnia, 71, 80, 82, 132, 228, 248, 249, 290, 291
hypogammaglobulinemia, 174, 185
hypokalemia, 290
hyponatremia, 166
hypoperfusion, 67, 128, 227, 247
hypoplasia, pulmonary, 91, 97, 112
hypoproteinemia, 101, 156
hypoprothrombinemia, 156
hyposensitization, 119, 120, 134-135
hypotension, 74, 79, 131, 235, 237, 247, 290, 294
hypothalamus, 22
hypoventilation, 66, 67, 68, 71, 76, 79, 81, 108, 109, 128, 228, 237, 238, 260, 262, 268, 289, 290
   myxedema, 79, 80
   obesity, 79, 80
   oxygen-induced, 132
hypovolemia, 132
hypoxemia, 63, 68, 70, 71, 76, 78, 79, 81, 268, 280, 290
   in ARDS, 248, 249
   in asthma, 128, 129, 130, 131-132, 133
   in bagassosis, 218
   in beryllium disease, 213
   in bronchiectasis, 155
   in COPD, 143, 144, 153
   in dermatomyositis, 262
   with flail chest, 239
   in hyaline membrane disease, 250-251
   in IDIPF, 253
   in kyphoscoliosis, 108, 109
   in lung cancer, 165
   with lung lavage, 278
   nocturnal, 293
   in PAP, 258
   progression of, 294
   in PSS, 260
   with pulmonary contusion, 247
   with pulmonary edema, 228
   and respiratory failure, 291
   in rheumatoid arthritis, 259
   in sarcoidosis, 254
   in SLE, 261
   and tracheal suctioning, 279
hypoxia, 75-76, 77, 78-79, 80, 81, 82, 153
   in asthma, 120, 132

hypoxia—continued
   in bronchitis, 149
   cerebral, 248, 251
   exercise, 291
   with flail chest, 239
   in hyaline membrane disease, 250
   in kyphoscoliosis, 108, 109
   with pulmonary edema, 237

I

idiopathic diffuse interstitial pulmonary fibrosis (IDIPF), 253-254, 259, 262
idiopathic pulmonary hemosiderosis (IPH), 257
ileus, 156, 294
iliac crest, 6, 9
immune processes, 120-122, 254-255
immunization
   influenza, 181
   pneumonia, 176
   tuberculosis, 199, 200, 201
   see also vaccines
immunoassay, 130
immunoblasts, 27
immunodeficiency, 185, 197, 198
immunoelectrophoresis, 147
immunofluorescence, 183
immunoglobulins, 119, 120, 121, 122, 134-135, 254, 255, 259
immunosuppressive therapy, 134-135, 183, 184, 185, 191, 197, 261, 263
impedance plethysmography, 222, 224-225
inclusions, 130
   cytoplasmic, 259
   osmiophilic, 40
indicator dilution technique, 61
indomethacin, 120, 256
infarction
   myocardial, 227
   pulmonary, 100, 227, 228, 230, 263
infection
   asthma and, 119, 121, 124, 125, 126
   bacterial, 134, 152, 190-191, 261
   and bronchogenic cysts, 113
   and COPD, 151-152, 286
   and cystic fibrosis, 156, 157
   cytomegalovirus, 183
   disseminated, 183
   fungal, 168, 192-198, 261
   hemorrhagic pulmonary, 198
   initial (primary) tuberculous complex, 201
   and mechanical ventilation, 294
   metastatic, 176
   parasitic, 130
   parenchymal, 165
   pneumonias caused by, 174-187
   recurrent bronchial, 144
   and respiratory failure, 291
   respiratory tract, 109, 111, 119, 128, 180, 241
   with SLE, 261
   and tracheostomy, 277
   viral, 146, 147, 152, 183
infertility, 156
infiltrates, pulmonary, 196, 198, 211, 212, 215, 227, 254, 259

infiltrates—continued
   cellular, 181, 253
   inflammatory, 120, 137, 183
   mononuclear, 182, 183, 185
   nodular, 180, 182
   patchy alveolar, 168
   pneumonic, 186, 192, 193, 201
inflammation
   with abscess, bronchiectasis, carcinoma, foreign bodies, 281
   endobronchial, visualization of, 281
   necrotizing, of arteries, 263
   periarticular, 167
   with tuberculosis, 200, 281
   see also infiltrates, inflammatory
influenza, 151, 178, 179-181, 186
inhalation tests, 134
insomnia, 293
inspiration
   diaphragmatic action and, 12, 38
   and dynamic compliance, 57
   and elastic fibers, 40
   muscles of, 12, 36, 38, 47, 48, 50, 51
   in quiet breathing, 50
   and work of breathing, 58
inspiratory capacity (IC), 48, 49, 127, 267
inspiratory reserve volume (IRV), 48, 49, 127, 141
insulin secretion, 167
intercostal spaces, 7, 8, 11, 13, 21, 130, 173, 240, 244, 284
intermittent positive pressure breathing (IPPB), 116, 132, 152, 239, 269, 270, 286, 287, 291
interstitial lung disease, 97, 103, 168, 198, 258
   diffuse, 100, 253-254, 259, 262
interstitium, 29, 30, 31, 165, 253, 262
intestines
   carcinoma of, 165, 168, 281
   herniation of, 101, 110
intubation
   nasogastric, 240, 276, 294
   nasopharyngeal, 274
   thoracostomy, 241, 243, 244, 245, 246
   thoracotomy, 245, 284
   tracheal, 91, 116, 117, 118, 132, 133, 238, 239, 258, 274, 275, 276, 277, 279, 280
iodine, radioactive, 95, 223, 228, 229
iontophoresis, 156-157
iron; iron oxide, 212, 214, 257, 259, 261
irradiation, 163, 164
irritant receptors, 22, 76, 77, 79, 80, 123
ischemia
   cerebral, 251
   myocardial, 130
   pulmonary, 248
isoetharine, 131, 132, 134, 270
isoniazid, 202, 206, 207, 261
isoproterenol, 63, 122, 123, 124, 130, 132, 134, 270
Isovitalex, 184
isovolume pressure-flow curves, 55, 59

membranes—*continued*
oronasal, 35, 38
oropharyngeal, 34
plasma, 30, 31, 74
protein, 179
thyrohyoid, 37, 117
and transcapillary exchange, 236
meningitis, 82, 191, 194
aseptic, 183, 186
pneumococcal, 176, 177
tuberculous, 201, 203
meningoencephalitis, 183, 186
mental retardation, 183
meperidine hydrochloride, 280
mercury strain gauge
plethysmography, 224-225
mesenchyme, 35, 36, 40
mesentery, esophageal, 40
mesotheliomas, 100, 101, 171, 173,
211
mesothelium, 39, 156
metabolites, 82, 121, 124
metalloproteins, 219
metals, reactions to, 125, 212, 213
metaplasia
airways, 252
epithelial, 212, 213
goblet cell, 126
squamous cell, 136, 137, 159
metaproterenol, 131, 270
methenamine-silver stain, 185
methotrexate, 174, 253
methyl xanthine, 124, 125
metyrapone, 166
microcephaly, 183
microembolism, 248
microfilaments; microtubules, 30
Micropolyspora faeni, 216, 218
microvilli, 40
migration inhibitory factor (MIF),
255
milk-leg, 227
Miller laryngoscope, 275
minocycline, 190, 191
miosis, 163
mites, 120
mitochondria, 27, 30, 31
mitosis, 26, 160, 170
mitral valve disease, 237
Mobin-Uddin umbrella filter, 234
monoamine oxidase, 73
monocytes, 255
mononucleosis, 183, 186
Morgagni, foramen of, 101, 110
morphine, 81, 274
mouth, airway resistance in, 52
mucin production, 162, 169
mucopolysaccharides, 29, 130
Mucor stolonifer, 218
mucosa, 23, 113, 116, 136
lesions of, 213, 254, 256
visualization of, 280
mucous plugs, 115, 126, 127, 136,
139, 278
mucoviscidosis (cystic fibrosis),
129, 130, 154, 156-157
mucus, 53, 60
decreased, 125
excessive, 111, 119, 121, 122, 124,
126, 250
impaction of, 130
Mueller-Hinton medium, 184
Müller maneuver, 90
multiple sclerosis, 82

mummy disease, 218
mumps, 254
muscles
abdominal, 3, 6, 7, 8, 10, 11, 12,
47, 48, 76, 153
accessory, 43, 47, 119, 120, 288
anterior thoracic wall, 6-7
atrophied, 262
cervical, 10, 40
compensatory contraction of, 286
constrictor, 117
deltoid, 6, 7, 9
diaphragmatic, 38, 40, 47
digastric, 117
erector spinae, 11
esophageal, 23
gastrocnemius, 220
geniohyoid, 117
hyoglossus, 117
hypothenar, 167
infrahyoid, 40
infraspinatus and supraspinatus, 9,
11
inspiratory and expiratory, 3, 36,
57, 59
intercostal, 6, 7, 8, 10, 11, 20, 21,
47, 75, 76, 77, 262
intervertebral, 10
latissimus dorsi, 6, 7, 9, 11, 297,
298
levator scapulae, 7, 9, 10
lingual, 40
mylohyoid, 37, 117
oblique, 3, 6, 7, 9, 10, 11, 47, 48
omohyoid, 6, 7, 117
parasternal intercartilaginous, 47
pectoralis, 6, 7, 11, 296
pharyngeal, 262
platysma, 118
in polyarteritis nodosa, 263
psoas, 12, 199
quadratus lumborum, 12
rectus abdominis, 3, 6, 7, 11, 47,
48
respiratory, 47-48, 50, 51, 52, 54,
58, 59, 76, 80, 82, 127, 288
rhomboideus, 9-10, 11, 297, 298
sacrospinalis, 9, 10
scalene, 5, 7, 8, 10, 18, 20, 21, 32,
47
serratus, 5, 6, 7, 9, 10, 11, 297,
298
smooth, 25, 36, 53, 122, 123, 124,
125, 127
soleus, 220
splenius capitis, cervicis, 9, 10
sternalis, 6, 7
sternocleidomastoid, 6, 7, 9, 47,
128
sternothyroid and sternohyoid, 6, 7,
8, 117
strap, 40, 276, 295
striated, 38
stylohyoid, 117
subclavius, 5, 6, 7, 20, 21
subscapularis, 10, 11
teres major and minor, 9, 10, 11
thoracic, 6-7, 9-10, 11
thyrohyoid, 117
trachealis, 23
transversus abdominis, 6, 8, 10, 12,
47, 48
transversus thoracis, 7, 8, 11
trapezius, 6, 9, 11, 297, 298

muscles—*continued*
vertebrocostal, 10
wasting of, in Pancoast's syndrome,
163
muscular dystrophy, 82
mushroom picker's disease, 216,
218
myasthenia; myasthenia gravis, 82,
167, 172, 301
mycelia; mycelioma, 194, 198
mycobacteria, 203, 205, 206, 207,
209
Mycobacterium
intracellulare, 205, 209
kansasii, 205, 206, 207, 209
tuberculosis, 199, 200, 202, 206,
207, 254, 255
Mycoplasma pneumoniae, 174, 186
myelin, tubular, 29, 30
myelitis, transverse, 186
myelomas, 174, 227, 238
myocarditis, 180, 182, 186
myofibrils, 124
myoglobinuria, 180
myopathy, 134, 167, 254, 256
myositis, 262
myotome, somite, 39, 40
myringitis, 186
myxedema, 79, 80

N

narcotics, 235, 237
nasal cannula or catheter, 91, 279,
292, 293
nasal turbinates (conchae), 3
nasogastric tube, 240, 276, 294
nasopharynx, 3
visualization of, 280
nasotracheal or nasopharyngeal
intubation, 274, 275, 277, 279
nausea, 166, 191
nebulizers, 134, 152, 269-271, 294
neck, 4
innervation of, 40
posterior triangle of, 6, 9
necrosis
aseptic, 134
cell, 121
focal (fibrinous), 181, 261
ischemic, 116
tuberculous, 200
neon, 65
nephritis, 182, 261
nephrosis, 237
nerves
accessory, 9, 10
adrenergic, 22, 121, 122-123, 124
afferent and efferent, 22, 75, 76-77,
121, 123
autonomic, 22, 36, 63, 123
cardiac, 21
cervical, 6, 7, 9-10, 12, 38, 40
cholinergic, 22, 121, 123, 125
in control of breathing, 76-77
cranial, 9, 77
cutaneous, 9, 11
destruction of, in Pancoast's
syndrome, 163
diaphragmatic, 12, 40
dorsal and ventral roots and rami of,
11
of epithelium, 26
glossopharyngeal, 22, 75, 77

nerves—*continued*
hypoglossal, 40
intercostal, 5, 6, 7, 8, 10, 11, 20,
21, 75, 76, 82, 238
intraepithelial, 25
irritant reflex, 76, 77
joint, 76, 77
laryngeal, 18, 20, 21, 117
motor, 27, 38
myelinated, 25
nociceptive alveolar, 76, 77
nonmyelinated, 25, 26
olfactory, 77
parasympathetic, 22, 36, 63
peripheral, 172
phrenic, 7, 8, 12, 18, 20, 21, 38,
39, 40, 75, 76, 77, 82, 298, 299
of pulmonary blood vessels, 63
recurrent, 18, 20, 21, 163, 299
seventh, 254, 256
sinus, 77
spinal, 11, 38
splanchnic, 12, 18, 20, 21
subcostal, 11
submucosal gland, 27
supraclavicular, 7
sympathetic, 11, 12, 18, 20, 21, 22,
36, 63, 82, 121, 122, 123, 124,
125, 163, 172
thoracic, 6, 7, 9, 10, 11, 20, 21, 77
trigeminal, 22
ulnar, 167
vagus, 12, 18, 20, 21, 22, 75, 76,
77, 121, 123, 124, 125, 163, 299
neuraminidase, 179, 180
neurilemomas, 172
neurofibromas, 172, 301
neurohormones, 122
neuromuscular disorders, 48, 167
neuromyopathy, carcinomatous, 161,
167
neurons
medullary, 77
motor, 76, 77
respiratory, 75, 76-77, 78, 79, 80
neuropathy, 167
neutrophil chemotactic factor, 124
neutrophils, 124, 127, 129, 180, 186,
253
New Guinea lung, 218
nickel, 158, 212
nicotinamide-adenine dinucleotide
phosphate (NADPH), 72
nitrofuran, 253
nitrofurantoin, 174
nitrogen, 145, 268
to test distribution of ventilation,
49, 60, 61, 65, 66, 68
nitrogen dioxide, 215, 237
nitrogen washout, 49, 141
Nocardia, 198, 258
asteroides, 174, 183, 191
brasiliensis; caviae; madurae, 191
nocardiosis, 191
nodules, pulmonary, 86, 97-99, 100,
168
in adenocarcinoma, 162
Caplan's, 209
hemosiderin-impregnated, 257
interstitial, 100
lymphoid, 257
multiple, 193
necrobiotic, 99
p, 210

nodules—*continued*
  in pulmonary siderosis, 212
  rheumatoid, 259
  in silicosis, 208, 209
  subcutaneous, 254
nonrebreathing mask, 292
norepinephrine, 22, 63, 122, 123, 124
nose
  airway resistance in, 52
  catheterization of, 91, 279, 292, 293
  external and internal, 3
  lesions of, 196, 263
  polyps of, 119, 126, 129, 133
  receptors in, 22
notches
  cardiac, 13, 15, 39
  jugular, 4
  suprasternal, 4, 13, 276
notochord, 39
nuchal line, 9, 10
5'-nucleotidase, 31
nucleotides, cyclic, 123-124
nutrition, 133, 151, 152, 155, 185, 294

O

obesity, 52, 79, 80, 82, 220
obstruction
  airway, 58, 59, 60, 79, 81, 111, 120, 126-128, 129, 130, 131, 132, 134, 145-147, 157, 239, 242, 267, 272, 293
  blood flow, 64, 100, 220, 237, 257 (*see also* embolism; thrombosis)
  bronchial, 68, 97, 98, 100, 115, 119, 132, 154, 159, 218, 241, 271-273, 280, 281
  endotracheal or tracheostomy tube, 294
  esophageal, 111
  intestinal, 156, 294
  and jaundice, 156
  with pneumonitis, 160, 161
obturators, 291
occupational risks and diseases, 82, 128, 129, 133, 144, 151, 158, 173, 195, 198, 208-218, 259
oidiomycin, 254
oleic acid, 72, 205, 207
oligemia, 100
olive oil, 246
omentum, 38, 110
"Ondine's curse," 78
open-circuit nitrogen washout technique, 49
optochin (Taxos P) test, 174
organelles, 29
oronasal membrane, 35, 38
oropharynx, 3, 34, 274, 277
orotracheal intubation, 274, 275, 277
orthopnea, 215
osteoarthropathy, hypertrophic pulmonary, 167, 171
osteoporosis, 134
osteosarcoma, 168
osteotomy (sternal), 107
ostium of auditory tube, 3
ovary, choriocarcinoma of, 168
overhydration, 237, 249
overinflation (*see* hyperinflation)

overtransfusion, 237
oxalacetate, 72
oxidant injury, 72
oximetry, ear, 278, 291
oxygen
  ambulatory and home use of, 293
  breathing 100%, 68-69, 292
  control of, in ventilation, 75, 80, 81
  diffusion of, 64, 65, 79, 80, 143
  for measuring flow rates, 59, 60, 61
  in MEFR tests, 145, 146
  partial pressures of, 64, 72, 268, 289-290
  in single-breath test, 141, 145
  in spirometry, 49
  supplemental, 239, 247, 248, 275, 278, 280, 290, 292, 293
  tensions (pressures) of, 228, 248, 251, 258, 268, 289-290, 291
  transport of, 69-70
oxygenation, 144, 202, 215, 242, 248, 278, 279, 291, 294
  reduced, 251
  therapeutic, 152, 153, 251
oxygen-carbon dioxide exchange, 3, 19, 31, 34, 41, 42, 47, 65-69, 72, 236, 268
  see also gas exchange
oxygen therapy, 131, 132, 181, 182, 215, 231, 232, 244, 254, 286
  in acute respiratory failure, 291
  administration of, 292
  in asthma, 132
  in cardiorespiratory failure, 109
  continuous and short-term, 293, 294
oxygen toxicity, 237, 248, 249, 294
oxyhemoglobin dissociation curve, 68, 69-70, 290, 291
ozone, 72

P

pacinian corpuscles, 77
pain afferents, 77
palate, primitive, 35
palatine process, 38
palmitic acid, 250
palsy, seventh nerve, 254
Pancoast's syndrome, 159, 163
pancreas, 74
  carcinoma of, 166, 220
  cystic fibrosis of, 129, 130, 154, 156-157
  in polyarteritis nodosa, 263
pancreatitis, 100, 237, 248, 290
Papanicolaou stain, 158, 185
paper mill worker's disease, 218
papilledema, 129, 242
paprika slicer's disease, 218
Papuan lung, 218
para-aminosalicylic acid (PAS), 127, 206
Paracoccidioides brasiliensis; paracoccidioidomycosis, 196
paralysis
  mechanical ventilation for, 294
  in sarcoidosis, 256
paraneoplastic syndromes, 161
paraplegia, 167
paraquat, 72
parasitic infestations, 121
parathormone, 166
parathyroids, 36, 172

parenchyma, lung, 62, 165
  destruction of, 138, 147, 178
  scarred, 169, 177
  tumors of, 171
paresthesias, 163, 167
parotid gland enlargement, 256
partial pressures of gases, 64, 65, 69, 72, 268, 289-290
partial rebreathing mask, 292
patch tests, 213
pectus carinatus; pectus excavatum, 107
pelvic inflammatory disease, 226
penetrating wounds, 238, 240, 242, 243, 244
penicillin, 134, 155, 184, 186, 190
  allergy to, 126
  penicillin G, 189
  resistance to, 175
Penicillium, 218
pentamidine isethionate, 185
pentose shunt, 72
Peptostreptococcus; Peptococcus, 174
perfusion, 73
  cephalization of, 100
  disturbances of, 67, 128, 227, 247, 251
  see also ventilation-perfusion ratio
perfusion scan, 95, 96, 97, 128, 228
pericarditis, 182
  lupus, 261
  purulent, 176, 177
pericardium, 3, 18, 20, 21, 35, 296, 298, 299, 301
  bare area of, 13
  fibrous, 12
  serous, 39
  tuberculous spread to, 199
perichondritis, 116
perichondrium, 25, 296
pericytes, 30
periodic acid-Schiff (PAS) stain, 258
peripheral neuromuscular disease, 256
peritonitis, pneumococcal, 176
perivascular sheath, 298, 299
personality changes, 109
Petit, trigone of, 9
6-P-gluconate, 72
pH, 75, 78, 129, 268, 289, 290
  changes in, 131-132
phagocytes, 72, 212, 214
  see also macrophages
pharyngitis, 186
pharynx, 3, 18, 34, 52, 91, 263, 275, 280
phenformin, 290
phenylbutazone, 256
phlebitis, 220, 223, 225, 227
  see also thrombophlebitis
phlebography (venography), 94, 221, 222, 225, 229
phlegmasia alba dolens, 227
phlegmasia cerulea dolens, 220
phosgene, 72, 215, 237
phosphate buffer, 205, 207
phosphodiesterase, 124, 125, 133
phospholipids, 41, 42, 219, 233, 250, 258
photochromogens, 205
photometric clot timer, 233
Phycomycetes, 174, 198
phytohemagglutinin (PHA), 255

pickwickian syndrome, 80
pigeon breast, 107
pigeon breeder's disease, 216, 218
pigmentation, increased, 166
Pitressin snuff, 218
pituitary snuff disease, 218
planography, 88-89, 189
plaques, 211, 231, 254
plasma, 31, 42, 65
  bicarbonate levels in, 82
  oxygen and carbon dioxide transport in, 69, 70, 71
  clotting factors in, 219, 233
  donors and recipients of, 223
plasmin, 221
platelets, 219
plethysmography, 49-50, 141
  body, 53, 61, 134, 267
  impedance, 222, 224-225
  mercury strain gauge, 224-225
pleura, 3, 14, 15, 23, 28, 100
  canals of, 36-37, 38, 39
  "cobblestoned," 253
  costal, 12, 13, 14, 18, 20, 21
  costodiaphragmatic recess of, 12, 13, 14, 100
  cupola of, 3, 13, 14, 20, 21
  development of, 38-39
  diaphragmatic, 3, 12, 13, 14, 18, 20, 21
  herniation of, 110
  lesions of, 95, 100-101, 102-103
  lymphatic drainage of, 32-33
  mediastinal, 3, 12, 13, 18, 20, 21
  parietal, 3, 12, 14, 18, 20, 21, 39, 100, 173, 242, 246, 296, 298, 301
  pericardial, 3, 12, 20, 21
  reflected, 13, 14
  tuberculous spread to, 199
  visceral, 3, 14, 18, 19, 21, 35, 39, 40, 100, 114, 171, 173, 242, 246, 260
  see also effusions, pleural
pleurisy, 129, 203, 261, 263
pleuritis, 227, 259, 260
  fibrinopurulent, 177
  lupus, 261
pleuropericarditis, 186
pleuropneumonialike organisms (PPLO), 100, 186
plexuses
  brachial, 6, 7, 9, 10, 18, 20, 21, 163
  capillary, 28
  cervical, 7, 12
  esophageal, 18, 20, 21
  lymphatic, 32, 33
  pulmonary, 22
pneumatoceles, 178
pneumoconiosis, 100, 129, 208-215
  benign, 212
  coal worker's, 210
  mineral, 214
  rheumatoid, 209
Pneumocystis carinii, 174, 183, 185, 258
pneumocystosis, 185
pneumocytes, 40, 41, 42, 43, 52, 72, 236, 250
pneumomediastinum, 95, 130, 241, 251
pneumonectomy, 297-298, 299
pneumonia, 97, 108, 109, 129, 130, 170, 174, 238, 248, 261

sputum—*continued*
  in cystic fibrosis, 156
  examination of, 158, 204-205, 206, 207
  in legionnaires' disease, 184
  with lung tumors, 159, 160, 171
  mucoid, 130
  in PAP, 258
  in pneumonia, 177, 182
  in pneumoconiosis, 191, 194, 198, 209, 210, 211
  and postural drainage, 287
  purulent, 113, 114, 119, 129, 130, 154, 155, 157, 175, 177, 178, 180, 188, 190, 203, 215
  tuberculous, 203, 204-205, 206
stab wounds, 238, 240, 243, 244
staphylococci, 129, 156, 157
Staphylococcus
  aureus, 174, 176, 178, 180, 188
  epidermidis, 178
Starling resistor, 63
Starling's law, 236, 237
stasis, venous, 226, 227, 229, 234
status asthmaticus, 100, 119, 120, 125, 126, 127, 130, 131-133, 135, 290
  management of, 132-133
stenosis
  mitral, 100, 181
  pulmonary, 73, 111
  subglottic, 290
  tracheal, 116, 117, 277
stereoscopy, 87
sterility, 157
steroids, 198, 218, 239
  see also corticosteroids
sternotomy, 117
sternum, 3, 4, 5, 6, 7, 8, 11, 12, 20, 39, 102, 296
  angle of, 4, 13, 20
  bifid, 107
  depressed, 107
  fractured, 238, 239, 247
  sternum-splitting thoracotomy, 301
Stevens-Johnson syndrome, 186
stiff lung syndrome, 239, 248
stimulation, excitatory and inhibitory, 22, 122
stomach, 13, 14, 18, 38
  herniation of, 101, 110, 240
stomodeum, 34, 35
streptococci, 174, 188
Streptococcus pneumoniae and pyogenes, 151, 174, 180
streptomycin, 206, 207
stretch receptors, 22, 76, 77
stroma, 25, 34, 35, 39
subacute cerebellar degeneration, 167
suberosis, 218
substance of anaphylaxis, slow-reacting (SRS-A), 121, 122, 124, 125
suctioning
  bronchofiberscopic, 152, 278
  nasotracheal and orotracheal, 132, 152, 277, 279
  underwater-seal, 285
  ventilator, 294
sugar cane, 174
  see also bagasse; bagassosis
sulcus, costophrenic, 12, 13, 14, 100
sulfadiazine, 191, 196

sulfonamides, 191, 196
sulfur dioxide, 215
surface tension, 41, 42, 43, 52, 53
surfactant (surface-active layer), 29, 30, 40, 41-42, 52, 53, 65, 228, 236, 252, 258
  abnormalities of, 97
  loss of, 248
surfactant deficiency syndrome, 250-252
surgery
  advisability of, and perfusion scanning, 97
  for bronchiectasis, 155
  cardiac, 78
  and chylothorax, 246
  for diaphragmatic injury, 240
  for embolism, 230, 231, 234
  for emphysema, 115, 153
  for hemothorax, 244
  for hernia, 110
  for lung sequestration, 114
  for lung tumors, 159, 160, 162, 163, 169, 170, 171, 295, 296, 301
  open-heart, 301
  for pectus excavatum (or carinatum), 107
  to prevent pulmonary embolism, 234
  segmental, 300
  thrombosis and embolism due to, 226, 227, 229, 235
  tracheal, 111, 117, 118
  in tuberculosis, 207
  see also specific procedures
sweating, 119, 120, 156, 188, 191, 203
sweat test, 130, 156-157
Swyer-James anomaly, 97
sympathicoblastoma, 172
syncope, 227, 231, 232
syndactyly, 107
synovial cavities, 5
synovitis, 261
syphilis, 164, 172, 261
systemic lupus erythematosus
  (*see* lupus erythematosis, systemic)

T

tachycardia
  in asthma, 119, 120, 129, 130
  with congenital diaphragmatic hernia, 110
  in cor pulmonale, 228, 231
  in PAP, 258
  in pneumonia, 175
  with pulmonary contusion, 247
tachypnea, 79
  in asthma, 127, 128-129
  in COPD, 148
  in hyaline membrane disease, 251
  in IPH, 257
  with mechanical ventilation, 294
  in pneumonia, 175, 178, 184, 185
  with pulmonary contusion, 247
  with pulmonary embolism, 227, 232, 236, 237
  with reaction to metals, 212, 213
  in rheumatoid arthritis, 259
talc, 259
tamponade, 244, 251
tanned red cell test, 221

tantalum, 91, 118
tartrazine, 120
Taxos P test, 174
tea grower's disease, 218
tears, 156
technetium, 95, 223, 228
telangiectasia, 170, 171
tendons, central, 12
tent, oxygen, 292
teratomas, 172, 301
terbutaline, 132, 134
testes
  carcinoma of, 168
  degenerative changes in, 213
tetany, 294
tetracycline, 134, 155, 184, 186, 190, 194, 197
tetralogy of Fallot, 112
thatched roof disease, 216, 218
Thermoactinomyces saccharii and vulgaris, 216, 218
thermodilution technique, 61
thiacetazone, 206
thiourea, 72
thoracentesis, 101, 173, 176, 244, 245, 246
thoracic wall
  abnormalities of, 101-102, 107
  anterior, 6-8
  arteries and veins of, 7-8
  dorsal aspect of, 9-10
  elastic properties of, 52, 54
  floating, 239
  injuries to, 100, 238, 242, 243, 247, 248, 249
  lymphatic drainage of, 8
  muscles of, 3, 6-7, 9-10
  nerves of, 7, 11
thoracostomy, 241, 243, 244, 245, 246
thoracotomy, 117, 158, 173, 241, 244, 284, 295, 296, 297, 299, 300
thorax, 3, 12, 20-21
  bony, 4, 43
  ducts of, 7, 8, 12, 18, 20, 21
thrombin, 219, 221
thrombocytes, 73
thrombocytopenia, 261
thromboembolism, 91, 97, 219, 220, 234
  see also embolism
thrombolytic agents, 231
thrombophlebitis, 220, 230
  clinical manifestations of, 220
  diagnosis of, 221, 222, 223
  fibrinogen scan for, 220, 221, 222, 223, 225
  leg, 226, 228-229
  migratory, 167
  pelvic, 226
  and phlebography, 221, 222
  and plethysmography, 224-225
  and ultrasonography, 224
thromboplastin, 219, 233, 235
thrombosis, 82, 180
  leg vein, 220, 221, 222, 223, 224, 225, 226, 232
thromboxanes, 124
thymomas, 95, 102, 166, 172, 301
thymus, 15, 20, 21, 36, 102, 301
thyroid, 13, 18, 34, 35, 36, 82, 116, 168, 172, 276
  blockade of, 223

thyroid—*continued*
  cricothyroid stab, 274
  deficiency of, 80
  and mediastinoscopy, 295
  tumors of, 168, 301
thyroid diverticulum, 34
thyroxine, 30, 42
tidal volume, 48, 49, 58-59, 60, 66, 77, 78, 108, 109, 141, 145, 248, 260, 262, 267, 268, 271, 278
time constants, 57
tine test, 204
T-lymphocytes, 255
T-N-M risk factors, 295
tobacco fumes, 125, 126, 133
  see also smoking
tobacco grower's disease, 218
tobramycin, 177
toluene diisocyanate, 125, 129
tomography, 88-89, 90, 112, 116, 158, 171
tongue, 3, 35, 36, 38, 91
  innervation of, 40
  lesions of, 192, 196
Torula histolytica; torulosis, 197
total eosinophil counts, 130
total lung capacity (TLC), 48, 49, 51, 54, 55, 59, 60, 108, 109, 140-141, 143, 145, 149, 218, 253, 267, 268, 270
trachea, 3, 13, 15, 19, 20, 102, 301
  airway resistance in, 52
  anomalies of, 111
  cartilages of, 23, 34, 37, 53, 111
  development of, 34-35, 36, 37, 38
  deviated, 110, 113, 115, 160, 244, 254
  epithelium of, 26
  erosion of, 116, 117
  intubation of, 91, 116, 117, 118, 132, 133, 238, 239, 258, 274, 275, 276, 277, 279, 280, 294
  irritant receptors in, 22
  lymph nodes of, 32, 33
  and mediastinoscopy, 295
  plastic reconstruction of, 118
  relations of main bronchi and, 18
  resection and anastomosis of, 117
  ruptured, 241, 242
  stenosis of, 116, 117, 277
  structure of, 23
  submucosal gland openings in, 27
  turbulence in, 55
  visualization of, 278, 280, 281, 283
  wall of, 23
tracheitis, 213
tracheobronchial lavage, 278
tracheobronchial tree, innervation of, 22
tracheobronchitis, 186
tracheobronchomegaly, 154
tracheography, 116
tracheomalacia, 116, 277
tracheostomy, 117, 118, 238, 239, 242, 274, 276, 277, 292, 294
tranquilizers, 129
transamination reaction, 219
transplantation, 183, 185
Trendelenburg position, 287
Trichophyton, 198, 254
trichterbrust, 107
triiodothyronine, 77
trimethoprim-sulfamethoxazole, 185

trophozoites, 185
truncus arteriosus, 34, 35, 39
trypsin, 147
tuberculin sensitivity, 213
tuberculin test, 203-204, 205, 254-255
tuberculosis, 89, 97, 101, 163, 164, 198, 300
  and bronchiectasis, 154-155
  inflammation with, 200, 281
  and lung abscess, 189
  miliary, 100, 169, 201, 203, 204
  pathology of, 200-203
  and pneumoconiosis, 209-210, 212
  primary, 102, 172
  progressive, 203
  reactivated, 202, 203
  sputum examination and culture in, 204-205, 206, 207
  transmission and dissemination of, 199-200, 202
  treatment of, 206-207
  tuberculin test, 203-204, 205, 254-255
tubes
  Carlens, 258
  multifenestrated, 284
  pleural drainage, 284, 285
  T, 292, 294
  see also intubation
tubules, mucous and serous, 27
tumors, 33, 82, 97, 99, 100, 154
  benign, 171, 300
  brain, 109
  bronchogenic, 158-170
  carcinoid, 73, 166, 170
  "dumbbell," 301
  epithelial, 173
  esophageal, 90
  fibrous, 173
  gastrointestinal tract, 166
  "iceberg," 170
  laryngeal, 128
  mediastinal, 128, 172, 281, 301
  metastatic, 99, 100, 101, 102, 168
  multiple primary, 211
  neurogenic, 102, 172
  pleomorphic, 170
  removal of, 159, 160, 162, 163, 169, 170, 171, 295, 296, 301
  salivary gland, 168, 170
  staging of, 295
  teratoid, 102, 172, 301
  thymic, 102
  tracheal, 128, 129
  vascular, 171, 301
  of vertebral column, 102
  see also carcinomas
tungsten, 212
turbulence, 54-55, 56, 59
turkey handler's disease, 218
tympany, 188
Tzanck cells, 182

U

ulceration
  avascular, 116
  with bowel disease, 183
  peptic, 134
ultrasonography, 89, 224, 225, 229, 287

underwater-seal drainage, 241, 243, 244, 245, 284, 285
uremia, 71, 82, 249
urinalysis, 261
urine
  in cystic fibrosis, 156
  decreased osmolality of, 166
urticaria, 120
uveitis, 254, 256
uveoparotid fever, 254

V

vaccines; vaccination, 151
  allergy to, 126
  bacterial, 134
  BCG, 207
  influenza, 181
  for pneumonia, 176
  viral, 134
vagotomy, 123, 167
vallecula, 275
valley fever fungus, 194
Valsalva maneuver, 90
varicella-zoster pneumonia, 179, 182
vasculitis, 99, 260, 263
  granulomatous, 235
  lupus, 261
  systemic, 129
vas deferens, atresia of, 156
vasoactive substances, 73, 124, 248
  precursors of, 74-82
vasoconstriction, 22, 63, 73, 74, 108, 121, 123, 144, 149, 237, 250
vasodilation, 22, 63, 109, 123, 124, 172
vasospasm, 220
Veillonella, 174
veins
  antecubital, 223
  axillary, 7
  azygos, 8, 12, 15, 18, 20-21, 25, 28, 94, 164, 246, 298
  brachiocephalic (innominate), 8, 15, 18, 20, 21, 32, 33, 164, 246, 301
  bronchial, 25, 28, 68
  cephalic, 6, 7
  common cardinal, 34, 37, 38, 39
  distended, 144, 148
  epigastric, 7, 8, 11
  esophageal, 12
  femoral, 164, 222, 224, 225, 226
  gonadal, 226, 230, 234
  hemiazygos, 8, 12, 20, 21, 114
  iliac, 164, 224, 226
  intercostal, 5, 8, 11, 20, 21, 164, 301
  internal thoracic (internal mammary), 7, 8, 12, 164, 296
  intersegmental, 300
  jugular, 7, 8, 18, 32, 164
  leg, thrombosis of, 220, 221, 222, 223, 224, 225, 226, 232
  musculophrenic, 7, 8
  pelvic, 226, 230
  pericardiacophrenic, 8, 12, 18, 20, 21
  peripheral, 223, 226
  peroneal, 225
  popliteal, 224, 226
  portal, 73
  pressure in, 61, 62, 63

veins—continued
  pulmonary, 15, 18, 20, 21, 25, 28, 32-33, 35, 69, 90, 114, 237, 248, 249, 298, 299
  saphenous, 220, 226
  segmental, 16
  and shunting, 68, 69
  soleal, 220, 221, 225, 226
  subclavian, 3, 5, 7, 8, 10, 18, 20, 21, 32, 163, 164
  subcostal, 8
  surgery on, 234
  thebesian, 68, 69
  thoracic, 7-8, 164
  thyroid, 276
  tibial, 224, 225, 226
  uterine, 226, 235
  varicose, 91, 220, 227
  vertebral, 8
  yolk sac, 34
  see also vena cava
vena cava
  distortion of, 244
  grooves for, 15
  inferior, 12, 18, 20, 39, 40, 224, 234
  superior, 8, 15, 18, 20, 90, 94, 246, 298, 301
  superior vena cava syndrome, 164
  surgery for, 230, 234
venography (phlebography), 94, 102, 221, 222, 225
ventilation
  alveolar vs dead-space, 108
  apparatus for, 50-59
  arterial tension and, 75-76
  distribution of, 57-58, 59-60, 268
  failure of, 132, 133
  mechanical, 132, 133, 144, 231, 239, 244, 247, 248, 269-270, 277, 278, 279, 280, 290, 292, 293, 294
  minute, 52, 59, 66, 78, 109, 270
  neural theory of control of, 77
  and oxygen–carbon dioxide exchange, 65-66
  at sea level or high altitudes, 76
  see also breathing;
    hyperventilation;
    hypoventilation; respiration
ventilation-perfusion ratio ($\dot{V}C/\dot{Q}C$), 67, 68
  imbalance in, 128, 131-132, 165, 228, 239, 243, 248, 249, 253, 268, 289, 290
ventilation scan, 95, 96, 97, 228
ventral respiratory groups (VRG), 76
Venturi mask, 152, 291, 292, 293
vertebrae, 11, 12, 20, 21, 39, 85, 301
  articulation of ribs with, 5
  cervical, 9, 10, 18
  lumbar, 9, 10
  sacral, 9
  thoracic, 4, 9, 10, 12, 13, 14, 15, 18, 20, 21, 23, 39
vertigo, 167
vestibule, nasal, 3
vincristine, 161
viremia, 182
viruses
  adenovirus, 174, 179, 186
  coxsackie, echovirus, herpes simplex, 179

viruses—continued
  cytomegalovirus, 179, 183, 186
  influenza and parainfluenza, 174, 179, 180, 181
  measles, 179
  pneumonias caused by, 100, 174, 179-183, 253
  respiratory syncytial, 174, 179
  varicella-zoster, 179, 182
visual defects, 164, 183, 242
  see also eyes
vital capacity (VC), 48, 49, 55, 58, 59, 108, 109, 127, 139-140, 141, 145, 146, 149, 155, 211, 215, 218, 239, 245, 253, 257, 258, 262, 267, 268, 294
vitamins, 72, 112, 156, 219, 233
vocal cords, 3, 275
  visualization of, 277, 280, 281, 283
Vollmer patch, 204
vomiting, 130, 166, 184, 191, 248
volumes, lung, 48-51
  and airway resistance, 53
  closing, 60, 61, 145-146
  isoflow, 59
  measurement of, 49-50
  minute, 149
  pressure and, 54, 56-59
  relationship of airflow and, 55-56
  static, 140
  volume-dependent tests, 145-146
  see also specific volumes and subdivisions

W

warfarin, 219, 229, 230, 232, 233
water
  in air, 65
  interstitial, 236, 237
  lost in respiration, 41
  surface tension of, 41, 43
weakness, 148, 155, 166, 218, 260, 262
wedge resection, 300
Wegener's granulomatosis, 168, 263
weight loss, 191, 195, 203, 218, 253, 258
wet lung, 248
wheat flour sensitivity, 129
wheat thresher's lung, 216, 218
wheezing, 87, 119, 120, 128, 129, 149, 161, 170, 171, 180, 198, 215, 257, 263
work of breathing, 58-59, 60, 108, 128, 132

X

xenon, 95, 228, 280
xiphoid process, 4, 6, 7, 8, 12, 107, 271, 272

Y

Yersinia pestis, 174

Z

Ziehl-Neelsen staining, 204, 206
zymogens, 219

Information on
CIBA COLLECTION
Volumes

Since the publication of its first volume in 1953, THE CIBA COLLECTION OF MEDICAL ILLUSTRATIONS has enjoyed an enthusiastic reception from members of the medical community. The remarkable illustrations by Frank H. Netter, M.D. and text discussions by leading specialists make these books unprecedented in their educational, clinical, and scientific value.

Volume 1   **NERVOUS SYSTEM**
"... a beautiful bargain ... and handsome reference work."
Psychological Record

Volume 2   **REPRODUCTIVE SYSTEM**
"... a desirable addition to any nursing or medical library."
American Journal of Nursing

Volume 3/I   **DIGESTIVE SYSTEM (Upper Digestive Tract)**
"... a fine example of the high quality of this series."
Pediatrics

Volume 3/II   **DIGESTIVE SYSTEM (Lower Digestive Tract)**
"... a unique and beautiful work, worth much more than its cost."
Journal of the South Carolina Medical Association

Volume 3/III   **DIGESTIVE SYSTEM (Liver, Biliary Tract and Pancreas)**
"... a versatile, multipurpose aid to clinicians, teachers, researchers, and students ..." *Florida Medical Journal*

Volume 4   **ENDOCRINE SYSTEM and Selected Metabolic Diseases**
"... another in the series of superb contributions made by CIBA ..."
International Journal of Fertility

Volume 5   **HEART**
"The excellence of the volume ... is clearly deserving of highest praise."
Circulation

Volume 6   **KIDNEYS, URETERS, AND URINARY BLADDER**
"... a model of clarity of language and visual presentation ..."
Circulation

Volume 7   **RESPIRATORY SYSTEM**
"... far more than an atlas on anatomy and physiology. Frank Netter uses his skills to present clear and often beautiful illustrations of all aspects of the system ..."
British Medical Journal

In the United States, copies of all CIBA COLLECTION books may be purchased from the Medical Education Division, CIBA Pharmaceutical Company, Division of CIBA-GEIGY Corporation, Summit, New Jersey 07901. In other countries, please direct inquiries to the nearest CIBA-GEIGY office.